NURSING ASSISTANT

A Nursing Process Approach

Barbara R. Hegner, MSN, RN
Professor Emerita
Nursing and Life Science, Long Beach City College (CA)

Esther Caldwell, MA, PhD
Consultant in Vocational Education (CA)

Contributing Author:
Joan F. Needham, MSN, RN
Consultant and Educator
for Long-Term Care and Gerontology (IL)

Delmar Publishers

an International Thomson Publishing company I(T)P®

Albany • Bonn • Boston • Cincinnati • Detroit • London • Madrid
Melbourne • Mexico City • New York • Pacific Grove • Paris • San Francisco
Singapore • Tokyo • Toronto • Washington

NOTICE TO THE READER

Cover Design: Charles Cummings Advertising/Art, Inc.

Cover Photos: Stock Studios, Thomas Stock

Delmar Staff:

Publisher: Susan Simpfenderfer
Acquisitions Editor: Dawn Gerrain
Developmental Editor: Marjorie A. Bruce
Marketing Manager: Darryl Caron
Marketing Coordinator: Nina Lontrato
Editorial Assistant: Donna L. Leto
Team Assistant: Sandra Bruce

Production Manager: Wendy A. Troeger
Project Editor: Elizabeth LaManna
Production Coordinator: John Mickelbank
Art and Design Coordinator: Vincent S. Berger

COPYRIGHT © 1999
Delmar is a division of Thomson Learning. The Thomson Learning logo is a registered trademark used herein under license.

Printed in the United States of America
5 7 8 9 10 XXX 05 04 03 02 01

For more information, contact Delmar, 3 Columbia Circle, PO Box 15015, Albany, NY 12212-0515; or find us on the World Wide Web at http://www.delmar.com

International Division List

Japan:
Thomson Learning
Palaceside Building 5F
1-1-1 Hitotsubashi, Chiyoda-ku
Tokyo 100 0003 Japan
Tel: 813 5218 6544
Fax: 813 5218 6551

Australia/New Zealand
Nelson/Thomson Learning
102 Dodds Street
South Melbourne, Victoria 3205
Australia
Tel: 61 39 685 4111
Fax: 61 39 685 4199

UK/Europe/Middle East:
Thomson Learning
Berkshire House
168-173 High Holborn
London
WC1V 7AA United Kingdom
Tel: 44 171 497 1422
Fax: 44 171 497 1426

Latin America:
Thomson Learning
Seneca, 53
Colonia Polanco
11560 Mexico D.F. Mexico
Tel: 525-281-2906
Fax: 525-281-2656

Canada:
Nelson/Thomson Learning
1120 Birchmount Road
Scarborough, Ontario
Canada M1K 5G4
Tel: 416-752-9100
Fax: 416-752-8102

Asia:
Thomson Learning
60 Albert Street, #15-01
Albert Complex
Singapore 189969
Tel: 65 336 6411
Fax: 65 336 7411

Spain:
Thomson Learning
Calle Magallanes, 25
28015-MADRID
ESPANA
Tel: 34 91 446 33 50
Fax: 34 91 445 62 18

Library of Congress Cataloging-in-Publication Data
Hegner, Barbara R.
   Nursing assistant: a nursing process approach / Barbara R. Hegner, Esther
Caldwell; contributing author, Joan F. Needham—8th ed.
     p. cm.
   Includes index.
   ISBN 0-8273-9063-7 (hard cover) / 0-8273-9058-0 (soft cover)
   1. Nurses' aides. 2. Care of the sick. I. Caldwell, Esther. II. Needham,
Joan Fritsch. III. Title.
   [DNLM: 1. Nurses' Aides. 2. Nursing Care. WY 193 H4644n 1998]
RT84.J45 1998
610.73'06'98—dc21
DNLM/DLC
for Library of Congress   98-9510
                        CIP

Contents

About the Authors   xi

Preface   xii

Acknowledgments   xiv

Features of This Book   xvi

SECTION 1

INTRODUCTION TO NURSING ASSISTING   1

Unit 1
Community Health Care   1

Introduction   2
Overview of Health Care   3
Needs of the Community   4
Community Health Care Services   4
Financing Health Care   7

Unit 2
Role of the Nursing Assistant   9

The Interdisciplinary Health Care Team   10
The Nursing Team   12
Organization of Nursing Care   12
Regulation of Nursing Assistant Practice   13
Lines of Authority   14
Guidelines for the Nursing Assistant   14
The Role and Responsibilities of the Nursing Assistant   16
Personal Vocational Adjustments   16
Personal Health and Hygiene   18

Unit 3
Consumer Rights and Responsibilities in Health Care   22

Consumer Rights   23
Responsibilities of Health Care Consumers   23

Unit 4
Ethical and Legal Issues Affecting the Nursing Assistant   30

Ethical Standards and Legal Standards   31
Ethics Questions   31
Respect for Life   31
Respect for the Individual   32
Patient Information   32
Tipping   33
Legal Issues   33

SECTION 2

SCIENTIFIC PRINCIPLES   39

Unit 5
Medical Terminology and Body Organization   40

Medical Terminology   41
Medical Word Parts   41
Body Organization   45
Anatomic Terms   45
Organization of the Body   47

Unit 6
Classification of Disease   54

Introduction   54
Disease   54
Major Conditions   55
Diagnosis   56
Therapy   58
Neoplasms   58
Body Defenses   59

SECTION 3

BASIC HUMAN NEEDS AND COMMUNICATION   63

Unit 7
Communication Skills   64

Introduction   65
Communication in Health Care   65
Communicating with Staff Members   66
Guidelines for Communicating with Patients   70
Communicating with Patients   70

Unit 8
Observation, Reporting, and Documentation   70

Introduction   77
Nursing Process   77
Making Observations   77
Reporting   86
Documentation   86
Guidelines for Charting   89

Unit 9
Meeting Basic Human Needs   92

Introduction   93
Human Growth and Development   93
Basic Human Needs   97

■ **Unit 10**
Developing Cultural Sensitivity   105
Introduction   106
Race, Ethnicity, and Culture   106
Traditions   111
Guidelines for Developing Cultural Sensitivity   112

SECTION 4

INFECTION AND INFECTION CONTROL   115

■ **Unit 11**
Infection   116
Introduction   117
Microbes   117
The Chain of Infection   119
Types of Infections   121
Body Flora   121
How Pathogens Affect the Body   121
Body Defenses   121
Immunity   122
Immunizations   122
Immunosuppression   122
Serious Infections in Health Care Facilities   122
Bacterial Infections   122
Viral Infections   125
Other Important Infections   126
Guidelines for Preventing Infections   127
Outbreak of Infectious Disease in a Health
Care Facility   127
Self-Care   128

■ **Unit 12**
Infection Control   130
Disease Prevention   131
Medical Asepsis   131
Guidelines for Maintaining Medical Asepsis   131
Handwashing   132
Procedure 1 Handwashing   132
Protecting Yourself   133
Standard Precautions   133
Guidelines for Standard Precautions   134
Guidelines for Environmental Procedures   135
Transmission-Based Precautions   137
Isolation Technique   141
Personal Protective Equipment   141
Procedure 2 Putting on a Mask   144
Procedure 3 Putting on a Gown   145
Procedure 4 Putting on Gloves   145
Procedure 5 Removing Contaminated Gloves   146
Procedure 6 Removing Contaminated Gloves,
Mask, and Gown   147
Procedure 7 Serving a Meal Tray in an
Isolation Unit   149
Procedure 8 Measuring Vital Signs in an Isolation
Unit   150

Procedure 9 Transferring Nondisposable
Equipment Outside of Isolation Unit   151
Procedure 10 Specimen Collection from
Patient in an Isolation Unit   151
Procedure 11 Caring for Linens in an
Isolation Unit   152
Procedure 12 Transporting Patient to and from
Isolation Unit   153
Disinfection and Sterilization   155
Sterile Procedures   156
Procedure 13 Opening a Sterile Package   156

SECTION 5

SAFETY AND MOBILITY   159

■ **Unit 13**
**Environmental and Nursing
Assistant Safety   160**
Introduction   161
The Patient Environment   161
Safety Measures   163
Fire Safety   166
Other Emergencies   168
Nursing Assistant Safety   168

■ **Unit 14**
Patient Safety and Positioning   174
Patient Safety   175
Guidelines for Preventing Patient Falls   175
Use of Physical Restraints   177
Guidelines for the Use of Restraints   178
Prevention of Other Incidents   179
Introduction to Procedures   179
Body Mechanics for the Patient   181
Moving and Lifting Patients   183
Procedure 14 Turning the Patient toward
You   183
Procedure 15 Turning the Patient Away from
You   184
Procedure 16 Moving a Patient to the Head
of the Bed   185
Procedure 17 Logrolling the Patient   186
Guidelines for the Use of Splints   191

■ **Unit 15**
The Patient's Mobility: Transfer Skills   193
Introduction   194
Types of Transfers   194
Guidelines for Safe Patient Transfers   194
Transfer Belts   195
Procedure 18 Applying a Transfer Belt   195
Procedure 19 Transferring the Patient from
Bed to Chair–One Assistant   196
Procedure 20 Transferring the Patient from
Bed to Chair–Two Assistants   199

OBRA 0.9 Procedure 21 Transferring the Patient from
Chair to Bed–One Assistant   200

OBRA 0.9 Procedure 22 Transferring the Patient from
Chair to Bed–Two Assistants   200

OBRA Procedure 23 Independent Transfer, Standby
Assist   202

Stretcher Transfers   202

Procedure 24 Transferring the Patient from
Bed to Stretcher   202

Procedure 25 Transferring the Patient from
Stretcher to Bed   203

OBRA 0.9 Procedure 26 Transferring the Patient with a
Mechanical Lift   204

Toilet Transfers   206

OBRA 0.9 Procedure 27 Transferring the Patient onto
and off the Toilet   206

Tub Transfers   207

OBRA Procedure 28 Transferring the Patient into
and out of the Bath Tub   208

Car Transfers   209

Procedure 29 Transferring a Patient into and
out of a Car   209

Unit 16
The Patient's Mobility: Ambulation   211
Ambulation   212
Assistive Devices   213
Guidelines for Safe Ambulation   213

OBRA 0.9 Procedure 30 Assisting the Patient to Walk
with a Cane and Three-Point Gait   215

OBRA 0.9 Procedure 31 Assisting the Patient to Walk
with a Walker and Three-Point Gait   216

The Falling Patient   217

OBRA 0.9 Procedure 32 Assisting the Falling Patient   217

Use of Wheelchairs   218

Guidelines for Wheelchair Safety   218

Positioning the Dependent Patient in a
Wheelchair   219

Wheelchair Activity   220

SECTION 6

MEASURING AND RECORDING VITAL
SIGNS, HEIGHT, AND WEIGHT   223

Unit 17
Body Temperature   224
Introduction   225
Temperature Values   225
Definition of Body Temperature   225
Temperature Control   226
Measuring Body Temperature   226
Clinical Thermometers   226

Guidelines for Using an Oral or Rectal
Thermometer   228

Guidelines for the Safe Use of a Glass
Thermometer   228

OBRA 0.9 Procedure 33 Measuring an Oral Temperature
(Glass Thermometer)   229

OBRA Procedure 34 Measuring Temperature Using a
Sheath-covered Thermometer   230

OBRA 0.9 Procedure 35 Measuring a Rectal Temperature
(Glass Thermometer)   232

OBRA 0.9 Procedure 36 Measuring an Axillary or Groin
Temperature (Glass Thermometer)   233

OBRA 0.9 Procedure 37 Measuring an Oral Temperature
(Electronic Thermometer)   233

OBRA 0.9 Procedure 38 Measuring a Rectal Temperature
(Electronic Thermometer)   234

OBRA Procedure 39 Measuring an Axillary
Temperature (Electronic Thermometer)   235

OBRA 0.9 Procedure 40 Measuring a Tympanic
Temperature   235

Procedure 41 Cleaning Glass Thermometers   237

Unit 18
Pulse and Respiration   240
Introduction   241
The Pulse   241

OBRA 0.9 Procedure 42 Counting the Radial Pulse   242
Respiration   242

0.9 Procedure 43 Counting the Apical-Radial Pulse 243

OBRA 0.9 Procedure 44 Counting Respirations   244

Unit 19
Blood Pressure   246
Introduction   247
Equipment   247
Measuring the Blood Pressure   248

Guidelines for Preparing to Measure Blood
Pressure   249

How to Read the Gauge   250

OBRA 0.9 Procedure 45 Taking Blood Pressure   250

Unit 20
Measuring Height and Weight   253
Weight and Height Measurements   254

Guidelines for Obtaining Accurate Weight
and Height Measurements   255

OBRA 0.9 Procedure 46 Weighing and Measuring the
Patient Using an Upright Scale   255

OBRA 0.9 Procedure 47 Weighing the Patient on a Chair
Scale   256

OBRA 0.9 Procedure 48 Measuring Weight with an
Electronic Wheelchair Scale   257

OBRA 0.9 Procedure 49 Measuring and Weighing the
Patient in Bed   257

SECTION 7

PATIENT CARE AND COMFORT MEASURES   261

Unit 21
Admission, Transfer, and Discharge   262
Introduction   263
Admission   263
Transfer   264
Discharge   264
Procedure 50 Admitting the Patient   264
Procedure 51 Transferring the Patient   267
Procedure 52 Discharging the Patient   268

Unit 22
Bedmaking   270
Introduction   271
Operation and Uses of Beds in Health Care Facilities   271
Bedmaking   272
Guidelines for Handling Linens and Making the Bed   273
Procedure 53 Making a Closed Bed   273
Procedure 54 Opening the Closed Bed   277
Procedure 55 Making an Occupied Bed   277
Procedure 56 Making the Surgical Bed   279

Unit 23
Patient Bathing   282
Introduction   283
Patient Bathing   283
Guidelines for Patient Bathing   284
Procedure 57 Assisting with the Tub Bath or Shower   284
Procedure 58 Bed Bath   286
Procedure 59 Partial Bath   291
Procedure 60 Female Perineal Care   292
Procedure 61 Male Perineal Care   293
Procedure 62 Hand and Fingernail Care   295
Procedure 63 Bed Shampoo   295
Dressing a Patient   297
Guidelines for Dressing and Undressing Patients   298
Procedure 64 Dressing and Undressing Patient   298

Unit 24
General Comfort Measures   302
Introduction   303
AM Care and PM Care   303
Oral Hygiene   304
Procedure 65 Assisting with Routine Oral Hygiene   304
Procedure 66 Assisting with Special Oral Hygiene   306

Procedure 67 Assisting Patient to Floss and Brush Teeth   306
Dentures   307
Procedure 68 Caring for Dentures   307
Back Rubs   308
Procedure 69 Backrub   309
Daily Shaving   310
Guidelines for Safety in Shaving   310
Procedure 70 Shaving a Male Patient   310
Daily Hair Care   311
Procedure 71 Daily Hair Care   312
Comfort Devices   312
Elimination Needs   313
Procedure 72 Giving and Receiving the Bedpan   313
Procedure 73 Giving and Receiving the Urinal   315
Procedure 74 Assisting with the Use of the Bedside Commode   316

SECTION 8

PRINCIPLES OF NUTRITION AND FLUID BALANCE   319

Unit 25
Nutritional Needs and Diet Modifications   320
Introduction   321
Normal Nutrition   321
Essential Nutrients   321
The Six Food Groups   322
Basic Facility Diets   324
Special Diets   326
Supplements and Nourishments   328
Fluid Balance   329
Changing Water   331
Feeding the Patient   331
Procedure 75 Assisting the Patient Who Can Feed Self   331
Procedure 76 Feeding the Dependent Patient   333
Alternative Nutrition   334

SECTION 9

SPECIAL CARE PROCEDURES   337

Unit 26
Warm and Cold Applications   338
Introduction   339
Therapy with Heat and Cold   339
Guidelines for Warm and Cold Treatments   339
Use of Cold Applications   340
Procedure 77 Applying an Ice Bag   340
Procedure 78 Applying a Disposable Cold Pack   342

Use of Warm Applications 342

Procedure 79 Applying an Aquamatic K-Pad® 343

Procedure 80 Performing a Warm Soak 344

Procedure 81 Applying a Warm Moist Compress 345

Temperature Control Measures 345

Procedure 82 Assisting with the Application of a Hypothermia Blanket 347

Unit 27
Assisting with the Physical Examination 349

Introduction 350
Positioning the Patient 350
Physical Examination 352

Procedure 83 Assisting with a Physical Examination 353

Unit 28
The Surgical Patient 355

Introduction 356
Pain Perception 356
Anesthesia 356
Surgical Care 357
Preoperative Care 357

Procedure 84 Shaving the Operative Area 359

During the Operative Period 360
Postoperative Care 360

Procedure 85 Assisting Patient to Deep Breathe and Cough 364

Procedure 86 Performing Postoperative Leg Exercises 366

Procedure 87 Applying Elasticized Stockings 366

Procedure 88 Applying Elastic Bandage 368

Procedure 89 Assisting Patient to Dangle 369

Guidelines for Assisting the Patient in Initial Ambulation 370

Unit 29
Caring for the Emotionally Stressed Patient 372

Introduction 373
Mental Health 373
Defense Mechanisms 373
Assisting Patients to Cope 374
The Demanding Patient 374
Alcoholism 375
Maladaptive Behaviors 376

Guidelines for Assisting the Patient Who is Depressed 378

Guidelines for Reality Orientation 380

Guidelines for Managing the Patient Who is Agitated 381

Unit 30
Death and Dying 384

Introduction 385
Five Stages of Grief 385
Preparation for Death 387
The Patient Self-Determination Act 387
The Role of the Nursing Assistant 388
Hospice Care 390
Physical Changes as Death Approaches 390
Postmortem Care 391
Organ Donations 392
Postmortem Examination (Autopsy) 392

Procedure 90 Giving Postmortem Care 392

SECTION 10

OTHER HEALTH CARE SETTINGS 395

Unit 31
Care of the Elderly and Chronically Ill 396

Introduction 397
Types of Long-Term Care Facilities 397
Long-Term Care Population 398
Legislation Affecting Long-Term Care 399
Role of the Nursing Assistant in a Skilled Care Facility 399
Effects of Aging 400
Nutritional Needs 403
Preventing Infections in Residents 403
Keeping Residents Safe 405
Exercise and Recreational Needs 405
General Hygiene 406
Guidelines for Bathing the Elderly 407
Mental Changes 408
Caring for Residents with Dementia 408
Guidelines for Activites of Daily Living for Residents with Dementia 411
Guidelines for Reality Orientation 413

Unit 32
The Organization of Home Care: Trends in Health Care 416

Introduction 417
Providers of Home Health Care 417
Benefits of Working in Home Health Care 418
Source of Referral 418
Payment for Home Health Care 418
The Home Health Care Team 418
The Assessment Process 419
Liability and the Nursing Assistant 420
Recordkeeping 420
Guidelines for Avoiding Liability 420
Time Management 421
Working with Families 424

Unit 33
The Nursing Assistant in Home Care 426

The Home Health Caregiver   427
The Home Health Assistant and the Nursing
Process   427
Characteristics of the Home Care Nursing
Assistant and Homemaker Assistant   427
Home Health Care Duties   428
Safety in the Home   429
Elder Abuse   430
Guidelines for Supervising Self-Administration
of Medications   430
Infection Control   430
Housekeeping Tasks   431

Unit 34
Subacute Care   435

Description of Subacute Care   436
Special Procedures Provided in the Subacute
Care Unit   436
Guidelines for Caring for Patients with
Intravenous Lines   439
Procedure 91 Changing a Gown on a Patient
with a Peripheral Intravenous Line in Place   439
Pain Management Procedures   440
Caring for Patients with Tracheostomies   440
Caring for the Patient Receiving Dialysis
Treatments   441
Oncology Treatments   442

SECTION 11

**BODY SYSTEMS, COMMON DISORDERS,
AND RELATED CARE PROCEDURES   445**

Unit 35
Integumentary System   446

Integumentary System Structures   447
Skin Functions   447
Aging Changes   447
Skin Lesions   448
Guidelines for Preventing Pressure Ulcers   452

Unit 36
Respiratory System   458

Introduction   459
Structure and Function   459
Upper Respiratory Infections   460
Chronic Obstructive Pulmonary Disease   460
Malignancies   461
Diagnostic Techniques   462
Special Therapies Related to Respiratory Illness   462
Procedure 92 Refilling the Humidifier Bottle   464
Collecting a Sputum Specimen   466
Procedure 93 Collecting a Sputum Specimen   466

Unit 37
Circulatory (Cardiovascular) System   469

Introduction   470
Structure and Function   470
Common Circulatory System Disorders   472
Peripheral Vascular Diseases   472
Guidelines for Caring for Patients with
Peripheral Vascular Disease   477
Heart Conditions   478
Blood Abnormalities   480
Diagnostic Tests   481

Unit 38
Musculoskeletal System   483

The Musculoskeletal System   484
Common Conditions   488
Guidelines for Caring for Patients with THA   492
Range of Motion   493
Procedure 94 Performing Range-of-Motion
Exercises (Passive)   494
Diagnostic Techniques   498

Unit 39
Endocrine System   500

Structure and Function   501
Common Conditions of the Thyroid Gland   502
Common Conditions of the Parathyroid Glands 503
Common Conditions of the Adrenal Glands   503
Diabetes Mellitus   503
Diagnostic Techniques   506
Blood Glucose Monitoring   506
Procedure 95 Testing Urine for Acetone:
Ketostix® Strip Test   507

Unit 40
Nervous System   509

Structure and Function   510
Common Conditions   516
Procedure 96 Caring for Eye Socket and
Artificial Eye   525
Guidelines for Caring for a Hearing Aid   526
Guidelines for Troubleshooting Hearing Aids   526
Procedure 97 Applying a Behind-the-Ear
Hearing Aid   526
Procedure 98 Removing a Behind-the-Ear
Hearing Aid   527
Procedure 99 Applying and Removing an
In-the-Ear Hearing Aid   528
Diagnostic Techniques   528

Unit 41
Gastrointestinal System   531

Introduction   532
Structure and Function   532
Common Conditions   533

Procedure 100 Collecting a Stool Specimen   536
Special Diagnostic Tests   537
Enemas   537
Procedure 101 Giving a Soap Solution Enema   538
Procedure 102 Giving a Commercially Prepared Enema   541
Procedure 103 Inserting a Rectal Suppository   542
Procedure 104 Inserting a Rectal Tube and Flatus Bag   544

Unit 42
Urinary System   546
Introduction   547
Structure and Function   547
Common Conditions   548
Responsibilities of the Nursing Assistant   549
Urinary Incontinence   550
Guidelines for Caring for the Patient with Incontinence   550
Diagnostic Tests   551
Procedure 105 Collecting a Routine Urine Specimen   551
Procedure 106 Collecting a Clean-Catch Urine Specimen   553
Procedure 107 Collecting a Fresh Fractional Urine Specimen   554
Procedure 108 Collecting a 24-Hour Urine Specimen   555
Procedure 109 Testing Urine with the Hemacombistix®   556
Renal Dialysis   556
Urinary Drainage   557
Procedure 110 Routine Drainage Check   558
Procedure 111 Giving Indwelling Catheter Care   558
Procedure 112 Emptying a Urinary Drainage Unit   560
Procedure 113 Disconnecting the Catheter   561
Procedure 114 Applying a Condom for Urinary Drainage   562
Procedure 115 Connecting a Catheter to a Leg Bag   563
Procedure 116 Emptying a Leg Bag   564

Unit 43
Reproductive System   567
Structure and Function   568
Conditions of the Male Reproductive Organs   571
Conditions of the Female Reproductive Organs   571
Sexually Transmitted Disease (STD)   573
Diagnostic Tests   574
Vaginal Douche   574
Procedure 117 Breast Self-Examination   575
Procedure 118 Giving a Nonsterile Vaginal Douche   576

SECTION 12

EXPANDED ROLE OF THE NURSING ASSISTANT   579

Unit 44
Rehabilitation and Restorative Services   580
Introduction to Rehabilitation and Restorative Care   581
Reasons for Rehabilitation/Restorative Care   582
The Interdisciplinary Health Care Team   582
Principles of Rehabilitation   583
Complications from Inactivity   583
Restorative Programs   584
Guidelines for Implementing Restorative Programs   586

Unit 45
Obstetrical Patient and Neonate   589
Introduction   590
Prenatal Care   590
Preparation for Birth   591
Prenatal Testing   591
Labor and Delivery   591
Cesarean Birth   594
Postpartum Care   594
Toileting and Perineal Care   595
Breast Care   595
Neonatal Care   595
Discharge   598

Unit 46
Pediatric Patient   600
Introduction   601
Pediatric Units   601
Developmental Tasks   601
Procedure 119 Admitting the Pediatric Patient   602
Caring for Infants (Birth–1 Year)   602
Procedure 120 Weighing the Pediatric Patient   604
Procedure 121 Changing Crib Linens   605
Procedure 122 Changing Crib Linens (Infant in Crib)   606
Procedure 123 Measuring Temperature   607
Procedure 124 Determining Heart Rate (Pulse)   608
Procedure 125 Counting Respiratory Rate   609
Procedure 126 Measuring Blood Pressure   609
Procedure 127 Bottle-Feeding the Infant   609
Procedure 128 Burping (Method A)   611
Procedure 129 Burping (Method B)   612
Guidelines for Ensuring a Safe Environment for Infants   612
Caring for Toddlers (1–3 Years)   612
Guidelines for Ensuring a Safe Environment for Toddlers   614

Caring for Preschool Children (3–6 Years)   615
Guidelines for Ensuring a Safe Environment for Preschoolers   615
Caring for School-Age Children (6 – 12 Years)   616
Guidelines for Ensuring a Safe Environment for the School-Age Child   617
Caring for the Adolescent (13–18 Years)   617
Guidelines for Ensuring a Safe Environment for Adolescents   619

Unit 47
Special Advanced Procedures   621
Introduction   622
Urine and Stool Tests   622
Procedure 130 Testing for Occult Blood Using Hemoccult® and Developer   622
Procedure 131 Testing for Occult Blood Using Hematest® Reagent Tablets   623
Procedure 132 Collecting a Urine Specimen Through a Drainage Port   624
Ostomies   625
Procedure 133 Giving Routine Stoma Care (Colostomy)   626
Procedure 134 Routine Care of an Ileostomy (With Patient in Bed)   628

SECTION 13

RESPONSE TO BASIC EMERGENCIES   631

Unit 48
Response to Basic Emergencies   632
Dealing With Emergencies   633
Guidelines for Responding to an Emergency   633
Being Prepared   634
First Aid   634
Emergency Care   634
Cardiac Arrest   634
Procedure 135 Adult CPR, One Rescuer   635
Procedure 136 Adult CPR, Two-Person   639
Choking   641
Procedure 137 Heimlich Maneuver— Abdominal Thrusts   642
Procedure 138 Assisting the Adult Who Has an Obstructed Airway and Becomes Unconscious   643
CPR and Obstructed Airway Procedures for Infants   644
CPR and Obstructed Airway Procedures for Children   644

Procedure 139 CPR for Infants   644
Procedure 140 Obstructed Airway: Conscious Infant   646
Procedure 141 Obstructed Airway: Unconscious Infant   647
Procedure 142 CPR for Children, One Rescuer 648
Procedure 143 Child with Foreign Body Airway Obstruction   648
Other Emergencies   649
Bleeding   649
Shock   650
Fainting   650
Heart Attack   651
Brain Attacks   651
Seizures   652
Electric Shock   652
Burns   652
Orthopedic Injuries   653
Accidental Poisoning   653

SECTION 14

MOVING FORWARD   657

Unit 49
Employment Opportunities and Career Growth   658
Introduction   659
Objective 1: Self-Appraisal   659
Objective 2: Search for All Employment Opportunities   659
Objective 3: Assemble a Proper Resume   660
Objective 4: Validate References   660
Objective 5: Make Specific Applications for Work   660
Objective 6: Participate in a Successful Interview 663
Objective 7: Accept a Job   663
Objective 8: Keep the Job   664
Objective 9: Continue to Grow throughout Your Career   664
Objective 10: Resign Properly from Employment   665

Appendix
Guidelines for Infection Control in Health Care Personnel (CDC, 1998)   667

Glossary   673

Index   693

About the Authors

BARBARA R. HEGNER

Barbara Robinson Hegner, RN, MSN, is a graduate of a three-year diploma nursing program where direct and total care was the focus. She earned a BSN at Boston College and an MS in nursing from Boston University, with a minor in biologic sciences. She is Professor Emerita of Nursing and Life Sciences at Long Beach City College, Long Beach (CA).

Throughout her professional career, she has had a deep interest in both hospital-based and long-term care nursing. She continues to update her nursing knowledge and skills and has kept performance levels current with nursing practice. She is an active participant in clinical symposia.

It has long been Ms. Hegner's belief that to ensure the rights and well-being of all patients and residents requires the care of competent, caring nursing assistants under the supervision of professional nurses. The nursing assistants who provide this care should be thoroughly trained and consistently encouraged, evaluated, and given the opportunity for continued learning. Providing the tools to prepare these health care providers in the most effective and efficient way is the goal of *Nursing Assistant, A Nursing Process Approach,* eighth edition. She is the author of the following texts, also from Delmar Publishers: *Geriatrics, A Study of Maturity,* fifth edition, and *Assisting in Long-Term Care,* third edition.

JOAN F. NEEDHAM

Joan Fritsch Needham, MSEd, RNC, is a contributing author to the eighth edition of *Nursing Assistant, A Nursing Process Approach.* She also graduated from a three-year diploma nursing program. She received her BS from the College of Saint Francis and her MS from Northern Illinois University. She is certified by the American Nurses Association in Gerontological Nursing. Ms. Needham was Director of Education at a long-term care facility where she was responsible for staff development, curriculum development and instruction for basic and advanced nursing assistant training, and development and instruction in continuing education courses for licensed nurses. In addition, she is a part-time instructor at a community college for nursing assistant and nursing continuing education courses.

She contributed to *Assisting in Long-Term Care,* second and third editions (Delmar), is the coauthor of the *Pocket Reference for the Long-Term Care Nursing Assistant* (Delmar), and is the author of *Gerontological Nursing—A Restorative Approach* (Delmar) and *Plans of Care for Specialty Practice, Gerontological Nursing* (Delmar).

Preface

INTRODUCTION

The passage of the Omnibus Budget Reconciliation Act (OBRA) of 1987, which included the Nursing Home Reform Act, was the first federal legislation to address standards for certification of nursing assistants as health care providers in long-term care. This legislation has influenced both the education and practice of all nursing assistants.

Following the enactment of OBRA, the National Council of State Boards of Nursing Inc. developed the Nurse Aide Competency Evaluation Program as the guideline for evaluating the training of nursing assistants to meet the specific needs of health care consumers. Individual states have developed training programs that meet, and in many cases, exceed the minimum standards of the evaluation program.

Nursing assistants are important members of the nursing team (one part of the interdisciplinary health care team that plans and provides care to clients). Nursing assistants make valuable contributions to the nursing process that the professional nurse follows in assessing the client's needs, planning interventions, implementing care, and evaluating outcomes. Nursing assistants must be helped to see the vital role their accurate observations, reporting skills, and careful attention to instructions plays in the overall success of the nursing care plan. Only then can they recognize the full value of their role as part of the nursing team.

Previous editions of this best-selling text emphasized the importance of treating those entrusted to care as total individuals who possess dignity, have value, and deserve respect. The continuing goal of this text and supplement package is to provide the tools that instructors can use to train nursing assistants to meet high standards of care. This will enable them to help clients achieve a desirable level of comfort, restoration, and wellness while ensuring their rights as health care consumers.

THE FUTURE

The ways in which health care is provided in the United States continue to change. Emphasis continues to be placed on maintaining wellness, limiting length of stay in acute care facilities, controlling costs through managed care, providing short- and long-term rehabilitation and restorative care in more cost-effective settings, and increasing home care services. In addition, the population of the United States is aging, with the greatest increase in the number of people over 65. As a result, restorative care and home care services will be major components in health care. Nursing assistants will provide much of this service. It is essential that nursing assistants be prepared to assume these vital responsibilities.

EIGHTH EDITION

Numerous revisions were made in the 8th edition to keep pace with the evolution of health care. New health care settings, new and improved technology, shorter acute care stays, an aging population, and drug resistant microorganisms are some of the factors that are changing the ways in which care is provided. These factors also affect the way in which nursing assistants provide care.

The 8th edition of *Nursing Assistant* was also revised to achieve a better organization of content, more consistency between units, less repetition of content, and an improved reading level.

The following updated and enhanced content addresses the changing character of nursing assistant responsibilities.

- New content was added on the role of the multiskilled health care worker on the interdisciplinary health care team

- New unit 3 on consumer rights and responsibilities in health care, including content on financing health care

- Unit 4 presents separate clients' rights, patients' rights and residents' rights for comparison and contrast

- Unit 5 was reorganized to cover basic body organization and the elements of medical terminology. Anatomy and physiology content is now found in individual body system units

- Greater emphasis on the direct nursing care provided by nursing assistants with specific guidelines for various patient care situations

- Nursing Assistant Challenge provided at the end of each unit to help learners develop critical thinking skills

- Expanded unit 7 on communication skills to provide guidelines for communicating with patients with sight impairment, hearing impairment, dementia, aphasia, agitation, etc.

- Content in unit 9 on meeting basic human needs now stresses growth and development from infancy through old age with the characteristic needs for each group

- New unit 10 on cultural diversity covers how cultural influences affect the client's expectations from health care and reactions to it, as well as the effect of cultural practices

- Units 11 and 12 were expanded and up-dated to reflect the latest CDC guidelines and OSHA recommendations; also includes information on reducing environmental contamination through the use of the one-glove technique and the latest CDC recommendations (1997/1998) for the immunization of health care workers

- Unit 13 provides expanded content on environmental and nursing assistant safety, including new content on ergonomics; safety issues are stressed in each unit

- Unit 14 provides expanded content on patient safety and positioning

- Separate units on patient transfers (15) and ambulation (16) highlight these important aspects of nursing assistant practice

- Unit 31 on care of the elderly and chronically ill was reorganized to focus on this population. Content that also applied to other populations of patients was moved to the appropriate units

- Content on home care was expanded and divided between two units: 32 on the organization of home care and 33 on the nursing assistant in home care

- New unit 34 on subacute care discusses the need for this type of care as sicker patients are discharged from hospitals, where this care can be found, and typical nursing assistant responsibilities in providing care in this setting

- Body systems units in Section 11 cover basic anatomy and physiology of the system, common conditions, diagnostic tests, nursing assistant actions and related procedures.

- In unit 35 on the integumentary system, content on pressure ulcers was updated to reflect guidelines from the Agency for Health Care Policy and Research (AHCPR)

- Expanded and updated unit 44 on rehabilitation and restorative services

- Obstructed airway and CPR procedures for adults, infants and children were added to unit 48 on response to basic emergencies

- The Appendix summarizes infection control guidelines for health care personnel (CDC, 1998)

EXTENSIVE TEACHING/ LEARNING PACKAGE

The complete supplement package was developed to achieve two goals:

1. To assist students in learning essential information to permit them to become certified and function as skilled nursing assistants

2. To assist instructors in planning and implementing their instructional program for the most efficient use of time and other resources

Each supplement has been extensively revised to reflect text changes.

Student Workbook

The comprehensive workbook reinforces the text content. It is recommended that the student complete each workbook unit to confirm understanding of essential content.

The workbook content includes:

- Tips on how to study more effectively

- Organization by units with student activities to increase comprehension. Each unit consists of objectives to focus the content for the student, a unit summary to point out key topics, nursing assistant alerts that provide key actions with an explanation of the benefit resulting from the action, and various exercises (review questions, vocabulary exercises and games, and clinical situations).

- Student Performance Record — alphabetical listing of 143 text procedures to monitor student completion of return demonstrations

- Flash cards provide a review of basic medical terms, including combining forms, prefixes, and suffixes.

Instructor's Manual

The Instructor's Manual provides the following support:

- An extensive list of resource materials

- A list of health care and aging-related organizations providing free or low-cost educational materials

- Curriculum syllabus for a typical 75–90 hour nursing assistant program

- Organized by corresponding text unit: instructor objectives, suggested activities, and answers to unit review questions

- Answers to student workbook exercises

- Section tests with answers

- Comprehensive final examination with answers

- Extra bank of test questions (with answers) to simplify preparation of tests or to provide additional testing material for advanced students

- Procedures Evaluation Form that can be duplicated for each student as a checklist of progress in successfully demonstrating procedures; essential OBRA procedure skills are identified as an aid in monitoring student progress
- Transparency masters
- The Manual is available as a separate item or as part of the Instructor's Resource Kit.

Computerized Test Bank

Computerized testbank (Windows) with more than 2,000 questions that will give the instructor an expanded capability to create tests. The testbank is available as a separate item or as part of the Instructor's Resource Kit.

Instructor's Resource Kit

This supplement provides the instructor with resources to simplify the planning and implementation of the instructional program. It integrates the use of the text, Student Workbook, Instructor's Manual, and video series to help the instructor develop an efficient instructional plan.

The complete Instructor's Resource Kit includes the following list of sections, plus the complete Instructor's Manual and the computerized testbank.

Section content:

- Section A — Teaching Methods and Strategies provides tips on teaching adult learners, including English as a second language (ESL) students
- Section B — Teaching Resources includes a listing of *Delmar's Nursing Assisting Video Series,* other audiovisual aids, software resources, reference texts, models and charts, media sources, and a listing of professional health organizations.
- Section C — course syllabi for 70 to 90 hour, 120-hour, 300-hour, and 600-hour programs. Each syllabus outlines the number of hours for didactic work and clinical experience and relates these to the use of *Nursing Assistant, A Nursing Process Approach, 8E.*
- Section D — Lesson Plans in which the supplemental materials and the text are related into a cohesive plan for presenting each topic

- Section E — Unit Outlines highlight the essential topics for each unit. Suggested activities provide a means of generating student interest and interaction in class to reinforce learning
- Section F — English-Spanish Flash Cards show common terms and simple phrases in English and Spanish to facilitate communication in the workplace. ESL students can use the flash cards to improve English skills. English speaking students will find them useful in communicating with Spanish-speaking colleagues, patients, and residents
- Section G — Computerized Test Bank

Delmar's Nursing Procedures Video Series

Delmar's Nursing Assisting Video Series, third edition, is a series of 22 videos, which contain 144 segments and 104 essential clinical skills. Many of the procedures are core procedures used in acute care, long-term care, and home care situations. Other procedures are designed to meet the unique needs of the elderly in long-term care. The videos average 30 minutes in length and are cross-referenced with symbols in the text and various supplements to help instructors integrate them into their teaching plans.

The videos were developed by health care professionals based on requests from our textbook users. The procedures and activities shown on the videos recognize the nursing assistant of the 1990s as a skilled professional who works as an important member of the interdisciplinary team under the supervision of a licensed nurse.

Tape 5 on infection control and tape 21 on isolation skills were recently revised to reflect the latest CDC guidelines on standard precautions and transmission based precautions.

Acknowledgments

Each new edition brings with it the pleasant task of acknowledging the contributions of a number of individuals.

We particularly want to thank Joan Fritsch Needham, RN, MSN, who, as contributing author, played a crucial role in the 7th and 8th editions of the text. Ms. Needham draws from her many years' experience in staff development (including the training of nursing assistants) in a long-term care facility, as well as her responsibilities at a community college for training programs for nursing assistants and multiskilled workers. Ms. Needham is also responsible for the revision of the Instructor's Manual to accompany the text.

We also wish to thank Saratoga Hospital, Saratoga Springs, NY for allowing our photo team to conduct part of the photo shoot for the 8th edition on site. Special thanks to Denise Clyne for making the arrangements and for gathering equipment and supplies used in the shoot.

Special thanks are due to the photographer, Thomas Stock, and his staff from Stock Studios of Saratoga Springs, NY. Using a digital camera, the photo crew was able to review each shot immediately on a monitor, restage the shot if required, and obtain the exact image needed. Mr. Stock's attention to detail, creativity, and humor were critical factors in the success of the photo shoot.

Reviewers

The revision was aided by a dedicated group of instructors who reviewed content at different stages of the revision process. For their valuable suggestions and corrections, we thank:

Barbara Acello, MS, RN, Innovations in Health Care, Denton, TX

Suzann Balduzzi, BSN, MSED, Western Wisconsin Technical College, La Crosse, WI

Patricia Bittinger, RN, MS, Salina Area Vocational Technical School, Salina, KS

Betty Fields Brisbin, Duval County School Board, Jacksonville, FL

Hannah Dixon, RN, PhD, Penn Valley Community College, Kansas City, MO

Kathleen Hess, RN, MS, Antonelli Medical and Professional Institute, Pottstown, PA 19464

Janet Knight, RN, Davis Supply Technical Center, Kaysville, UT 84037

Patricia A. Morganroth, MSN, RN, Cincinnati State Technical & Community College, Cincinnati, OH

Bertha A. Mowatt, RN, BSN, Montcalm Community College, Sidney, MI

Anne E. Simms, Albuquerque Technical-Vocational Institute, Albuquerque, NM 87106

Glenda Stapf, MS, RN, James Logan High School, Union City, CA

David Wagner, Camelot College, Baton Rouge, LA

Features of This Book

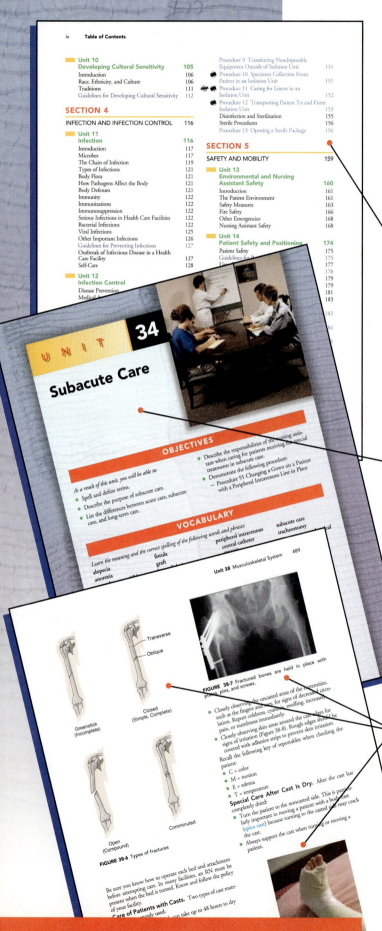

iv   Table of Contents

Unit 10
Developing Cultural Sensitivity   105
Introduction   106
Race, Ethnicity, and Culture   106
Traditions   111
Guidelines for Developing Cultural Sensitivity   112

SECTION 4

INFECTION AND INFECTION CONTROL   116

Unit 11
Infection   116
Introduction   117
Microbes   117
The Chain of Infection   119
Types of Infections   121
Body Flora   121
How Pathogens Affect the Body   121
Body Defenses   121
Immunity   122
Immunizations   122
Immunosuppression   122
Serious Infections in Health Care Facilities   122
Bacterial Infections   122
Viral Infections   125
Other Important Infections   126
Guidelines for Preventing Infections   127
Outbreak of Infectious Disease in a Health Care Facility   127
Self-Care   128

Unit 12
Infection Control
Disease Prevention
Medical

Procedure 9 Transferring Nondisposable Equipment Outside of Isolation Unit   151
Procedure 10 Specimen Collection From Patient in an Isolation Unit   151
Procedure 11 Caring for Linens in an Isolation Unit   152
Procedure 12 Transporting Patient To and From Isolation Unit   153
Disinfection and Sterilization   155
Sterile Procedures   156
Procedure 13 Opening a Sterile Package   156

SECTION 5

SAFETY AND MOBILITY   159

Unit 13
Environmental and Nursing Assistant Safety   160
Introduction   161
The Patient Environment   161
Safety Measures   163
Fire Safety   166
Other Emergencies   168
Nursing Assistant Safety   168

Unit 14
Patient Safety and Positioning   174
Patient Safety   175
Guidelines for P   175
Li   177
178
179
179
181
183
183
84

The eighth edition of *Nursing Assistant, a Nursing Process Approach* has been carefully designed and updated to make the study of nursing assistant tasks and responsibilities easier and more productive. For best results, you may want to become familiar with the features incorporated into this text and accompanying learning tools.

Table of Contents

For each unit, the table of contents lists the unit title, major topic headings, general guidelines for specific areas of care and topics of importance to the nursing assistant, and patient care procedures. As appropriate, icons are used with the procedures to identify:

- Essential OBRA procedures that students must master for certification

- Procedures for which there is a corresponding segment on *Delmar's Nursing Assisting Video Series, 3rd edition*

Unit Opening Page

Each unit opening page contains objectives and vocabulary terms.

The **objectives** help you know what is expected of you as you read the text. Your success in mastering each objective is measured by the review questions at the end of each unit.

The **vocabulary** list alerts you to new terms presented in the unit. When each term is first used in the unit, it is highlighted in boldface and color. Each term is defined at this point in the unit. Read the definition of the term and note the context in which it is used so that you will feel comfortable in using the term. Note that the glossary at the back of the book also defines these highlighted terms.

Photographs and Line Drawings

Numerous color illustrations and photos, including more than 100 new photos taken for this edition, help to clarify and reinforce the unit content. Many figures are used in the procedures to help you visualize critical steps. Full color anatomy drawings help you to locate body components and understand body organization.

Guidelines

The table of contents identifies guidelines included in units. These guidelines highlight important points that you need to remember for specific situations or types of care. They are presented in an easy to use format that you can refer to repeatedly until you know the actions you must take when confronted with the situation.

Procedures

The text contains 143 clinical procedures in a step-by-step format. Each procedure reminds you to perform the beginning procedure actions. A list of equipment and supplies needed for the procedure is provided. Any notes or cautions about performing the procedure are given. The steps take you carefully through the procedure, emphasizing at all times the need to work safely and to protect the patient's privacy. At the end, you are reminded of the procedure completion actions.

Some or all of the following icons may be used in the procedures:

- **OBRA** to indicate an essential procedure required for certification
- **gloves** to indicate the need to observe standard precautions and wear personal protective equipment
- **video** to indicate that there is a companion video segment for the procedure in *Delmar's Nursing Assisting Video Series, 3rd edition*
- **note** to indicate important considerations in the performance of the procedure
- **caution** to make you aware of special concerns or practices

The **note** and **caution** icons are also used through out the text to relate to specific content.

Review and Testing Material

Unit Reviews

A variety of review questions at the end of each unit test your understanding of the unit content. Each review contains a **Nursing Assistant Challenge** that presents a typical clinical situation and asks questions about your response to the situation. These questions require you to integrate what you have learned to arrive at an appropriate solution or set of actions.

For additional activities and exercises to reinforce your learning, refer to the Student Workbook. Your instructor may also give you additional questions and tests from the Instructor's Manual, Instructor's Resource Kit or the Computerized Test Bank that accompany the text.

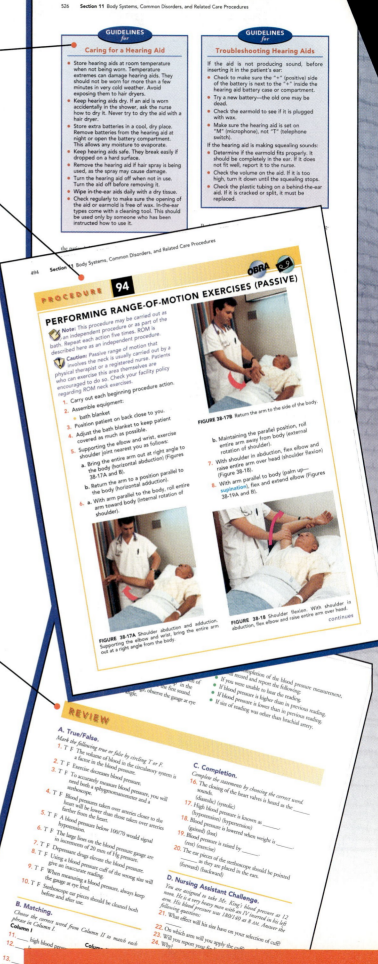

Introduction to Nursing Assisting

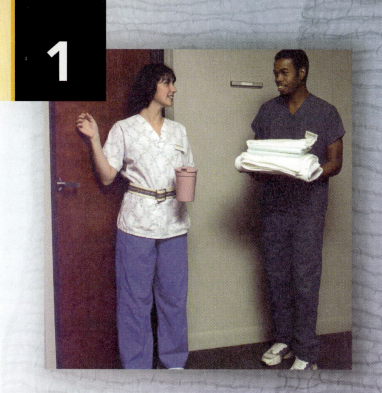

UNIT 1
Community Health Care

UNIT 2
Role of the Nursing Assistant

UNIT 3
Consumer Rights and Responsibilities in Health Care

UNIT 4
Ethical and Legal Issues Affecting the Nursing Assistant

U N I T **1**

Community Health Care

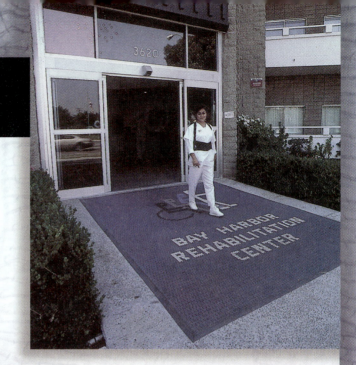

As a result of this unit, you will be able to:

- Spell and define terms.
- List the five basic functions of health care facilities.
- Describe four changes that have taken place in health care in the last few years.
- Describe the differences between short-term care and long-term care.
- Name the departments within a hospital.
- Describe the functions of the departments within a hospital.
- Explain three ways by which health care costs are paid.

VOCABULARY

Learn the meaning and the correct spelling of the following words and phrases:

acute illness	hospice	pathology	prenatal
chronic illness	hospital	patient	psychiatric
client	managed care	patient focused care	rehabilitation
community	Medicaid	pediatric	resident
facility	Medicare	physical therapy	skilled care facility
health care consumer	obstetric	post-anesthesia recovery	speech therapy
health maintenance	occupational therapy	(PAR)	
organization (HMO)	orthopedic	postpartum	

INTRODUCTION

Nursing assistants play an important role in the care of people who are ill or injured. The care you give to these persons will be done under the direction and supervision of licensed, professional health care workers, such as doctors and nurses. Care is provided in various types of health care facilities. The term **facility** refers to the place in which care is given. A **hospital** is a complex organization that provides a full range of health care services. Highly sophisticated equipment and treatments are available. A **skilled care facility** provides care to persons whose conditions are stable but who require monitoring, nursing care, and treatments. All health care facilities have five basic functions:

1. Providing services for the ill and injured (Figure 1-1).
2. Preventing disease.
3. Promoting individual and community health.
4. Educating health care workers (Figure 1-2).
5. Promoting research in medicine and nursing.

OVERVIEW OF HEALTH CARE

Emphasis is placed on **patient focused care**. This means that each patient is a unique individual and has different needs. Attention must be given to the physical, mental, and emotional aspects of the person's being if that person is to lead a fulfilling and satisfying life.

Many changes have occurred in health care within the last few years. There are several reasons for these changes:

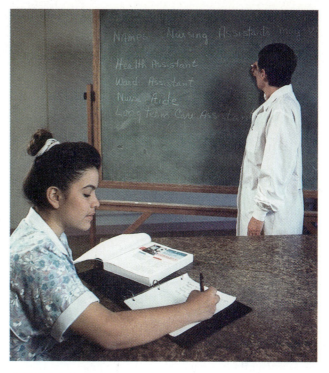

FIGURE 1-2 Health care facilities provide education for health care workers.

● People are living longer. As people age, the need for health care increases, so more services are needed (Figure 1-3).
● Advanced technology means that more lives are saved. Although life is maintained, some of these individuals will need continuing health care.

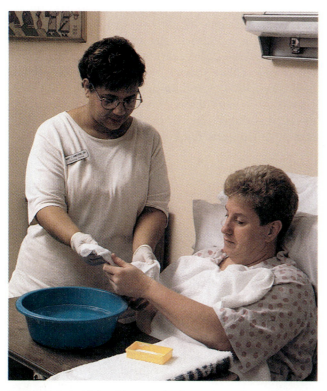

FIGURE 1-1 All health care facilities provide services for the ill and injured.

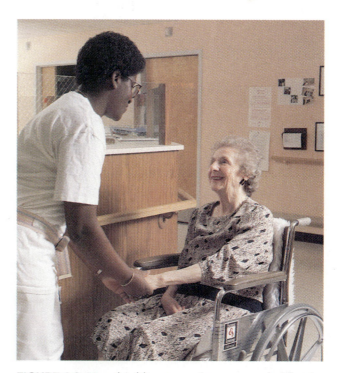

FIGURE 1-3 More health care services are needed for the growing elderly population.

- The cost of health care has increased tremendously because of the demand for services and because of the technology.
- Science has created many ethical (moral) questions that must be answered by health care providers and health care consumers.

To reduce the cost of health care, patients are discharged earlier from hospitals. These patients may still require health care. This care can be given more economically in skilled care facilities and in the patient's home. More diagnostic tests and procedures are provided in outpatient facilities, to further decrease costs. Surgicenters, urgent care centers, and clinics are examples of such facilities. It is less expensive, for example, to receive treatment for a throat infection in an urgent care center than in a hospital emergency room.

Most health care is paid for with insurance. Insurance companies use managed care to provide the services in the most efficient manner at the lowest cost. Briefly, this means that the insurance company will:

- Require approval by the insurance company before certain procedures or diagnostic tests are done.
- Negotiate with specific physicians, hospitals, pharmacies, and other care providers to render services at a lower cost to the company's members.
- Approve only a certain number of days of hospitalization for specific diagnoses. A woman giving birth, for example, may be allowed up to 48 hours of hospitalization.
- Require that specific procedures be done on an outpatient basis rather than having the patient admitted to the hospital.

NEEDS OF THE COMMUNITY

People who live in a common area and share common health needs form a community. Provisions for disposal of wastes, assurance of safe drinking water, availability of healthful foods, protection from disease, and health care are important to every person within a community. Public health laws regulate these services and are enforced by government agencies.

Health care is needed throughout life. The care may be short-term or long-term and includes:

- Preventive care
  - Prenatal care (care of the mother during pregnancy).
  - Well baby checkups and immunizations.
  - Health education to teach individuals how to avoid disease and injury.
  - Physical examinations throughout life.
- Emergency care
  - Short-term care given for sudden illness or injury.
- Surgery
  - To repair an injured body or remove a diseased organ.
- Rehabilitation
  - To help a patient to regain abilities after illness or injury.

- Long-term care
  - For patients who have chronic or incurable conditions.
- Hospice care
  - For patients who are dying and their families.

Persons receiving health care are called health care consumers. They are also identified by the type of care they need:

- Patient is a term used for persons in acute care facilities such as hospitals.
- Client is a term used for persons receiving care in their own homes.
- Resident is usually a term for people in skilled care (long-term) facilities.

COMMUNITY HEALTH CARE SERVICES

There are basically two types of health care facilities: those that provide short-term care and those that provide long-term care (Table 1-1). Short-term care is given to patients who have a routine or minor problem, such as a urinary tract infection. The care may be given in the physician's office, an outpatient clinic, or an urgent care center. Uncomplicated surgeries, such as hernia repair, are short-term and may be done in a surgicenter. Hospitals provide short-term care for acute illnesses. An acute illness or injury comes on suddenly and requires intense, immediate treatment. Heart attacks, severe burns, strokes, and uncontrolled diabetes are examples of acute conditions.

Long-term care is necessary for persons who have chronic conditions. A chronic illness is one that is treatable but not curable and is expected to require lifelong care. This care may be given in a skilled care facility, adult day-care setting, respite care facility, assisted living facility, or the patient's home (Figure 1-4). Cardiovascular disease (heart and blood vessels), Alzheimer's disease, multiple sclerosis, Parkinson's disease, and diabetes are chronic illnesses. Additional information for long-term care is given in Section 10.

TABLE 1-1 TYPES OF HEALTH CARE FACILITIES	
Short-Term Care	**Long-Term Care**
Hospitals	Skilled Care Facilities
Urgent Care Facilities	Adult Day Care
Surgicenters	Assisted Living Facilities Rehabilitation Centers Psychiatric Hospitals
Outpatient Clinics	Respite Care
Psychiatric Hospitals	
Physician's Offices	Home Care

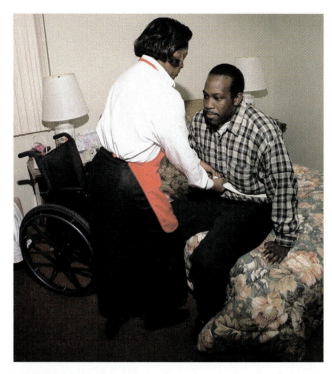

FIGURE 1-4 Health care is often given in the client's home.

Hospitals

Most hospitals are licensed to care for patients of all ages and for patients with a variety of problems. Some hospitals take care of patients with special conditions or care for specific age groups:

- Pediatric hospitals care only for children from birth to 18 years of age.
- Psychiatric hospitals provide care for persons with mental illness.
- Rehabilitation hospitals provide services to patients after an acute illness or injury.

Hospital Organization

Hospitals are organized in ways that provide the most efficient delivery of service. Major departments are established within each facility to meet the needs of patients with specific conditions (Figure 1-5). These units provide nursing care 24 hours a day, 7 days a week.

- Medical department: cares for patients with medical conditions such as pneumonia or heart disease.
- Surgical department: cares for patients before, during, and after surgery. There are many operating rooms where surgical procedures are performed, and a post-anesthesia recovery (PAR) room where patients are closely monitored for several hours after surgery.
- Pediatric department: cares for sick or injured children.
- Obstetric department: cares for newborns and their mothers. This department includes the labor and delivery unit, the postpartum unit (for mothers who have given birth), and the nursery for the newborns (Figure 1-6).

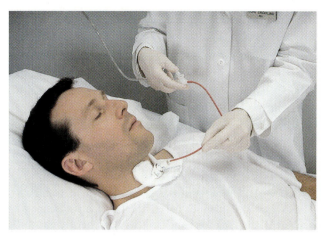

FIGURE 1-5 Facilities are organized to meet the needs of patients with specific conditions.

- Emergency department: cares for victims of trauma or of natural disasters (tornadoes, for example), or medical emergencies.
- Critical care department: cares for seriously ill patients who require constant monitoring and care.

Larger hospitals have many specialized units staffed by nurses and therapists who have been trained to care for persons with specific problems such as cancer, cardiovascular disease, or kidney disease, or for those requiring orthopedic (bones and muscles) surgery. Specialized health care workers provide direct or indirect services to the patients in these units. These units include:

- Dietary services. A registered dietitian plans the meals for all patients and provides educational services to patients on special diets. The hospital's food service department prepares meals and delivers them to patients.
- Pharmacy services. Registered pharmacists prepare and provide all medications and intravenous therapy solutions.
- Diagnostic services.
  - Pathology (study of disease). Physicians and technicians perform diagnostic tests on specimens taken from body tissue to help the doctor make a diagnosis.
  - Diagnostic imaging and radiology. Physicians and technicians take x-rays and do other specialized pro-

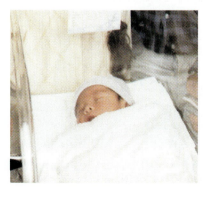

FIGURE 1-6 The obstetric department cares for mothers and newborns.

cedures to help make a diagnosis.

- Rehabilitation services.
    - **Physical therapy** assists patients to regain mobility skills.
    - **Occupational therapy** helps patients to regain self-care skills.
    - **Speech therapy** helps patients to regain the ability to communicate and works with patients diagnosed with swallowing disorders.
- Social services. Staff members provide counseling for patients and their families, help needy families get financial assistance, plan for patient discharge, and arrange for patient transfers from one facility to another (Figure 1-7).
- Environmental services.
    - Housekeeping department is responsible for the overall cleaning of the hospital (Figure 1-8).
    - Maintenance cares for and repairs equipment.
    - Laundry services provide and clean all hospital linens.
- Business services are responsible for patient billing, employee payroll, and other financial concerns.
- Medical records department transcribes and catalogs all patient records.
- Volunteers provide services free of charge and perform tasks such as delivering mail and flowers, running the gift shop, directing visitors, and raising funds for the facility (Figure 1-9).
- Pastoral care helps patients meet their religious needs and provides counseling.

Patients may be transferred from one unit to another within a hospital. For example, a patient having surgery will go from the operating room to the PAR room and then to the surgical nursing unit.

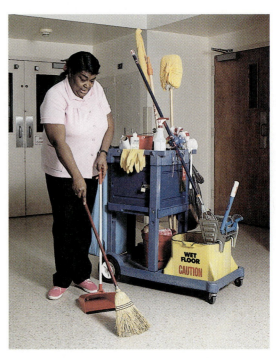

FIGURE 1-8 The housekeeping department keeps the facility clean.

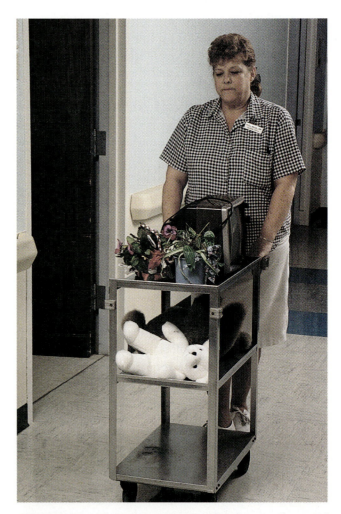

FIGURE 1-9 Volunteers provide many hours of unpaid labor.

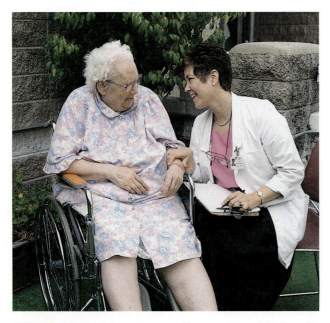

FIGURE 1-7 Social services staff are responsible for discharge planning.

FINANCING HEALTH CARE

Health care is paid for by:

- Insurance. Employers may offer a group insurance plan or persons may buy individual insurance. Premiums are costly—employers may pay all or a portion of the cost of a group insurance plan. Health maintenance organizations (HMO) are one type of prepaid insurance.
- Out-of-pocket payments by the health care consumer who has no insurance or for expenses not covered by insurance.

- Medicare is a federal government program that pays a portion of health care costs for persons 65 years and over and for younger persons who are permanently disabled and who qualify for the benefit.
- Medicaid is a state and federal government program that pays health care costs for persons of any age who do not have financial resources for health care.

Cost containment is a priority, which means that the maximum benefit of health care must be achieved for every dollar spent. Each care provider must do everything possible to avoid waste and to keep expenditures down.

REVIEW

A. True/False.

Mark the following true or false by circling T or F.

1. T F Nursing assistants work under the supervision of licensed professional health care workers.
2. T F Hospitals provide a full range of health care services.
3. T F Skilled care facilities provide care to persons who require monitoring, nursing care, and treatments.
4. T F The only function of a health care facility is to provide services for the ill and injured.
5. T F Patient focused care means treating all patients as unique individuals.
6. T F Patients can remain in the hospital until they feel well enough to go home.
7. T F Persons receiving care in the hospital are called residents.
8. T F People who live in a common area and share common health needs form a community.
9. T F Many procedures and treatments are done on an outpatient basis in an effort to reduce costs.
10. T F A chronic illness comes on suddenly and is usually curable.

B. Multiple Choice.

Select the one best answer for each problem.

11. The general term used for a person needing health care is
    a. patient.
    b. resident.
    c. health care consumer.
    d. health care provider.
12. Psychiatric hospitals provide care only to
    a. children.
    b. persons with mental illness.
    c. persons with contagious diseases.
    d. dying persons.
13. Health care facilities
    a. provide services for the ill and injured.
    b. provide education for health workers.
    c. promote research in medicine and nursing.
    d. all of these.
14. Health care has changed because
    a. there is less demand for services.
    b. people are living longer.
    c. the death rate is decreasing.
    d. all of these.
15. Hospice care is provided to patients who
    a. are dying.
    b. need rehabilitation.
    c. need surgery.
    d. are pregnant.
16. Managed care means that insurance companies may
    a. require approval by the company before certain procedures or diagnostic tests are done.
    b. negotiate with specific health care providers to render services at a lower cost.
    c. approve only a certain number of days of hospitalization.
    d. all of these.
17. The obstetrics department of the hospital cares for patients
    a. with heart disease.
    b. before, during, and after childbirth.
    c. with conditions of the bones and muscles.
    d. who are mentally ill.

18. Social services provides
    a. nursing care 24 hours a day.
    b. diagnostic testing.
    c. counseling for patients.
    d. all of these.
19. Environmental services includes
    a. laundry.
    b. housekeeping.
    c. maintenance.
    d. all of these.
20. One type of prepaid health care insurance is
    a. Medicare.
    b. Medicaid.
    c. health maintenance organization.
    d. out-of-pocket payment.

C. Word Choice.

Choose the correct word from the following list to complete each statement in questions 21–30.

hospitals	physical therapy
Medicare	prenatal
occupational therapy	residents
pathology	skilled care facility
patient focused care	surgicenter

21. A _____ provides care to persons whose conditions are stable but require monitoring, nursing care, and treatments.
22. _____ are complex organizations that provide a full range of health care services.
23. _____ is given when the patient is considered a unique individual with specific needs.
24. _____ care is given to a mother during her pregnancy.
25. Persons living in a skilled care facility are usually called _____.
26. Uncomplicated surgeries may be performed in a _____.
27. _____ means the study of disease.
28. _____ helps patients regain self-care skills.
29. _____ helps patients regain mobility skills.
30. A federal program that pays health care costs for persons 65 years of age and older is called _____.

D. Nursing Assistant Challenge.

Mrs. Hernandez is pregnant with her first child. She wants to do everything she can to make sure that she has a safe and uncomplicated pregnancy, labor, and delivery, and that her baby is healthy. Consider how Mrs. Hernandez will move through the health care system to achieve this goal.

31. What is the first type of care that Mrs. Hernandez needs to help her meet the goal of an uncomplicated pregnancy?
32. In your community, where is this type of care provided?
33. What programs are offered to pregnant women in your community?
34. From which hospital departments do you think Mrs. Hernandez will receive services when she delivers her baby?
35. After the baby is born, what health care will the baby need?

U N I T 2

Role of the Nursing Assistant

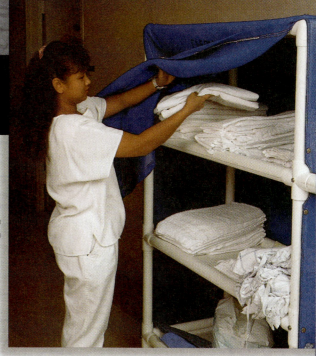

As a result of this unit, you will be able to:

- Spell and define terms.
- Identify the members of the interdisciplinary health care team.
- Identify the members of the nursing team.
- List the job responsibilities of the nursing assistant.
- Make a chart showing the lines of authority an assistant follows.
- List the rules of personal hygiene and explain the importance of a healthy mental attitude.
- Describe the appropriate dress for the job.
- Describe the importance of good human relationships.
- List the ways to build productive working relationships with staff members.

VOCABULARY

Learn the meaning and the correct spelling of the following words and phrases:

attitude
burnout
cross-trained
interdisciplinary health
  care team

interpersonal
  relationships
licensed practical nurse
  (LPN)
licensed vocational
  nurse (LVN)

Nurse Aide
  Competency
  Evaluation Program
  (NACEP)
nursing assistant
nursing team

Omnibus Budget
  Reconciliation Act
  (OBRA)
registered nurse (RN)
scope of practice

THE INTERDISCIPLINARY HEALTH CARE TEAM

The nursing assistant is an important member of the **interdisciplinary health care team**. This team includes the patient, members of his or her family, the physician, the nursing team, and other specialists trained to meet both general and specific patient needs (Figure 2-1). The physician names the condition or illness (makes a diagnosis) and prescribes treatment. Physicians frequently specialize in one area of medical practice. Table 2-1 lists medical specialties, the name for the physician who practices each specialty, and a description of the care provided by each specialist.

The **nursing team** provides skilled nursing care. The team consists of registered nurses, licensed practical (or vocational) nurses, and nursing assistants. Registered nurses plan and direct the nursing care of patients in cooperation with the physician's orders. All members of the team provide direct patient care.

Care provider specialists who may also be part of the team include the dietitian, physical therapist, occupational therapist, speech therapist, respiratory therapist, and pharmacist. Table 2-2 provides details of the training and certification or

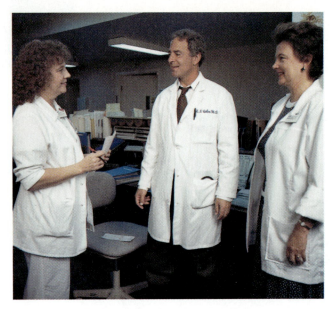

FIGURE 2-1 Each member of the team has special skills. For example, the physician (center) writes orders for medical care. The registered nurse (left) plans and coordinates the nursing care. The social worker (right) helps the patient find ways to manage social and financial problems.

TABLE 2-1 MEDICAL SPECIALTIES

Specialty	Physician	Type of Care
Allergy	Allergist	Diagnoses and treats patients with hypersensitivities
Cardiovascular Diseases	Cardiologist	Diagnoses and treats patients with disorders of the heart and blood vessels
Dermatology	Dermatologist	Diagnoses and treats patients with disorders of the skin
Gastroenterology	Gastroenterologist	Diagnoses and treats patients with disorders of the digestive system
Gerontology	Gerontologist	Specializes in diagnosing and treating disorders of the aging person
Gynecology	Gynecologist	Diagnoses and treats disorders related to the female reproductive tract
Hematology	Hematologist	Diagnoses and treats patients with disorders of the blood and blood-forming organs
Internal Medicine	Internist	Diagnoses and treats patients with disorders of the internal organs
Neurology	Neurologist	Diagnoses and treats patients with disorders of the nervous system
Obstetrics	Obstetrician	Specializes in providing care to women during pregnancy, childbirth, and immediately thereafter
Oncology	Oncologist	Diagnoses and treats people with cancerous tumors
Ophthalmology	Ophthalmologist	Diagnoses and treats patients with disorders of the eyes
Pediatrics	Pediatrician	Diagnoses, treats, and prevents disorders in children
Psychiatry	Psychiatrist	Diagnoses and treats disorders of the mind
Radiology	Radiologist	Diagnoses and treats disorders with x-rays and other forms of imaging technology
Urology	Urologist	Diagnoses and treats disorders of the urinary tract and male reproductive tract

TABLE 2-2 INTERDISCIPLINARY HEALTH CARE TEAM MEMBERS

Each of these disciplines requires a specified course of study (usually a minimum of a college degree and clinical training). Most require either licensing by a state agency or certification from a professional association. Requirements may vary from state to state for some disciplines.

Patient	The most important member of the interdisciplinary team. The patient has input into the planning and implementation of care. The family may participate with the patient or in place of the patient if the patient is unable to do so.
Physician	Licensed by the state to diagnose and treat disease and to prescribe medications. Many specialty areas within medicine require additional education.
Registered Nurse (RN)	Licensed by the state to make assessments and plan, implement, and evaluate nursing care. Supervises other nursing staff and may coordinate the interdisciplinary health care team. Many specialty areas within nursing require additional education.
Licensed Practical Nurse (LPN or LVN)	Licensed by the state to provide direct patient care under the supervision of a registered nurse. Called licensed vocational nurse in Texas and California.
Nursing Assistant	Has completed at least 75 hours of a state-approved course and is certified to provide direct patient care under the supervision of a registered nurse.
Specialty Services	
Respiratory Therapist	Licensed to evaluate and treat diseases and problems associated with breathing and the respiratory tract.
Occupational Therapist	Licensed to provide rehabilitative services to evaluate and treat persons with physical injury or illness, psychosocial problems, or developmental disabilities. Occupational therapy assistants and aides have completed specified courses of study and work under the supervision of a physical occupational therapist.
Orthotist	Licensed by the state to design and fit braces and splints for the extremities.
Physical Therapist	Licensed by the state to provide rehabilitative services to evaluate and treat persons with physical injury or illness, psychosocial problems, or developmental disabilities. Physical therapy assistants and aides have completed specified courses of study and work under the supervision of a physical therapist.
Social Worker	Licensed by the state to assess and provide services for the nonmedical, psychosocial needs of patients.
Chaplain	Provides services to meet the spiritual needs of patients.
Support Services	
Pharmacist	Licensed by the state to fill prescriptions for medications as ordered by the physician. Acts as information resource to nurses and physicians for updates on new medications and for maintaining safe drug therapy for patients.
Dietitian	Licensed by the state to assess nutritional needs and provide food services for patients.

In addition to these members of the interdisciplinary health care team, other employees in the health care facility provide services that benefit patients.

- Administrator—Provides general administration and supervision.

- Environmental services—Maintain a clean and comfortable environment.

- Volunteers—Provide personal services such as delivering mail, doing errands, and providing reading materials.

licensure requirements for the members of the health care team mentioned here, as well as others.

THE NURSING TEAM

The Registered Nurse

The **registered nurse** (**RN**) becomes registered by passing a required examination given by the state. The nurse has a four-year college education with a baccalaureate degree, or an associate in applied science degree from a two-year community college or technical school program, or a diploma from a hospital school of nursing. Because they have taken and successfully passed a licensing examination and are registered, all of these nurses use the initials RN after their names.

Registered nurses have been educated to assess, plan for, evaluate, and coordinate the many aspects of patient care. Registered nurses teach patients and their families about good health practices. They also provide nursing care and supervise any duties they delegate to others.

Nurses may specialize in a specific area of nursing practice. Some of the common nursing specialties are:

- Maternal and child health
- Anesthesiology
- Gerontology
- Oncology
- Administration
- Public health
- Teaching
- Telemetry
- Surgery
- Home care
- Cardiac care
- Independent practice (nurse practitioner)
- Research
- Infection control

The Licensed Practical/Vocational Nurse

The **licensed vocational** or **licensed practical nurse** has generally completed a 1-year to 18-month training program and has passed a national licensure examination administered by the state. She or he is identified by the initials LVN or LPN. This nurse works under the supervision of the registered nurse, a physician, or a dentist. The LPN is able to provide most of the care when the patient's nursing needs are not complex, and also assists the RN in more complicated situations.

The Nursing Assistant

The **nursing assistant** is trained to assist with the care of patients under the supervision of either an RN or an LPN (Figure 2-2). Because the assistant's responsibilities and skills are not as great as those of the RN or LPN/LVN, the

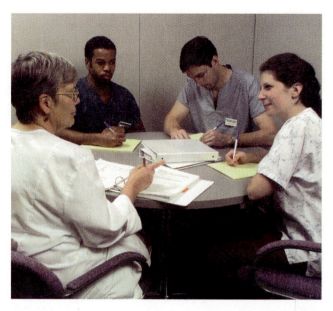

FIGURE 2-2 The nursing team provides direct care under the direction of the professional nurse.

basic training period is shorter. However, growth and learning will continue throughout your career as a caregiver. In the health care facility, the assistant is called by one of the following names:

- Patient care attendant
- Nurse's aide
- Home health aide
- Nursing assistant
- Health care assistant
- Ward attendant
- Patient care technician

ORGANIZATION OF NURSING CARE

Nursing care may be organized in one of four ways:

1. Primary nursing
2. Functional nursing
3. Team nursing
4. Patient focused nursing

The nursing assistant has a functional role in each.

Primary Nursing

In primary nursing, care is given by a registered nurse. This nurse is responsible for an assigned patient's care for that patient's entire hospitalization. Licensed staff and assistants help with the care when the RN is not actually on duty. The nurse plans the nursing care, teaches, carries out treatments, gives direct nursing care, and plans for the patient's discharge. Patients appreciate primary nursing because it enables them to relate directly to one specific nurse. Each RN is assigned to and responsible for six to eight patients in the primary nursing situation.

Functional Nursing

Functional nursing is a task-oriented way to organize care service. It is an older method that is once again being used more frequently. In this service organization, the charge nurse is the one person responsible for all patients. All other staff members are assigned specific tasks, such as giving medications, administering treatments, or providing hygienic care.

Patients may find this type of nursing confusing because many people are involved in their care. However, some facilities feel that this method uses available, qualified personnel to best advantage.

Team Nursing

Team nursing is one of the most common methods of delivering nursing care. In this system, a registered nurse team leader determines the nursing needs of all the patients assigned to the team for care. Team members receive instructions and assignments from, and report back to, the team leader.

The team approach is successful when:

- Team members understand the philosophy, goals, and purposes of restorative care. Restorative care helps patients reach their highest possible level of functioning.
- Team members understand their responsibilities.
- All team members, including the patient, and family members if the patient desires, attend the care plan conference.

Patient Focused Care

The goals of patient focused care are to:

- Limit the number of people involved in patient care.
- Contain costs.
- Meet patients' needs efficiently.

Staff members are prepared as multiskilled workers by cross-training them to perform special skills. This training allows the staff members to carry out selected duties that are usually performed by other workers, such as drawing blood, giving special treatments, working in specialty departments, and using more sophisticated instruments to perform tests. For example, a multiskilled nursing assistant may be **cross-trained** to draw blood, give respiratory treatments, or perform an electrocardiogram. These tasks can be done without calling a technician from another department or moving the patient out of the unit.

You can be an effective member of the interdisciplinary team by:

- Recognizing the importance of all team members.
- Appreciating each member's contribution to the team.
- Learning as much as possible about the patients and their families, to help you understand their feelings and concerns.
- Attending care plan conferences and giving the team your observations and ideas.
- Attending in-service training sessions to increase your knowledge.
- Becoming cross-trained, if possible, to increase your skills.
- Cooperating with other team members to provide patient focused care.

REGULATION OF NURSING ASSISTANT PRACTICE

Nursing assistants must understand the scope of the specific tasks they will be expected to carry out. They should also know the state regulations that govern their clinical practice. Federal regulations for the training and certification of nursing assistants require that all states spell out the duties and responsibilities of the assistant, as well as the basic education and level of competency required for practice.

In 1987, a federal law was passed that regulates the education and certification of nurse aides. The law is called the **Omnibus Budget Reconciliation Act** (**OBRA**). OBRA includes statements from the Department of Health and Human Services and the Health Care Financing Administration that established the minimum requirements for nurse aide competency evaluation programs.

Effective October 1, 1990, all persons working as nurse aides had to complete a competency evaluation program or approved course. The actual training and education of nursing assistants is under individual state jurisdiction, guided by federal regulations.

The National Council of State Boards of Nursing, Inc., then developed the **Nurse Aide Competency Evaluation Program** (**NACEP**). NACEP meets the requirements of OBRA. NACEP is a guide for individual programs that register and award credentials to nurse aides. NACEP specifies the minimum skills to be achieved. Programs may exceed these minimums.

Nursing assistants who wish to be certified must complete a minimum of 75 hours of theory and practice. Some states require a minimum of 80 to 120 program hours in written or oral and clinical skills in several areas. These areas include:

- Basic nursing skills
- Basic restorative services
- Mental health and social service needs
- Personal care skills
- Resident rights
- Safety and emergency care

Other regulations that guide nursing assistant practice require:

- Completion of a competency evaluation program by October 1, 1990, of all persons working as nurse aides prior to July 1989.
- At least three opportunities for noncertified nurse aides to meet requirements.
- Completion of a new training and competency program by persons who wish to work as aides but who have not performed nursing or nurse-related services for pay for a

continuous 24-month period after completing a training and competency evaluation program.

- Continuing education (12 to 48 hours per year, in some states).

The OBRA regulations are important because they:

- Give nursing assistants recognition through registration.
- Help define the scope of nursing assistant practice.
- Assure better uniformity of care provided by nursing assistants.
- Promote educational standards for nursing assistants.

Be sure you are familiar with any specific state regulations or laws that relate to your role as an assistant.

LINES OF AUTHORITY

Nursing assistants receive their assignments from the team leader or charge nurse, nurse manager, or unit manager. When they finish their assignments, they report to this same person. This represents the assistant's immediate line of authority and communication.

If the hospital is a large one, the assistant may work with a team whose leader is a licensed practical nurse or a registered nurse. In this case, the assistant's immediate superior is the team leader. The team leaders receive their instructions from the charge nurse. The charge nurse is responsible for the total care of a certain number of patients. Sometimes this includes all the patients on a wing, a unit, or a floor of the facility. Supervisors are responsible for several charge nurse units. They receive their authority and direction from the director of nursing. Health care facilities vary in the complexity of their staffing.

Assistants should learn the lines of authority in their health care facility, as shown in Figure 2-3. As a student, your

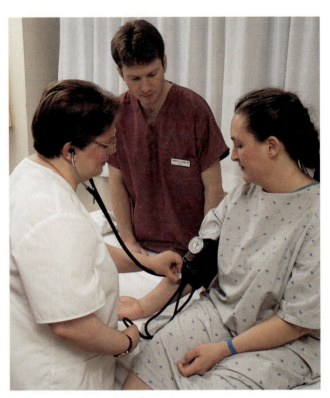

FIGURE 2-4 Always ask for clarification if you are unsure how to proceed.

immediate authority is your teacher or the person designated as your supervisor.

The physician directs the patient's medical care. The registered nurse carries out the physician's orders and plans the patient's nursing care. The authority for nursing care passes from the registered nurse supervisor to the charge nurse, to the team leader, and then to the nursing assistant. When you accept the responsibility for an assignment, you must fully understand the assignment and be capable of handling it. *If there is any doubt, you should discuss it with the team leader or charge nurse* (Figure 2-4).

GUIDELINES FOR THE NURSING ASSISTANT

Only perform tasks you have been trained to do. If you are unsure how to carry out a procedure that was part of your training program, inform the nurse. Do not feel embarrassed. It is better to ask for clarification and supervision than to make an error and injure a patient.

Seeking Higher Authority

Sometimes a report you make to your immediate supervisor is not taken seriously. It seems to fall on deaf ears. Make very sure of your facts and try again to make your supervisor understand. If you fail and your information is very important, you can move up the chain of command.

For example, if you report that a person is being harmed by inattention by a coworker, but your supervisor does not lis-

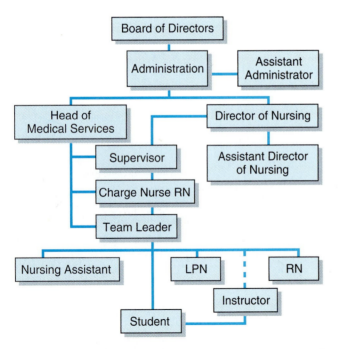

FIGURE 2-3 Lines of authority for patient care (one typical model; there are others).

ten to your report of the situation, for your patient's safety you must try again. If the second attempt also fails, the next step is to bring the problem to the attention of the next level of authority. This situation should not occur often if there are good staff relations, but it can happen.

Scope of Practice

Scope of practice means the skills the nursing assistant is legally permitted to perform by state regulations. If another health care worker asks you to perform a task that is clearly out of your scope of training, such as giving medications, be prepared to refuse. Explain in a courteous manner that this is a task for which you have not been technically or legally prepared. Report the incident to your charge nurse so that your scope of duties can be clearly understood by all staff members.

For the same reason, nursing assistants do not take orders from doctors or tell families about the contents of patient care plans or records. These actions are not within the scope of nursing assistant functions.

Nevertheless, be willing to learn new skills under the close supervision of your nurse. If the new skill is within the scope of nursing assistant practice, this will increase your ability to provide good, safe nursing care. If, for example, your nurse suggests a new way to lift a patient that is different from the way you learned in your program, listen and watch carefully as the instruction is given. Seek supervision as you practice the new technique until both you and your supervisor feel you can do it safely on your own.

TABLE 2-3 TYPICAL JOB DESCRIPTION FOR A NURSING ASSISTANT

Nursing assistants commonly participate in the nursing process by carrying out the activities listed. Note: Use standard precautions while providing care.

1. Assist with patient assessment and care planning.
   a. Check and record vital signs
   b. Measure height and weight
   c. Measure intake and output
   d. Collect specimens
   e. Test urine and feces
   f. Observe patient response to care given
   g. Report and record observations

2. Assist patients in meeting nutritional and elimination needs.
   a. Check food trays
   b. Pass food trays
   c. Feed patients
   d. Provide fresh drinking water and nourishments
   e. Assist with bedpans, urinals, and commodes
   f. Empty urine collection bags
   g. Assist with colostomy care
   h. Give enemas
   i. Observe feces and urine

3. Assist patients with mobility.
   a. Turn and position
   b. Provide range-of-motion exercises
   c. Transfer to wheelchair or stretcher
   d. Assist with ambulation

4. Assist patients with personal hygiene and grooming.
   a. Bathe patients
   b. Provide nail and hair care
   c. Give oral hygiene
   d. Provide denture care
   e. Shave male patients
   f. Assist with dressing and undressing

5. Assist with patient comfort and anxiety relief.
   a. Protect patient privacy and maintain confidentiality
   b. Keep call bell within patient's reach
   c. Answer call bells promptly
   d. Provide orientation to the room or unit and to other patients and visitors
   e. Assist patients with communications
   f. Protect personal possessions
   g. Provide diversional activities
   h. Give back rubs
   i. Prepare hot and cold applications

6. Assist in promoting patient safety and environmental cleanliness.
   a. Use side rails and restraints appropriately
   b. Keep patient unit clean and clutter-free
   c. Make beds
   d. Clean and care for equipment
   e. Carry out isolation precautions
   f. Observe oxygen precautions
   g. Assist in keeping recreational and nonpatient areas clean and free of hazards
   h. Participate in fire drills and patient evacuation procedures

7. Assist with unit management and efficiency.
   a. Transport patients
   b. Take specimens to lab
   c. Assist with special procedures
   d. Do errands as required
   e. Assist with cost-containment measures

Courtesy of Eileen Cowart, Director of Education, International Career Institute, Panama City, FL

THE ROLE AND RESPONSIBILITIES OF THE NURSING ASSISTANT

The nursing assistant works directly with the patient, giving physical care and emotional support. This care is always given under the direction of the registered nurse. The nursing assistant has an important role and can contribute much to the patient's comfort. Observations made during the delivery of care are reported to the nurse and are recorded on the patient's chart.

Tasks commonly assigned to nursing assistants are listed in Table 2-3. Remember that not all health care facilities assign the same tasks to nursing assistants.

Not everyone can be a nursing assistant. Nursing assistants are special people: they are interested in others, they take pride in themselves, and they are willing to learn the skills necessary to care for those who are ill.

This interest in and caring for people can be a valuable asset to the entire nursing team. You are the person whom the patient sees most often. This means that you have the chance to observe and hear many things which the other team members will not. By transmitting these observations to your charge nurse, you are likely to give the other team members a valuable insight into the patient's illness and attitude toward that illness. For example, you may see that the patient's attitude toward the attending doctor or nurse is much less relaxed than it is with you, the nursing assistant. For that same reason, the patient is far more likely to tell you of "minor complaints" that may not be minor at all. Competent, caring nursing assistants make a valuable contribution to the comfort and safety of the patients.

PERSONAL VOCATIONAL ADJUSTMENTS

You will have to make a certain amount of personal adjustment to your new work situation. Health care facility rules and orders from supervisors must be obeyed promptly, even if you do not agree with them. Rules are written for the protection and welfare of both the patient and the health care provider. You must also learn to accept constructive criticism and profit by it. It means you are willing to learn and grow.

How mature you are shows in many other ways. You demonstrate:

- Dependability and accuracy by reporting for duty on time (Figure 2-5) and completing your assignments carefully.
- Respect for your coworkers and the place you share together on the nursing team when you are ready to help.
- Understanding of human relationships by being empathetic, patient, and tactful with others.

Interpersonal Relationships

Interpersonal relationships are simply interactions between people. You develop interpersonal relationships with everyone you know. Some are deep and lasting, and some are only

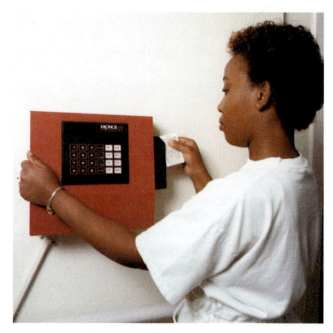

FIGURE 2-5 Reporting for duty on time demonstrates dependability.

casual. But to some degree, you react to others and they react to you. Friendship is a good example of an interpersonal relationship that is satisfactory to two people.

Much of the satisfaction that a nursing assistant gets from work comes from the quality of the relationships that are developed with other staff members and patients. Some people call this the ability to get along with others.

Similarly, good relationships with others begin with your own personality and attitudes. If you are a warm and accepting person with positive attitudes, others will respond in the same way. If you walk down the street and someone smiles at you, without thinking, your reaction is to smile back. Most human relationships are like this.

It is not necessary for you personally to like someone else to be pleasant and cooperative with them as you carry out your duties (Figure 2-6).

Attitude

Perhaps the most important single characteristic that you bring to your job is your attitude. Your attitude is developed throughout your lifetime, and it is shaped by the experiences you have had. Some people think having an "attitude" means being negative or opinionated, but all people show attitude through their behavior. Sometimes the attitude demonstrated is good and sometimes it is poor.

All the other characteristics described are an outer reflection of your inner feelings—of your attitude toward yourself and others. Your attitude should reflect:

- Courtesy
- Cooperation
- Emotional control
- Empathy (understanding)

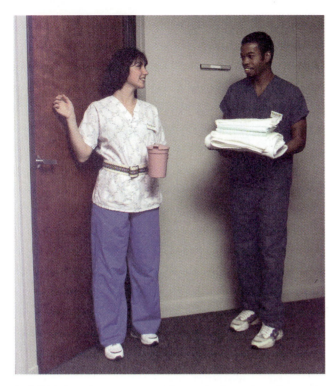

FIGURE 2-6 Keeping a positive attitude makes the workplace more pleasant.

- Tact
- Sympathy

Patients have the right and need to be cared for in a calm, unhurried atmosphere by people with a caring attitude.

Patient Relationships

Patients come in all sizes and shapes and ages: young, old, and in between. Some have major, complicated illnesses. Others have physical problems that can be helped with rest and medication. Some patients are in the health facility to begin their lives. Others will end their lives there. A good nursing assistant shows empathy for the patient by being eager to serve and by using a gentle touch.

Every patient entering a health care facility presents a unique set of problems and concerns to the staff. These problems and concerns are important. As you compare the conditions of many patients in your own mind, however, it might seem that one has more serious problems than another. Because patients do not share your knowledge, they will not know this. Never forget that, to the patient, her or his own problems are the most important.

Meeting the Patient's Needs

Patients' personalities are shaped by their life experiences, which are now complicated with illness. Their social, spiritual, and physical needs must continue to be met even though they are in a different, more confined setting. The restrictions imposed by illness limit, to some degree, their ability to satisfy these needs through the normal channels.

This is naturally frustrating and puts great strain on the patient's ability to establish and maintain good interpersonal relationships.

Some patients become irritable, complaining, and uncooperative because of:

- Fears about their diagnosis, disfigurement, disability, and death
- Pain
- Unrealistic perceptions of activities around them
- Uncertainties about the future
- Worries about family
- The loss or lack of social support systems
- Dependence on others
- Financial concerns

Offer emotional support (Figure 2-7), listen carefully, and report these concerns to the nurse.

Meeting the Family's Needs

Families and friends are very concerned when one of their loved ones is in a health care facility and, indeed, may have a life-threatening illness. This put stress in their lives too. They need to be reassured. Their anxiety sometimes makes them demanding and uncooperative.

The nursing assistant who understands human behavior makes allowances for these stresses and realizes that ill people, coworkers, and families under stress may be touchy and not always on their best behavior. This is why sensitivity and awareness of the needs of others are most important at this time (Figure 2-8). It is in these situations that patience and tact are most needed. Sometimes just quietly listening to another or rephrasing your sentences can change an entire interaction. Try to be aware not only of the words used but also of the body language. As with words, clues such as the tone of a voice or a hand movement reveal much about the inner feelings of other people. Always keep in mind that people are three-dimensional. They are physical beings, emotional beings, and social beings.

Staff Relationships

You are part of the staff of a health care facility. All of you share a single goal: to help the patient. This single purpose welds you together into a unit that must work smoothly if your goal is to be accomplished. Good interpersonal rela-

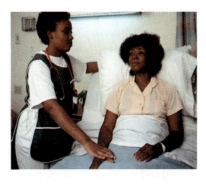

FIGURE 2-7 The worried patient responds to a gentle touch.

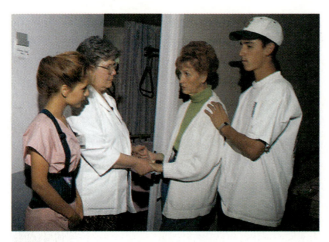

FIGURE 2-8 Concerned family members need the support of the staff.

tionships will make your working hours satisfying and productive. Good relationships can be formed if you:

- Remember that each of you has a specific role to fulfill and jobs to carry out.
- Do not overstep your authority or criticize others.
- Listen to instructions from your supervisor carefully. Phrase questions about your assignment in such a way that your supervisor knows you are looking for clarification—not challenging authority.
- Remember that your tone of voice and body language can change the message you are trying to convey.
- Promptly carry out orders and report any work you are unable to finish.
- Offer help to others and accept help when you need it. Coworkers can often help one another when a task is particularly difficult or physically taxing (for example, lifting a heavy patient or moving equipment). Simply being available when another member of the team gets behind in his or her work is a great help.
- Have a cheerful, positive attitude. This is as important for staff members' relationships as it is in establishing rapport (sympathetic understanding) with patients.
- Extend the same dignity and courtesy to every staff member that you would to patients.
- Always keep your common goal in mind. Recognize coworkers as important members of the total team.

Professional and personal adjustments are made easier if the nursing assistant:

- Understands and follows facility policies and procedures.
- Treats patients, coworkers, and visitors with respect.
- Practices proper hygiene and grooming, good nutrition, and stress reduction.

PERSONAL HEALTH AND HYGIENE

Good personal grooming is essential, because the assistant is in close contact with patients (Figure 2-9). Because the work

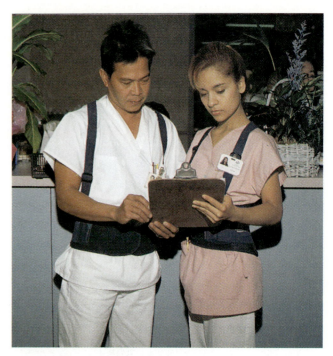

FIGURE 2-9 Nursing assistants who are well groomed show pride in themselves and in their careers.

of the assistant, although rewarding, can be physically challenging, it is important that all body odors be controlled. The nursing assistant is often the last to know that he or she has bad breath or body odor. A daily shower or bath and the use of an antiperspirant/deodorant are essential. The mouth and teeth must be kept clean. The nursing assistant should also recognize that strong perfumes, aftershave lotions, and cigarette odors are often offensive to patients.

Hair and fingernails should be kept short and clean. If nail polish is used, it should be clear, not colored.

Stockings and socks should be freshly laundered. Shoes and shoelaces should be cleaned daily. Fatigue will be lessened if shoes give proper support to the feet and are well-fitted.

Jewelry is not part of the nursing assistant's uniform, as it is a ready medium for bacterial growth. Jewelry may also injure the patient or the assistant, especially if the patient is confused or is a young child. Long, dangling earrings can be especially dangerous to the assistant because they are easily caught in linen or pulled out by a combative patient. Most health care agencies do permit members of the nursing staff to wear wedding rings, small earrings, and watches with second hands. The watch is used to monitor the condition of patients and to measure vital signs.

Uniforms

Many health care facilities allow health care workers great leeway in selecting the type and style of their uniforms. Traditionally, patients were able to identify the various types of health care workers by their uniforms, including caps. Today, it can be very difficult to distinguish between a physical therapist, registered nurse, physician, or social worker. It is no wonder that newly admitted patients are often confused as to whom they should approach for information or help. To help avoid this confusion, some states and many health care facilities require personnel to wear a name badge or photo identification tag at all times while on the job.

If your health care facility requires that you wear a uniform, you should wear it only while you are on duty. If your health care agency does not provide facilities for changing your uniform before and after going on duty, be sure to wear a cover-up as you travel to and from work so you will not spread germs. When you get home, remove your uniform, fold it inside out, and put it into the laundry. This helps keep the dirtiest part of your uniform away from the other clothes in the laundry. Wearing a fresh uniform every day should become a habit. It should be clean and in good condition. Torn hems and missing buttons should be repaired and replaced.

Above all, remember that your patients' safety and comfort are your main concerns. Try to keep in mind their needs and feelings. After all, would you feel confident if you were ill and the assistant caring for you had long fingernails that could scratch you, or that could collect dirt and possibly infect your surgical incision? How would you feel if the assistant who was preparing you for surgery kept having to push the hair out of his eyes? Or if the assistant assigned to give you a back-rub wore clanking bracelets on her wrists?

Remember, too, that how you look reflects the pride you have in yourself and in your work. Well-groomed nursing assistants who pay attention to the details of their person and appearance show others, especially their patients and coworkers, that they are likely to have the same pride and caring attitude in their work. If you are well groomed and have good personal habits, patients will feel more secure and confident, and other staff members will regard you as mature and reliable. As you develop good health habits, you become a role model for your family, friends, and coworkers.

Reducing Stress

Your work as a nursing assistant is physically and emotionally demanding because you must give so much of yourself to those in your care. To stay healthy and do your best, you will need:

- Sufficient rest
- Good nutrition
- Satisfying leisure activities (Figure 2-10)
- Ways to reduce stress

Burnout is total mental, emotional, and sometimes physical exhaustion. Burnout is common among those working in health care facilities. You can reduce the stress that leads to burnout by balancing your work with rest and recreation.

Some facilities offer programs to help employees reduce stress. Group discussions, exercise programs, and special counseling are available for general stress management and to meet special circumstances, such as when a patient dies or when individual interstaff conflicts arise. Death is always a possibility, but the staff usually focus on improvement and

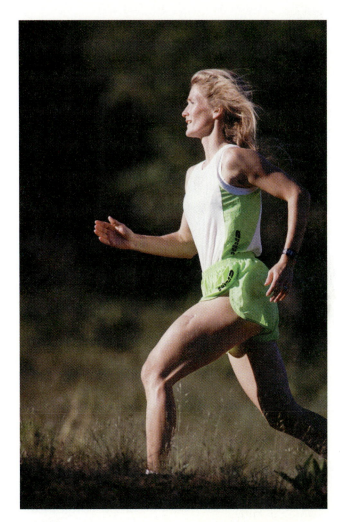

FIGURE 2-10 Work should be balanced with recreational exercise.

recovery. The loss of a patient, especially a child, can be very stressful. Caring for an abused child can take a great toll on the staff as they try to work with the child and family.

Occasionally personality conflicts are aggravated by the daily close contact. Stress caused by these situations can often be handled through a stress management group discussion.

Personal Stress Reduction

You can learn personal stress-reducing techniques. Food, alcohol, or other drugs are used by some people to reduce stress, but these substances can cause serious health problems. For example, some people use chemicals or drugs to reduce stress. This is dangerous because chemicals and drugs alter the body's chemistry, causing serious changes to thought and behavior. In some cases, drug use becomes addictive and can cause death.

There are better and safer ways to prevent burnout and relieve stress. To reduce stress:

- Talk to your supervisor; a team conference may help.
- Try sitting for a few moments with your feet up.
- Shut your eyes and take some deep breaths.

- With your eyes shut, picture a special place you like and, in your mind, take yourself there.
- Take a warm, relaxing bath.
- Listen to some quiet music.
- Carry out a specific relaxation exercise.
- Make yourself a cup of herbal tea and drink it slowly.

- Exercise.
- Devote time to hobbies such as sewing, painting, wood-working, or playing a musical instrument.
- Go for a walk.
- Take advantage of available stress reduction programs.

REVIEW

A. True/False.

Mark the following true or false by circling T or F.

1. T F The registered nurse plans and directs the nursing care of patients.

2. T F Interdisciplinary health care providers act as a team.

3. T F The LVN has completed a four-year college-based program.

4. T F The nursing assistant gives physical care and emotional support to patients under the direction of the registered nurse.

5. T F The nursing assistant is an important member of the nursing team.

6. T F Patients enjoy primary nursing because it allows them to relate directly to one specific registered nurse.

7. T F Team nursing is a common way of providing patient care.

8. T F It is all right to perform a task even if you are unsure.

9. T F Nursing assistants are special people.

10. T F Nursing assistants should be willing to learn and practice new skills under the supervision of the nurse.

11. T F Caring about people is a valuable asset for a nursing assistant.

12. T F It is not important for the nursing assistant to be well groomed.

13. T F Patients may find strong perfumes or aftershave lotions offensive.

14. T F Hair and fingernails should be kept short and clean.

15. T F It is all right to wear your uniform when you go food shopping.

16. T F How you look reflects the pride you feel in yourself.

17. T F Patient safety and comfort are main concerns for all caregivers.

18. T F Being a nursing assistant can be very stressful.

19. T F Smoking and eating are the best ways to reduce stress.

20. T F One of the most important characteristics you bring to your job is a positive attitude.

B. Multiple Choice.

Select the one best answer for each question.

21. The interdisciplinary team member who writes the orders for patient care is the
    a. dentist.
    b. social worker.
    c. physician.
    d. dietitian.

22. The nursing care approach that is task-oriented is
    a. primary nursing.
    b. functional nursing.
    c. team nursing.
    d. focused patient care.

23. A nursing assistant who has a question regarding an assignment should properly ask the
    a. physician.
    b. charge nurse.
    c. physiotherapist.
    d. administrator.

24. A patient tells you that he has difficulty making a fist because his hand feels weak. He did not mention the fact to the nurse. You must
    a. ignore it. The patient should have told the nurse.
    b. tell another assistant.
    c. tell the nurse.
    d. tell the physician.

25. You demonstrate maturity by
    a. rushing assignments.
    b. being disrespectful to coworkers.
    c. "bending" the rules.
    d. reporting for duty on time.

C. Matching.

Match the interdisciplinary team member and his or her function.

26. _____ Licensed to fill prescriptions for medications.

27. _____ Qualified to test hearing and prescribe.

28. _____ Licensed to provide services to meet spiritual needs.

29. _____ Licensed to fit and design braces and splints for extremities.

30. _____ Licensed to provide rehabilitative services and to evaluate and treat persons with physical injury or illness, psychosocial problems, or developmental disabilities.

a. orthotist
b. pharmacist
c. chaplain
d. occupational therapist
e. audiologist

D. Completion.

Complete the following.

31. Why is it improper for nursing assistants to take orders directly from the physician? _____

32. The benefits of a nurse aide certification are:

a. _____

b. _____

c. _____

d. _____

E. Nursing Assistant Challenge.

Read each clinical situation and answer the questions.

33. Enrique is given his assignment and has questions.

a. He must check his assignment with _____.

b. One of his assignments is to bathe patients. Is this appropriate? _____

c. One of his assignments is to give medications. Is this appropriate? _____

34. Felicia once worked as a part-time assistant to an elderly woman but was never certified as a nursing assistant. What can you tell her about the requirements?

a. Is a competency evaluation program required? _____

b. How many opportunities are there to meet requirements? _____

c. How much continuing education is required once certification is granted? _____

35. Peggy reported for duty wearing bracelets, long earrings, and pale pink nail polish. Her uniform was clean and crisp but the hem was hanging down on one side. Her shoes were dirty. State ways in which her appearance can be improved.

Consumer Rights and Responsibilities in Health Care

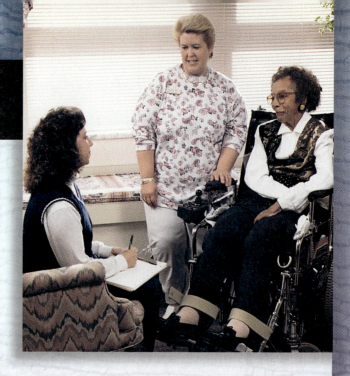

As a result of this unit, you will be able to:
- Spell and define terms.
- Explain the purpose of health care consumer rights.
- Describe six items that are common to Resident's Rights, the Patient's Bill of Rights, and the Client's Rights in Home Care.
- List three specific rights from each of the three documents.
- Describe eight responsibilities of health care consumers.

Learn the meaning and the correct spelling of the following words and phrases:

advance directives	corporal punishment	informed consent	Patient's Bill of Rights
Client's Rights	grievance	involuntary seclusion	Resident's Rights

CONSUMER RIGHTS

All citizens in the United States have certain rights (for example, the right to vote) that are guaranteed by law. Health care consumers have rights to ensure that they will receive quality patient care. There are different documents for patient rights, depending on where care is given. In each setting, if the health care consumer is unable to read or understand the document, it is given to the person's family. A copy of the **Resident's Rights** is given each person before he or she is admitted to a skilled care facility (Figure 3-1). The rights of residents in skilled care facilities were legislated by the federal government in the Omnibus Budget Reconciliation Act (OBRA) of 1987. The resident must sign a form indicating that the resident and/or the resident's family have received the document. The **Patient's Bill of Rights** is given to patients upon admission to a hospital. Persons receiving care in their homes are given a copy of the **Client's Rights** by the nurse on the first visit to the home. The client is asked to sign a form indicating that he or she received the document.

All persons working in health care should be familiar with the document that pertains to the facility they work in. Supporting the rights of the health care consumer contributes to more effective care. Each of these documents is

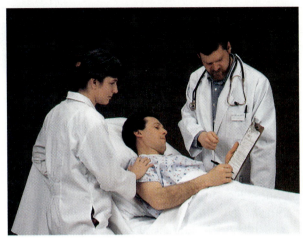

FIGURE 3-2 Informed consent must be obtained from the patient before certain procedures are performed.

similar and emphasizes the right of the patient, resident, or client to:

- Be treated in a respectful, dignified manner—this includes the right to privacy and to confidentiality.
- Have the benefit of open and honest communication with caregivers.
- Have a role in decision making for treatment choices and planning of care. **Informed consent** means that the consumer gives permission for care or procedures after full disclosure of the purpose of the care or procedure, the benefits, and any risks involved with the care or procedure (Figure 3-2).
- Be advised of their rights about **advance directives** (a document that gives instructions about the consumer's wishes for treatment if the consumer is unable to communicate).
- Receive continuity of care.
- Be informed of resources for resolving conflicts or grievances. A **grievance** is a situation in which the consumer feels there are grounds for complaint.

Each rights document is presented at the end of this unit (Figures 3-3, 3-4, and 3-5).

RESPONSIBILITIES OF HEALTH CARE CONSUMERS

Providing for the rights of the consumer will not ensure quality care unless consumers are willing to fulfill certain responsibilities. These responsibilities include:

- maintaining personal health care records so information is readily available when it is needed
- communicating openly and honestly with the physician and other caregivers and being willing to give a complete health and family history
- providing information regarding past hospitalizations and medications

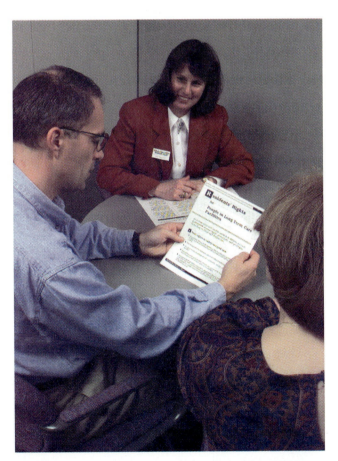

FIGURE 3-1 Residents are given a copy of the Resident's Rights before being admitted to a skilled care facility.

Resident's Rights

This is an abbreviated version of the Resident's Rights as set forth in the Omnibus Budget Reconciliation Act. This document must be given to all residents and/or their families prior to admission to a long-term care facility.

1. The resident has the right to free choice, including the right to:
   - choose an attending physician
   - full advance information about changes in care or treatment
   - participate in the assessment and care planning process
   - self administration of medications if the resident is assessed as being able to do so
   - consent to participate in experimental research
2. The resident has the right to freedom from abuse and restraints, including freedom from:
   - physical, sexual, mental abuse
   - **corporal punishment** (the use of physical force) and **involuntary seclusion** (isolating a resident without a medical reason)
   - physical and chemical restraints
3. The resident has the right to privacy including privacy for:
   - treatment and nursing care
   - receiving/sending mail
   - telephone calls
   - visitors
4. The resident has the right to confidentiality of personal and clinical records.
5. The resident has the right to accommodation of needs including:
   - choices about life
   - receiving assistance in maintaining independence

6. The resident has the right to voice grievances.
7. The resident has the right to organize and participate in family and resident groups.
8. The resident has the right to participate in social, religious, and community activities including the right to:
   - vote
   - keep religious items in the room
   - attend religious services
9. The resident has the right to examine survey results and correction plans.
10. The resident has the right to manage personal funds.
11. The resident has the right to information about eligibility for Medicare/Medicaid funds.
12. The resident has the right to file complaints about abuse, neglect, or misappropriation of property.
13. The resident has the right to information about advocacy groups.
14. The resident has the right to immediate and unlimited access to family or relatives.
15. The resident has the right to share a room with the spouse if they are both residents in the same facility.
16. The resident has the right to perform or not perform work for the facility if it is medically appropriate for the resident to work.
17. The resident has the right to remain in the facility except in certain circumstances.
18. The resident has the right to use personal possessions.
19. The resident has the right to notification of change in condition.

FIGURE 3-3 Resident's Rights

A Patient's Bill of Rights

Introduction

Effective health care requires collaboration between patients and physicians and other health care professionals. Open and honest communication, respect for personal and professional values, and sensitivity to differences are integral to optimal patient care. As the setting for the provision of health services, hospitals must provide a foundation for understanding and respecting the rights and responsibilities of patients, their families, physicians, and other caregivers. Hospitals must ensure a health care ethic that respects the role of patients in decision making about treatment choices and other aspects of their care. Hospitals must be sensitive to cultural, racial, linguistic, religious, age, gender, and other differences as well as the needs of persons with disabilities.

The American Hospital Association presents *A Patient's Bill of Rights* with the expectation that it will contribute to more effective patient care and be supported by the hospital on behalf of the institution, its medical staff, employees, and patients. The American Hospital Association encourages health care institutions to tailor this bill of rights to their patient community by translating and/or simplifying the language of this bill of rights as may be necessary to ensure that the patients and their families understand their rights and responsibilities.

Bill of Rights*

1. The patient has the right to considerate and respectful care.

2. The patient has the right to and is encouraged to obtain from physicians and other direct care givers relevant, current, and understandable information concerning diagnosis, treatment, and prognosis.

   Except in emergencies when the patient lacks decision making capacity and the need for treatment is urgent, the patient is entitled to the opportunity to discuss and request information related to the specific procedures and/or treatments, the risks involved, the possible length of recuperation, and the medically reasonable alternatives and their accompanying risks and benefits.

   Patients have the right to know the identity of physicians, nurses, and others involved in their care, as well as when those involved are students, residents, or other trainees. The patient also has the right to know the immediate and long-term financial implications of treatment choices, insofar as they are known.

3. The patient has the right to make decisions about the plan of care prior to and during the course of treatment and to refuse a recommended treatment or plan of care to the extent permitted by law and hospital policy and to be informed of the medical consequences of this action. In case of such refusal, the patient is entitled to other appropriate care and services that the hospital provides or transfer to another hospital. The hospital should notify patients of any policy that might affect patient choice within the institution.

4. The patient has the right to have an advance directive (such as a living will, health care proxy, or durable power of attorney for health care) concerning treatment or designating a surrogate decision maker with the expectation that the hospital will honor the intent of that directive to the extent permitted by law and hospital policy.

   Health care institutions must advise patients of their rights under state law and hospital policy to make informed medical choices, ask if the patient has an advance directive, and include that information in patient records. The patient has the right to timely information about hospital policy that may limit its ability to implement fully a legally valid advance directive.

5. The patient has the right to every consideration of privacy. Case discussion, consultation, examination, and treatment should be conducted so as to protect each patient's privacy.

These rights can be exercised on the patient's behalf by a designated surrogate or proxy decision maker if the patient lacks decision-making capacity, is legally incompetent, or is a minor.

A Patient's Bill of Rights was first adopted by the American Hospital Association in 1973. This revision was approved by the AHA Board of Trustees on October 21, 1992.

FIGURE 3-4 A Patient's Bill of Rights. *Courtesy of American Hospital Association, copyright 1992*

6. The patient has the right to expect that all communications and records pertaining to his/her care will be treated as confidential by the hospital, except in cases such as suspected abuse and public health hazards when reporting is permitted or required by law. The patient has the right to expect that the hospital will emphasize the confidentiality of this information when it releases it to any other parties entitled to review information in these records.

7. The patient has the right to review the records pertaining to his/her medical care and to have the information explained or interpreted as necessary, except when restricted by law.

8. The patient has the right to expect that, within its capacity and policies, a hospital will make reasonable response to the request of a patient for appropriate and medically indicated care and services. The hospital must provide evaluation, service, and/or referral as indicated by the urgency of the case. When medically appropriate and legally permissible, or when a patient has so requested, a patient may be transferred to another facility. The institution to which the patient is to be transferred must first have accepted the patient for transfer. The patient must also have the benefit of complete information and explanation concerning the need for, risks, benefits, and alternatives to such a transfer.

9. The patient has the right to ask and be informed of the existence of business relationships among the hospital, educational institutions, other health care providers, or payers that may influence the patient's treatment and care.

10. The patient has the right to consent to or decline to participate in proposed research studies or human experimentation affecting care and treatment or requiring direct patient involvement, and to have those studies fully explained prior to consent. A patient who declines to participate in research or experimentation is entitled to the most effective care, that the hospital can otherwise provide.

11. The patient has the right to expect reasonable continuity of care when appropriate and to be informed by physicians and other caregivers of available and realistic patient care options when hospital care is no longer appropriate.

12. The patient has the right to be informed of hospital policies and practices that relate to patient care, treatment, and responsibilities. The patient has the right to be informed of available resources for resolving disputes, grievances, and conflicts, such as ethics committees, patient representatives, or other mechanisms available in the institution. The patient has the right to be informed of the hospital's charges for services and available payment methods.

The collaborative nature of health care requires that the patients, or their families/surrogates, participate in their care. The effectiveness of care and patient satisfaction with the course of treatment depend, in part, on the patient fulfilling certain responsibilities. Patients are responsible for providing information about past illnesses, hospitalizations, medications, and other matters related to health status. To participate effectively in decision making, patients must be encouraged to take responsibility for requesting additional information or clarification about their health status or treatment when they do not fully understand information and instructions. Patients are also responsible for ensuring that the health care institution has a copy of their written advance directive if they have one. Patients are responsible for informing their physicians and other caregivers if they anticipate problems in following prescribed treatment.

Patients should also be aware of the hospital's obligation to be reasonably efficient and equitable in providing care to other patients and the community. The hospital's rules and regulations are designed to help the hospital meet this obligation. Patients and their families are responsible for making reasonable accommodations to the needs of the hospital, other patients, medical staff, and hospital employees. Patients are responsible for providing necessary information for insurance claims and for working with the hospital to make payment arrangements, when necessary.

A person's health depends on much more than health care services. Patients are responsible for recognizing the impact of their life-style on their personal health.

Conclusion

Hospitals have many functions to perform, including the enhancement of health status, health promotion, and the prevention and treatment of injury and disease; the immediate and ongoing care and rehabilitation of patients; the education of health professionals, patients, and the community; and research. All these activities must be conducted with an overriding concern for the values and dignity of patients.

FIGURE 3-4 *continued*

Client's Rights in Home Care

The persons receiving home health care services or their families possess basic rights and responsibilities.

These include:

The right to:

1. be treated with dignity, consideration and respect
2. have their property treated with respect
3. receive a timely response from the agency to requests for service
4. be fully informed on admission of the care and treatment that will be provided, how much it will cost, and how payment will be handled
5. know in advance if you will be responsible for any payment
6. be informed in advance of any changes in your care
7. receive care from professionally trained personnel, to know their names and responsibilities
8. participate in planning care
9. refuse treatment and to be told the consequences of your action
10. expect confidentiality of all information
11. be informed of anticipated termination of service
12. be referred elsewhere if you are denied services solely based on your inability to pay
13. know how to make a complaint or recommend a change in agency policies and services

The responsibility to:

1. remain under a doctor's care while receiving services
2. provide the agency with a complete health history
3. provide the agency all requested insurance and financial information
4. sign the required consents and releases for insurance billing
5. participate in your care by asking questions, expressing concerns, stating if you do not understand
6. provide a safe home environment in which care is given
7. cooperate with your doctor, the staff, and other caregivers
8. accept responsibility for any refusal of treatment
9. abide by agency policies which restrict duties our staff may perform
10. advise agency administration of any dissatisfaction or problems with your care

FIGURE 3-5 Client's Rights in Home Care

- informing the physician and other caregivers if they anticipate problems with following prescribed treatment
- accepting responsibility for learning how to manage their own health (Figure 3-6)
- asking for clarification if they do not fully understand instructions or explanations
- living a healthy lifestyle and avoiding unnecessary risks of illness or injury
- accepting financial responsibility for payment of health care and providing information for insurance claims

The rights of health care consumers have both a legal and an ethical basis. Legal and ethical aspects are discussed in Unit 4.

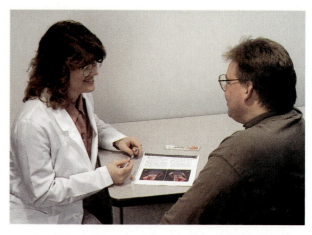

FIGURE 3-6 Patients are responsible for learning how to manage their own health.

REVIEW

A. True/False.

Mark the following true or false by circling T or F.

1. T F The rights of health care consumers are important only to patients in hospitals.
2. T F All United States citizens have certain rights that are guaranteed by law.
3. T F The Client's Bill of Rights is given to persons receiving home care.
4. T F The Patient's Bill of Rights was legislated by the OBRA of 1987.
5. T F Health care consumers in any setting have the right to prepare advance directives.

B. Multiple Choice.

Select the one best answer for each problem.

6. Resident's Rights are given to persons before they are admitted to
   a. home care.
   b. a skilled care facility.
   c. the hospital.
   d. none of the above.
7. All types of consumer rights state that the consumer has the right to
   a. be treated in a respectful, dignified manner.
   b. open and honest communication with caregivers.
   c. have a role in decision making for treatment choices.
   d. all of the above.

8. The purpose of advance directives is to
   a. allow individuals to give instructions about their care should they become unable to do so.
   b. give individuals the right to choose their caregivers.
   c. provide a resource for resolving conflicts.
   d. permit the physician to prescribe treatment without conferring with the individual.
9. Health care consumers are responsible for
   a. communicating openly and honestly with the physician and other caregivers.
   b. providing information about hospitalizations and medications.
   c. learning how to manage their health.
   d. all of the above.

C. Completion.

Choose the correct word from the following list provided to complete each statement in questions 10–15.

advance directive	involuntary seclusion
grievance	privacy
informed consent	respect

10. _____ means that the consumer gives permission for care or procedures after full disclosure.
11. A _____ exists when the consumer feels there are grounds for complaint.
12. A document that gives instructions about the consumer's wishes for treatment if the consumer is unable to communicate is called a[an] _____.
13. Isolating a resident without a medical reason is called _____.

14. By not opening and reading the consumer's mail, you are allowing the consumer the right to _____.

15. All health care consumers have the right to be treated with _____.

D. Nursing Assistant Challenge.

Mr. Delmonico was admitted to General Hospital for surgery to repair a fractured hip. After a few days in the hospital, he will be transferred to Memorial Nursing Center, a skilled care facility, for additional rehabilitation. After discharge from Memorial, it is expected that he will need home care for four to six weeks. Briefly explain how the different rights of each document will affect Mr. Delmonico's care.

16. Consider Mr. Delmonico's diagnosis and the services he will need for recovery. Which aspects of the Patient's Bill of Rights are especially important to his hospital care?

17. Discuss the statements in the Residents' Rights document that pertain specifically to rehabilitation and independence.

18. For which items in the Clients' Rights would the nursing assistant be responsible?

Ethical and Legal Issues Affecting the Nursing Assistant

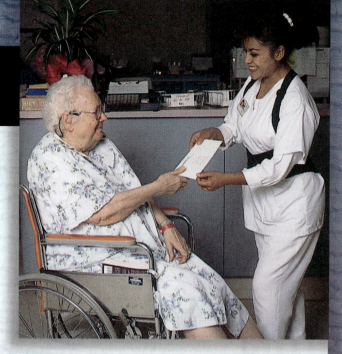

ETHICAL STANDARDS AND LEGAL STANDARDS

Each day, as you carry out your work and relate to patients, coworkers, families, and others from the community, you will be faced with decisions to make about your actions. Some of these decisions involve the moral right or wrong of an action. Other decisions involve the legality of your behavior.

Two sets of rules help govern these moral and legal actions you will take. They are:

1. **Ethical standards**. These are guides to moral behavior. People who give health care voluntarily agree to live up to these standards. When these rules are not followed, the nursing assistant fails to live up to the promise to give safe, correct care and to do no harm.

2. **Legal standards**. These are guides to lawful behavior. When laws are not obeyed, the nursing assistant may be prosecuted and found **liable** (held responsible) for injury or damage. Legal guilt can result in the payment of fines or imprisonment.

The ethical standards and legal standards are established to assure that only safe, quality care is given. Following these standards also protects the caregiver. Sometimes the rules that govern moral actions and the laws that govern legal actions cover the same area.

ETHICS QUESTIONS

Probably at no other time in history have the questions of medical ethics been under such scrutiny. Questions health care providers ask include:

- When is life gone from a person on life support systems?
- How much lifesaving or resuscitation effort should be given in situations of terminal illness?
- When does human life actually begin?
- How much assistance should be given to the conception process?
- Should the body organs of a brain-dead person be harvested for transplants for the living?
- Does an unborn baby have rights?
- Is assisting a patient during or after an abortion right or wrong?
- Is euthanasia (assisted death) ever justified?
- Should animals be used in research of potential value to human life?
- Should food and water be withheld to speed death when the patient has expressed the desire to have this action performed?
- Who makes decisions about removing life support systems when there is no direct expression of the patient's wishes or there is conflict within the family?
- How will a choice be made when two or more people could benefit from an organ transplant but only one organ is available?

- How should the limited money available be spent when many serious disease conditions need to be researched?
- Who has the final authority over whether a woman will carry a pregnancy to term?
- Should marijuana be used for medicinal purposes?

Many facilities have ethics committees that advise the staff on ethical matters. The members of the ethics committees often include staff, clergy, interested community members, and advocates for the sick and elderly.

The committee usually does not make recommendations for specific cases. Instead, the committee reviews the ethical problems and principles involved to help guide the staff and family.

Respect for patients and their wishes is the primary concern. Part of this respect for life is shown by having patients actively involved in decisions about their care and future.

As a nursing assistant, you will take directions from the legal and ethical guidelines established by your facility.

RESPECT FOR LIFE

One of the most basic rules of ethics is that life is precious. Everyone involved in the care of patients has the promotion of health and the quality of life as primary goals (Figure 4-1).

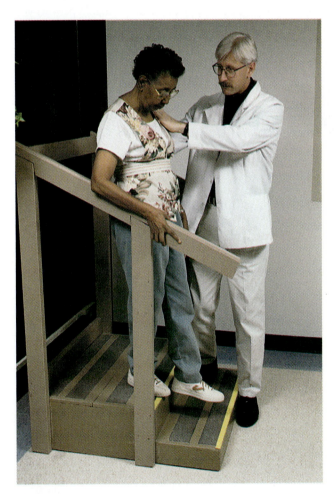

FIGURE 4-1 Promoting health and the quality of life is a primary goal.

Death, however, is a natural progression of life. When death is certain, the objective is to keep the dying person comfortable. Today, there is a greater appreciation of individual wishes and the quality of life expected. One fact remains clear—the major responsibility of medicine and all members of the health care team is to maintain quality of life and make comfortable those whose lives are limited.

RESPECT FOR THE INDIVIDUAL

Respect for each patient as a unique individual is another ethical principle. This uniqueness is demonstrated by differences in:

- age
- race
- religion
- culture
- attitudes
- background
- response to illness

You may find the differences that make the patient so special also make dealing with the patient challenging or difficult. If you respect each patient as a valuable person, you can learn to accept and work with each one in the best possible way.

PATIENT INFORMATION

The ethical code asserts that information about patients is privileged and must not be shared with others (Figure 4-2).

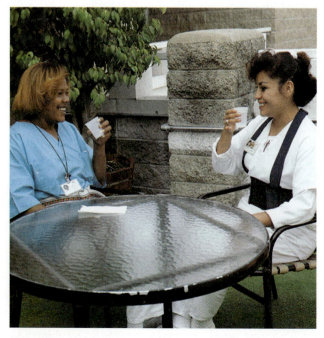

FIGURE 4-2 Information about patients is confidential and must not be discussed casually with others.

1. Discuss patient information only in appropriate places.
   a. It is unwise to discuss a patient's condition while in the patient's room, even if the patient is unresponsive. The patient may be able to hear everything that is said. This could cause the patient unnecessary worry.
   b. Never discuss the patients in your care with your family or in the community.
   c. Never discuss the patients during lunch or coffee breaks, even with your coworkers.
2. Discuss information only with the proper people.
   a. At times you will be approached by others requesting information about a patient. For example, you might be asked for such information by other patients, family members, or members of the public, such as newspeople.
   b. Discuss patients and their personal concerns only with your supervisor during conference or report. Make sure you will not be overheard by visitors or other patients.
   c. You will learn to evade inquiries tactfully by:
      - Stating that you do not know all the details of the treatment or the patient's condition.
      - Redirecting inquirers to the proper authority.
      - Firmly, but politely, indicating that you do not have the authority to provide the answers they seek.
3. Refer patient requests for information about laboratory results, the patient's condition, or course of the illness to the nurse or doctor.
4. Let the nurse or doctor relay information about a patient's death. Never give information concerning the death of a patient to the patient's family. When done with tact, a refusal of this kind is rarely resented by the family.
5. Follow the ethical code to ensure respect of the patient's personal religious beliefs. People of all faiths or beliefs and those with no proclaimed faith are admitted for care. These differences must be respected. You show your respect when you:
   a. Inform the nurse of requests for clergy visits.
   b. Know correct information about the type of chaplain services available in your facility.
   c. Know if a chapel is open for use by patients and families.
   d. Respectfully treat the patient's religious articles, such as a Bible, crucifix, Koran, or holy pictures.

When the clergy visits (Figure 4-3), you should:

a. Be helpful and courteous.
b. Escort the clergyperson to the patient's bedside.
c. Draw the curtains or close the door for privacy.
d. Leave the room.

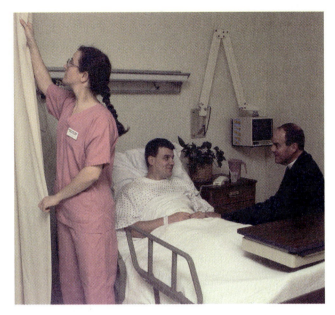

FIGURE 4-3 A visit from clergy or other members of the religious community can be reassuring and helpful to the patient.

TIPPING

If you follow the ethical code, the service you give will depend on need. It will *not* depend on the patient's race, creed, color, or ability to pay. There is no place for tipping within the health care system (Figure 4-4).

Patients are charged for the services they receive while in the hospital. The salary you are paid is included in that charge.

Sometimes patients will offer a "little something" to you. A firm but courteous refusal of the money is usually all that is necessary to assure the patient of your meaning.

As you can see, the ethical code assures that the patient is treated with dignity and respect in ways that always promote safe care.

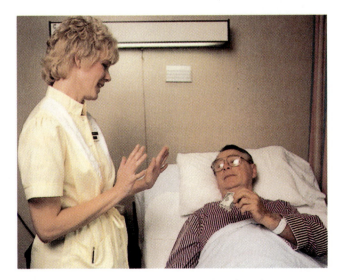

FIGURE 4-4 Tips must be courteously refused.

LEGAL ISSUES

Laws are passed by governments (local, state, and federal) and are to be obeyed by citizens. Anyone who fails to obey a law may be liable (responsible) for fines or imprisonment.

You need not fear breaking these laws if you are careful to:

- Stay within your scope of practice and do not overstep your authority.
- Do only those things that you have been taught and that are within the scope of your training.
- Carry out procedures carefully and as you were taught.
- Keep your skills and knowledge up to date.
- Request guidance from the proper person before you take action in a questionable situation.
- Always keep the safety and well-being of the patient foremost in your mind, and act accordingly.
- Make sure you thoroughly understand directions for the care you are to give.
- Perform your job according to facility policy.
- Stay within OBRA guidelines.
- Maintain in-service requirements of OBRA.
- Do no harm to the patient.
- Respect the patient's belongings (property).

Situations you must avoid are negligence, theft, defamation, false imprisonment, assault and battery, abuse, and invasion of privacy.

Negligence

Nursing assistants are trained care providers and are expected to perform in certain ways. When a nursing assistant fails to give care that is expected or required by the job, that assistant is guilty of **negligence**.

You would be guilty of negligence if you injured a patient by:

- Not performing your work as taught. For example, a patient is burned by an enema solution that you prepared and was too hot.
- Not carrying out your job in a conscientious manner. For example, your facility has a policy that bed rails must be up at night, but in your hurry you fail to secure the bed rails as ordered; the patient falls and is injured.

Theft

Taking anything that does not belong to you makes you guilty of **theft**. If you are caught, you will be liable. The article taken need not be expensive to be considered stolen.

If you see someone stealing something and do not report it, you are guilty of **aiding and abetting** the crime.

Because of the nature of their work, people working in facilities must be honest and dependable. Despite careful screening, dishonest people are sometimes hired and things do disappear. These range from washcloths, money, and patients' personal belongings to drugs.

Sometimes workers are reluctant to report things that they see other people doing. Remember, however, that you are responsible for your own actions and must take the proper actions. For a nursing assistant, the opportunities for poor practice, illegal activities, and neglect are ever present. Resist the temptation to lower your standards. Honesty and integrity are the hallmarks of the sincere and conscientious nursing assistant.

Defamation

If you make false statements about someone to a third person and the character of the first person is injured, you are guilty of **defamation**. This is true if you make the statement verbally (**slander**) or in writing (**libel**). For example, if you inaccurately tell a coworker that a patient has AIDS, you have slandered that patient. If you write the same untrue information in a note, you are guilty of libel.

False Imprisonment

Restraining a person's movements or actions without proper authorization constitutes unlawful or **false imprisonment**. For example, patients have the right to leave the hospital *with or without* the physician's permission. You may not interfere with this right. If you do interfere, you will be guilty of false imprisonment.

If you learn of a patient's intention to leave the hospital without permission, inform your supervisor. The supervisor will handle the situation.

Using physical restraints, or even threatening to do so, in order to make a patient cooperate can also constitute false imprisonment. Restraints may be in the form of physical devices or chemical agents. A physical restraint is any device that:

- A patient cannot easily remove.
- Restricts a patient's movement.
- Does not allow the patient normal access to his or her own body.

Examples of physical restraints include:

- Wrist/arm and ankle/leg restraints
- Vests
- Jackets
- Hand mitts
- Geriatric and cardiac chairs
- Wheelchair safety belts and bars

Bed rails are considered physical restraints if they meet the definition listed.

Psychoactive medications are considered chemical restraints because they affect the patient's mobility. The use of restraints is discussed further in Unit 14 on safety.

Sometimes it is necessary to support and restrain the movement of patients. Supports and restraints cannot be used without a physician's order. This order indicates the extent of restraint or support to be used and the reason for it.

Assault and Battery

Assault and battery are serious legal matters. **Assault** means intentionally attempting to touch the body of a person or even threatening to do so. **Battery** means actually touching a person without that person's permission.

The care we give is given with the patient's permission or **informed consent**. This means the patient must know and agree to what we plan to do before we start. Consent may be withdrawn at any time. For example, you are assigned to give a patient a warm foot soak. Despite your explanation of the reasons for the order, the patient refuses. You may not force the patient to submit. To do so would make you guilty of battery. To threaten the patient by telling her or him that you will get others to assist you if she or he refuses is to commit assault.

Either situation could make you liable for legal charges. You can avoid this legal pitfall by:

- Informing the patient of what you plan to do.
- Making sure the patient understands.
- Pausing before starting, to give the patient an opportunity to refuse.
- Reporting refusal of care to supervisor and documenting the facts.
- Never carrying out a treatment on your own against the patient's wishes.

Abuse

Abuse of a patient (doing harm to a patient) violates ethical principles and makes you liable for legal prosecution. Ethical standards require that you do no harm to patients. Legal standards enforce this through laws, with subsequent penalties if you are found guilty.

Abuse is defined as any act that is nonaccidental and causes harm to the patient. Some forms of abuse are subtle but nevertheless cause the patient physical harm or mental anguish. Abuse can occur in several forms, including verbal, sexual, physical, and mental abuse and involuntary seclusion.

Verbal abuse may be directed toward the patient or expressed about the patient. You are guilty of verbally abusing a patient if you:

- Use profanity (swearing) in dealing with the patient.
- Raise your voice in anger at the patient.
- Call the patient unpleasant names.
- Tease or embarrass the patient.
- Use threatening or obscene gestures.
- Make written threats or abusive statements.
- Use inappropriate words to describe a person's race or nationality.

Sexual abuse is the use of physical means or verbal threats to force a patient to perform sexual acts. Examples of sexual abuse include:

- Tormenting or teasing a patient with sexual gestures or words.
- Touching a patient in a sexual way.

- Suggesting that the patient engage in sexual acts with you.

Physical abuse does actual physical harm to the patient. Examples of physical abuse include:

- Handling a patient roughly (Figure 4-5).
- Hitting, slapping, pushing, kicking, or pinching the patient.
- Performing the wrong treatment on the patient, such as ambulating a patient who should remain in bed.
- Neglecting to turn the patient, causing the circulation to be impaired.
- Failing to perform proper exercises, so that the patient experiences pain when unused joints are finally moved.
- Failing to ensure that the patient has food and water.
- Failing to carry out proper patient hygiene, such as not shaving the patient on a regular basis.

Psychological abuse includes:

- Making the patient fearful of you, such as threatening not to respond when the patient calls.
- Threatening the patient with harm.
- Threatening to tell something to others that the patient does not want known.
- Making fun of or belittling the patient in any way (Figure 4-6). Calling the patient by names such as "honey" and "grandma" is another way of belittling the patient.
- Calling the attention of others to a patient's behavior.

Involuntary seclusion is the separation of a patient from other patients against the patient's will. Examples of involuntary seclusion are:

- Shutting the door to the patient's room when the patient is confined to bed and wants the door open.

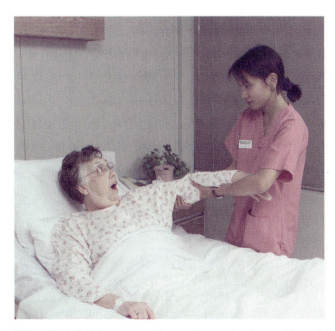

FIGURE 4-5 Pulling roughly on the patient's arm constitutes physical abuse.

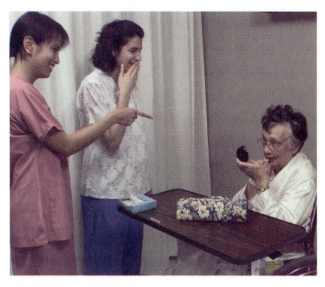

FIGURE 4-6 It is psychological abuse to make fun of a patient in any way.

- Continually placing a patient's gerichair far from others.
- Leaving a patient without a form of communication, such as a signal cord or call bell.

Separation may be permitted if it is part of a therapeutic plan to reduce agitation. The decision to use seclusion must be made by the nurse. This form of seclusion requires accurate documentation and a plan of care. The seclusion must be effective. Note: When describing a patient's behavior, avoid the use of words such as *uncooperative, belligerent,* or *hostile.* Instead, describe the exact actions that you observed. Often, so-called uncooperative behavior is a problem caused by faulty communication on the part of the health care provider. People should not be unfairly labeled.

Abuse by Others

If you suspect that a person in your care is being abused by others, discuss this matter with your supervisor. Laws require a health care provider who suspects abuse to report the situation so the patient can be protected. In some states, a person who does not report the abuse is held as guilty as the abusing person.

It may be difficult to understand why anyone would abuse a person who is weak or infirm, but it happens. A few people may take satisfaction out of feeling that they have control of others. Most abuse, however, probably originates in feelings of frustration or fatigue.

Anyone can be abused, but the old and the young are the most vulnerable. Usually, the caregiver or a family member is the abuser.

- Some families provide loving, capable care for older, dependent relatives for many years without assistance. After providing care for a long period, they may be physically and emotionally exhausted and may also have depleted their financial resources.
- In some cases, a long family history exists of one spouse abusing the other.

- Self-abuse may occur when a disabled person is unable to adequately carry out activities of daily living and is unwilling to accept help.

It is not the responsibility of the nursing assistant to determine if an individual has been abused or what type of abuse has been inflicted. It *is* the nursing assistant's responsibility to report to the nursing supervisor any signs or symptoms that might be the result of abuse. This includes:

- Statements of the patient that reflect neglect or abuse.
- Unexplained bruises or wounds.
- Signs of neglect such as poor personal hygiene.
- A change in personality.

Remember, these do not necessarily indicate that the person is being abused. However, they may indicate a need for further investigation by your supervisor. Any observed abusive behavior toward patients, whether inside or outside a facility, must be reported to the appropriate authority.

When Your Patience Is Stressed

If you feel that your own tolerance level is being tested, you need to find ways to safeguard the patient and release your own stress. You might:

- Try to identify the exact cause of your irritation.
- Talk with your supervisor about your feelings.
- Consider asking to be assigned to another patient.
- Try to reduce your overall stress and fatigue so you bring a more positive, patient attitude to your job.
- Request counseling through an employee assistance program.

Invasion of Privacy

Patients have a right to have their person and personal affairs kept **confidential**. To do otherwise is an **invasion of privacy**. Invading the privacy of another is against the law. You can protect the patient's privacy by:

- Protecting the patient from exposure of the body.
- Knocking and pausing before entering a room.
- Drawing curtains when providing care.
- Leaving while visitors are with the patient.
- Not listening as patients make telephone calls.
- Abiding by the rules of confidentiality.
- Not trying to force a patient to accept your personal beliefs or views.

REVIEW

A. Multiple Choice.

Select the one best answer for each question.

1. You overhear another assistant raise his voice when speaking to Mrs. Ryan. The assistant is guilty of
   a. negligence.
   b. theft.
   c. abuse.
   d. invasion of privacy.

2. Mr. Deonne offers you two dollars for picking up a newspaper for him. Your response should be to
   a. ignore the money and pretend not to see it.
   b. take the money—you earned it.
   c. report the matter to the supervisor.
   d. politely refuse because tipping is not allowed.

3. Mr. Chan's daughter is visiting and wants to know what her father's blood pressure reading is. Your best response is to
   a. tell her.
   b. say you don't know.
   c. refer her to the nurse.
   d. refer her to another assistant who measured blood pressure this morning.

4. You observe another assistant slipping a patient's rosary into her pocket. Your response is to
   a. know you are not required to do anything.
   b. report the matter to your supervisor.
   c. tell the patient.
   d. tell the patient's family.

5. You notice that every time a patient makes a telephone call, one nursing assistant stands so that she can hear the conversation. That assistant is guilty of
   a. invasion of privacy.
   b. defamation.
   c. negligence.
   d. libel.

B. True/False.

Mark the following true or false by circling T or F.

6. T F A patient may not refuse any treatment prescribed by the physician.

7. T F You may learn much about a patient's personal life as you provide care.

8. T F Lunchtime is the best time to discuss your patients with others.

9. T F When a person dies, you should call and inform the family.

10. T F If you accept a tip, you are guilty of abuse.

11. T F Your patient has an order to encourage fluid intake, and you fail to do this. You are guilty of negligence.

12. T F You forget to put side rails up when ordered, and a patient falls. You are guilty of negligence.

13. T F Failure to report your observation of an illegal act makes you guilty of aiding and abetting the action.

14. T F Leaving a patient unnecessarily exposed is an invasion of the patient's privacy.

15. T F Jackets, belts, vests, and straps can be considered unlawful restraints.

16. T F Ethics relates to moral rights and wrongs of behavior.

17. T F Anxiety can sometimes make a person very demanding.

18. T F It is not always easy to keep the basic rule of ethics in mind when you witness a patient suffering.

19. T F People give up their right to privacy when they are admitted to health care facilities.

20. T F You add to a patient's sense of security when you use terms of endearment like "honey."

21. T F Your primary purpose is to help the patient by assisting the nursing staff.

22. T F If an error occurs as you give care, it is important to report it immediately.

23. T F Patients should not question the cost of care.

24. T F Every patient has the right to considerate, respectful care.

25. T F You should knock and pause before entering a patient's room.

26. T F It is all right for you to give your evaluation of the patient's condition to the patient himself.

27. T F Honesty and integrity are the hallmarks of a conscientious nursing assistant.

28. T F You should report all requests for clergy visits to the doctor.

29. T F If a patient resists you, you may apply restraints to make sure the treatment is given.

30. T F Patients may not be subjected to either verbal or physical abuse.

C. Nursing Assistant Challenge.

In each of the following situations, describe the correct nursing assistant action.

31. Ms. Harvey is dying. Her doctors believe that she will live only a few days. What is your responsibility to this patient? _____

32. Mrs. Wybok insists on saying her prayers every morning just as breakfast is ready. _____

33. Mr. Bishop's daughter asks you what medicine the doctor ordered for her father's heart condition. _____

Scientific Principles

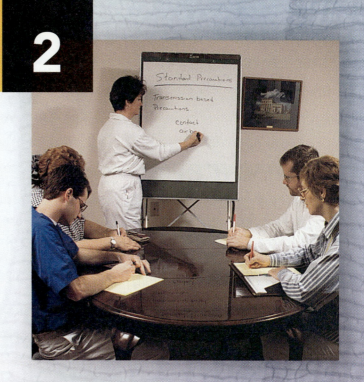

UNIT 5
Medical Terminology and Body Organization

UNIT 6
Classification of Disease

Medical Terminology and Body Organization

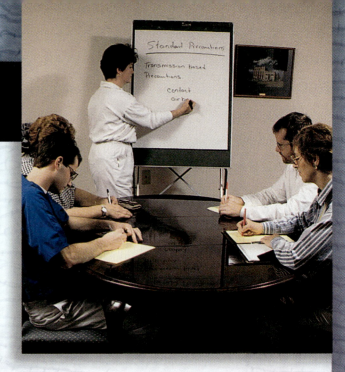

As a result of this unit, you will be able to:

- Spell and define terms.
- Recognize the meanings of common prefixes, suffixes, and root words.
- Build medical terms from word parts.
- Write the abbreviations commonly used in health care facilities.
- Describe the simple to complex organization of the body.
- Name four types of tissues and their characteristics.
- Name and locate major organs as parts of body systems, using proper anatomic terms.

VOCABULARY

Learn the meaning and the correct spelling of the following words and phrases:

abbreviation	distal	muscle cell	quadrant
anatomic position	dorsal	muscle tissue	serous membrane
anatomy	epithelial cell	nerve cell	skeletal muscle
anterior	epithelial tissue	nervous tissue	smooth muscle
cardiac muscle	health	organ	suffix
cavity	inferior	pericardium	superior
cell	lateral	peritoneum	synovial membranes
combining form	medial	physiology	system
connective tissue	membranes	pleura	tissue
connective tissue cell	meninges	posterior	umbilicus
cutaneous membrane	mucous membrane	prefix	ventral
disease	mucus	proximal	word root

MEDICAL TERMINOLOGY

Medical science and health care have a special language called *medical terminology* or the language of health care. In this language, the terms are formed by building on common word parts (Figure 5-1). Terms are developed by combining:

- **Word root**—the foundation of a medical term. A word root usually, but not always, refers to the part of the body or condition that is being treated, studied, or named by the term.
- **Combining form**—a vowel may be added to the end of the word root to make it easier to form medical words. This combination of the word root and vowel is called a combining form.
- **Prefix**—word part added to the beginning of a word to change or add to its meaning.
- **Suffix**—word part added to the end of a word to change or add to its meaning.
- **Abbreviation**—shortened form of a word (often letters). You already know the abbreviation RN (registered nurse). You will soon become familiar with additional abbreviations that are common to the world of medicine and health care.

Each health care facility also has special abbreviations that it uses (Figure 5-2). Check with the procedure or policy manual of your facility to determine which abbreviations have been approved for use. A good medical dictionary is also a helpful tool.

MEDICAL WORD PARTS

Word Roots

Familiarity with the important word parts comes from study and repeated usage. You will gain experience with the word parts as you practice reporting and charting, and by communicating with your coworkers.

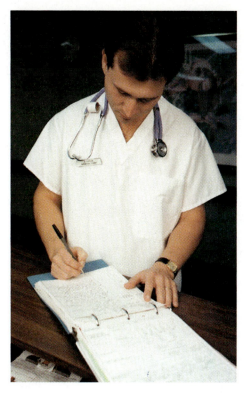

FIGURE 5-2 A knowledge of medical terminology will help make charting and recordkeeping easier.

A single medical word root can sometimes be placed in different parts of a word and still have a specific meaning. For example, the root *cyte* means cell:

- *cyt*ology—the study of cells
- a leuko*cyte*—a white blood cell
- poly*cyt*osis—an illness in which there are too many red and white blood cells

No matter where the form *cyte* occurs in a medical word, it refers to cells. It may be a prefix, a suffix, or a root word.

Word roots are often derived from Greek or Latin. For example, the word root *nephro* is derived from the word for kidney. This root may be used to form a variety of medical terms. For example:

- Nephroma—a tumor of the kidney
- Nephrectomy—surgical excision of the kidney
- Nephroptosis—a kidney dropped out of place

Give special attention to the exercises and activities in this unit. Learning the new words and parts of words in this unit will make it easier for you to recognize meanings of medical terms.

Table 5-1 lists combining forms (word roots plus vowel) pertaining to body parts. Other common combining forms are shown in Table 5-2.

Prefixes and Suffixes

Many medical words have common beginnings (prefixes) or common endings (suffixes). By learning some of the more common prefixes (Table 5-3) and suffixes (Table 5-4), you can put together many new words.

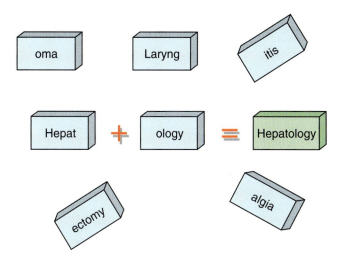

FIGURE 5-1 New words can be formed by combining prefixes and suffixes.

TABLE 5-1 COMBINING FORMS RELATING TO BODY PARTS

Combining Form	Meaning	Example	Meaning
abdomin (o)	abdomen	abdominal	portion of body between the thorax and pelvis
aden (o)	gland	adenoma	a glandular tumor
arthr (o)	joint	arthritis	inflammation of a joint
bronch (i) (o)	bronchus bronchi	bronchiectasis	one of the larger passages conveying air to and within the lungs becomes abnormally enlarged
cardi (o)	heart	cardialgia	pain in the region of the heart
cephal (o)	head	cephaloma	soft or encephaloid tumor
cerebr (o)	brain	cerebrovascular accident	another name for a stroke
chol (e)	bile	cholecystitis	inflammation of the gallbladder
col (o)	colon, large intestine	colectomy	excision of the colon
crani (o)	skull	craniotomy	opening of the skull
cyst (o)	bladder, cyst	cystitis	inflammation of the bladder
cyt (o)	cell	cytology	study of cells
dent (i) (o)	tooth	dentist	person licensed to practice dentistry
dermat (o)	skin	dermatitis	inflammation of the skin
enter (o)	small intestine	enteritis	inflammation of the intestines
gastr (o)	stomach	gastritis	inflammation of the lining of the stomach
hem (o)	blood	hematuria	discharge of blood in urine
hepat (o)	liver	hepatitis	inflammation of the liver
hyster (o)	uterus	hysterectomy	surgical removal of the uterus
laryng (o)	larynx	laryngectomy	partial or total removal of the larynx by surgery
mast (o)	breast	mastitis	inflammation of the breast
my (o)	muscle	myalgia	muscular pain
nephr (o)	kidney	nephrolithiasis	presence of renal calculi (kidney stones)
neur (o)	nerve	neuropathy	any disease of the nervous system
ot (o)	ear	otitis media	inflammation of the middle ear
pharyng (o)	throat, pharynx	pharyngitis	inflammation of the pharynx
pneum (o)	lung, air, gas	pneumonectomy	resection of lung tissue
proct (o)	rectum	proctoscopy	rectal exam with a proctoscope
psych (o)	mind	psychology	study of human behavior
pulm (o)	lung	pulmonary	pertaining to the lungs
py (o)	pus	pyogenic	producing pus
rect (o)	rectum	rectocele	hernial protrusion of part of the rectum into the vagina
thorac (o)	chest	thoracotomy	opening of the chest
trache (i) (o)	trachea	tracheotomy	incision of the trachea for exploration
ur (o)	urine, urinary tract, urination	urinalysis	analysis of the urine
urin (o)	urine	urinometer	an instrument for determining the specific gravity of urine

TABLE 5-2 COMBINING FORMS NOT RELATED TO BODY PARTS

Combining Form	Meaning	Example	Meaning
fibr (o)	fiber	fibroma	tumor composed mainly of fibrous or fully developed connective tissue
glyc (o)	sugar	glycemia	sugar in the blood
gynec (o)	woman, female	gynecology	branch of medicine dealing with diseases of the reproductive organs in women
hydr (o)	water	hydrocephalus	enlargement of the cranium caused by abnormal accumulation of fluid
lith (o)	stone	lithiasis	formation of stones in any hollow structure of the body
ped (o)	child	pediatric	pertaining to diseases of children
py (o)	pus	pyogenic	producing pus
thromb (o)	clot	thrombosis	formation of blood clots inside a blood vessel
tox (o), toxic (o)	poison	toxemia	presence in the blood of toxic (harmful) products

TABLE 5-3 COMMON PREFIXES

Prefix	Meaning	Example	Meaning
a-	without	asepsis	without infection
brady-	slow	bradycardia	slow heart rate
dys-	pain or difficulty	dysuria	painful urination
hyper-	above, excessive	hypertension	high blood pressure
hypo-	low, deficient	hypotension	low blood pressure
pan-	all	pandemic	widespread epidemic
poly-	many	polyuria	excessive urine
post-	after	postoperative	after surgery
pre-	before	premenstrual	before the menses
tachy-	fast	tachycardia	pulse rate above normal

TABLE 5-4 COMMON SUFFIXES

Suffix	Meaning	Example	Meaning
-ectomy	removal of	appendectomy	removal of the appendix
-itis	inflammation of	hepatitis	inflammation of the liver
-gram	record	electrocardiogram	record produced by electrocardiography
-emia	blood	anemia	lacking sufficient quality or quantity of blood
-logy	study of	hematology	study of blood
-oma	tumor	fibroma	a tumor containing fibrous tissue
-otomy	incision	tracheotomy	incision of trachea
-plegia	paralysis	hemiplegia	paralysis of one side of the body
-pnea	breathing, respiration	apnea	temporary cessation of breathing
-scope	examination instrument	otoscope	instrument for inspecting or auscultating the ear
-scopy	examination using a scope	proctoscopy	rectal exam with a proctoscope

Common Abbreviations

Table 5-5 lists abbreviations and their meanings. They have been grouped according to most common usage for easier learning. Other abbreviations will be presented in following units where they find their greatest application.

TABLE 5-5 COMMON ABBREVIATIONS

Body Parts

abd	abdomen
ax	axillary
bld	blood
GI	gastrointestinal
GU	genitourinary
lt	left
os	mouth
sh	shoulder
vag	vagina, vaginal

Diagnosis

AFB	acid fast bacillus
AIDS	acquired immune deficiency syndrome
AKA	above knee amputation
AMI	acute myocardial infarction
ASHD	arteriosclerotic heart disease
BKA	below knee amputation
c̄	with
CA	cancer
CBC	complete blood count
CHD	coronary heart disease
CHF	congestive heart failure
COPD	chronic obstructive pulmonary disease
CVA	cerebrovascular accident; stroke
DJD	degenerative joint disease
FUO	fever of unknown origin
Fx	fracture
HBV	hepatitis B virus (infection)
HIV	human immunodeficiency virus (infection)
IDDM	insulin dependent diabetes mellitus
IH	infectious hepatitis
KS	Kaposi's sarcoma
LBP	low back pain
MI	myocardial infarction (refers to the death of tissues due to loss of blood supply)
MRSA	methicillin resistant *Staphylococcus aureus*
MS	multiple sclerosis
NB	newborn
NIDDM	noninsulin dependent diabetes mellitus
NSU	nonspecific urethritis
PID	pelvic inflammatory disease
PVD	peripheral vascular disease
RF	renal failure
s̄	without
SDAT	senile dementia of Alzheimer's type
STD	sexually transmitted disease
TIA	transient ischemic attack
URI	upper respiratory infection
UTI	urinary tract infection

Patient Orders and Charting

a	before
ADL	activities of daily living
ad lib.	as desired
adm	admission
ADT	admission, discharge, transfer
amb	ambulate, ambulatory
ASAP	as soon as possible
as tol	as tolerated
B.M., bm	bowel movement
B/P	blood pressure
B.R.	bed rest
BRP	bathroom privileges
BSC	bedside commode
c̄	with
cath	catheterize
CBC	complete bed bath
CBR	complete bed rest
cl liq	clear liquid
C/O	complains of
CP	care plan
DAT	diet as tolerated
DC, D/C	discontinue
disch	discharge
DNR	do not resuscitate
DR	doctor
drg	dressing
DSD	dry, sterile dressing
Dx	diagnosis
E	enema
FM	flow meter
FU	follow-up
GT	gastrostomy tube
HOB	head of bed
HOH	hard of hearing
ht	height
Hx	history
I & O	intake and output
irrig	irrigation
isol	isolation
IV	intravenous
lg	large
liq	liquid
N/C	no complaints
neg	negative
NPO	nothing by mouth
N & V	nausea and vomiting
NVD	nausea, vomiting, diarrhea
O₂	oxygen
OOB	out of bed
O	oral
per	by
p.o. (per os)	by mouth
preop	preoperative
p.r.n.	whenever necessary
pt	patient; pint (500 mL)
Px	prognosis (prog)
q.s.	sufficient quantity
qt	quiet
R	rectal
rehab	rehabilitation
resp	respiration
rt (R)	right, routine
RT	respiratory therapy
Rx	treatment
s̄	without
sm	small
spec	specimen
SSE	soapsuds enema
ST	speech therapy
stat	at once
Sx	symptoms
TPN	total parenteral nutrition
TPR	temperature, pulse, respiration

continues

TABLE 5-5 *continued*

TWE	tap water enema	**Places or Departments**		WA	while awake	

TWE	tap water enema
Tx	treatment
Ty	tympanic
ung.	ointment (oint)
VRE	vancomycin-resistant enterococcus
V.S.	vital signs
w/c	wheelchair
wt	weight

Physical and History

DOB	date of birth
FH	family history
LMP	last menstrual period
L & W	living and well
M & F	mother and father
MH	marital history
NB	newborn
PI	present illness
PMH	past medical history
R/O	rule out
UCD	usual childhood diseases
UK	unknown
WDWN	well-developed, well-nourished
WNL	within normal limits
YOB	year of birth

Tests

ABG	arterial blood gas study
CBC	complete blood count
FBS	fasting blood sugar
H & H	hemoglobin and hematocrit
UA	urinalysis

Places or Departments

CS	central supply
DR	delivery room
ED/ER	emergency department or emergency room
EENT	eye, ear, nose, throat
ICCU	intensive coronary care unit
Lab	laboratory
MRD	medical record department
OPD	outpatient department
OR	operating room
OT	occupational therapy
PAR	post-anesthesia room
Peds	pediatrics
PT	physical therapy
RR	recovery room

Time Abbreviations

a.c.	before meals
AM	morning
b.i.d.	twice a day
h.s.	hour of sleep (bedtime)
noc, noct	night
p	after
p.c.	after meals
PM	evening or afternoon
qd	every day
qh	every hour
q4h	every four hours
q.i.d.	four times a day
qm (qAM)	every morning
qn	every night
qod	every other day
t.i.d.	three times a day

Roman Numerals

I	1
II	2
III	3
IV	4
V	5
VI	6
VII	7
VIII	8
IX	9
X	10

Measurements and Volume

cc	cubic centimeter
mL	milliliter
L	liter
>	greater
<	lesser
$\overline{ss}$	one-half

Weight/Height

kg	kilogram
lb	pounds
in	inches

Temperature

F	Fahrenheit
C	Celsius
°	degree

Sumbols

♂	male
♀	female
@	at

BODY ORGANIZATION

All nursing care is directed toward helping patients reach optimum health and independence. **Health** is a state of well-being in which all parts of the body and mind are functioning properly. **Disease** is any change from the healthy state. Disease takes many forms. Medical science is the study of disease and its effects on the human body. These effects are easier to understand when you have a clear picture in your mind of a normal and properly functioning body. The first step is to understand the organization of the body.

ANATOMIC TERMS

The **anatomy** (structure) and **physiology** (function) of the body are most easily understood and learned if they are studied in an orderly manner. Special terms are used to describe the relationship of one body part to another.

Whenever we describe the relationship of the body parts, keep in mind the **anatomic position** (Figure 5-3), which is:

- Standing erect with feet together or slightly separated
- Facing the observer
- Arms at the sides with the palms forward

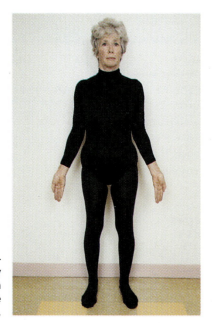

FIGURE 5-3 All references to body parts are made in relationship to the anatomic position.

In our own minds, we should always position the body in this way before describing any body part or area. This gives everyone the same frame of reference.

Notice as you look at a patient's body or the pictures in the book that you are seeing a mirror image of yourself. The patient's right side is opposite to your left and your left is opposite to the right of the patient or the picture.

Descriptive Terms

Imaginary lines drawn through the body (Figure 5-4) can provide us with other reference terms.

- A line drawn down the center of the body from head to foot divides the body into equal right and left sides. Note that the body has the same parts on either side. For example, there is an arm, a leg, an eye, and half of a nose on each side of the line.
- Parts close to this line are **medial** to the line.
- Parts farther away from the line are **lateral** to the line.

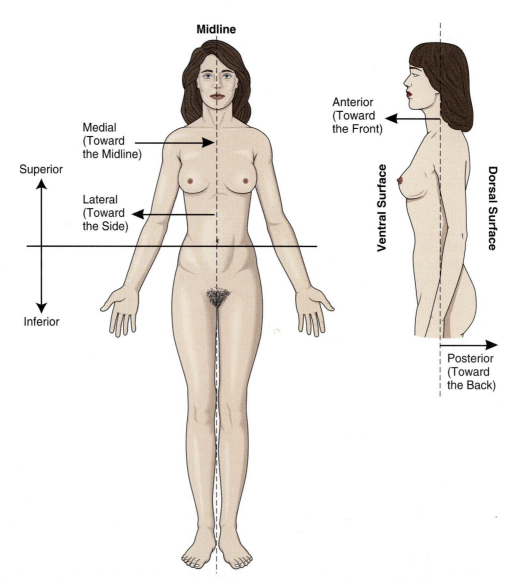

FIGURE 5-4 Imaginary lines can be used to section the body to make it easier to locate parts.

For example, in the anatomic position, the thumbs are more lateral to the line and the little fingers are more medial to the line.

Another line drawn parallel to the floor divides the body into upper and lower parts. This line can be drawn at any level on the body as long as it is parallel to the floor.

● Parts located above this line are **superior** to the line.
● Parts located below this line are **inferior** to the line.

For example, if the line is drawn between the knees and ankles, the knees are superior to the ankles and the ankles are inferior to the knees.

A third line can be drawn to divide the body into front and back.

● Parts in front of this line are **anterior** or **ventral** to the line.
● Parts in back of this line are **posterior** or **dorsal** to the line.

Points of Attachment

The arms and legs are called the *extremities* of the body. The arms are attached to the body at the shoulders. The legs are attached to the body at the hips. Two terms are used to describe the relationship between the parts of the extremities and their points of attachment to the body.

● **Proximal**—means closest to the point of attachment
● **Distal**—means farthest away from the point of attachment

Because the upper arm is closest to the shoulder, where it is attached, this part is described as *proximal* when compared to the fingers, which are farthest away. The fingers are *distal* or farthest away from the point of attachment of the upper extremity.

Abdominal Regions

The abdomen is divided into four **quadrants**, with the **umbilicus** (navel) at the central point (Figure 5-5A). The abdomen can also be divided into nine regions (Figure 5-5B). Knowing these regions will be important as you report and document your observations.

ORGANIZATION OF THE BODY

All parts of the body are interdependent. The basic unit of the body is the **cell**. Groups of similar cells are organized into **tissues**. Different tissues form **organs**. The organs are organized into **systems** that perform the body functions.

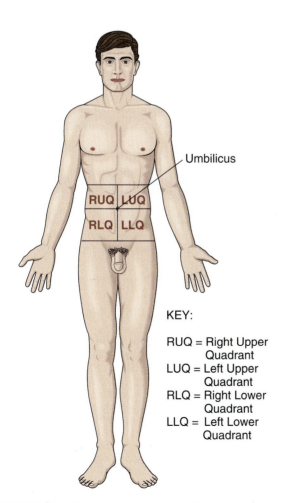

FIGURE 5-5A The abdominal quadrants

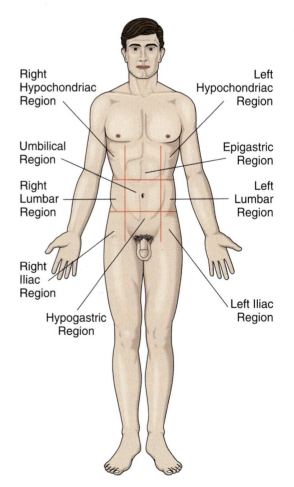

FIGURE 5-5B The abdomen can also be divided into nine regions.

Cells

Each cell performs the same basic functions that the total body performs, but on a smaller scale. These functions are breathing (respiration), reproduction, nutrition, and excretion (eliminating wastes). Some cells perform different kinds of work necessary for the body as a whole to function. Some of the various specialized types of cells are:

- Epithelial cells
- Nerve cells
- Muscle cells
- Connective tissue cells

Epithelial cells, which are very close together, form protective coverings and sometimes produce body fluids.

Nerve cells carry electrical messages to and from the different parts of the body, coordinating activities and making us aware of changes in the environment.

Muscle cells are special in their ability to shorten or lengthen, changing their shape and the position of parts to which they are attached. They also surround body openings, such as the mouth, to control the size of these openings.

Connective tissue cells are present throughout the body in many different types. They support and connect body parts.

Tissues

Groups of similar cells are organized into tissues. The basic tissue types are:

- Epithelial tissue
- Connective tissue
- Nervous tissue
- Muscle tissue

Epithelial tissue is specialized in its ability to absorb, secrete (produce) fluids, excrete (eliminate) waste products, and protect.

Nervous tissue forms the brain and spinal cord and the nerves throughout the body. This tissue is also found in the special sense organs such as the eyes, ears, and tastebuds. The activities of the rest of the body are directed and coordinated through the nervous tissues.

Three kinds of **muscle tissue** are found in the body:

- **Skeletal muscle** is attached to bones for movement.
- **Cardiac muscle** forms the heart wall.
- **Smooth muscle** (visceral) forms the walls of body organs such as the stomach and intestines.

Connective tissue forms blood, bone, and fibrous and elastic tissues to hold the skin on the body, attach muscles to bones, and support delicate cells throughout the body. Generally, connective tissues support and form connections for other tissue types.

Organs

Each organ is made up of more than one kind of tissue and performs special functions that contribute to the function of the body systems. Some organs, like the kidneys, are found in pairs. Some single organs contribute to more than one system. For example, the pancreas contributes secretions to both the endocrine and digestive systems.

Systems

The body has 10 major body systems. Table 5-6 lists the organs that contribute to the function of each system. Notice that some organs are included with more than one system.

TABLE 5-6 SYSTEMS OF THE BODY

System	Function	Organs
Cardiovascular	Transports materials around the body; carries oxygen and nutrients to the cells and carries waste products away; part of the immune system that provides protective cells and chemicals to fight current infections and protect against future infections	Heart, arteries, capillaries, veins, spleen, lymph nodes, lymphatic vessels, blood, lymph
Endocrine	Produces hormones that regulate body processes	Pituitary gland, thyroid gland, parathyroid glands, thymus gland, adrenal glands, testes, ovaries, pineal body, islets of Langerhans in pancreas
Gastrointestinal (Digestive)	Digests, transports food, absorbs nutrients, and eliminates wastes	Mouth, esophagus, pharynx, stomach, small intestine, large intestine, salivary glands, teeth, tongue, liver, gallbladder, pancreas
Integumentary	Protects the body from injury and against infection, regulates body temperature, eliminates some wastes	Skin, hair, nails, sweat and oil glands

continues

TABLE 5-6 *continued*

System	Function	Organs
Skeletal	Supports and protects body parts, produces blood cells, acts as levers in movement	Bones, joints
Muscular	Protects organs by forming body walls, forms walls of some organs, assists in movement by changing position of bones at joints	*Smooth* muscles—form walls of organs *Skeletal* muscles—attached to bones *Cardiac* muscles—form wall of heart
Nervous	Coordinates body functions	Brain, spinal cord, spinal nerves, cranial nerves, special sense organs such as eyes and ears
Reproductive	Reproduces the species, fulfills sexual needs, develops sexual identity	*Male:* Testes, epididymis, urethra, seminal vesicles, ejaculatory duct, prostate gland, bulbourethral glands, penis, spermatic cord *Female:* Breasts, ovaries, oviducts, uterus, vagina, Bartholin glands, vulva
Respiratory	Brings in oxygen and eliminates carbon dioxide	Sinuses, nose, pharynx, larynx, trachea, bronchi, lungs
Urinary	Manages fluids and electrolytes of body, eliminates liquid wastes	Kidneys, ureters, urinary bladder, urethra

For example, the ovaries contribute to the endocrine system by producing female hormones and to the reproductive system by producing the egg.

Membranes

Membranes are sheets of epithelial tissues supported by connective tissues. Membranes:

- Cover the body
- Line body cavities
- Produce some body fluids

Important membranes include:

- Mucous membranes
  - Produce a fluid called mucus
  - Line body cavities that open to the outside

Because the respiratory, digestive, and genitourinary systems all open to the outside, they are lined with mucous membranes. The eyelids are also lined with a mucous membrane; a mucous membrane covers the eyeballs.

- Synovial membranes
  - Produce synovial fluid
  - Line joint cavities

The synovial fluid is a clear fluid resembling the white of an egg. It reduces the friction between the bones of active joints and the tendons.

- Serous membranes
  - Produce serous fluid
  - Cover the organs and line the closed cavities of the body

Serous fluid reduces friction as the organs work and move. Important serous membranes are the:

- Pericardium—surrounds the heart
- Pleura—surrounds the lungs and lines the thoracic cavity
- Meninges—cover the brain and spinal cord and line the dorsal cavity
- Peritoneum—covers the digestive organs and lines the abdominal cavity
- Cutaneous membrane (skin)
  - Protects the body
  - Covers the entire body
  - Helps to control body temperature
  - Eliminates wastes through sweat glands
  - Produces vitamin D when exposed to sunlight

Special epithelial cells in this membrane, called glands, secrete perspiration and oils.

Cavities

The body seems like a solid structure, but cavities (spaces) within it contain the organs. Table 5-7 lists the two main cavities, the dorsal cavity and the ventral cavity. Each of these cavities is lined by and divided into other cavities by serous membranes. These other cavities are also listed in the table, as are the organs contained in each.

Figure 5-6 is a simple drawing of the location of these cavities.

TABLE 5-7 BODY CAVITIES AND THE ORGANS CONTAINED WITHIN EACH CAVITY		
Cavity	**Organs**	
Dorsal Cavity		
Cranial	Brain, pineal body, pituitary gland	
Spinal	Nerves, spinal cord	
Ventral Cavity		
Thoracic	Lungs, heart, great blood vessels, thymus gland	
Abdominal Peritoneal	Stomach, small intestine, most of large intestine, liver, gallbladder, pancreas, spleen	
Pelvic	*Male*	*Female*
	Seminal vesicles, prostate gland, ejaculatory ducts, urinary bladder, urethra, rectum	Uterus, oviducts, ovaries, urinary bladder, urethra, rectum
Retroperitoneal space	Kidneys, adrenal glands, ureters	

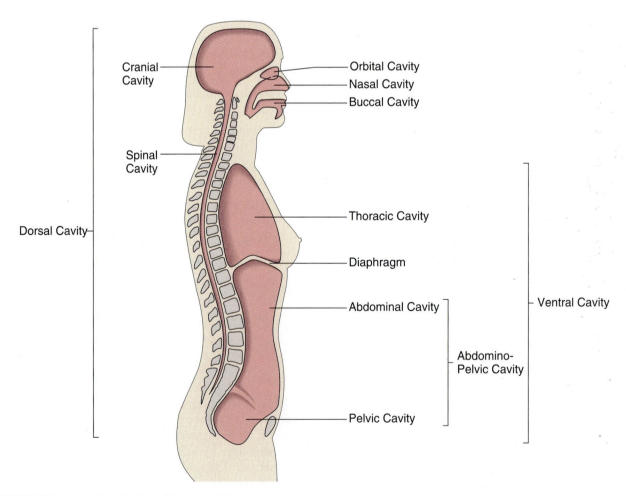

FIGURE 5-6 Lateral (side) view of body cavities

REVIEW

A. Matching.

Match the abbreviations in Column I with their meanings in Column II.

Column I

1. _____ a.c.
2. _____ b.i.d.
3. _____ OR
4. _____ p.r.n.
5. _____ p.o.
6. _____ stat
7. _____ h.s.
8. _____ c̄
9. _____ ung.
10. _____ s̄

Column II

a. three times a day
b. whenever necessary
c. hour of sleep
d. before meals
e. operating room
f. by mouth
g. after meals
h. without
i. twice a day
j. at once
k. ointment
l. with

B. Matching.

Match the prefixes in Column I with their meanings in Column II.

Column I

11. _____ ur (o)
12. _____ cardi (o)
13. _____ chol (e)
14. _____ dermat (o)
15. _____ gastr (o)
16. _____ ot (o)
17. _____ ped (o)
18. _____ pneum (o)
19. _____ my (o)
20. _____ pharyng (o)

Column II

a. bile
b. ear
c. lung
d. child
e. muscle
f. pharynx
g. stomach
h. larynx
i. heart
j. urine
k. chest
l. skin

C. Define the following medical terms.

Then circle the prefix that you have learned.

21. dysuria _____
22. apnea _____
23. craniotomy _____
24. hypertension _____
25. tachycardia _____

D. Define the following medical terms.

Then circle the suffix that you have learned.

26. neuralgia _____
27. apnea _____
28. appendectomy _____
29. hematology _____
30. fibroma _____

E. Write the medical term that means the following.

31. dropped kidney _____
32. examination of the rectum using an instrument _____
33. incision into thorax _____
34. inflammation of the stomach _____
35. white blood cell _____

F. In each of the following, circle the prefix and underline the suffix.

36. anemia
37. neuritis
38. pharyngitis
39. pandemic
40. tracheotomy

G. Measurements.

Print the abbreviations for the following.

41. milliliter
42. kilogram
43. pound
44. Fahrenheit
45. inches

H. Print the Roman numerals for each of the following.

46. 2 _____
47. 5 _____
48. 6 _____
49. 9 _____
50. 10 _____

I. Multiple Choice.

Select the one best answer for each question.

51. When describing the relationship of the hand to the elbow, you should refer to it as being
    a. proximal.
    b. posterior.
    c. distal.
    d. anterior.

52. The appendix is located in which quadrant of the abdomen?
   a. URQ
   b. LRQ
   c. ULQ
   d. LLQ

53. Which membrane covers the lungs?
   a. Pleura
   b. Pericardium
   c. Peritoneum
   d. Meninges

54. Which organs are located in the dorsal cavity?
   a. Heart and liver
   b. Kidney and spleen
   c. Brain and spinal cord
   d. Uterus and testes

55. Which organ pumps blood throughout the body?
   a. Lungs
   b. Heart
   c. Liver
   d. Adrenal glands

56. Which organ is part of the skeletal system?
   a. Ureters
   b. Sternum
   c. Gallbladder
   d. Testes

57. The breasts are part of which system?
   a. Muscular
   b. Urinary
   c. Cardiovascular
   d. Reproductive

58. Membranes that line body cavities that open to the outside are called
   a. mucous membranes.
   b. mucus membranes.
   c. serous membranes.
   d. fibrous membranes.

59. The eye and ear are part of which system?
   a. Endocrine
   b. Nervous
   c. Cardiovascular
   d. Digestive

60. The endocrine system
   a. reproduces the species.
   b. brings in oxygen.
   c. transports blood.
   d. produces hormones.

J. True/False.

Mark the following true or false by circling T or F.

61. T F   The urinary bladder and gallbladder are the same structures.

62. T F   The pancreas functions in both the digestive and endocrine systems.

63. T F   Muscular tissue enables the body to move.

64. T F   Structures of different tissues acting together to carry out a specific function are called organs.

K. Nursing Assistant Challenge.

Examine the sample care plan and use your understanding of medical science and terminology to define each medical term and abbreviation used on the plan.

1.	**Patient Name** Bruce Tratt	**Age** 47	**Rel** Prot	#876-3291-7		
2.	**Physician** R. Morgan M.D.	**Dx** Splenomegaly—Diabetes Mellitus				
3.	**Orders**					
4.	**Preop orders** 3/18 on call for OR @ 8 am 3/19					
5.	Stat CBC, ABG, FBS					
6.	UA					
7.	NG Tube @ 6 am 3/19					
8.	Foley cath this pm.					
9.	Surg Prep.					
10.	NPO p̄ midnight					
11.	SSE @ HS.					
12.	Amb ad Lib. this pm.					
13.						
14.	Anesthesiologist will call preop medication orders.					
15.						

Classification of Disease

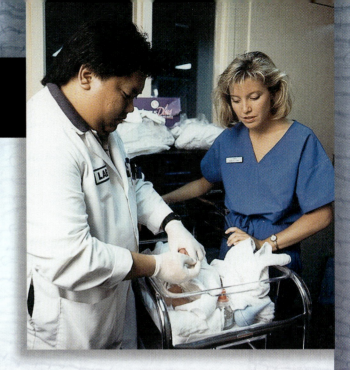

As a result of this unit, you will be able to:
- Spell and define terms.
- Define disease and list some possible causes.
- List six major health problems.
- Identify disease-related terms.
- Distinguish between signs and symptoms.
- List ways in which a diagnosis is made.
- Describe malignant and benign tumors.
- List six major health problems.

Learn the meaning and the correct spelling of the following words and phrases:

acute disease	etiology	malignant	protocol
antibodies	genetic	medical diagnosis	risk factors
autoimmune	hypersensitivity	metastasize	sarcoma
benign	immune response	neoplasm	signs
carcinoma	infection	noninvasive	symptoms
cachexia	inflammation	obstruction	therapy
chronic disease	invasive	predisposing factor	trauma
complication	ischemia	prognosis	tumor
congenital			

INTRODUCTION

The nurse values your observations and uses them when making evaluations and planning nursing care for patients, as part of the nursing process. The better you understand the basic principles of disease, the more accurate information you can provide.

DISEASE

The body is a complex chemical factory that depends upon all of its parts to perform efficiently. It is subject to external and internal forces and stress that can threaten its ability to function properly (Figure 6-1).

Disease is any change from a healthy state. The disease (illness) may be a change in structure or function, or it may be the failure of a part of the body to develop properly. Each illness has

- An **etiology**—cause of the illness or abnormality.
- A usual set of indications that the illness is in progress. These are called signs and symptoms.
- A usual course or disease progression.
- A **prognosis** or probable outcome of the process.

Predisposing factors to disease are general conditions, such as malnutrition, that may contribute to the development of illness. Some diseases have related risk factors. **Risk factors** are specific behaviors or conditions that tend to promote certain diseases (Figure 6-2). For example, smoking is a risk

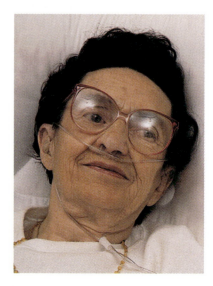

FIGURE 6-2
Advanced age is a predisposing factor to the development of some illnesses.

factor that increases the likelihood that the person will develop lung disease. Other risk factors and associated diseases include:

- Excess weight—high blood pressure, strokes, heart attack
- Poor nutrition—infections
- Lack of exercise—osteoporosis
- High-fat, low-fiber diet—cancer of the colon
- Unprotected sex—hepatitis, AIDS, gonorrhea
- Family history—breast cancer, heart disease, diabetes mellitus

A young child who is malnourished and underweight is much more likely to develop an infection than one who is well nourished. The germs causing the infection are the actual cause of the illness, but the age and nutritional state of the child contribute to the development of the infectious process. Table 6-1 lists common causes of disease (both external and internal) and a number of risk factors for disease.

Signs and Symptoms

Signs of a disease can be seen by others. The color or condition of the skin is an example of a sign of disease (Figure 6-3). **Symptoms** are felt by the patient, who tells us about them. Pain is a symptom common to many illnesses (Figure 6-4).

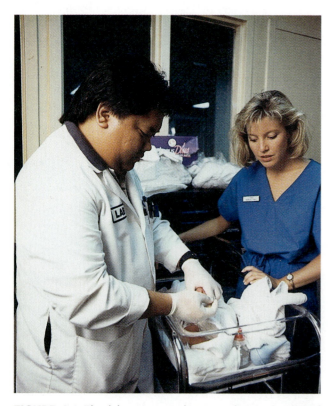

FIGURE 6-1 The laboratory technician takes a sample of blood from the heel of this neonate. A test will be performed to determine if the baby has a congenital condition called phenylketonuria (PKU) (a metabolic condition).

TABLE 6-1 COMMON CAUSES OF DISEASE AND PREDISPOSING FACTORS

External Etiology	Internal Etiology	Predisposing Factors
traumas	metabolic disorders	age
radiation	congenital abnormalities	malnutrition
microorganisms	tumors	heredity
chemical agents		previous illness

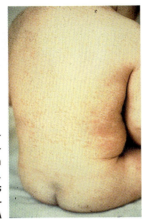

FIGURE 6-3 Note the maculopapular rash that is characteristic of the lesions (skin changes) of measles (rubeola). *Photo courtesy of the Centers for Disease Control and Prevention, Atlanta, GA*

The Course (Pattern) of Disease

The development and course of different illnesses vary greatly. **Acute disease** progresses rapidly and lasts for a predictable period, and then the person recovers (or dies). For example, the signs and symptoms of an infected finger may develop rapidly and last a relatively short period. Then, as the body controls the process, recovery is seen.

A **chronic disease** often has periods when the patient experiences the signs and symptoms and periods when evidence of the disease is less pronounced or disappears altogether. Rheumatoid arthritis is such a disease. At times the affected joints are red, hot to the touch, swollen, and painful. At other times, the signs and symptoms seem to go away.

Complications

A **complication** makes the original condition more serious. For example, if a child has measles and develops pneumonia (a serious lung condition), the pneumonia is a complication that makes it more difficult for the child to recover.

MAJOR CONDITIONS

Some of the major conditions or illnesses that can affect the body's ability to function are:

- **Ischemia**—the lack of adequate blood supply to a body tissue, which prevents delivery of the essential oxygen and nutrients. For example, a blood clot (thrombus) that has formed within a blood vessel wall can block the blood vessel.
- **Congenital** abnormalities—abnormalities that are present at birth (Figure 6-5). Some abnormalities occur while the baby is growing in the mother's uterus. Examples include:
  - Spina bifida—a defect in the formation of the vertebral column
  - Cleft lip—an imperfection in the formation of the upper lip
  - Agenesis of a kidney—one kidney fails to develop, so the baby is born with only one functioning kidney
  - Talipes (club foot)—the child's foot is turned or twisted out of its normal position

Some abnormalities are due to defects in the **genetic** information passed from the parents to the child. Examples include:

- Sickle cell anemia—the red blood cells are improperly formed so they do not maintain their normal disc shape
- Color blindness—the person is unable to distinguish between certain colors
- Hemophilia—there is a lack of an important blood component needed for proper blood clotting.

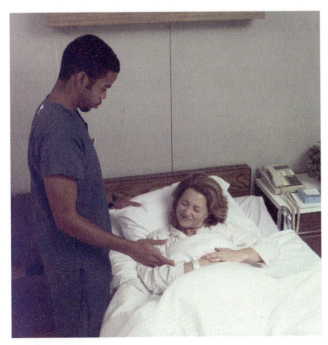

FIGURE 6-4 Sometimes the patient experiencing the symptom of pain shows this through body language.

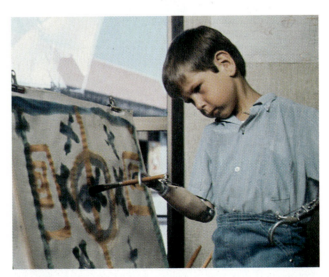

FIGURE 6-5 This child has phocomelia. His hands did not develop before birth because a drug taken by his mother during early pregnancy interfered with limb development. *Photo courtesy of the March of Dimes—Birth Defects Foundation*

- **Infection**—Infectious organisms or their products cause infection, including pneumonias, scarlet fever, and abscesses. Inflammation usually is part of the infectious process.
- **Inflammations** that develop for reasons other than infection include:
  - **Autoimmune** reactions—Mechanisms that are designed to protect the body turn against the body and cause damage, resulting in conditions such as rheumatoid arthritis (RA), systemic lupus erythematosus (SLE), and multiple sclerosis (MS).
  - **Hypersensitivity** reactions—Allergic types of reactions such as hay fever, skin rashes, and asthma.
  - Irritations—May be caused by seeds in the intestinal tract or stones in the gallbladder or kidney.
- Metabolic imbalances—Conditions of fluid and electrolyte imbalance include malnutrition, edema, scurvy, alcoholism, and diabetes mellitus.
- **Obstruction**—Tubes throughout the body carry a variety of materials that must continue to flow. Obstructions impede the flow. Examples of obstructions include blood clots in blood vessels, stones in the bile ducts or the kidneys, and blockages that occur when the tube structures become twisted, as in an intestinal obstruction.
- **Trauma**—Injuries that cause tissue damage resulting from a blow to the body, such as an auto accident. Exposure to unusual pressure or extremes of temperature also causes trauma.
- Neoplasm—The word **neoplasm** means new growth. It is another term for **tumor**. Neoplasms are an important kind of disease. There are two types of neoplasms: benign or nonmalignant tumors and malignant tumors. Sometimes benign tumors can change and become malignant. People with a malignant tumor or a malignancy are said to have cancer. Neoplasms are discussed further later in this unit.

DIAGNOSIS

The **medical diagnosis** (the process of identifying and naming the disease) is made by the physician. To do this, the patient is examined, a history of previous illness is taken and reviewed, and various laboratory tests are performed. The physician compiles the information, matches it to possible diseases, and then names the process to establish the medical diagnosis.

Diagnostic Studies

Laboratory tests (Figure 6-6) and diagnostic studies give the physician valuable information for naming the disease process and for planning the proper treatment for the patient. The nursing staff prepares the patient for the ordered tests and cares for the patient after the tests are completed. The nursing assistant helps give this care and may be assigned to collect certain specimens.

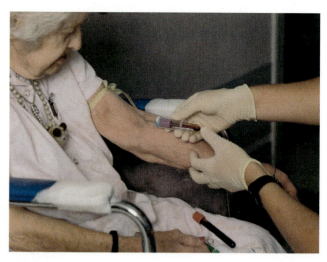

FIGURE 6-6 Blood tests give much information about the chemistry of the body and contribute to a correct medical diagnosis.

Protocols are standards of procedure and care developed for the preparation and care of the patient for each test or study. Protocols must be followed carefully to achieve satisfactory results. Improper patient preparation can result in:

- Inability to perform the test
- Inaccurate test results
- Delayed diagnosis
- Increased costs
- Increased patient anxiety
- Slower recovery

Noninvasive Tests

Some tests and studies are **noninvasive**. This means the techniques used do not break the skin or damage body tissues. For example, x-rays do not break the skin, but do give information about internal body structures. Commonly ordered noninvasive tests include:

- Ultrasound—sound waves are bounced against the body to measure variations in tissue density (Figure 6-7). For example, the Doppler ultrasound probe measures the blood flow in blood vessels. Sonograms of a pregnant woman's uterus give information about the growing fetus.
- Thermography—measures the temperature in different body tissues. Thermograms of the breast indicate increased temperature in tumorous tissue.
- X-ray and fluoroscopy—use short-wavelength electromagnetic radiation to examine internal tissues. X-ray techniques are sophisticated. One of the newest techniques is computerized axial tomography (CT scan or CAT scan). This procedure gives a three-dimensional view of the internal structures of the body. A computer records and prints out information.
- Magnetic resonance imaging (MRI)—an imaging technique that provides excellent pictures (images) with minimal risk to the patient (Figure 6-8). The body is

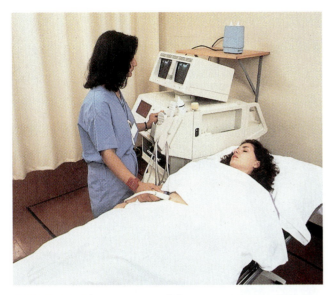

FIGURE 6-7 The sonogram of the uterus gives useful information about the fetus.

placed in a strong magnetic field. Radio frequency pulses cause certain chemicals (ions) in body tissues to change position. When the radio waves are discontinued, the ions return to their original positions. As they go back to normal, the energy given off is recorded. All of this occurs without the patient feeling any of it.

● Recording of the electrical activity occurring in different body organs. A recording of this activity is made on paper or on a screen for viewing. Such examinations include:

— Electrocardiogram (EKG or ECG) to record electrical activity of the cardiac cycle
— Electroencephalogram (EEG) to record electrical activity of the brain

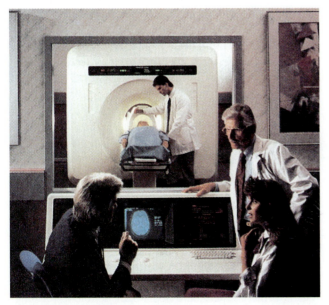

FIGURE 6-8 An MRI provides much detail during scans of portions of the body. *Courtesy of GE Medical Systems*

— Electromyogram (EMG) to record electrical activity of muscles.

Invasive Tests

Some tests and studies actually penetrate body surfaces and thus are known as invasive tests. Examples of invasive tests include taking tissue samples, introducing contrast media, and probing deeply into body cavities.

A sternal puncture is a procedure in which a needle pierces the sternum to draw a sample of blood-producing cells. For some invasive examinations, iodine dyes, barium compounds, or air may be introduced into a body cavity to produce contrast when making recordings and pictures.

Most of these invasive techniques are carried out in special areas, such as laboratories, that are specifically designed for this purpose. Also, patient specimens usually are examined in laboratories.

Some special invasive procedures include:

● Direct visualization procedures—to examine body parts with instruments (scopes) introduced into the body. For example, the proctoscope, inserted in the anus, allows direct observation of the interior rectum. Other direct visualization procedures are:

— Cystoscopy to observe the bladder
— Laryngoscopy to observe the larynx
— Sigmoidoscopy to observe the colon

● Dye studies—dyes are introduced into the body to outline body parts so that they will show up on x-rays. Some examples are:

— Upper GI series (barium swallow)—the patient swallows a barium solution and then x-rays or fluoroscopy show the structures highlighted.
— Lower GI series (barium enema)—the patient is given the barium rectally. The patient holds the solution while x-rays are taken.
— Myelogram—dye is introduced into the spinal canal and then x-rays are taken.

● Cardiac catheterization—a catheter (small sterile tube) is introduced into the vascular system and delivers a dye. As the catheter is moved through the blood vessels and heart chambers, a monitor shows the dye flowing through this system.

Other Techniques

Chemical and microscopic studies examine samples of various body tissues and secretions. Getting some samples requires invasive procedures. Other sampling requires non-invasive procedures. The most common samples are:

● Blood
● Urine
● Sputum from the lungs
● Cultures from infected tissues
● Gastric secretions
● Feces (Figure 6-9)

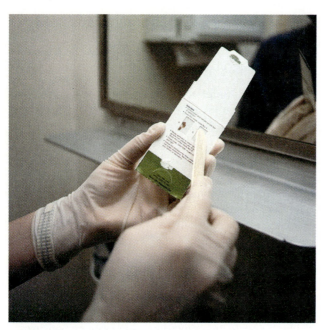

FIGURE 6-9 Stool specimens may be taken and examined for occult (hidden) blood.

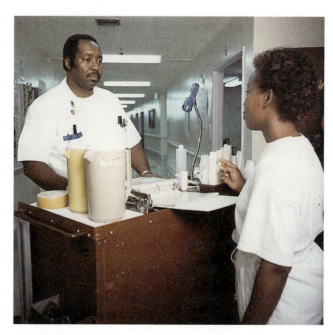

FIGURE 6-11 The nursing assistant reports the patient's complaint of pain to the registered nurse, who will administer the pain reliever ordered by the physician.

THERAPY

Once the medical diagnosis is confirmed, it is possible to predict the course of the disease and a probable prognosis (likely outcome or course of the disease process). Then the most appropriate **therapy** (treatment) is determined.

There are four basic approaches to therapy. They may be used alone or in different combinations.

1. Surgery: This form of therapy may remove unhealthy tissue (Figure 6-10), replace unhealthy parts, or repair injured, malformed, or congenitally defective areas.

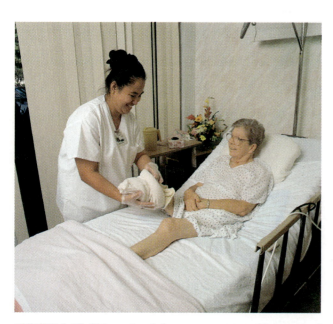

FIGURE 6-10 This patient's leg was amputated because of peripheral vascular disease.

Prostatectomies remove unhealthy prostate glands. Coronary bypasses replace blocked arteries with other arteries. Herniorrhaphies repair weakened muscle walls.

2. Chemotherapy: This form of therapy uses drugs and chemicals to promote and improve body functions and to control pain (Figure 6-11). For example, the patient with a fever is given an antipyretic, such as aspirin, to reduce the temperature.

3. Radiation: This form of therapy uses controlled radioactivity or x-rays to destroy tumor cells.

4. Supportive (palliative) care: This form of therapy is designed to support the patient's body in its attempt to stay healthy or return to health. For example, positioning a person upright makes it easier for him to breathe when he is having an asthmatic attack. Pain control, rest, proper nutrition, fluid intake, and good hygiene all aid the body's own attempt to control the effects of illness.

NEOPLASMS

Tumors can affect almost any organ of the body. In tumors, cells do not follow the normal laws of growth and reproduction and may not stay within the normal boundaries. Excess numbers of cells and abnormal cells crowd out the normal cells and compete with them for nutrients.

Types of Tumors

Different types of tumors are more common among certain groups of people. Children have more tumors of the nervous system, urinary system, and hematopoietic (blood-forming) system. Adults have more tumors of the reproductive organs, lungs, and colon.

The two major types of tumors are classified as benign or malignant. Each type has its own characteristics.

Benign or nonmalignant tumors:

- Usually grow slowly
- Do not spread
- Are usually encapsulated (surrounded by a capsule)
- Do not cause death unless located in a vital area such as the brain
- Are usually named by stating the part of the body involved and adding the suffix -oma. For example, *osteoma* names a benign bone tumor.

Malignant tumors or cancerous growths:

- Grow relatively rapidly
- Spread to other body parts (**metastasize**)
- If untreated, cause death
- May be named sarcoma or carcinoma or have special names like leukemia.
  - **Carcinomas** are spread primarily by way of the lymph system to the lymph nodes. They occur more commonly in people over 40 years of age.
  - **Sarcomas** are spread primarily by way of the bloodstream. They occur more commonly in people under 40 years of age.

Early Detection

Early detection of cancer can often result in a cure. The sooner the cancer is found, the higher the rate of cure. Pain is not usually an early symptom.

Early Signs and Symptoms. Early signs and symptoms of malignancies include:

Change in bowel or bladder habits

A sore that does not heal

Unusual bleeding or discharge

Thickening or lump in breast or elsewhere

Indigestion or difficulty in swallowing

Obvious change in wart or mole

Nagging cough or hoarseness

 Note: The first letters of these early signs and symptoms spell **CAUTION**.

Late Signs and Symptoms. Late signs and symptoms of malignancies include:

Fever of unknown origin

Cachexia or general wasting of the body tissues with loss of weight

Anemia

Pain due to pressure, obstruction, and ischemia

Hormonal irregularities

Inflammations of the skin

BODY DEFENSES

The body has a natural line of defense against disease. These defenses include:

- Unbroken skin and mucous membranes, which act as mechanical barriers
- Mucus, which traps foreign particles, and cilia (small hairlike structures), which propel them out of the body
- The acidity of certain body secretions such as perspiration, saliva, and stomach juices, which slows the growth of microorganisms
- White blood cells, which surround and destroy anything foreign that enters the body
- Inflammation
- The immune response

Inflammation

The process of inflammation, which we often associate with infections such as boils and abscesses, is really an important part of the body's natural defenses. When anything foreign enters the body, small blood vessels (capillaries) in the area get bigger (dilate), bringing more blood to the infected part. In the blood are white blood cells and other protective substances. Fluid (serum) and white blood cells pass through the capillary walls into the area and a wall is gradually built up around the foreign object. As the white blood cells try to destroy the invader, pressure builds up to force the material to the surface of the body. The inflammatory process takes place to some extent in the body whenever injury occurs. The signs and symptoms of acute inflammation are:

- Redness
- Swelling
- Heat
- Loss of function

Immune Response

Immune response (immunity) protects the body against specific infections by producing special chemicals called **antibodies**. For example, a person exposed to the measles virus may become ill with the disease. After recovery, the antibodies formed by the person against the measles virus will protect him from becoming sick again with the same disease.

Vaccines (altered germs or their products) may be given before exposure to a disease. The body can then produce antibodies before actual exposure occurs.

REVIEW

A. Matching.

Match the statements in questions 1–10 with the correct terms in the list a–j.

1. _____ Probable outcome
2. _____ Color of the skin
3. _____ Cause of disease
4. _____ Noncancerous tumor
5. _____ Pain as reported by the patient
6. _____ Illness with sudden onset and short course
7. _____ Injury
8. _____ Inflammation
9. _____ Condition transmitted from one generation to another
10. _____ Cancer

   a. acute
   b. benign
   c. a natural body defense
   d. etiology
   e. genetic
   f. malignancy
   g. prognosis
   h. sign
   i. symptom
   j. trauma

B. Fill-In.

For each of the items in questions 11–15, mark which is a sign and which is a symptom.

11. _____ dry, flushed skin
12. _____ nausea
13. _____ dizziness
14. _____ rapid pulse
15. _____ elevated temperature

C. Matching.

Match the abnormality with its classification by matching Column I with Column II.

Column I

16. _____ abscessed tooth
17. _____ adenosarcoma
18. _____ renal stones
19. _____ thrombosis
20. _____ strep throat
21. _____ frostbite
22. _____ osteoma
23. _____ rheumatoid arthritis
24. _____ spina bifida
25. _____ sickle cell anemia

Column II

a. ischemia
b. congenital
c. infectious
d. inflammation
e. metabolic imbalance
f. trauma
g. neoplasm
h. obstruction

D. True/False.

Mark the following true or false by circling T or F.

26. T F The medical diagnosis is made by the supervising nurse.
27. T F Nursing assistants may be assigned to collect certain specimens.
28. T F Protocols are drugs given in diagnostic testing.
29. T F Proper patient preparation contributes to the success of diagnostic testing.
30. T F Improper patient preparation may cause faulty results.
31. T F Ultrasound is used to give information about a growing fetus.
32. T F Thermography uses radio waves to test the electrical current of tissues.
33. T F An upper GI series is an x-ray of the lower intestinal tract.
34. T F Nursing assistants may be asked to deliver specimens.
35. T F Nursing assistants may contribute to the diagnostic testing process by offering emotional support to the patient.

E. Completion.

Write out the early signs of possible malignancies.

36. C _____
37. A _____
38. U _____
39. T _____
40. I _____
41. O _____
42. N _____

F. Nursing Assistant Challenge.

Read each clinical situation and answer the questions.

43. Your patient is 82 years old, poorly nourished, and has a diagnosis of pneumonia.
   a. Name two factors that might predispose your patient to pneumonia. _____ _____
   b. Will these factors make recovery more or less difficult? _____
   c. How would you classify the illness pneumonia? _____

44. Your patient is six years old and has a broken leg. He also has a condition that he inherited from his parents. This condition makes his bones brittle so they break more easily.

a. What word would you use to describe his inherited condition? _____

b. What term would you use to classify his inability to make strong bones? _____

c. Do you think this kind of injury might occur often? _____

45. Your patient is 45 years old, 40 pounds overweight, and gets little exercise. Her diagnosis is high blood pressure. She is scheduled for an ECG.

a. What factors might contribute to her diagnosis? _____ _____

b. For what conditions is she at risk? _____

c. What information will the ECG provide? _____

Basic Human Needs and Communication

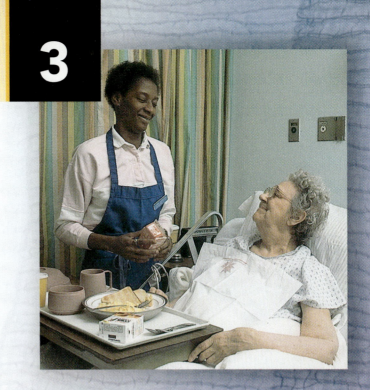

UNIT 7
Communication Skills

UNIT 8
Observation, Reporting, and Documentation

UNIT 9
Meeting Basic Human Needs

UNIT 10
Developing Cultural Sensitivity

Communication Skills

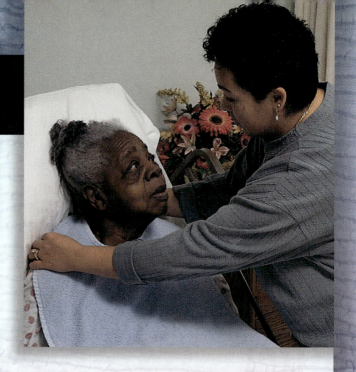

As a result of this unit, you will be able to:

- Spell and define terms.
- Explain the types of verbal and nonverbal communication.
- Describe and demonstrate how to answer the telephone while on duty.
- Describe four tools of communication for staff members.
- Describe the guidelines for communicating with patients with aphasia, impaired hearing, impaired vision, and disorientation.

Learn the meaning and the correct spelling of the following words and phrases:

aphasia	communication	nonverbal	sign language
assignment	disorientation	communication	staff development
body language	ethnic	organizational chart	symbols
braille	medical chart	shift report	verbal communication
care plan	memo		

INTRODUCTION

Communication is a two-way process. It is the way in which information—whether facts or feelings—is shared. For communication to happen, both a "sender" and a "receiver" of the information are needed. Information can be sent orally, in writing, and through body language. Nursing assistants communicate with their patients (Figure 7-1), with visitors, with their coworkers, and with their supervisors when they are working. As a nursing assistant, you will need to receive and send information about your:

- Observations and care of patients
- Interactions with patients and visitors
- Patients' feelings

This information is received and sent through the process of communication.

COMMUNICATION IN HEALTH CARE

Communication between staff members must be effective if the patients are to receive the safest and best care. Communication with your patients and their visitors is also important. You and your patients must understand each other. There are three things needed for successful communication. They are (1) a sender, (2) a clear message, and (3) a receiver.

Verbal Communication

Verbal communication uses words. They may be spoken or written. Written communication may depend upon the use of symbols. Traffic signs are an example of symbols. You will use words to explain to patients what you plan to do in carrying out a procedure and how they can help. Your nurse or team leader will use words to explain your assignment. You will use words to report your observations (Figure 7-2). You will use words to answer visitors' questions. Choose words carefully so that your message is clear. Tone of voice, choice of words, and hand movements give clues to the real meaning of the message. Listen carefully to the message and watch the sender's facial expressions.

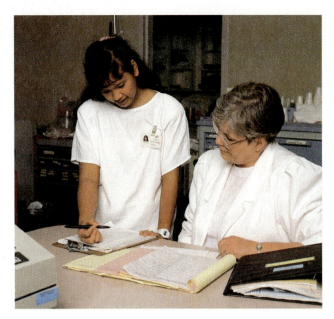

FIGURE 7-2 Verbal communication is used to report your observations.

Nonverbal Communication

Nonverbal communication is a message that is sent through the use of one's body, rather than through speech or writing. This kind of communication, called body language, can tell you a great deal (Figure 7-3). Often nonverbal messages send even stronger signals than verbal messages. A patient who is in pain may protect the affected area. Tears or an unwillingness to make eye contact with you may be a sign of depression. Some of the other ways your patients may "talk" to you through their body language include:

- posture
- hand and body movements
- activity level

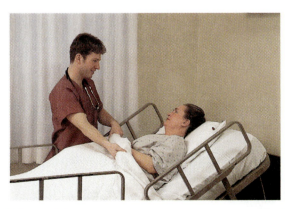

FIGURE 7-1 Nursing assistants communicate with their patients.

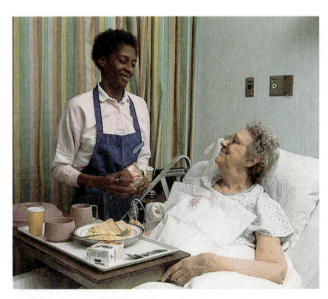

FIGURE 7-3 This patient is expressing positive body language.

- facial expressions
- overall appearance
- body position

COMMUNICATING WITH STAFF MEMBERS

In Unit 2 you learned that health care facilities have a line of authority and communication. The organizational chart is a guide for communication and spells out the line of authority. All facilities have an organizational chart that illustrates how each department relates to other departments. Some of the larger departments, such as nursing, have their own charts that indicate the line of authority within the department (Figure 7-4). As a nursing assistant, you will need to learn methods to communicate with other staff members in nursing and with members of other departments.

Oral Communications

Oral reports are used frequently to communicate information about patients. When you first come on duty, you will listen to the shift report. The nurse who worked the previous shift will report to oncoming staff. This report will include:

- changes in patients' conditions
- information about new patients
- names of patients who were discharged or died
- any incidents that occurred to patients
- new physicians' orders
- special events for the patients that will occur during your shift

Listen carefully to the report because it will help you plan your assignment (Figure 7-5). Your assignment tells you:

- which patients you will care for during your shift

- the procedures you will need to do for these patients

Your supervising nurse will then give you additional information about your assignment based on the shift report. This information may include orders to complete procedures for specific patients:

- take temperature, pulse, and respirations on designated patients
- obtain weights on designated patients
- allow a patient to remain in bed because of a change in condition
- make observations of a patient who has had a recent change of condition

During your shift, you will give oral reports to the nurse about procedures you have completed and observations you have made. At the end of the shift, you will summarize your assignment to the nurse so that the information can be included in the shift report to the employees coming on duty after you. When you leave the nursing unit for any reason during your shift, always report to the nurse before you go. Unit 8 gives additional information about oral reports.

Answering the Telephone

Many telephone calls come into a health care facility. Families call to inquire about the condition of a loved one. Physicians call frequently to leave new medical orders. The laboratory may call to give test results. Remember that nursing assistants are not allowed to take physicians' orders, to take results of diagnostic tests, or to give information to families. You must call the nurse to do this. If you answer the telephone:

- Identify the nursing unit: "third floor, north" for example.
- Identify yourself and your position: "Mary Smith, nursing assistant."
- Ask the caller's name and ask the caller to wait while you locate the person called.
- If the person is unavailable, take a message (Figure 7-6) and write down the following information:
  - date and time of call
  - caller's name and telephone number
  - message left by caller
  - whether the person is to return the call or whether the caller will telephone again later
  - your signature

Some facilities have more complex telephone systems. You will be taught how to transfer calls or to voice-page. Most facilities do not allow employees to make or receive personal telephone calls while they are on duty.

Written Communications Among Staff Members

In many situations, you and other staff members must rely on written communications. The ability to accurately read the communication is essential to the care of the patient.

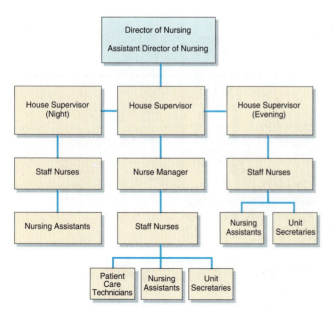

FIGURE 7-4 Organizational chart for nursing department.

CNA ASSIGNMENT SHEET DATE 4-18-XX

Rm.	Resident	Bath	Pos. Sched.	ROM	V.S.	WT.	B+B	ADL Prog.	Transfer	Safety
101^A	J. Damski	X	X	X			X	X	2+TB	X
101^B	G. Jones		X	X	X	X			Mech Lift	
102^A	C. Hernandez	X				X			Indep.	
102^B	R. Lattini	X	X	X			X		2+ TB	X
103	N. Goldberg	X			X	X	X		SBA	
104^A	M. Welch		X	X					Mech Lift	
104^B	L. Ordoni		X	X			X	X	1+TB	X
105	B. Brinzoski	X			X		X		Indep.	
106^A	A. Feinstein	X				X		X	1+TB	
106^B	D. Farmell		X	X	X		X	X	2+TB	
107	T. Green	X	X	X		X	X		2+TB	
108^A	H. Johnson	X	X	X	X			X	2+TB	
108^B	B. Miller		X	X		X			1+TB	X

FIGURE 7-5 The assignment sheet tells you what you need to do for your patients.

To J. Sampson ☐ URGENT

Date 4-29-XX Time 6:10 (A.M.) P.M.

WHILE YOU WERE OUT

From Dr. Olegna

Of Hillside Medical Center

Phone 123 555 1212

Area Code Number Ext.

Telephoned	X	Please call	
Came to see you		Wants to see you	
Returned your call		Will call again	

Message Call before noon-re: laboratory tests for Donelda Dirickson

Signed R. Samenetti, CNA

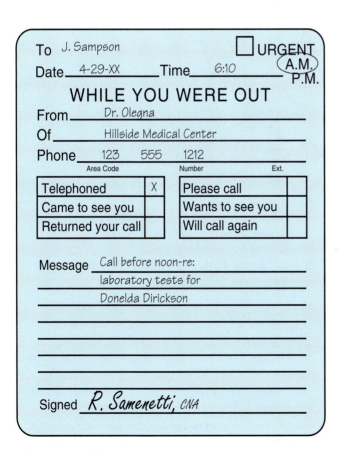

FIGURE 7-6 Telephone message

Memos

A **memo** (Figure 7-7) is a brief communication that informs or reminds employees of:

- changes in policies or procedures
- upcoming meetings or staff development programs

MEMO

Date: April 21, XXXX
From: Jane Sowalski, RN Director of Nursing
To: All nursing staff

Please note that the Nursing Procedure Manual has been updated and revised. The list of changes is attached. Please read the indicated procedures and sign the attached page.

Thank you.

FIGURE 7-7 Memos provide brief, important information.

- admission of new patients
- promotions of staff members

Be sure you know where memos are posted so that you will be aware of the facility activities.

Manuals

All facilities have several manuals that provide information about policies and procedures (Figure 7-8). These may include:

- Employee Personnel Handbook—Describes all personnel policies and benefits.
- Safety and Disaster Manual—Gives directions for actions to take in case of fire or other disasters.
- Procedure Manual—Gives directions on how all procedures should be performed for patients.
- Nursing Policy Manual—Describes rules and regulations pertaining to the care of the patients.

There may be other manuals for Infection Control and Quality Assurance. You are not expected to memorize all the information in these manuals, but you should know where they are kept on the nursing unit and be able to look up information when you need to.

Staff Development

Staff development is a process used to educate staff from all departments in the facility (Figure 7-9). Classes may be given to inform staff of:

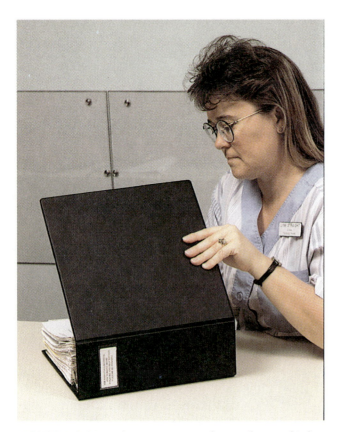

FIGURE 7-8 Manuals are a source of many forms of information.

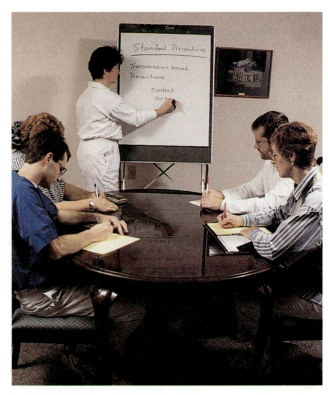

FIGURE 7-9 Nursing assistants need to participate in regular staff development.

- new rules and regulations
- new procedures
- recent health findings from research
- how to use new equipment

The Patient Care Plan

Each patient has a **care plan** that has been developed by the interdisciplinary health care team. Unit 8 presents more information on the patient care plan.

The Patient's Medical Chart

Each patient has a **medical chart** or record. The medical chart contains:

- the physician's medical orders for that patient: medications, treatments, diagnostic tests
- the medical history of the patient: summary of all past illnesses and surgeries
- results of physical examinations
- results of all diagnostic tests: blood tests and x-rays
- progress notes from the physician and from all disciplines involved in the patient's care: brief, periodic descriptions of the patient's condition and response to treatment
- assessments from all disciplines: the assessment identifies the patient's problems
- nursing notes: information that describes the patient's condition, nursing care that has been given, and the patient's response to the care

The information entered into the chart is called *documentation*. The chart is a legal document. It may be used to:

- determine payments by insurance companies
- determine settlement of lawsuits

Unit 8 gives instructions for documenting (making notations) on the patient's chart.

Other Methods of Communication

Modern technology has increased opportunities for communication. You will see computers at the nurses' station and throughout the building. Computers have many uses within health care facilities. They are used for:

- Writing letters, memos, policies, and procedures. Performing these tasks is called *word processing*.
- Compiling databases. A *database* may be developed for every patient and every employee within the facility. The database contains information such as name, address, telephone numbers, and social security number. The database allows the storage, retrieval, and manipulation of large amounts of information and simplifies procedures such as maintaining patient and personnel records.
- Doing mathematical calculations, which are performed with *spreadsheet programs*. These programs are used for budgeting and financial analysis.
- Communicating, using programs that allow computers to "talk" to each other over telephone lines, using special equipment called *modems*. Persons using this feature may be able to communicate with other computers within the facility or anywhere in the world. Messages can be sent via electronic mail (e-mail), equipment and supplies can be ordered, and information can be retrieved on just about any topic.

Most facilities will have at least one desktop computer in each department. In the nursing department, computers are used to document patient care, to maintain databases, to communicate with physicians' offices, and to maintain records of supplies and equipment. Some facilities have computers in every patient room. Nursing staff can then document appropriate information before they leave the bedside.

If you will be expected to use a computer and have had very little experience doing so, remember:

- Do not be intimidated by the computer. You have the ability to learn how to use one. You do not have to be a computer expert to use a computer.
- Learn from classes, from manuals, and from other users. Be creative and try to figure out some things on your own.
- Be patient, be determined, and don't panic. Do not be afraid to ask questions. You will not learn everything right away, but your confidence will grow by leaps and bounds as you master new tasks.

You will be given special training if you will be expected to use a computer (Figure 7-10).

Fax machines are common in health care facilities (Figure 7-11). They are used to send and receive information from physicians and laboratories.

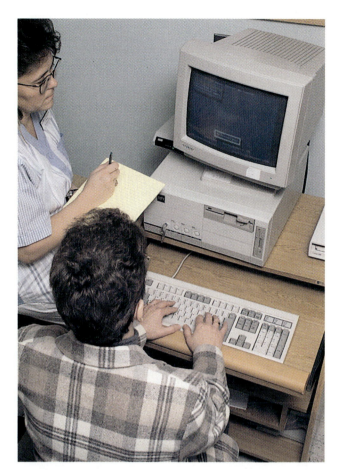

FIGURE 7-10 The use of computers in health care is increasing.

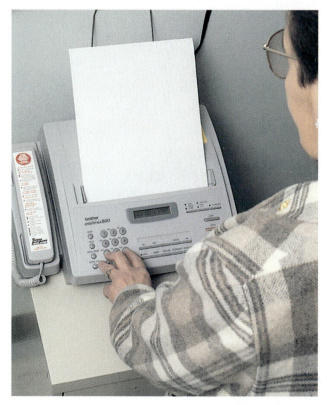

FIGURE 7-11 Fax machines are used throughout the health care facility.

GUIDELINES *for*

Communicating with Patients

1. Be sure you have the patient's attention.
2. Use nonthreatening words and gestures.
3. Speak clearly and courteously.
4. Use a pleasant tone of voice.
5. Use appropriate body language.
6. Be alert to the patient's needs to communicate with you—allow time for the patient to talk and respond. Show interest and concern (Figure 7-12).
7. Do not speak about the patient in front of the patient or other patients.
8. Do not interrupt the patient.
9. Reflect the patient's feelings and thoughts by rewording his or her statements into questions.
10. Ask for clarification if you are unsure of what the patient is saying.
11. Give the patient only factual information—not your personal feelings, opinions, or beliefs.
12. Information concerning the patient's condition, medications, and treatments should be given by the physician or nurse.
13. Do not argue with patients.

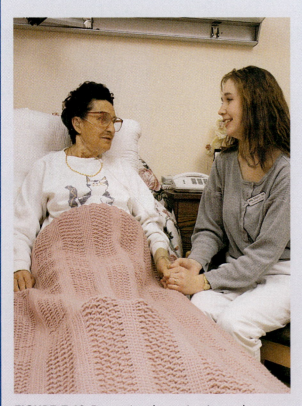

FIGURE 7-12 Recognize the patient's need to communicate with you.

COMMUNICATING WITH PATIENTS

The skill of communicating with patients will develop with experience. It is not always the words we choose that are important, but the way in which we say them. Tone of voice, facial expression, and even the way you touch a patient all communicate a sense of honest caring to the patient. Looking directly at the patient as you speak and addressing him or her respectfully by name are also indications of caring.

Listening actively is a special skill requiring more than just being physically present. When you listen actively, all of your attention is focused on the speaker. You maintain eye contact and do not interrupt while the other person is speaking. You ask questions that encourage the speaker to continue and respond to specific questions being asked. Follow these guidelines to communicate effectively with patients.

Communicating with Patients with Special Needs

There are many reasons why communication with patients may be impaired. The patient may:

- be hearing impaired
- be vision impaired
- have aphasia
- be disoriented
- be from a culture different than the nursing assistant's

These patients have special communication needs that should be addressed on the care plan. Always check the care plan before attempting to communicate with a patient with special communication needs. Specific approaches may be established for all staff members to use with the patient. Lack of consistency in the use of these approaches is confusing and frustrating to the patient.

Communicating with Hearing-Impaired Patients

1. Get the patient's attention first.
   - Make sure the patient sees you.
   - Touch the patient lightly to indicate that you wish to speak.
2. If the patient uses a hearing aid, be sure the patient is wearing it and that the hearing aid is on.
3. If the patient has a "good" ear, stand or sit on that side.
4. Don't chew gum, eat, or cover your mouth while talking.
5. Keep the light behind the patient, so your face can be clearly seen (Figure 7-13).
6. Face the patient; many hearing-impaired people can read lips or interpret your facial expressions.
7. Reduce outside distractions. Speak in a quiet, calm manner.

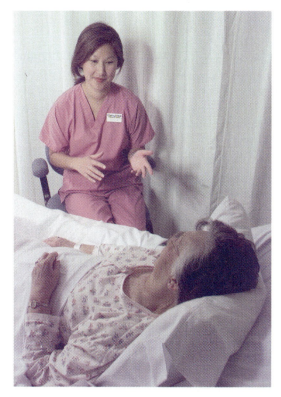

FIGURE 7-13 The light source should be behind the patient if she is hearing-impaired.

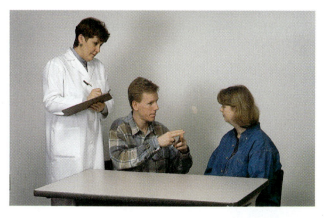

FIGURE 7-14 Communicating with sign language requires special skill and training.

8. Start conversations with a key word or phrase so the patient has some clues as to what you are saying (context).

9. Keep your voice pitch low.

10. Speak slowly, distinctly, and naturally.

11. Form words carefully, use familiar words, and keep sentences short.

12. Rephrase words as needed.

13. Avoid shouting, mouthing, or exaggerating words, or speaking very slowly. This only makes it harder for the patient to understand you.

14. Use facial expressions, gestures, and body language to help express your meanings.

15. Some hearing-impaired patients use **sign language**.
    — Signing depends upon hand and finger movements and facial expressions.
    — This is a skill that requires learning and practice (Figure 7-14).
    — There are different forms of sign language, just as there are different spoken languages.
    — There are some basic signs that may be helpful (Figure 7-15).

16. Patients who have been hearing impaired for several years may have speech that is difficult to understand.

17. Some hearing-impaired people are embarrassed to tell you when they do not understand you.

18. People who cannot hear may appear confused when they are not.

Communicating with Visually Impaired Patients

Visually impaired patients may have problems communicating because they are unable to see the sender or the sender's facial expressions and body language.

1. When approaching a visually impaired person, address the person by name and then touch lightly on the hand or arm to avoid startling.

2. After you speak to the patient, identify yourself and explain why you are there. "Hello, Mr. Smith. My

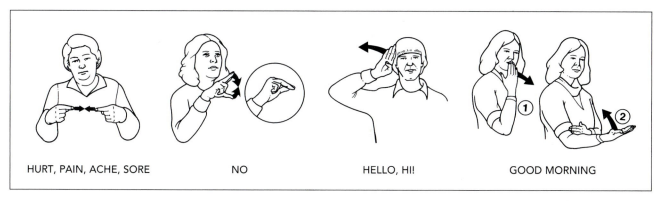

HURT, PAIN, ACHE, SORE   NO   HELLO, HI!   GOOD MORNING

FIGURE 7-15 Basic signs: Hurt, pain, ache, sore; No (repeat movement); Hello, Hi!; Good morning

name is Mary Jones and I would like to take your blood pressure."

3. Be specific when giving directions. "I am putting your call light on the right side of your bed".

4. When giving directions as to how to find an area in the building, tell the patient how many doors he or she will pass and when to turn right or left.

5. When you leave the patient, make sure you announce your departure. "I am leaving your room now. Can I get you anything else?"

6. Offer to read mail to visually impaired patients.

7. If the patient has a telephone, make sure he or she can use it. The patient can count the numbers on the dial to make calls.

8. Tactfully inform a visually impaired person if clothing is soiled, mismatched, or in need of repair.

9. Encourage the patient to listen to the radio or television to keep up with news and current events.

10. Make sure the patient is aware of talking book machines. Inform Social Services if the patient wishes to use one.

11. Describe the environment and objects around the patient so a frame of reference is established. This helps avoid disorientation related to vision impairment. Never change location of items or furniture without discussing it with the patient.

12. Some patients may read braille, a system that uses a series of raised dots to represent letters and words (Figure 7-16). The patient reads the letters and words by moving his or her fingertips over them.

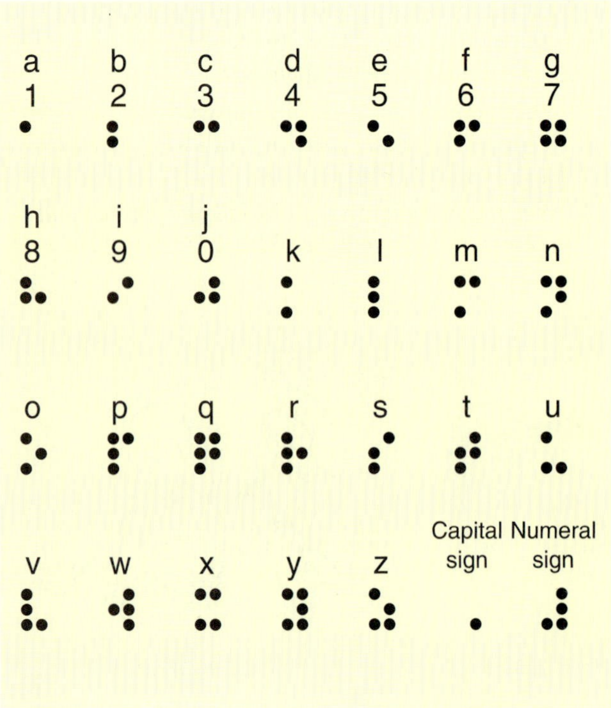

Communicating with Patients with Aphasia

Patients who have had a stroke or brain damage due to an injury may have aphasia. Aphasia means that the patient cannot understand spoken or written language, or cannot express spoken or written language, or both. Trying to communicate with patients with aphasia can be frustrating to both the patient and the caregiver.

1. Face the patient and make eye contact before speaking.

2. Say the patient's name and give a social greeting before asking questions or giving instructions.

3. Speak slowly and clearly. Use short, complete sentences.

4. Pause between sentences to allow the patient time to comprehend and interpret what you said.

5. Check the patient's comprehension before you proceed. Ask a question based on information you just gave the patient.

6. Use nonverbal cues to augment spoken communication. Use gestures, facial expressions, or pictures.

7. Ask questions that require only short responses or ones that can be answered nonverbally.

8. Repeat what the patient just said to help him or her keep focused on the conversation.

9. Find out if the speech therapist has devised methods of nonverbal communication, such as communication boards or picture books (Figure 7-17).

FIGURE 7-16 Many visually impaired persons use braille.

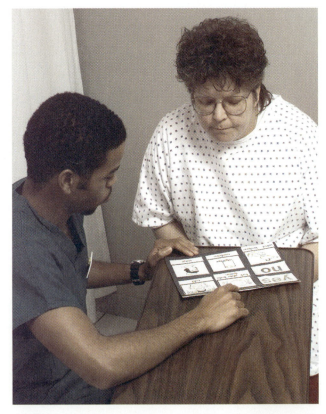

FIGURE 7-17 Communication boards or picture books may be used to communicate with patients with aphasia.

10. Do not avoid talking to a person with aphasia. Do not shout to try to make him understand.

11. If you sense frustration, let patient know that you are aware of the frustration. Suggest that you talk about something else for a while and then try again.

Communicating with Disoriented Patients

Some patients you care for may be disoriented. **Disorientation** means that the patient is confused about time, place (his physical location), or person (who he is). Disorientation can occur with Alzheimer's disease, stroke, or other disorders or injuries of the brain.

1. Begin conversation by identifying yourself and calling the patient by name. Do not ask the patient if he remembers you or if he knows who you are.

2. Talk to the patient at eye level and maintain eye contact.

3. Maintain a pleasant facial expression while you are talking and listening.

4. Place a hand on the patient's arm or hand, unless this causes agitation (Figure 7-18).

5. Make sure the patient can hear you. Avoid distractions of noise and activity.

6. Use a lower tone of voice.

7. Use short, common words and short, simple sentences.

8. Give the patient time to respond.

9. Ask only one simple question at a time. If you must repeat it, say it exactly the same.

10. Ask the patient to do only one task at a time.

11. Patients with dementia will eventually be unable to comprehend verbal communication.
    — Use pictures, and point, touch, or hand her things.
    — Demonstrate an action when you want her to complete a task.

12. The patient may use word substitutes. If these are consistent, find out what they mean. Use them yourself to see if the patient understands you better.

13. Avoid abstract, common expressions. For example, "You can hop into bed now" means just that to the patient.

14. Repeat the patient's last words to help him stay on track during conversation.

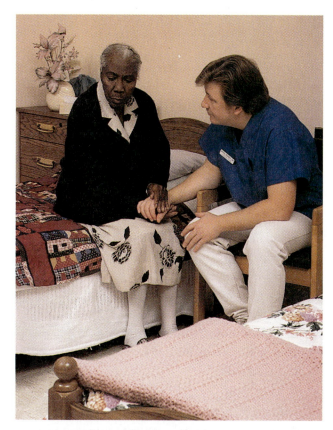

FIGURE 7-18 Placing a hand on the patient's arm or hand may be comforting to the patient.

15. Do not try to "make" the patient understand. Avoid lengthy explanations and excessive verbal communication. This tends to agitate most people with dementia.

16. Use nonverbal praise freely and always respect the patient's feelings.

Communicating with Patients of a Different Culture

The persons you care for may come from many different cultures or have different **ethnic** backgrounds. This means people who come from other countries and who have different customs, languages, and traditions. For example, in some countries it is considered a sign of disrespect to maintain eye contact when speaking with another person. If you are assigned to someone from a different ethnic background, you should be given specific communication guidelines.

REVIEW

A. Multiple Choice.

Select the one best answer for each question.

1. Successful communication requires a
   a. sender.
   b. message.
   c. receiver.
   d. all of these.

2. Verbal communication includes
   a. talking and listening.
   b. facial expressions.
   c. writing reports.
   d. using a fax machine.

3. Verbal communication is influenced by
   a. tone of voice.
   b. choice of words that are used.
   c. articulation.
   d. all of these.

4. Examples of nonverbal communication include
   a. reading and using the patient's care plan.
   b. answering the telephone.
   c. listening to shift report.
   d. conversing with patients.

5. A nursing assistant may give or take which information over the telephone?
   a. Report of a patient's condition
   b. Physician's orders
   c. Results of laboratory tests
   d. Name of person leaving the message

6. The shift report is given by the
   a. administrator.
   b. physician.
   c. nurse who worked the previous shift.
   d. director of nursing.

7. The purpose of the shift report is to
   a. give information about all the patients on the nursing unit.
   b. discuss the social activities of the staff.
   c. tell the nursing assistants when they are scheduled for days off.
   d. rest before starting work.

8. You must report to the nurse when you
   a. take a break or go to lunch.
   b. leave the nursing unit for any reason.
   c. have finished your shift.
   d. all of these.

9. One purpose of a memo is to inform staff of
   a. meetings or educational programs.
   b. patients' conditions.
   c. new physician's orders for specific patients.
   d. weather conditions.

10. Examples of manuals that are found on nursing units include
    a. procedure manual.
    b. disaster manual.
    c. infection control manual.
    d. all of these.

11. The patient's care plan provides information for
    a. the nursing assistant assignments.
    b. employee benefits.
    c. the procedure for fire drills.
    d. all of these.

12. The patient's medical record or chart is
    a. used only by the physician.
    b. used by all members of the interdisciplinary health care team.
    c. a temporary record.
    d. a report of the nursing assistant's competencies.

13. You may receive messages from the patient's
    a. body language.
    b. verbal statements.
    c. facial expressions.
    d. all of these.

14. If a patient is disoriented, it means that the patient is
    a. mentally ill.
    b. unaware of the environment and the time.
    c. unable to communicate with you.
    d. unable to hear.

15. Aphasia means that the patient
    a. has an infection of the respiratory tract.
    b. is hearing-impaired.
    c. is disoriented.
    d. is unable to speak or to understand the spoken language of others.

16. When working with hearing-impaired patients, you should
    a. speak in a calm, quiet manner.
    b. talk louder.
    c. avoid speaking if possible.
    d. speak very slowly.

17. When working with patients with aphasia, it is best to
    a. use only hand gestures to communicate.
    b. speak louder.

c. avoid communication if at all possible.

d. face the patient and make eye contact before speaking.

18. Patients who are visually impaired should

a. stay in their rooms to avoid getting lost in the facility.

b. have identification on their clothing so everyone realizes they are visually impaired.

c. learn to use sign language.

d. be given directions for locating various areas in the building.

19. When working with disoriented patients, you should

a. ask the patient if he or she remembers you or knows who you are.

b. try to make the patient understand you.

c. avoid distractions of noise and activity when communicating with them.

d. get as close as possible to the patient when talking or giving care.

20. Touching the patient can be a successful method of communication if you

a. are gentle and caring.

b. use appropriate gestures, facial expressions, and eye contact.

c. hold the patient's hand.

d. all of these.

B. Completion.

Choose the correct word from the following list to complete each statement in questions 21–30.

aphasia	medical chart
body language	memo
braille	nonverbal communication
care plan	shift report
disorientation	verbal communication

21. Persons who cannot express themselves verbally or understand verbal communication have _____.

22. Loss of recognition of time, place, location, or person is called _____.

23. The exchange of information given by the nurse going off duty to those coming on duty is called the _____.

24. The _____ is a legal document.

25. A brief, written message that provides information is a _____.

26. _____ is an example of nonverbal communication.

27. The record that contains a description of the patient's problems, the goals for resolving the problems, and the approaches used is the _____.

28. Sign language is an example of _____

29. Talking orally is _____

30. _____ is used by persons who are visually impaired.

C. Nursing Assistant Challenge.

Miss Johnson is one of your patients. She is in the hospital because she has a heart problem and is visually impaired. Miss Johnson can feed herself and can give her own bath, brush her teeth, and comb her own hair if she has adequate assistance. Think about suggestions presented in this unit for communicating with visually impaired persons.

31. What can you do to set up meal trays so that Miss Johnson can feed herself?

32. How can you prepare bath items so she can give herself her bath?

33. What can you do to enable her to comb her own hair and brush her teeth?

34. What other actions can you take to help this patient maintain as much independence as possible?

Observation, Reporting, and Documentation

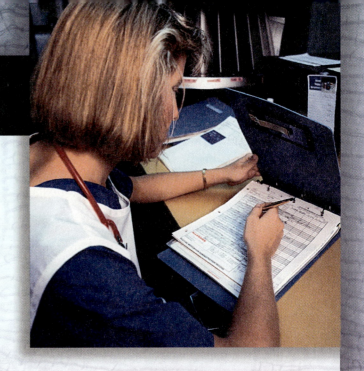

As a result of this unit, you will be able to:

- Spell and define terms.
- List the four components of the nursing process.
- Explain the responsibilities of the nursing assistant for each component of the nursing process.
- Describe two observations to make for each body system.
- Describe the purpose of the care plan.
- List three times when oral reports are given.
- Describe the information given when reporting.
- Describe the purpose of the patient's medical record.
- Explain the rules for documentation.

Learn the meaning and the correct spelling of the following words and phrases:

approaches	evaluation	Kardex	observation
assessment	flow sheet	nurse's notes	oral report
care plan conference	goal	nursing diagnosis	planning
charting	implementation	nursing process	subjective observation
document	intervention	objective observation	

INTRODUCTION

One of the responsibilities of the nursing assistant is to collect and communicate information about the patients. Information is collected by making observations of the patient. Information is communicated to other team members by reporting and documenting. The mechanism used to carry out these actions is called the **nursing process**.

NURSING PROCESS

The registered nurse is responsible for achieving patient focused care by using the nursing process. The nurse delegates responsibilities to other caregivers and coordinates the care in an effort to achieve this goal. The nursing process consists of four steps:

- Assessment
- Planning
- Implementation
- Evaluation

Assessment involves the collection of data (information) about the patient. The nurse coordinates assessment with other members of the interdisciplinary team. The data is entered on a special form contained in the patient's medical record (Figure 8-1). Information is obtained from:

- interviewing the patient
- the medical record
- the patient's family if the patient is unable to communicate
- physical examination (Figure 8-2)

The nursing assistant is responsible for collection of data by making and reporting observations. This is explained later in the unit. After the assessment is finished, the nurse analyzes the data, identifies the patient's problems, and formulates nursing diagnoses. A **nursing diagnosis** is the statement of a patient problem and the cause of the problem. For example, the nursing diagnosis may be impaired physical mobility (the problem) related to hemiplegia due to stroke (the cause of the problem). Table 8-1 gives a few examples of nursing diagnoses and what they mean.

Planning the care of the patient (developing a care plan) is done after the nursing diagnoses are made. The purpose of planning is to:

- identify possible solutions to the problems (nursing diagnoses).
- develop **approaches** (what team members are going to do) that will help the patient solve the problems. Approaches may also be called **interventions**.
- establish **goals** for the patient (a goal is an outcome) so that caregivers will know whether the approaches are successful and whether the problems are being resolved.

Planning may be done at a **care plan conference** (Figure 8-3). This is a meeting of the members of the interdisciplinary team who are directly involved with the care of the patient. The patient and/or the family (if the patient con-

sents) should be invited to attend the conference. The care plan developed at the conference contains a list of the nursing diagnoses, the approaches, and the patient's goals (Figure 8-4). The care plan may be kept in the patient's medical record or in a file called a **Kardex** (Figure 8-5) at the nurses' station. The nursing assistant is responsible for contributing information (observations) that will help the team develop a workable care plan. Some facilities invite nursing assistants to attend the care plan conference.

Implementation is the activation of the care plan. It means carrying out the approaches listed on the care plan in an effort to resolve the problems (nursing diagnoses) and to help the patient reach the goals (Figure 8-6). The approach states:

- who is going to carry out the approach
- when the approach is carried out
- how the approach is carried out

See Figure 8-4 for examples of approaches. The nursing assistant is responsible for knowing when and how the approach is to be carried out and for implementing the approach correctly.

Evaluation is the final step of the nursing process, but it is an ongoing procedure. The evaluation determines:

- whether the patient is reaching the goals on the care plan
- why the goals are not being reached, if the patient is not successful in obtaining the goals
- what should be done to assist the patient to reach the goals
- when goals are reached, they may be extended; for example if the patient reaches the goal of walking 200 feet, it may be increased to 250 feet

The nursing assistant is responsible for reporting to the nurse when the:

- approach cannot be carried out for any reason
- patient is having problems with the approach

MAKING OBSERVATIONS

An **observation** is information that is obtained by using one's senses: seeing, hearing, smelling, or feeling. This information can help the care team determine:

- A change in the patient's physical condition. *Example:* a patient with diabetes may be having an insulin reaction.
- A new condition that is developing. *Example:* a pressure ulcer may be noted.
- A change in the patient's mental condition. *Example:* a patient who has shown no signs of disorientation is now wandering about, saying he does not know where he is.
- A change in the patient's emotional condition. *Example:* a patient is crying and says she "does not want to continue living."
- The effectiveness of a medication or treatment. *Example:* a patient may be taking an antibiotic for a urinary tract infection. If the signs and symptoms of the infection are not going away, then the medication may not

NURSING ASSESSMENT   Patient Label
Instructions: Check mark indicates YES, no check mark indicates NO.
                Check ONLY appropriate box, unless otherwise indicated.

Informant: Family _____ Patient _____ Other _____

SECTION I   NEUROLOGICAL / COGNITIVE

#1 Oriented to
___ Person
___ Place
___ Time
___ None of the above

#2 Level of Consciousness
___ Alert ___ Lethargic
___ Responds appropriately
___ Unresponsive
___ Comatose

#3 Communication
___ Aphasic
___ Can read
___ Can write
___ Speaks clearly
___ Uses gestures
___ Attention span deficit
___ Hemianopsia

#4 Memory / Recall
___ Short term
___ Long term
___ Follows directions

#5 Eyes / Vision
___ Vision deficit
___ Macular degeneration
___ Glaucoma
___ Cataracts
___ Glasses
___ Contact lenses
___ Other
Pupil Reaction
          Right   Left
Brisk   ____ ____
Slow   ____ ____
None   ____ ____
___ Pupils equal round
___ Inflamed
___ Eye conditions (explain)
___ Cloudy iris
___ Date of last eye exam

#6 Hearing
___ Hearing deficit
___ Hearing aid: R ___ L ___
___ Ear drainage: R ___ L ___
___ Wax: R ___ L ___
___ Date of last hearing exam

#7 Behavior
___ Combative
___ Anxious
___ Depressed (Dx or Sx)
___ Angry
___ Insomnia
___ Alcohol use
___ Hx drug habits
___ Hx poor health maintenance / poor hygiene

#8 Miscellaneous
___ Headache
___ Numbness
___ Tingling
___ Tremors
___ Dizziness
___ Ear(s) ringing
___ Asymptomatic
Explain if checks:
_____
_____
_____

Comments:

SECTION II   INTEGUMENTARY / WOUND

#1 Appearance
___ Pale   ___ Normal
___ Flushed   ___ Good skin turgor
___ Mottled   ___ Tenting present
___ Cyanotic   ___ Other
___ Jaundiced

#2 Temperature
Lower extremities:
___ Hot ___ Warm ___ Cold
Upper extremities:
___ Hot ___ Warm ___ Cold

#3 Pain
___ Yes ___ No
 * If YES complete pain assessment form
Pain meds ordered ___ Yes ___ No

** Complete Pressure Ulcer Risk Assessment
** Complete Wound Assessment (if applicable)

Comments:

SECTION III   CIRCULATORY

#1 Vitals
Pulse
P – Palpable
N – Nonpalpable
Radial R ___ L ___
Pedal R ___ L ___
Radial pulse (record)
_____ Right _____ Left
Blood Pressure (Record)
_____ Right _____ Left
Temperature (Record) _____
Respirations (Record) _____

#2 Cardiac Rhythm
___ Regular ___ Irregular
___ Strong ___ Weak
___ Palpatations

#3 Edema (Use Key)
___ Right Upper Extremity
___ Left Upper Extremity
___ Right Lower Extremity
___ Left Lower Extremity
___ Sacral
___ Ascites

#4 History of:
___ Chest pain
___ Syncope
___ Epitaxis

___ Pacemaker

KEY: 0 = Absent   2+ = Mild (< 1/2")   4+ = Severe (> 1")
        1+ = Slight (< 1/4")   3+ = Moderate (1/2" – 1")

Comments:

SECTION IV   RESPIRATORY

#1 Breath Sounds
___ Clear all lobes R ___ L ___
___ Wheeze R ___ L ___
___ Crackles R ___ L ___
___ Diminished R ___ L ___
___ Equal bilaterally R ___ L ___
___ Abnormal R ___ L ___

#2 Breathing effort:
___ Easy
___ Labored
___ Uses accessory muscles

#3 Cough
___ Nonproductive
___ Productive (explain)
_____

#4 History of:
___ Dyspnea
___ On exertion
___ Without exertion
___ Orthopnea
___ Smoking ___ # packs / day
___ Chews (explain)
_____

#5 Miscellaneous
___ Trach
___ Oxygen Rx
___ Nebulizer
___ Respiratory therapy

Comments:

FIGURE 8-1 The assessment form is used to document the data collected about the patient.

SECTION V ELIMINATION GASTROINTESTINAL

#1 Mouth
___ Normal ___ Abnormal
Glands
___ Normal ___ Abnormal
___ Own teeth
___ Broken teeth
___ Dentures
Upper ___ Full ___ Partial
Lower ___ Full ___ Partial

Comments:

#2 Bowels _____
___ Bowel sounds present
___ Colostomy
___ Hemorrhoids
___ Rectal bleeding
___ Rectal prolapse
___ Hernia
___ Continent
___ Incontinent ___ Total ___ Occasional
___ Smears
___ Diarrhea
___ Constipated

#3 Bowel Program
___ Maintenance
___ Training
___ Uses incontinent garments
___ Dri–pride
___ Dri–pride pad
___ Other
___ Ostomy (type)

#4 Miscellaneous
___ Laxative / Freq _____
___ Suppository / Freq _____
___ Enema / Freq _____
___ Abdominal distension
___ Abdomen soft
___ Abdomen hard
___ Abdominal tenderness
___ G–tube
___ N / G tube
___ Other (explain)
_____

SECTION VI URINARY

#1 Urine Appearance
___ Clear ___ Cloudy
___ Yellow
___ Amber
___ Hematuria

Comments:

#2 Symptoms
___ Frequency
___ Burning
___ Urgency
___ Dribbling
___ Nocturia
___ Hx UTI

#3 Elimination
___ Continent
___ Incontinent
Night
___ Occasional
___ Total
Day
___ Occasional
___ Total
Evening
___ Occasional
___ Total
___ Cath / size _____
___ Ostomy / type _____

#4 Bladder Program
___ Maintenance
___ Training
___ Uses incontinent garment
___ Dri–pride
___ Dri–pride pad
___ Other

SECTION VII REPRODUCTIVE

#1 Male (Genitalia)
___ Urethral discharge / drainage
___ Swelling
___ Abnormalities

Prosthesis: _____

Comments:

#2 Female (Breast)
___ Discharge / drainage
___ Breast masses
___ Nipples
___ Mastectomy
R ___ L ___
___ Menopausal
___ Menses

#3 Female (Genitalia)
___ Itching
___ Redness
___ Abnormal bleeding
___ Discharge / drainage
___ Atrophy
___ Prolapse
___ None

SECTION VIII MUSCULOSKELETAL

Indicate: RUE, LUE, BUE, RLE, LLE, BLE
___ Joint stiffness
___ Swelling
___ Tremors
___ Contractures
___ Amputation
___ Internal rotation
___ External rotation
___ Shortening
___ Asymptomatic
Comments:

Miscellaneous
___ Quadriplegia
___ Hemiplegia
___ Paraplegia
___ Hand grasps equal
___ Hand grasps unequal
___ Weakness R ___ L ___
___ Generalized left sided weakness
___ Generalized right sided weakness

Signature & Date

_____
_____
_____
_____
_____

Signature & Date

_____
_____
_____
_____
_____

FIGURE 8-1 *continued*

BODY CHECK

Complete Upon Admission / Significant Change of Condition / Per Policy

Height _____

Weight _____

Allergies: _____

_____

_____

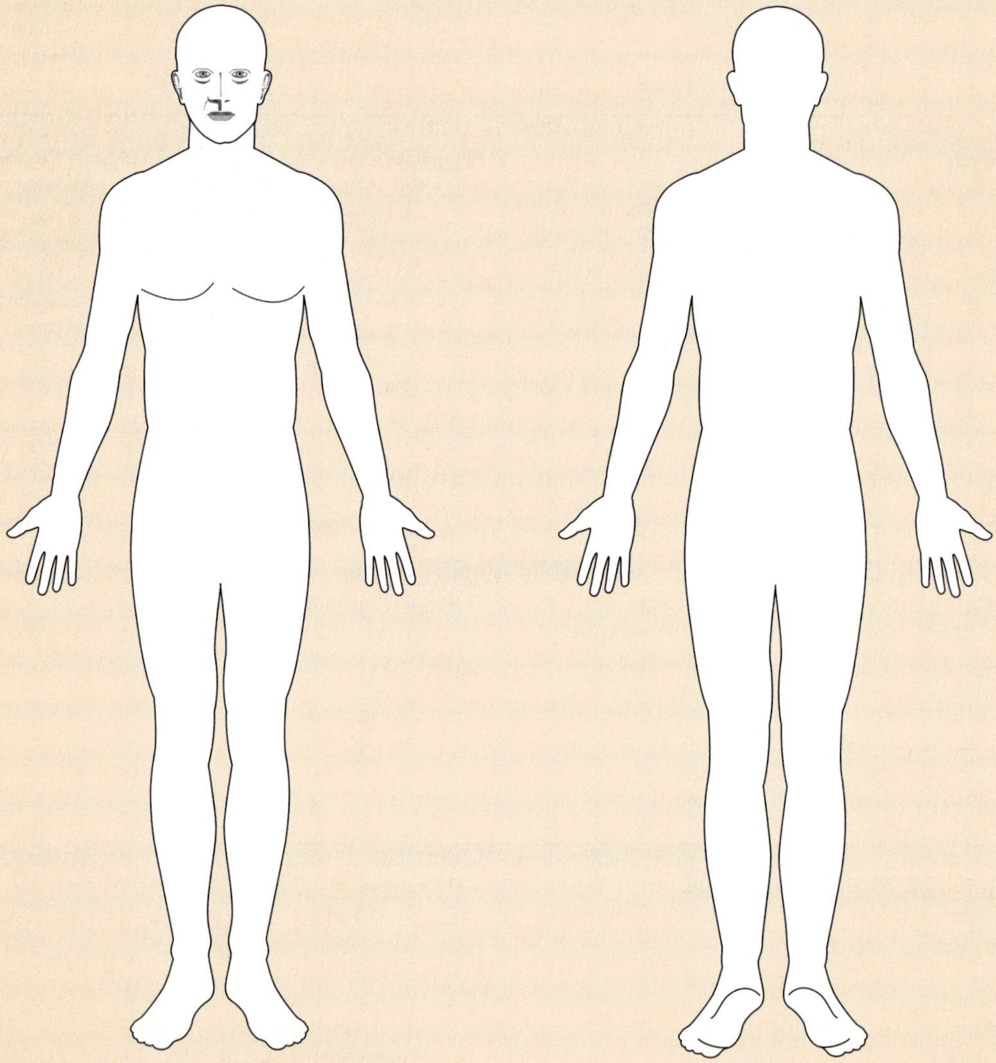

Initial body check completed by: _____   Date: _____

Note on body check:

Scars	**Feet / Ankles**
Moles	Corns
Petechiae	Callouses
Incision (s) (suture line)	Bunions
Bruises	Other
Rash	If yes or if diabetic, complete foot assessment
Skin tear (s)	
Pressure ulcer (s)	
Stasis ulcer (s)	
Surgical site (s)	
Surgical drain site (s)	

FIGURE 8-1 *continued*

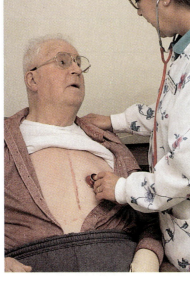

FIGURE 8-2 The nurse gathers information by doing a physical assessment of the patient.

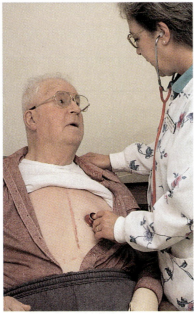

FIGURE 8-3 The patient's care plan is developed at a care plan conference.

TABLE 8-1 EXAMPLES OF NURSING DIAGNOSES AND OBSERVATIONS TO MAKE	
Nursing Diagnosis	**Observations to Make**
Altered nutrition; less than body requirements	• Food/fluid intake • Weight loss • Inability to eat • Pain in abdomen or mouth • Sores in mouth
Constipation	• Lack of bowel movement or hard, dry stools • C/O feeling full
Altered urinary elimination	• Incontinence, urgency, painful urination
Decreased cardiac output	• Changes in B/P, irregular pulse, fatigue, difficulty breathing
Risk of aspiration	• Difficulty in swallowing, depressed cough and gag reflex, reduced level of consciousness
Impaired skin integrity	• Redness or destruction of skin
Impaired verbal communication	• Inability or difficulty with speaking, difficulty breathing, disorientation
Ineffective individual coping	• Change in usual communication patterns • C/O inability to cope or meet basic needs • Change in behavior
Impaired adjustment	• Disbelief, anger, inability to solve problems
Impaired physical mobility	• Ability to move in bed, range of motion, balance, coordination, endurance
Activity intolerance	• Fatigue, weakness, shortness of breath • Irregular pulse
Sleep pattern disturbance	• C/O not sleeping • Changes in behavior or speech
Anxiety	• Shakiness, quivering voice, increased movements • Poor eye contact, helplessness

MARYSVILLE SKILLED CARE FACILITY	CARE PLAN	02/06/1999
		FORM # 280L

PROBLEM	SHORT TERM GOAL	APPROACH
(1) Potential for impaired skin integrity a) Related to altered circulation in legs b) Related to flexion contracture of neck ONSET TARGET RESOLVE 02/06/99 05/07/99 / /	(1) Will remain ulcer free (legs) through 5/7/99 ONSET TARGET RESOLVE 02/06/99 05/07/99 / / (2) Skin intact lower neck through 5/7/99 ONSET TARGET RESOLVE 02/06/99 05/07/99 / /	(1) R.N. check legs q a.m. DISC: NSG (2) Elevate legs when up in w/c. DISC: NA (3) Wash and dry area b.i.d. DISC: NA (4) Apply 4 x 4 to separate skin surfaces. DISC: NSG NA (5) Use Mycalog cream for increased redness prn. DISC: NSG
(2) Alteration in comfort a) Related to impaired circulation b) Related to joint pain ONSET TARGET RESOLVE 02/06/99 05/07/99 / /	(1) 2 nocs/week without leg cramps by 5/7/99 ONSET TARGET RESOLVE 02/06/99 05/07/99 / / (2) States relief of pain with heat packs through 5/7/99 ONSET TARGET RESOLVE 02/06/99 05/07/99 / /	(1) Administer Procardia as ordered and assess effectiveness. DISC: NSG (1) Heat packs to neck, shoulder, knees 5x/wk. DISC: RA

PHYSICIAN / ALT. PHYSICIAN	PHONE NO.	ALLERGIES / NOTES				
WASHINGTON, JAMES M.D. KEELEY, JANICE M.D.	(555) 555-8888	PENICILLIN, ASPIRIN				
PATIENT	STATION / ROOM / BED	ADMISSION NUMBER / DATE	SEX	DATE OF BIRTH	CARE PLAN DATE	PAGE #
JAMES, FIONA	NORTH-122-B	33652 10/18/1995	F	(75) 02/28/1923	02/06/1999	1

FIGURE 8-4 The care plan describes the patient's problems, the approaches used to resolve the problems, and the patient's goals.

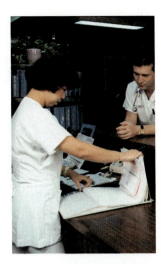

FIGURE 8-5 Care plans may be kept in a Kardex at the nurses' station.

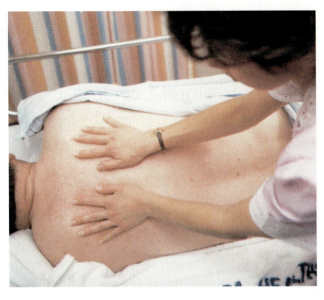

FIGURE 8-7 The nursing assistant observes for bruises or breaks in the skin while giving a backrub.

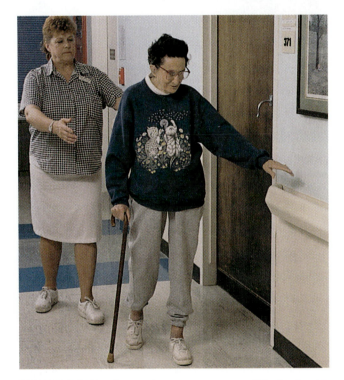

FIGURE 8-6 Nursing assistants are responsible for implementing many of the approaches on the care plan.

— the patient crying
— a change in the way the patient walks
- Your *ears* to *hear* observations:
  — wheezing when the patient breathes
  — pulse or blood pressure with a stethoscope
  — comments from the patient, such as "I am very tired today"
- Your *nose* to *smell* observations:
  — body odor
  — stool or urine when the patient is incontinent
- Your *hands and fingers* to *feel* observations:
  — a lump under the patient's skin (Figure 8-8)

be effective and the physician will need to change the order.

There are two types of observations: subjective and objective. An **objective observation** is one that is factual or measurable in some way. For example, blood in the urine is factual. Blood pressure, temperature, pulse, and respirations are measurable. A **subjective observation** is a statement or complaint made by the patient. For example, "I have a headache," or "I feel sick to my stomach" are subjective observations.

You make observations by using your senses.

- You use your *eyes* to *see* observations:
  — blood in the urine
  — bruises or breaks in the skin (Figure 8-7)

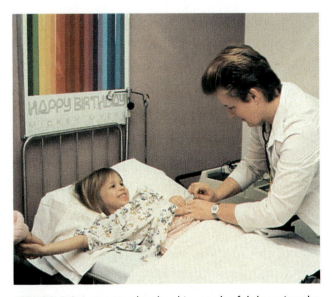

FIGURE 8-8 Lumps under the skin may be felt by using the sense of touch. *Photo courtesy of Henrietta Egleston Hospital for Children, Atlanta, GA. Photograph by Ginger Lovering*

— radial pulse

— warmth or coolness of the patient's skin

Remember that observations must be:

- accurate and timely
- reported to the nurse immediately
- documented in the patient's record, either by you or the nurse

Making Initial Observations

To make accurate observations, you must first know what is expected or normal for an individual. For this reason, baseline information is collected when the patient is admitted to the facility. If you help admit a patient, make observations while you are completing your assignment. It is especially important to note any possible signs of injury or skin breakdown. Think of the body systems as described in the following list. This information will give you a basis for making future comparisons. For example, one patient may have a blood pressure of 110/68 on admission. If you take the patient's blood pressure later and it is 140/88, you should report this to the nurse, because this is not the usual blood pressure for this person. Try to establish a routine way of making observations. Keep in mind the age and known illnesses of the patients. It may be helpful to think of each body system and note the following:

- Integumentary system (skin, nails)
  - Color: flushed, pale, jaundiced (yellow color), or cyanotic (bluish, ashen, gray color); nails pale, pink, or cyanotic.
  - Temperature: warm, hot, cool.
  - Moisture: dry, moist, perspiring.
  - Abnormalities: rashes, bruises, scars, pressure ulcers, areas of redness.
- Musculoskeletal system (muscles, bones, joints)
  - Posture: stooped, curled up in bed, straight.
  - Mobility: ability to move in bed, to get out of bed, to stand, to walk, and to maintain balance.
  - Range of motion: ability to move all joints (Figure 8-9).
- Circulatory system (heart, blood vessels, blood)
  - Pulse: strength, regularity, rate.
  - Skin: (see integumentary system).
  - Nails: (see integumentary system).
  - Blood pressure.
- Respiratory system (nose, throat, trachea, bronchi, lungs)
  - Respirations (breathing): rate, regularity, depth, difficulty in breathing, shortness of breath upon exertion or while still, wheezing or crackling heard.
  - Cough: frequency; dry, loose, productive. Color and consistency of sputum (if any).
- Nervous system (brain, spinal cord, nerves)
  - Mental status: orientation to time, place, person. Ability to make verbal or nonverbal responses.

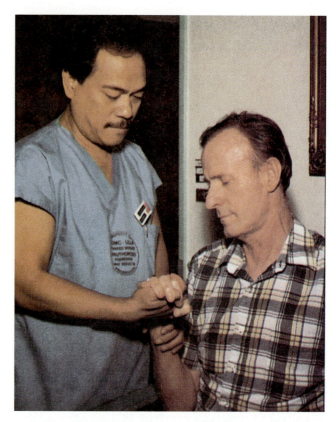

FIGURE 8-9 Report to the nurse if there is a change in the patient's ability to move the joints.

- Senses (eyes, ears, nose, sense of touch)
  - Eyes: reddened, drainage, pupils equal in size.
  - Ears: drainage.
  - Nose: drainage, bleeding.
  - Sense of touch: ability to feel pressure and pain.
- Urinary system (kidneys, ureters, bladder, urethra)
  - Urination: frequency, amount, color, clarity, presence of blood or sediment (Figure 8-10); ability to hold urine, incontinence.
  - Pain on urination (dysuria).
- Digestive system (mouth, teeth, throat, esophagus, stomach, large and small intestines, gall bladder, liver, pancreas)

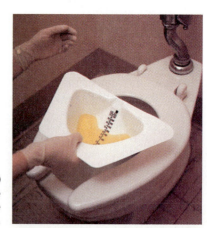

FIGURE 8-10
Examine the urine before disposing of it.

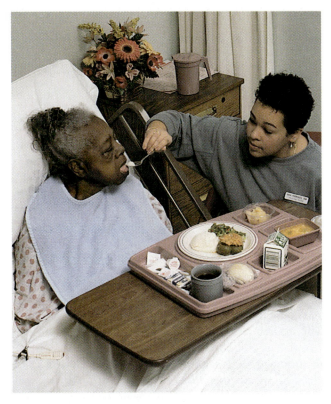

FIGURE 8-11 Observe the amount of fluids and food consumed.

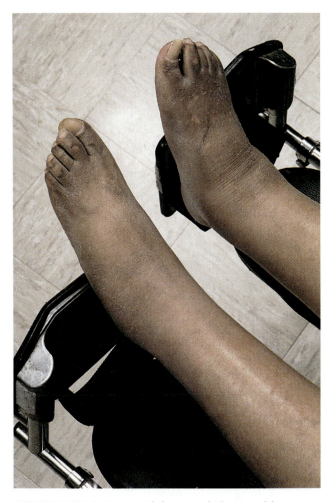

FIGURE 8-12 Patients with heart or kidney problems may have edema of the lower extremities.

— Appetite: amount of fluids and food consumed (Figure 8-11), tolerance to foods, belching or burping.

— Eating: difficulty chewing or swallowing.

— Nausea and/or vomiting.

— Bowel elimination: Frequency, amount, consistency, color of stools; diarrhea, constipation, incontinence, flatus; difficulty in passing stool.

● Endocrine system (glands)

— Signs and symptoms of diabetes (hypoglycemia, hyperglycemia).

● Reproductive system (male and female internal and external sex organs)

Female

— Breasts: condition of nipples, presence of lumps, discolorations.

— Menstrual periods: frequency, amount and character of bleeding; cramping.

— Vaginal drainage: amount, odor, and character.

Male

— Testes: lumps.

— Penis: amount and character of drainage.

In addition to the body systems observations, you also need to note facts related to pain, behavior, and function.

● Pain: location, type of pain (sharp, dull, aching), constant or intermittent or related to specific activities, time pain started

● Behavior: actions, conduct

● Function: ability to move about and complete tasks such as bathing

It is important that you be very factual in reporting observations of pain and behavior. Never try to judge whether a patient really has pain or how severe it is. Some individuals are very expressive about pain and others are very stoical (they try not to show their discomfort). A person's culture may also affect the response to pain. Never compare patients. One person may seem to have more pain than another person with the same diagnosis. It is not appropriate to think that they should both respond in the same way.

When reporting behavior, avoid using "labels" based on your judgment of the patient. Report only what you see and hear.

There are additional observations to make that are related to the patient's medical diagnoses. For example, if a patient has a kidney condition, you would look for edema (swelling) of the face, hands, and ankles (Figure 8-12). You would also monitor the person's fluid intake and output. You will learn more about observations related to medical diagnoses as you study these conditions.

In some situations, you may be expected to report "normal" observations. This information tells the nurse and physician

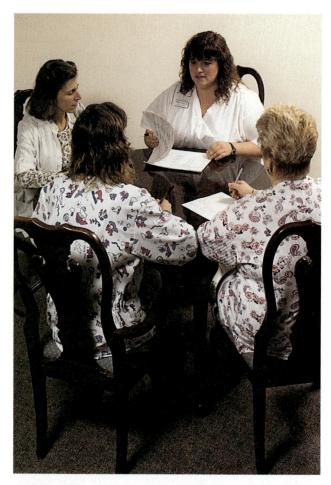

FIGURE 8-13 A report is given by the nurse who worked the previous shift.

whether the patient's condition is improving. For example, if a patient has had a respiratory tract infection and the signs and symptoms have diminished, it is important to report "no coughing or respiratory distress is noted."

REPORTING

Giving an **oral report** is a method used to relay information from one person to another. The nursing assistant may participate in oral reports several times on a shift. Oral reports are given by the:

- nurse going off duty to the staff coming on duty (Figure 8-13) (in some facilities the nurse may give a report only to the charge nurse of the oncoming shift)—this is called a shift report
- nursing assistant to the nurse when leaving the nursing unit for any reason (such as lunch break)
- nursing assistant to the nurse at the end of the shift
- nursing assistant to the nurse if any unusual or new observations are made

Be specific when you report your observations. If you are relaying a subjective observation (something the patient has told you), repeat it exactly the way the patient told it to you. Here are some examples:

- Mr. Jones in 249 says it hurts every time he urinates.
- Mrs. Goldberg was wandering around in the hall and said she did not know where she was.

To report objective observations, state your measurement or fact:

- Mrs. Dominick's blood pressure is 142/86.
- Mr. Hernandez only ate 50 percent of his meal at lunch time.

When you report off duty at the end of your shift, report to the nurse:

- the condition of each of the patients you were assigned to
- the care you gave each patient
- observations you made while giving care

DOCUMENTATION

In some facilities you may be expected to record your observations on the patient's medical record (chart) (Figure 8-14). The medical record is a **document**. A document is a legal record. The process of recording the patient's care, response to treatment, and progress in the patient's chart is called **charting** or *documentation*. Nursing assistants may document on **flow sheets** (Figure 8-15) in the chart or on the

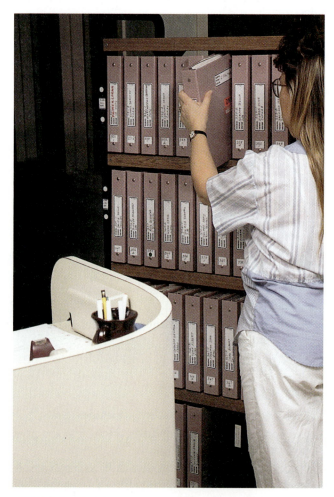

FIGURE 8-14 Observations are recorded on the patient's medical record.

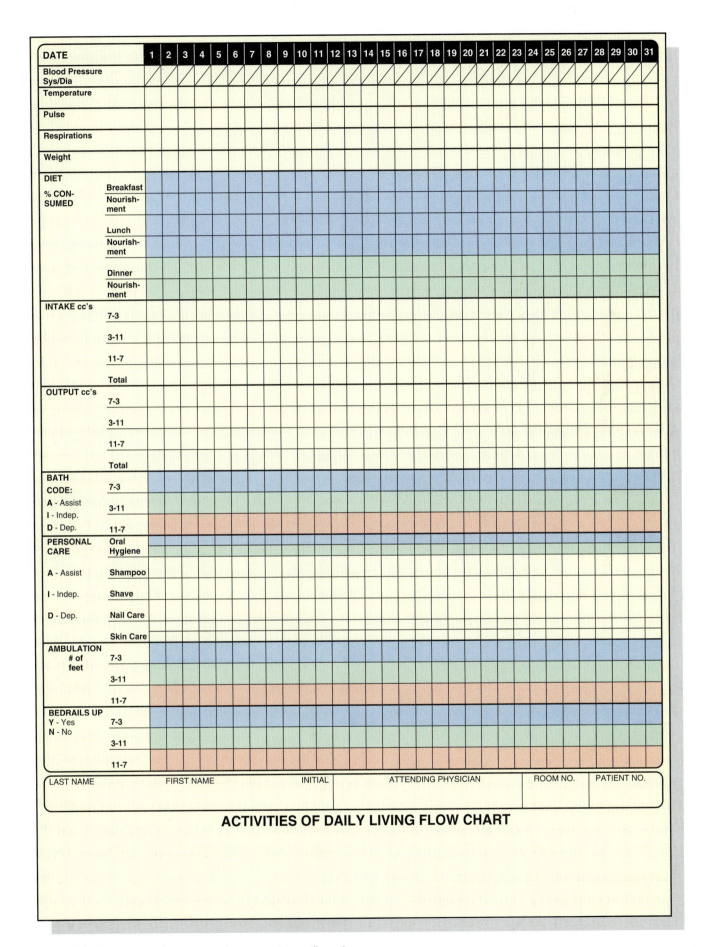

FIGURE 8-15 You may be expected to record on a flow sheet.

DATE		1	2	3	4	5	6	7	8	9	10	11	12	13	14	15	16	17	18	19	20	21	22	23	24	25	26	27	28	29	30	31
UP IN CHAIR	7-3																															
A - Assist	3-11																															
I - Indep. D - Dep.	11-7																															
ROM Exercises	7-3																															
A - Active P - Passive	3-11																															
POSITION **changed**	7-3																															
A - Assist	3-11																															
I - Indep. D - Dep.	11-7																															
BLADDER **ACTION**	7-3																															
C - Continent	3-11																															
I - Incontinent F - Foley # x's	11-7																															
BOWEL **ACTION**	7-3																															
C - Continent	3-11																															
I - Incontinent # x's	11-7																															
CONSISTENCY	7-3																															
L - Liquid S - Soft formed	3-11																															
H - Hard formed	11-7																															
PERI CARE	7-3																															
A - Assist	3-11																															
I - Indep. D - Dep.	11-7																															
RESTRAINT P - Pelvic W - Waist	7-3																															
B - Belt G - Geri Chair	3-11																															
Check q 1/2 Hr. Release q 2 hrs.	11-7																															
Nursing **Assistant's** **Initials**	A.M.																															
	P.M.																															
	NOC.																															
Licensed **Nurse** **Initials**	A.M.																															
	P.M.																															
	NOC.																															

Nursing Assistant's Initials and Signature

_____ _____ _____ _____
_____ _____ _____ _____
_____ _____ _____ _____

Licensed Nurse Initials and Signature

_____ _____ _____ _____
_____ _____ _____ _____
_____ _____ _____ _____

LAST NAME	FIRST NAME	INITIAL	ATTENDING PHYSICIAN	ROOM NO.	PATIENT NO.

FIGURE 8-15 *continued*

NURSE'S PROGRESS NOTES

DATE AND TIME	NURSING CARE NOTES	SIGNATURE
3-16-XX	2200 Found lying on floor beside bed. Responds verbally. States was "trying to get to the bathroom." Nurse notified immediately_____	C. Simmons CNA
	2205 ROM satisfactory. Denies having pain. No injuries noted. Assisted back to bed. Call light within reach. Instructed to use call light when having to go to B.R. Pulse 86, strong and regular. B/P 136/84. Oriented to time, place, person. Incontinent after fall. Pajamas chgd._____	
	2300 Sleeping s̄ distress_____	B. Selici RN
3-17-XX	2400-0200 Sleeping soundly. Respirations regular. Pulse 78 strong and regular._____	
	0230 Awake. c/o "arthritis pain" in both hips. Acetaminophen tabs ı̄ı̄ given with water. Assisted to bathroom. Voided large amt. clear urine.	
	0230-0630 Slept soundly. Pulse 72 strong and regular. B/P 128/80. T 98⁶(O). Denies pain anywhere. No other c/o distress._____	P. Hernandez RN
3-17-XX	~~2400 Up to B.R. c̄ assistance~~_____ Error ES	E. Seldes LPN

FIGURE 8-16 The nurse's notes are a record of all nursing care given to the patient.

nurse's notes (Figure 8-16) (sometimes called nurse's progress notes). The charting must:

- address the problems listed in the patient's care plan
- describe the approaches (interventions) listed in the care plan and note whether the interventions are effective
- indicate the progress the patient is making toward meeting the goals on the care plan

Charting Guidelines

A patient's medical record (chart) is a legal document and may be used in court as evidence. It is important that everything be correct and legible. All charting and records must be in clear, simple, and accurate language. Entries must be printed or written carefully so that there can be no misunderstanding of the meaning. If you follow the established rules of charting, there will be no problem.

Each chart relates only to one patient, so it is unnecessary to use the term *patient* or to use the patient's name. Use phrases rather than full sentences, and do not make erasures or leave empty spaces on the record. All entries are made in black ink because the chart is a permanent record; no erasable ink or correction fluid is allowed.

If you use medical terms in your charting, make sure you are using the correct words and that spelling is correct. Use a medical dictionary if you are not sure. Abbreviations are allowed, but they must be on the approved list of your facility. Do not make up your own abbreviations. You must chart only for yourself and only when the procedure or assignment has been completed.

The time of entry must be noted when the entry is made. Most health care facilities use international time (Table 8-2) to avoid confusion between A.M. and P.M. With international time, the 24 hours of each day are identified by the numbers 0100 (1:00 A.M.) through 2400 (12:00 A.M., midnight). The last two digits indicate the minutes of each hour (from 01 to

59). Thus, 0101 would be one minute after 1:00 A.M.; 1210 would be ten minutes after 12 P.M. (noon); 1658 would be 4:58 P.M., and so on.

Many health care facilities are using flow sheets for documenting patient care. Flow sheets save nursing time and simplify the documentation process. However, there are some things you should be aware of to avoid problems:

- Understand what you are supposed to be documenting. Read the flow sheet carefully.

GUIDELINES *for*

Charting

- Check for: right patient, right chart, right room
- Fill out new headings completely
- Use correct color of ink
- Date and time each entry
- Chart entries in correct sequence
- Make entries brief, objective, and accurate
- Print or write clearly
- Spell each word correctly
- Leave no blank spaces or lines between entries
- Do not use the term *patient*
- Do not use ditto marks
- Sign each entry with first initial, last name, and job title
- Make corrections by drawing one line through entry; then print the word "error" on the line and your initials above

TABLE 8-2 INTERNATIONAL TIME			
Standard Clock	**Int'l. Time**	**Standard Clock**	**Int'l. Time**
AM 12 midnight	2400	PM 12 noon	1200
1	0100	1	1300
2	0200	2	1400
3	0300	3	1500
4	0400	4	1600
5	0500	5	1700
6	0600	6	1800
7	0700	7	1900
8	0800	8	2000
9	0900	9	2100
10	1000	10	2200
11	1100	11	2300

- Never initial any procedure or observation that you did not do.
- Initial for the right procedure, on the right day, on the right shift.
- Your complete signature must on each flow sheet, usually at the bottom of the page.
- Remember that flow sheets are legal records just like the other forms in the medical record.

REVIEW

UNIT REVIEW

A. True/False.

Mark the following true or false by circling T or F.

1. T F The nursing process is a method used by the nurse to supervise the work of others.
2. T F The nursing assistant is responsible for completing an assessment on all patients.
3. T F Assessment involves the collection of data.
4. T F A statement of a patient's medical condition is called a nursing diagnosis.
5. T F An approach is sometimes called an intervention.
6. T F The patient's goal is called an outcome.
7. T F The care plan is developed at the care plan conference.
8. T F Nursing assistants are not responsible for the development or implementation of the care plan.
9. T F Taking a patient's weight is an example of an objective observation.
10. T F The patient's chart is a legal document.

B. Multiple Choice.

Select the one best answer for each question.

11. The purpose of the nursing process is to
    a. make a medical diagnosis.
    b. achieve patient focused care.
    c. make assignments.
    d. cure illness.

12. Assessment may involve
    a. interviewing the patient.
    b. talking to the patient's family.
    c. reading the patient's medical record.
    d. all of these.

13. The statement of a patient's problem and its cause is called

  a. a medical diagnosis.

  b. an approach.

  c. an assessment.

  d. a nursing diagnosis.

14. The purpose of evaluation is to determine whether the

  a. patient is reaching the goals on the care plan.

  b. physician has made the right medical diagnosis.

  c. nursing assistant is performing assignments.

  d. all of these.

15. The purpose of making observations is to

  a. note any change in the patient's condition.

  b. determine the effectiveness of medication or treatment.

  c. note a new condition developing.

  d. all of these.

16. An example of an objective observation is that the patient

  a. complains of abdominal pain.

  b. says she is feeling sad.

  c. has a pulse of 72.

  d. says she is not hungry.

17. When you offer to give Mrs. Jones a bath, she says, "Get out of here and don't come back." You report this to the nurse and say

  a. "Mrs. Jones told me to get out of her room and to not come back."

  b. "Mrs. Jones is angry today."

  c. "Mrs. Jones is not cooperating with me."

  d. "Mrs. Jones does not want a bath today."

18. The form on which nurses enter daily information about the patient is called the

  a. care plan.

  b. nurse's notes.

  c. assignment sheet.

  d. document.

19. Charting should always be

  a. done in ink.

  b. done after the procedure is completed and not before.

  c. signed by the person who did the charting.

  d. all of these.

20. In international time, midnight would be called

  a. 12:00 AM

  b. 2400

  c. 1200

  d. 12:00 PM

C. Nursing Assistant Challenge.

Mr. Fensten is a 47-year-old patient on the medical floor. He has had a stroke. These events occur while you are taking care of him:

- He has trouble walking because of hemiplegia (paralysis) on the right side of his body and almost falls while you are walking him to the bathroom.
- he refuses to eat his breakfast.
- He throws the washcloth across the room when you help him with his bath.
- His B/P is 146/88.
- He smiles and hugs his wife when she comes to visit.
- You do range-of-motion exercises on all joints without any problem.
- You notice a persistent reddened area on his coccyx (tailbone).

For each of these observations, write out the documentation exactly as you would on the patient's medical record.

Think about these observations and consider how many examples of verbal and nonverbal communication are given.

Are there any situations that involve Mr. Fensten's rights as a patient? If so, describe them.

Meeting Basic Human Needs

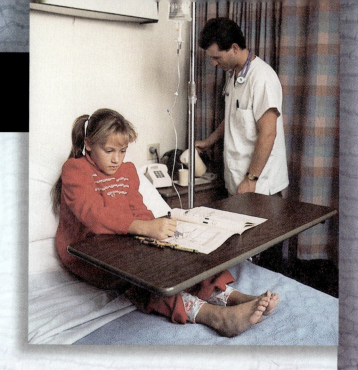

As a result of this unit, you will be able to:

- Spell and define terms.
- Describe the stages of human growth and development.
- List five physical needs of patients.
- List four reasons why patients have difficulty sleeping.
- Define self-esteem.

- Describe how the nursing assistant can meet the patient's emotional needs.
- Discuss methods of dealing with the fearful patient.
- List nursing assistant actions to ensure that patients have the opportunity for intimacy.
- List the guidelines to assist patients in meeting their spiritual needs.

Learn the meaning and the correct spelling of the following words and phrases:

adolescence	growth	personality	sexuality
bisexuality	heterosexuality	preadolescence	tasks
celibate	homosexuality	reflex	tasks of personality
coitus	intimacy	self-esteem	development
continuum	masturbation	self-identity	toddler
development	neonate		

INTRODUCTION

Each of us has things that we need to live successfully. These are called *needs* simply because we cannot get along without them. When a patient is admitted to the hospital, his or her needs come too. The difference now is in the way those needs are expressed and fulfilled. Expression and fulfillment have to be different because of the hospital environment and the illness. Remember that the basic needs remain the same, regardless of how they are expressed or how they have to be met because of an individual's level of development or state of health.

HUMAN GROWTH AND DEVELOPMENT

Human beings change as they age, through the processes of growth and development. **Growth** involves the changes that take place in the body. It is usually measured by height and weight and degree of system maturation. **Development** involves the changes that take place on a social, emotional, and psychological level. Developmental levels are shown in behavior and interpersonal skills.

People move from one level of development to the next (Table 9-1). At each level, they change in both the way they look and the way they think and act (Figure 9-1). Each level presents tasks that must be mastered before the person can move on to the next level.

The **tasks** to be mastered are those things that lead to healthy and satisfactory participation in society. The tasks are defined by the needs of the individual and the pressures of society.

Sometimes growth spurts occur and developmental skills must catch up. Both growth and development progress from simple to complex. Each depends on the other to achieve the

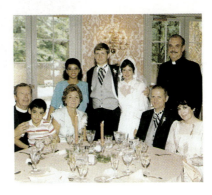

FIGURE 9-1 The characteristics of the different age groups are reflected in this group picture.

orderly progression. For example, a child cannot be toilet trained until the nerve pathways have matured.

Growth and development follow a set of basic principles of progression.

- There is a continuous movement from simple to more complex. For example, baby sounds progress to speech patterns.
- Development and growth move from head to feet and from torso to limbs. The infant first raises the head, then sits, stands, and finally walks.
- Each stage of development has a specific set of tasks that the person must master before he or she can successfully move on to the next level. For example, the child learns to catch big balls before she can catch a baseball.
- Progression moves forward in an orderly manner, but the rate varies for each person. There are growth spurts in the preschool and teen years, but not all children grow to the same extent or at the same rate.
- Growth patterns progress at their own individual rate.

Neonatal and Infant Period (Birth to Two Years)

The neonatal and infant period extends through the first two years of life. It is a time of rapid physical growth and development (Table 9-2). The infant gradually learns to:

- Sit
- Crawl
- Stand
- Take first steps

Other changes also occur during this period:

- Emotional attachments move from self-awareness and parental or caregiver attachment toward ties with other family members.
- Systems that are relatively immature at birth become more stabilized.
- Alertness and activity increase.
- Teeth appear (erupt).
- Food intake progresses from milk to solid food.
- Verbal skills begin to develop.

The mother or primary caregiver of the infant is the central figure of emotional attachment. Growth and development progress so rapidly that changes can be seen each month.

TABLE 9-1 STAGES OF GROWTH AND DEVELOPMENT	
Neonate	Birth to 1 month
Infancy	1 month to 2 years
Toddler	2 years to 3 years
Preschool	3 years to 5 years
School Age	5 years to 12 years
Preadolescent	12 years to 14 years
Adolescence	14 years to 20 years
Adulthood	20 years to 50 years
Middle Age	50 years to 65 years
Later Maturity	65 years to 75 years
Old Age	75 years and beyond

TABLE 9-2 HEIGHT/WEIGHT FOR THE FIRST YEAR OF LIFE (BOYS)

Age (Months)	Height (Inches)	Weight (Pounds)
Birth	20	7–8
1 Month	21¼	7½
2 Months	22½	10
3 Months	23¾	11½
4 Months	24¾	12½
5 Months	25½	14
6 Months	26	15
7 Months	26¾	16¾
8 Months	27½	18
9 Months	28	19
10 Months	28½	20
11 Months	29	20¾
12 Months	29½	21½

Remember that the figures are averages only.

The **neonate** (newborn) (Figure 9-2):

- Weighs 7–8 pounds
- Is approximately 20–21 inches long
- Has a head that seems disproportionately large compared to the body
- Has skin that is wrinkled, thin, and red

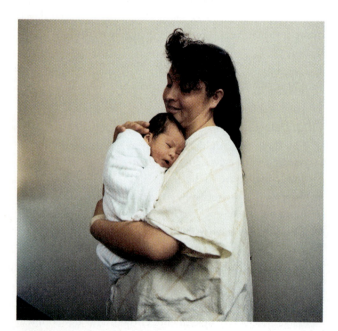

FIGURE 9-2 Newborn infant (neonate)

- Has an abdomen that seems to stick out (protrude)
- Has dark blue eyes

In the newborn, the:

- Conversion of cartilage to bone (ossification) is not complete. This can be seen in the soft spots (fontanels) and suture lines (joints) of the skull.
- Nervous system is not fully developed, so muscular activities are uncoordinated.
- Vision is not clear, but hearing and taste are developed. Certain **reflexes** (automatic responses) are also developed. They are the:
  - Moro reflex—when a loud noise startles the infant, the arms are spread across the chest, the legs are extended, and the head is thrust back. This response is also called the *startle reflex*.
  - Grasp reflex—touching the infant's palm causes the fingers to flex in a grasping motion.
  - Rooting (sucking) reflex—stroking the cheek or side of the lips stimulates the infant to turn its head in the direction of the stroking. This is important in finding the nipple to suck the milk.
- Diet is milk or milk substitute.
- Routine is largely sleeping, eating, and eliminating.

The neonate is completely dependent on the caregiver for all needs. The infant is unable to support her head, so the newborn must be handled carefully and be well supported when held.

The three-month-old infant:

- Has gained enough muscular coordination to hold her head up and raise her shoulders.
- Has lost the Moro, rooting, and grasp reflexes.
- Produces real tears.
- Can follow objects with his eyes.
- Can smile and coo at the caregiver.

The six-month-old infant:

- Has learned to roll over.
- Can sit for short periods of time.
- Holds things with both hands and directs them toward his mouth.
- Responds with verbal sounds when a caregiver speaks.
- Is beginning to cut front teeth.
- Eats finger foods and strained fruits and vegetables.
- Recognizes family members.
- Develops fear of strangers.

The nine-month-old infant:

- Crawls and may begin to stand when supported.
- Has more teeth erupt.
- Can respond to her name.
- Says one- and two-syllable words such as "mama."
- Shows a preference for right- or left-hand control.
- Eats junior baby foods.

The one-year-old infant:

- Understands simple commands such as "No."
- Begins to take steps—supported at first, then independently.
- Eats table foods and can hold her own cup.
- Weighs three times what he weighed at birth (refer to Table 9-2).

Toddler Period (Two to Three Years)

The toddler period is a busy, active phase. It is a time when exploration and investigation are the main activities. It is also a period in which motor abilities develop (Figure 9-3) and vocabulary and comprehension increase.

During this period, the toddler:

- Learns to control elimination.
- Begins to become aware of right and wrong.
- Often reacts with frustration and negative responses to attempts at socialization and discipline as she becomes more aware of herself as a separate person.
- Tolerates brief periods of separation from the mother, but the mother still remains the source of security and comfort.
- May play in the company of other children but with no interaction. This age group is very possessive. "No" and "mine" are a major part of their vocabularies.

Reaching the end of this period, the toddler is able to:

- Walk and run.
- Display motor (manual) skills that include feeding himself and riding toys.
- Put words together and speak more clearly. The average vocabulary of a two-year-old is about 300 words.
- Play near others, but is not able to interact in play with children of the same age (peers).

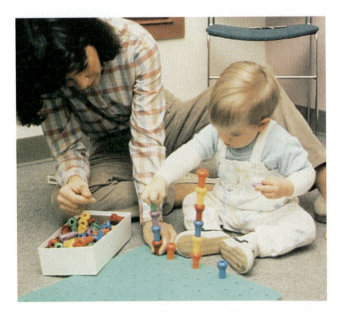

FIGURE 9-3 The toddler begins to develop gross motor skills. *Photo courtesy of Henrietta Egleston Hospital for Children, Atlanta, GA. Photograph by Ginger Lovering*

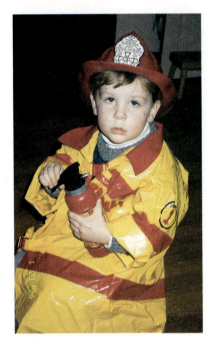

FIGURE 9-4 The preschooler expands his awareness of the world around him.

Preschool Years (Three to Five Years)

The three- to five-year-old (Figure 9-4) builds on the motor and verbal skills developed as a toddler. During this period, the preschooler:

- Grows less reliant on the mother. Children in this age group begin to recognize their position as members of the family unit and their uniqueness from other members.
- Develops rivalries with siblings and develops greater attachments to the father or alternate caregiver.
- Gradually increases cooperative play.
- Improves language skills and asks many questions.
- Develops a more active imagination.
- Becomes more sexually curious.

By the end of this period, children have become far more socialized than they were as toddlers. They are more cooperative. They seem almost eager to follow established rules within limits. They enjoy interacting with family members and peers.

School-Aged Children (6 to 12 Years)

The school-aged child (Figure 9-5):

- Is able to communicate.
- Has developed small (fine) motor skills. With these skills, the child is able to master tasks such as writing.
- Develops an increased sense of self.
- Establishes peer relationships.
- Reinforces proper social behavior through games, simple tasks, and play.
- Chooses sex-differentiated friends.
- Joins groups like Scouts. This serves to further identify the individual as a person of a particular gender.

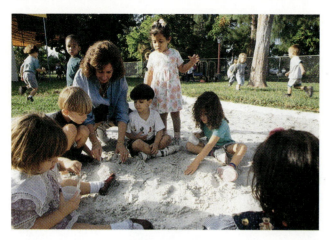

FIGURE 9-5 School-aged children like to play in peer groups.

- Begins to show concern for other living things (Figure 9-6).

Preadolescent (12 to 14 Years)

Preadolescence is a transitional stage. It is a period of great uncertainty. During this period:

- Hormonal changes stimulate the secondary sex characteristics.
- The individual feels on the threshold of tremendous change, though not yet in a period of sexual functioning.
- Mood swings and feelings of insecurity are common.
- There is a growing awareness of and interest in the opposite sex.

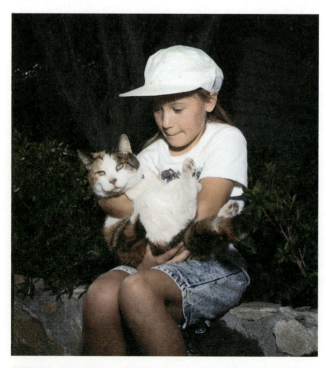

FIGURE 9-6 Young children learn to reach out and have concern for others.

- Arms and legs seem out of proportion to the rest of the body.

Adolescence (14 to 20 Years)

Adolescence is marked by:

- The gradual development of sexual maturity.
- A greater appreciation of the individual's own identity as a male or a female person.
- Conflicting desires for the freedom of independence and the security of dependence. Because of these conflicting desires, this is often a troublesome period.
- The establishment of personal coping systems and the ability to make independent judgments and decisions.
- Gradual success in mastering the developmental tasks of the age. The adolescent is able to make comparisons between the values she has been taught and reality.

Adulthood (20 to 50 Years)

Early adulthood is marked by:

- Independence and personal decision making.
- The choice of a mate.
- Establishment of a career and family life.
- Optimal health.
- The choice of friends to form a support group.

Middle Age (50 to 65 Years)

Middle age is associated with:

- Final career advancement, ending in retirement.
- Children who were reared during the period of adulthood leaving home to enter their own adult period.
- Health that is usually still at good levels, though some slowing may be seen.
- More time that can be spent on leisure activities.
- More time and money to pursue personal interests.
- Revitalizing one's relationship with a mate.
- Enjoying grandchildren.
- For some middle-aged persons, being a member of the "sandwich" generation—caring for both their own parents and their children or grandchildren.

Later Maturity (65 to 75 Years)

Later maturity is marked by:

- A gradual loss of vitality and stamina.
- Physical changes that signal the aging process. For example, sight and hearing diminish.
- Chronic conditions that develop and persist.
- A period of gradual losses: loss of mate, friends, self-esteem, some independence.
- Examination of a lifetime.
- More time to pursue personal interests.
- Fewer responsibilities related to raising a family and holding a job.
- Increased wisdom.

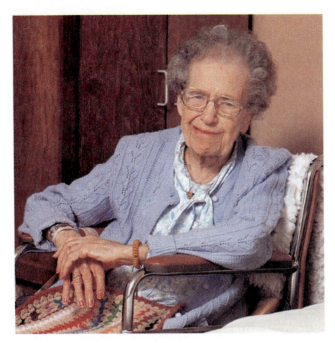

FIGURE 9-7 Physical status may decline during old age.

Old Age (75 Years and Beyond)

Old age is frequently characterized by:

- Failing physical health and growing dependency (Figure 9-7).
- The need to deal with illness, loneliness, loss of friends and loved ones, and the realization of mortality.

Success in this final period depends on the mechanisms of coping that the older adult has developed over the years. The extent of available emotional and physical support is also important.

Aging is a gradual process that begins at birth. Old age can be a period of development and enjoyment.

BASIC HUMAN NEEDS

Developmental skills and physical growth may vary during the life span. The basic human needs, however, are much the same for every individual.

Basic human needs are the things and activities required by all persons to successfully and satisfactorily live their lives. The needs are the same for all people at all ages. Cultural backgrounds influence the way in which individuals express these basic needs. *Culture* refers to those customs and practices that are common to groups of people that become ingrained beliefs, habits, and responses. Culture embraces language, dietary habits, health practices, expressions of spirituality, and ways of celebrating. These cultural patterns are part of the uniqueness of each individual and must be considered when providing for the person's care.

Abraham Maslow and Erik Erikson are two leaders in the field of human behavior. They have helped us understand the basic needs and how people go about satisfying them.

Personality

Exactly how each person goes about satisfying personal psychological needs reflects his personality. **Personality** is the sum of ways we react to the events in our lives. It is gradually formed through experience and molded by cultural heritage.

Erikson suggested that our personalities are formed as we mature from infancy to old age. He believed that we pass through eight growing stages in search of who we really are (**self-identity**). During each stage, there are choices to be made before moving on to the next task. He called these the **tasks of personality development** (Table 9-3).

Maslow described human needs as physical, psychological, and sociological. He placed the needs on a **continuum** in which physical needs had to be satisfied first. The psychological or sociological needs can be met only after the physi-

---

TABLE 9-3 TASKS OF PERSONALITY DEVELOPMENT ACCORDING TO THE STAGES DEFINED BY ERIKSON

Physical Stage	Year of Occurrence	Tasks to Be Mastered
Oral-sensory	Birth–1 year (infant)	To learn to trust (Trust)
Muscular-anal	1–3 years (toddler)	To recognize self as an independent being from mother (Autonomy)
Locomotor	3–5 years (preschool years)	To recognize self as a family member (Initiative)
Latency	6–11 years (school-age years)	To demonstrate physical and mental skills/abilities (Industry)
Adolescence	12–18 years	To develop a sense of individuality as a sexual human being (Identity)
Young Adulthood	19–35 years	To establish intimate personal relationships with a mate (Intimacy)
Adulthood	35–50 years	To live a satisfying and productive life
Maturity	50+ years	To review life's events and examine how they have influenced the development of a unique individual (Ego integrity)

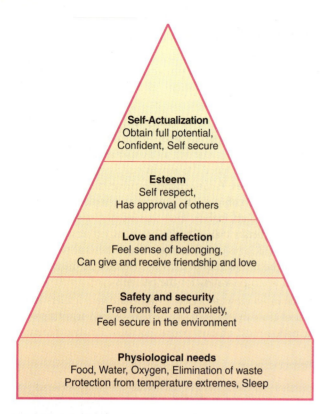

FIGURE 9-8 Maslow's hierarchy of needs

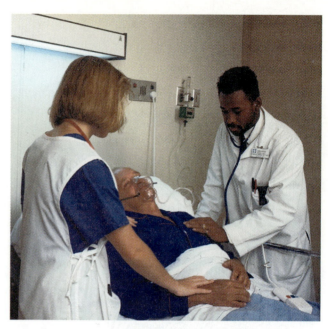

FIGURE 9-9 Some patients may need additional oxygen.

cal needs have been satisfied (Figure 9-8). The progression of needs is called a *hierarchy of needs*.

Physical Needs

The most basic human needs are physical needs. They include:

- Nutrition
- Rest
- Oxygen
- Shelter
- Elimination
- Activity
- Sexuality

Illness at any age creates stresses that make meeting the needs a challenge for both patient and caregivers.

Meeting the Patient's Physical Needs

You will need to provide for the physical needs of your patients. These are the need to be sheltered, to breathe, to eat, to sleep, and to eliminate waste products.

Shelter. In the health care facility, the need to be sheltered is met when the proper environment is maintained. Some examples include making sure that:

- A comfortable room temperature is maintained
- Needed repairs are reported, such as a leaking faucet.

Oxygen. Most of us take breathing for granted. We hardly give it more than a passing thought until it becomes difficult. There are many reasons why people have trouble

breathing. When they do have difficulty, though, the need is always the same. The body cannot live without oxygen, which is found in the air. It may be necessary, therefore, to give the patient extra oxygen and moisture to ensure that body tissues receive enough oxygen. Oxygen delivered by cannula or mask may be used for this purpose (Figure 9-9). Sometimes this need can be met by adjusting the overbed table in such a way that the patient, supported by pillows, is able to lean on it.

Food. Patients may lose their appetites when they are in the hospital. Decreased appetite and intake of fluids may be due to:

- Inactivity
- Hospital odors
- Pain
- Fear and anxiety
- Types of food served
- Illness itself
- Age of the patient

Some patients have to be fed because of their condition. Some may be given only special foods. Some are unable to take food in the usual way. Some patients are given liquid nourishment through a tube that has been passed through the nose and into the stomach. Fluid replacement may also be given through a sterile tube into the veins.

Because patients receive nourishment in such a variety of ways, you need to see to the special needs of each individual. There are, however, some general points to keep in mind:

- Appetites improve when food is served at the proper temperature in pleasant surroundings.
- Bathroom doors should be closed and room deodorants used to get rid of unpleasant odors.
- Unneeded equipment should be removed from sight.

- Cultural preferences should be considered.
- Patients should be prepared by allowing them to wash hands and face. Help them sit up in bed or get out of bed, if permitted.
- The tray should be offered in a calm, pleasant manner, even if the food is not what you like. Even a bland diet offered in this way is more acceptable.
- Patients should be allowed to do as much as they are able for themselves. Be available, however, to assist if needed.

Sleep. Noise and pain are the main reasons patients have difficulty sleeping. You should:

- Control noise whenever possible.
- Handle equipment carefully.
- Reduce the volume on televisions.
- Limit conversation with coworkers.
- Use a lowered voice.
- Keep the door to the patient's room closed.

To help the patient fall asleep, a few extra moments of your time are well spent in giving a soothing backrub, providing a change of position, and making the bed neat. Sometimes medication is needed to help the patient sleep. The patient is completely prepared for sleep before the nurse gives the medication. By doing this, the patient will not have to be disturbed after being medicated.

Worry also plays a role in a patient's sleeplessness. Patients worry about many things, such as:

- What the future will bring
- How much the hospitalization will cost
- Who is taking care of their home and work responsibilities

You will not have the answers to all these pressing concerns. You can listen, however. Share these concerns with the nurse. This is not gossiping. The nurse and the other members of the staff may be able to help the patient solve the problems. With worries reduced, the patient will rest easier.

Elimination. To stay healthy, the body must be able to rid itself of perspiration, urine, and feces. Elimination is promoted by:

- Bathing, which helps get rid of perspiration and keeps the skin healthy.
- Encouraging the patient to drink six to eight glasses of fluids and, if possible, to eat foods high in fiber.
- Providing additional help, if needed, to relieve the patient's body of waste. A sterile tube (catheter) can be inserted into the urinary bladder to drain the urine out. The sterile catheter may be left in the bladder to provide constant drainage. The tube is then attached to a bag that collects the urine. Enemas, laxatives, and suppositories help the bowels get rid of solid wastes in the form of feces.
- Helping patients who are unable to use the usual toilet facilities, by providing them with bedpans, urinals, and bedside commodes.

Physical Activity. People, by nature, are active beings. When illness occurs, it often limits activity. Sometimes the patient must stay in bed for a long time. The staff must find ways to promote appropriate activity for these individuals. The capability of the patient and the goals of treatment must be kept in mind when the activity level of any patient is established.

The complications resulting from inactivity and actions to take to avoid these complications are presented in Unit 44.

Activity promotes improved functioning of all systems. Circulation and respiration are increased. Muscles, bones, and joints function more efficiently. The body as a whole responds in a positive way to activity.

When patients are unable to carry out activity, such as walking, getting into and out of bed, and using the bedpan or commode independently, you may have to help them (Figure 9-10). Be sure you are aware of the patient's limitations, as well as the degree and type of activity allowed. Encourage patients to do as much as possible, but do not allow them to become either overstressed or tired.

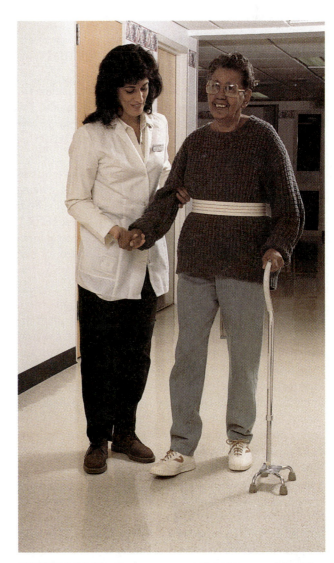

FIGURE 9-10 The patient may need assistance with ambulation.

Security and Safety Needs

If physical needs are not being met, the individual has no energy to be concerned about safety. For example, a mother whose children are starving may risk her life to provide food. Once physical needs are provided for, safety and security become priorities. Security and safety for patients are provided by:

- Maintaining a safe environment (see Units 13 and 14)
- Knowing how to respond to medical emergencies, such as patient falls
- Knowing how to respond to facility emergencies, such as fire
- Implementing the patient's care plan as indicated

Emotional Needs

The third and fourth levels of Maslow's hierarchy are related to emotional needs, including the need for love and belonging and the need for esteem. There is a need:

- To give love
- To feel love
- To be loved
- To be treated with respect and dignity
- To feel that self-esteem (our opinion of ourselves) is protected

All individuals—you, your coworkers, and your patients—have in their own minds an idea of how they appear and wish to appear to others. This idea is referred to as **self-esteem**. A person's self-esteem must be protected at all costs.

For example, a person might visualize and project to others the image of a very self-reliant person, capable of making important decisions and able to care for self and family. Suddenly that same person is scantily dressed in a hospital bed. A stranger is taking care of her most intimate physical functions. Even the times to eat and bathe are decided for her. This set of circumstances threatens even the most secure person's self-esteem.

How patients respond to this threat to their self-esteem depends on two things. First, it depends on how often the patient has had these feelings of helplessness before, and how well he has dealt with them. Second, it depends on you and your ability to appreciate those feelings.

One patient may feel frustrated and angry. He may not even know that these feelings are based on fear. The patient may act out these feelings by complaining about the hospital, the staff, roommates, you, or the food. In fact, every aspect of the care may be cause for complaint. Be open and receptive to these actions, recognizing the underlying feelings.

Still another patient may react quite differently to the same emotional stress. That person may be quiet and withdrawn. She may be completely cooperative and noncomplaining (Figure 9-11). The behavior shown is a false front. It hides the patient's feelings of not being able to cope with the situation. The nursing assistant must be aware of these feelings and the need for caring support.

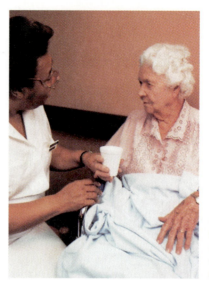

FIGURE 9-11
Patience may be needed to break through a wall of fear and frustration.

Intimacy and Sexuality

Intimacy is a feeling of closeness with another human (Figure 9-12). It is a relationship marked by feelings of love. It is an integral part of human response.

Sexuality is a lifelong characteristic that defines the maleness or femaleness of each person. This definition may be different for each person. All individuals are sexual, whether or not they have physical sexual relations. Sexuality has to do with the ability to develop relationships, to give of oneself to others, and to appreciate the giving by others. Intimacy is one aspect of sexuality.

Intimacy may be shared between friends or lovers. Also, a degree of intimacy is established when patient and caregiver learn they can trust and have confidence in each other.

Intimate relationships may be sexual and expressed in different ways. Humans express sexual intimacy depending on ori-

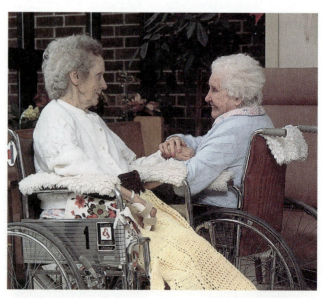

FIGURE 9-12 Most persons have a need for intimacy.

entation, preference, opportunity, and moral standards. Sexual behavior is a personal choice, but intimacy is an important aspect of the human sexual experience.

Each intimate relationship has an element of commitment. Sometimes this commitment includes a sexual aspect and sometimes it does not. For example, a loving couple may choose not to have sexual intercourse. Despite remaining celibate (no sexual intercourse), they still share an intimacy and commitment that is natural and fulfilling.

Being old, ill, or disabled does not diminish human sexuality. However, our society tends to associate youth, beauty, and physical agility with sexuality. By these standards, persons who are old or disabled are not considered to be sexual beings. It is important to remember that the person within a human being does not change. Although the hair is gray, or the body is not so agile, the person inside still has feelings and longing for love, affection, and intimacy. As a nursing assistant, there are several actions you can take to help patients maintain their sexuality:

- Give attention to the patient's grooming and appearance.
- Give sincere compliments on their appearance.
- Converse with patients on an adult level.

It is important to recognize that not everyone has the same orientation, preference, opportunities, or moral standards. This does not mean that differences make one person wrong and another right. As a caregiver, you must be understanding of others who do not share your personal views.

Some terms related to human sexual expression are:

- Heterosexuality—sexual attraction between opposite sexes.
- Homosexuality—sexual attraction between persons of the same sex. Female partners are called lesbians.
- Bisexuality—sexual attraction to members of both sexes.
- Masturbation—self-stimulation for sexual pleasure.

The range of ways to express love is enormous. Genital and nongenital caressing, exchange of loving gestures, talking, and touching are all ways love is expressed between people. Coitus (intercourse), although an enjoyable part of many relationships, is not always necessary for satisfaction.

Providing opportunities for patients to meet sexual and intimate needs in a health care setting is not always easy. However, there are some actions that nursing assistants can do to help patients meet these needs:

- Respect patients' privacy. Always knock and wait before opening a closed door.
- Speak before opening curtains drawn around the bed.
- Do not judge behaviors and preferences that are different from yours as wrong.
- Do not discuss personal sexual information about a patient with others.
- Provide privacy if a patient is masturbating.
- Discourage patients who make sexual advances to you. State in a calm, matter-of-fact way that you are not

interested and move on to other work. If a patient persists, report the matter to the nurse.
- Recognize that the need for intimacy is a basic human need that is expressed in many ways.

Human Touch

The need for human touch should not be overlooked. Pleasure and satisfaction are felt by a parent and child as they touch one another. The same human feelings are also experienced by adults.

As people grow older, they tend to reserve touching for intimate friends and family members. When circumstances change and opportunities for touching become fewer, people often feel deprived and lonely. This is especially true when one lives alone or is a resident in long-term care.

A friendly hug and smile, a pat on the shoulder, a clasp of a hand, and a backrub are ways that nursing assistants can satisfy the patient's need for human contact. Never force your attentions on a patient, but be open to nonsexual touching. It can mean much to the lives of those in your care.

Dealing with the Fearful Patient

The experienced nursing assistant does not take remarks personally. The assistant realizes that the patient's complaints and refusal to cooperate may be a way of saying, "I need to be reassured and protected." Give the patient an opportunity to talk. Listen carefully to everything that is said (Figure 9-13). You may be able to convince the fearful patient to assume some personal care whenever possible. If help in feeding, shaving, elimination, or other such personal matters is needed, act in a very gentle, efficient manner and assure the patient's privacy at all times.

To handle these situations successfully, the nursing assistant must:

- Recognize that this patient is a person with individual likes and dislikes.
- Give the quality of care that considers these likes and dislikes.

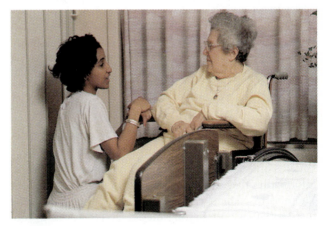

FIGURE 9-13 Successful communication is a two-way exchange.

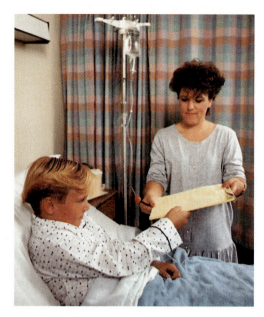

FIGURE 9-14 Activities help pass the time during convalescence.

- Help the patient find ways to fill the time while in the hospital (Figure 9-14). Boredom alone can lead to irritability. Some hospitals have volunteers who bring books and other activities directly to the bedside.

Patient Privacy

Patients in the hospital give up a good bit of control over their lives. They put their lives and well-being into the hands of caregivers. In exchange, patients assume that certain of their rights will be assured. These rights include the right to privacy.

Patients must feel certain that their privacy will be protected. Even though you perform the most intimate procedures for them, you must do so in a way that neither exposes them unnecessarily nor embarrasses them. Privacy may be provided by means of:

- Curtains or screens placed around the bed.
- Knocking and saying the patient's name before entering a room.
- Speaking to the patient before entering a screened area. Privacy must be provided for the patient who is:
  - Bathing
  - Using the bedpan
  - Receiving treatments
  - Being visited by clergy.

Be prompt at other times to recognize a patient's need for privacy and to provide it.

Patients must also be secure in knowing that personal information they share with you will not be told to others. You add to patients' sense of security if you always treat them with the courtesy you would extend to a guest in your home.

Understanding what patients are really trying to tell us is one of the most difficult parts of giving nursing care. When we are successful, it is probably the most rewarding. With this in mind, always remember to treat the patient as a unique individual.

Spiritual Needs

Spiritual beliefs are deeply held by some patients and disregarded by others. When beliefs are strongly held, they are apt to guide a patient's actions and responses in direct ways such as praying, reading religious writings, and participating in ceremonies and celebrations. Some personal items may have special religious significance and must be treated with respect.

Patients' spiritual needs are often greater when they are fearful and ill (Figure 9-15). Be prepared to act on requests for clergy visits and spiritual support. Do not impose your beliefs on the patient.

There is always the temptation to share your personal religious faith with others. This is especially true when the patient directly asks your opinion. To handle such a situation appropriately is a challenge. Here are some guidelines to assist you.

- Remember that each person has a right to believe in any faith system or to deny the existence of any beliefs.
- Listen to the patient's thoughts and keep them confidential.
- Your role is to reflect the patient's ideas. Do not try to convince the patient of your ideas. For example, if the patient asks you if you believe in God, reflect the patient's thinking with a statement such as "You have been thinking about God," or "Would you like to talk?"

The patient may want to visit with a familiar clergy member, or may ask about the chaplain or clergy service available at the health care facility.

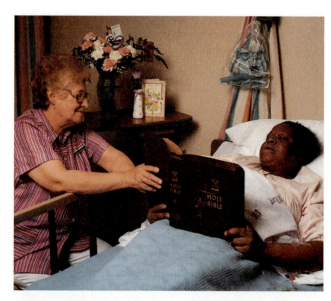

FIGURE 9-15 Spiritual needs may be greater during illness.

Some health care facilities ask clergy from the community to make visits to patients who want such a visit but who do not know a particular minister, priest, or rabbi. Larger facilities have chaplain educational residencies for people preparing for careers in the clergy. The residencies serve patients' spiritual needs while offering training for the chaplains.

Chapels are open in some facilities. Both visitors and ambulatory patients often find comfort in visiting them. Religious services are sometimes broadcast to patients' rooms from these chapels.

Know what services are available to your patients. When asked, share this information, but do not recommend any particular service. Patients should be free to make their own choices. You should always be ready and willing to support the choice.

Social Needs

When primary physical, psychological, and spiritual needs have been met, the person is free to pursue the third level of social needs and activities that are unique to the individual. These activities make one feel good as a person and increase self-esteem. They give a sense of accomplishment. Sociological needs are met by interactions with others and opportunities for free personal expression.

One of the most basic needs of all people is the need to understand others and to be understood. We achieve this sense of understanding when we communicate successfully with others. We usually try to communicate verbally. Sometimes we do this also by the:

- Words we choose
- Way we say the words
- Tone of voice
- Facial expression
- Form of touch

Even the way we stand or reach out says a lot. We know it is not always easy to find the right words to express our thoughts and feelings. Thus, caregivers must be constantly aware of the patient's need to communicate effectively, too.

Volunteers and visitors, as well as television and reading, can provide entertainment and diversion for the patient who is confined. Try to find out about your patients' special interests. Look for ways to support them in these interests.

If all care providers are interested and unhurried in talking with their patients, they make it easier for patients to say what they need. This approach also makes it easier for the staff to find proper ways to fulfill these needs.

REVIEW

A. True/False.

Mark the following true or false by circling T or F.

1. T F Growth and development go from the simple to the complex.

2. T F Body development proceeds from the head toward the feet.

3. T F All individuals move through the stages of growth.

4. T F Growth and development progression are interdependent.

5. T F Ossification of bones is not complete at birth.

6. T F The Moro reflex occurs when the infant's palm is touched.

7. T F The sucking reflex occurs when the infant is startled.

8. T F The three-month-old infant cries real tears.

9. T F The six-month-old infant can walk if well supported.

10. T F First teeth begin to erupt about the sixth month of life.

11. T F The one-year-old infant has progressed to eating table foods.

12. T F The toddler period finds children interacting freely and playing well with one another.

13. T F Between the ages of three and five years, the child seems to have an endless list of questions.

14. T F The school-aged child is interested in and chooses members of the same sex as close friends.

15. T F One of the developmental tasks of old age is to learn to deal successfully with loss.

16. T F Basic human needs are the same at all ages, but different ways must be found to satisfy them.

17. T F Erikson believed that one of the developmental tasks of infancy is learning to trust.

18. T F Erikson states that the developmental task of the middle years is to integrate life's experiences.

19. T F Patients who are fearful often behave in angry or frustrated ways.

20. T F Spiritual needs are part of basic human needs.

21. T F Culture has no influence over how basic human needs are met.

B. Matching.

Match the appropriate chronologic age to the life time period by matching Column I and Column II.

Column I	Column II
22. ____ old age	**a.** 65 years old
23. ____ adolescence	**b.** 16 years old
24. ____ later maturity	**c.** 7 years old
25. ____ school age	**d.** 35 years old
26. ____ adulthood	**e.** 80 years old

C. Multiple Choice.

Select the one best answer for each question.

27. Growth and development
    a. move from head to feet and from torso to limbs.
    b. involve continuous progression from simple to more complex actions.
    c. have a specific set of tasks that must be mastered in each stage.
    d. all of these.

28. The main activity (activities) of the toddler period is (are)
    a. exploration and investigation.
    b. cooperative play.
    c. establishing peer relationships.
    d. showing concern for others.

29. Preschoolers are
    a. less reliant on their mothers.
    b. able to join groups like Scouts.
    c. able to choose sex-differentiated friends.
    d. all of these.

30. The ways in which we react to the events in our lives are called
    a. personality.
    b. self-identity.
    c. tasks of personality development.
    d. hierarchy of needs.

D. Nursing Assistant Challenge.

Mrs. McClendon is a 35-year-old patient with a diagnosis of breast cancer. She has lost most of her hair and has no appetite as a result of chemotherapy. Mrs. McClendon has lost weight and has occasional severe pain. She has a husband and three young children. Consider the needs that all people have and think about Mrs. McClendon.

31. Which physical needs may be difficult to meet? What can the nursing staff do to help Mrs. McClendon meet these needs?

32. Do you think her need for safety and security will be met? What information do you have indicating that she has reason to feel fear and anxiety?

33. How might Mrs. McClendon's condition affect her relationship with her husband and children?

34. How do you think her sexuality may be affected?

35. Maslow states that human needs are on a hierarchy. Describe how this hierarchy may change throughout the day for Mrs. McClendon.

Developing Cultural Sensitivity

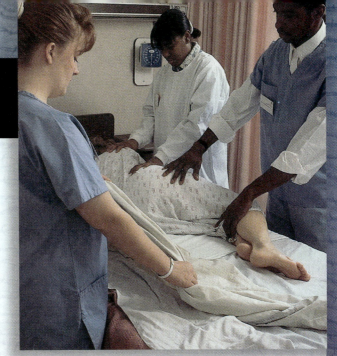

As a result of this unit, you will be able to:

- Spell and define terms.
- Name six major cultural groups in the United States.
- Describe ways the major cultures differ in their family organization, communication, need for personal space, health practices, religion, and traditions.
- List ways nursing assistants can develop sensitivity about cultures other than their own.
- State ways the nursing assistant can demonstrate appreciation of and sensitivity to other cultures.
- List ways the nursing assistant can help patients in practicing rituals appropriate to their cultures.

Learn the meaning and the correct spelling of the following words and phrases:

acupuncture	dialect	race	standard
amulet	ethnicity	ritual	stereotype
belief	mores	sensitivity	talisman
culture	personal space	spirituality	tradition

INTRODUCTION

America is a nation of people whose ancestors came primarily from other countries. Each group brought its own cultural heritage with its language, beliefs, and customs. These people are your patients. Each one is a unique individual whose development is the result of his or her own culture, current life-style and community participation, and personal experiences. As a health care provider, you are expected to show sensitivity to the individuality and cultural heritage of each patient. Sensitivity is the ability to be aware of and to appreciate the personal characteristics of others.

When members of different groups must live and work together in a community, it is easy for members of each group to form specific beliefs about the other groups. When these beliefs are rigid and are based on generalizations, they are called stereotypes. For example, others may view people of Asian heritage as present-focused (thinking about immediate rather than long-term goals), not self-expressive, and reluctant to make eye contact. These traits are stereotypes when applied to an entire group without consideration of the traditions of the group and individual characteristics. In contrast to these stereotypes, Van (whose heritage is Vietnamese) (Figure 10-1) is outgoing, looks directly at a person speaking to her, has a quick smile, and is future-oriented as she studies to become a health care provider.

Health care providers must be careful not to make assumptions about their patients based on stereotypes of the group of which the patient is a part. The longer a group is associated with the American culture, the less its members rely on the cultural values and traditions of the country of origin. Young immigrants and second- or third-generation residents of the United States are much closer to American culture than to the original culture. Older people and new immigrants tend to cling more closely to the customs of their homeland.

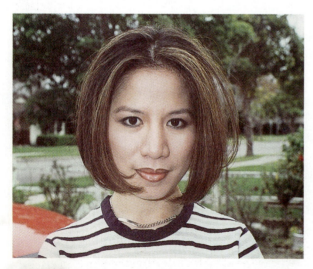

FIGURE 10-1 This young woman, whose parents were Vietnamese immigrants, has absorbed aspects of her parents' culture and the American culture in which she lives.

RACE, ETHNICITY, AND CULTURE

The terms *race, ethnicity,* and *culture* are used to describe groups of people. Race is the classification of people according to shared physical characteristics such as skin color, bone structure, facial features, hair texture, and blood type.

Ethnicity

Ethnicity refers to special groups within a race as defined by national origin and/or culture. Members of an ethnic group share common:

- Heritage
- National origin
- Social customs
- Language

Six ethnic groups predominate in the United States (see Table 10-1):

- Caucasians—those of European and Scandinavian descent
- African Americans—those of African, Haitian, or Dominican Republic descent
- Hispanics—those whose ancestors came from Spanish-speaking countries
- Asians/Pacific—those whose ancestors came from the islands and countries of the Pacific Rim
- Native Americans—those descended from one of the more than 600 tribes of North America
- Middle Easterners/Arabs—those whose ancestors came from Middle Eastern countries

Culture

Culture refers to the way a particular group views the world and the set of traditions that are passed on from generation to generation. Culture enforces the standards (rules) established by the group based on the values and beliefs of the group. Cultural differences among ethnic groups include:

- Family organization
- Personal space needs
- Communication
- Beliefs about health/illness and health care practices
- Religions
- Traditions

Cultural mores (customs) influence the way people will interact. Ethnicity and culture contribute to an individual's sense of self-identity as he or she relates to the group and to other cultures. Cross-cultural nursing recognizes the individual within an ethnic and cultural group and provides nursing care that assures cultural as well as individual acceptance and comfort.

Family Organization. Families form the basic cultural social groups, but their structure varies from culture to cul-

TABLE 10-1 MAJOR ETHNIC GROUPS IN AMERICA

Group	Some Countries and Areas of Origin	
Caucasian	England, Scotland, Ireland, Poland, Scandinavia, Italy, Russia	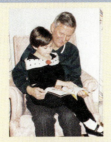
African American	Africa, Haiti, Jamaica, Dominican Republic	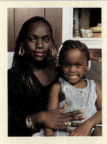
Hispanic	Cuba, Puerto Rico, Mexico, Latin and South America	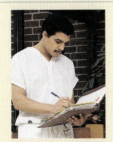
Asian/ Pacific	China, Japan, Philippines, Vietnam, Cambodia, Korea, Hawaii, Samoa	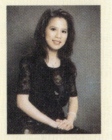
Native American	Hundreds of tribes, such as Cherokee, Apache, Navajo, Blackfoot, Inuit (Alaskan)	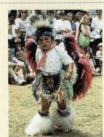
Middle Eastern	Egypt, Iran, Yemen, Palestine, Lebanon, Jordan, Saudi Arabia, Kuwait	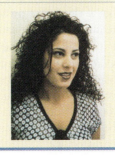

ture. The family organization determines who will be the decision makers and who is responsible for providing health care. In some families, the father or oldest male is the authority figure. In others, both the mother and father make decisions. In Hispanic and Middle Eastern families, the father is the dominant person, whereas in many African American households the mother has the strongest influence. In Caucasian families, the highest wage earner is often given the greatest respect and authority.

Health care may be a family responsibility. Figure 10-2A shows an extended family and Figure 10-2B a nuclear family. For example, in Asian families the elderly are given great respect, and caring for them is considered a duty and privilege by all family members. In Asian, Hispanic, and Native American cultures, extended families are common, and may include grandparents, aunts, and uncles. In these cases, caregiving is personal and shared by family members. Caucasian families tend to be structured as more independent units consisting of mother, father, and children. In this case, care of the elderly is more likely to be given over to others.

Personal Space Needs. **Personal space** refers to the actual physical closeness that one person is comfortable with during social interaction with others. Personal space can be invaded by standing too close to another person, patterns of eye contact, and touching.

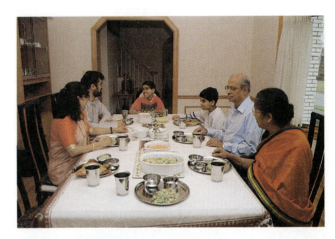

FIGURE 10-2A An extended family

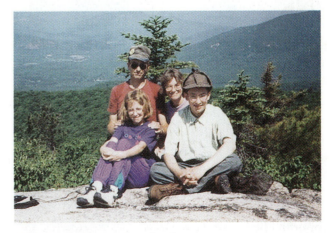

FIGURE 10-2B A nuclear family

TABLE 10-2 PERSONAL SPACE IS INTERPRETED DIFFERENTLY BY PEOPLE OF DIFFERENT CULTURES

Culture	Definition of Personal Space	Eye Contact
American	About 3 feet	Yes
Asian	Close, no contact	No
African American	Close	Yes
European	Distant	Yes
Native American	Distant	No
Hispanic	Close	Yes

Caucasians prefer to stand and speak at a distance of about 18 inches from one another. African Americans are comfortable standing closer to another person (5 to 10 inches). Space is important to Native Americans but has no specific boundaries. Asians tend to be uncomfortable if standing too close to another person.

Eye contact travels through the visual personal space and is interpreted differently by different cultures (Table 10-2). Asians consider eye contact inappropriate. The averted eyes and shifting gaze perceived as respectful in Asian cultures may be interpreted by Americans as inattention or insincerity. Members of Hispanic cultures make direct eye contact when speaking but consider prolonged contact disrespectful. The direct eye contact of Caucasians and African Americans may be considered an invasion of visual space by an Asian patient.

Touching a person is considered an invasion of personal space in some cultures. A handshake is traditional in the United States for both men and women. In Middle Eastern

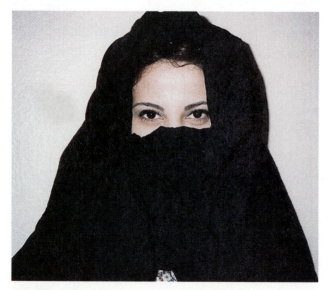

FIGURE 10-3 Traditional Muslim culture requires that women be completely veiled from head to toe.

countries, however, only men may greet other men in this manner. Greeting with handshakes and hugs is common in Hispanic cultures. Persons from Asian cultures are less likely to shake hands, especially with women.

Touching the body of another person may be even more restricted than the touching of hands in greeting. In Middle Eastern countries, men may not touch females who are not members of their immediate family. Uncovering the body is considered disrespectful in some cultures and is forbidden for women in others. For example, Muslim women may be completely veiled (Figure 10-3). Uncovering the shoulders of a person from India may be considered disrespectful. The mode of dress and body covering is very important to an individual's modesty. In some cultures, caregivers cannot care for members of the opposite sex.

As you care for patients from cultures other than your own, remember that the customs of the individual's culture greatly influence the acceptance of the person giving care and how the care is given, the amount of disrobing that is permitted, and the degree of touch that is comfortable for and accepted by the patient. Ask the nurse for guidance. You can also learn much about the patient's desires by watching the interactions of the patient with his or her family and with other staff members.

Communication. Touching and eye contact are nonverbal forms of communication. A common verbal language is one characteristic of an ethnic group. Silence may be an important part of the language. For example, some Native American groups consider silence to be essential to understanding. Silence does not always mean that the listener has not heard or is inattentive to the speaker.

An ethnic group may share a common language, but local terminology and usage may vary (a **dialect**). For example, Hispanic Americans may have originated in Puerto Rico, Mexico, Cuba, or Central or South America. The basic language of all of these people is Spanish, but there are many dialects depending on the country of origin or even a portion of a country. The Spanish you speak may differ in certain ways from the Spanish your patients speak.

Patients may be bilingual and speak both their native language and English. Some of your patients, however, may have only a minimal understanding of English. Older people and the newest immigrants will be most comfortable communicating in their own language. The desire to return to that which is familiar and most comfortable is especially important when people are ill or frightened. Communicating in a patient's own language adds greatly to his or her sense of security. It is helpful to have an interpreter present, but if this is not possible, some form of communication is required if good nursing care is to be given.

Patients are pleased when a caregiver can speak even a few words in the patient's own language. If many of your patients share a common language, it would be helpful for you to learn some common words and phrases. Remember, too, that body language, gestures, and facial expression can be used to express thoughts and words when verbal language is inadequate.

When communicating:

- Use a normal tone.
- Speak slowly.
- Use simple words.
- Look directly at the listener even if someone is interpreting (be sensitive to any discomfort this may cause the patient because of cultural variations).
- Try to obtain feedback from the patient to determine the level of understanding.

You may wish to go back to Unit 7 to review other ways to communicate.

Beliefs About Health, Illness, and Health Care Practices.

Beliefs are based on commonly held opinions, knowledge, and attitudes about the world and life. These beliefs will influence the person's feelings about illness and the kind of health care he will choose. Members of a culture share beliefs about:

- The nature and cause of illness
- Types of health care practices
- Their relationship to a higher power

People tend to view the causes of health and illness in one of three ways, or in a combination of these ways. Some people hold magical beliefs, in which the causes of illness are supernatural forces. Others hold scientific beliefs, relating health and illness to causes such as infectious agents, the wear and tear on the body caused by daily living and stress, environmental agents, or injury. Still others have holistic beliefs that view the person and the environment as continuously exchanging energy and matter with one another. In this belief system, the mind and body must be in harmony to ensure health.

Those who believe that illness and pain are a penance from a higher power, as punishment for wrongdoing, will be less willing to complain of suffering and to seek relief through medication and scientific medicine. They rely more on the use of charms, chants or holy words, and rituals. Some cultures turn to folk healers or shamans to help bring their bodies back into balance with nature. They believe that the imbalance is the cause of their discomfort. The balance is achieved by eating certain foods, taking natural medicines, or through the power of healing ceremonies.

Those who see illness as the result of environmental factors, infectious agents, or injury are more likely to seek scientifically based medical help. Asian cultures, which have traditional health and illness beliefs, use traditional medications such as herbs, acupuncture (placement of metal needles in the body), and mind-body practices such as tai chi and meditation to achieve balance and wellness.

Arabs who believe that some illnesses are the "Will of Allah" use amulets (charms against evil) and verses from the Koran (a holy book) written on turquoise stones to help them. Native Americans believe illness develops when the harmony between body, mind, and spirit is disrupted. Sand paintings are used in healing rituals to diagnose conditions and prescribe treatment. Hispanics believe that illness is caused when an imbalance exists in the four body fluids. They may use native healers, candles, prayers, and the wearing of medals as methods of treatment and to restore balance. Hot and cold conditions (illnesses) are identified and "hot" and "cold" foods and medicines, similar to those recognized in Asian cultures, are used in treatment. Cold remedies are given to balance a hot condition and vice versa. See Table 10-3 for hot and cold conditions and remedies. Table 10-4 lists some of the common belief systems related to health and illness.

Religious Practices.

Spirituality is the part of a person that gives a sense of wholeness by fulfilling the human need to feel connected with the world around one and to a power greater than oneself. For many, spirituality is expressed in religious practice. *Religion* is an organized system of belief in a deity (higher power). Spirituality and religion are products of an individual's cultural background and experience. Spiritual values and religious beliefs form the rules of what a person considers to be right or wrong.

Religious beliefs provide a person with guidelines for moral behavior. Religious preferences are highly personal and can

TABLE 10-3 HOT AND COLD CONDITIONS AND REMEDIES

Hot Conditions	Cold Conditions
Constipation	Cancer
Fever	Colds
Infections	Headache
Sore throat	Pneumonia
Ulcers	Tuberculosis
Cold Food Remedies	**Hot Food Remedies**
Dairy products	Cereals
Milk	Eggs
Lima beans	Beef
Vegetables	Oils
Honey	Spicy foods
Chicken	Wine
Raisins	
Cold Medical Remedies	**Hot Medical Remedies**
Bicarbonate of soda	Aspirin
Milk of magnesia	Cinnamon
Orange flower water	Cod liver oil
Sage	Garlic
	Penicillin

TABLE 10-4 BELIEF SYSTEMS RELATED TO HEALTH/ILLNESS

Culture	Related Concepts	Health Care Provider	Cause of Illness	Methods of Treatment
European Americans	Illness is not superficial, but can be influenced by poor health practices; disease is treatable and sometimes curable	Physician	• Punishment for sins • Self-abuse; outside forces such as germs	Diet, exercise, home remedies, medication, surgery, religious rituals, wearing amulets
Asian Americans	Body has two energy forces: *yang*, which is cold, and *yin*, which is hot (hot and cold do not refer to temperature); hot conditions are treated with cold foods and treatments; cold conditions are treated with hot foods and treatments	Traditional healers	• Imbalance between the positive (yang) energy and the negative (yin) energy that are found in the body • Overexertion	Herbs, hot foods for conditions associated with yin conditions and cold foods for conditions associated with yang conditions; home remedies and folk medicines
Hispanic Americans	Body contains four humors (fluids) that need to be balanced. Illness develops from imbalance. Humors are blood (hot, moist), phlegm (cold, moist), black bile (cold, dry), yellow bile (hot, dry)	Native healers (Jerbero, Curandera)	• Punishment from God for sins	Candles, prayers, wearing medals, hot and cold foods to restore balance of humors
Native Americans	Spiritual powers control body's energy; harmony must exist between body, mind, and spirit; illness results when harmony is disrupted	Medicine man, shaman	• Violation of taboo • Attack by witch or evil spirits • Do not believe in germ theory	Sandpanting to diagnose condition and determine treatment; elaborate rituals; carrying medicine bundles; wearing masks to hide from evil spirits
African Americans	Body, mind, and spirit must be in harmony for health; life is a process rather than a state; illness can occur if self-care is not taken	Folk practitioners, root workers	• Punishment from God • Spirits and demons	Prayer, diet, home remedies, wearing copper and silver bracelets, wearing talismans and amulets
Islamic Americans	Magico-religious; emotional distress; expressed as "heart disease"; feel responsible to visit and help ill; the individual has no control over life events, as good and evil usually are result of "Will of Allah"; male-dominated society with male children more highly valued than female children; may use female circumcision to ensure faithfulness and be accepted by the women; may resist medical direction	Traditional healers; physicians	Will of Allah; punishment for sins; various beliefs in causes such as imbalance of hot and cold; influence of an "Evil Eye"	Magico-religious; prayer; self-care and medical science; use amulets inscribed with verses from the Koran; turquoise stones; charm of a hand with five fingers to protect against the evil eye; male health professionals prohibited from touching or examining females; males may refuse health care from females

vary within a given culture. For example, Hispanics are traditionally Roman Catholic. However, it is not unusual to find a Protestant church of Hispanics in the same community. The major religions of the United States include:

● Protestantism (various denominations)
● Roman Catholicism
● Judaism
● Islam
● Hinduism

Religious items and **rituals** (solemn and ceremonial acts that reinforce faith) are especially meaningful to practitioners. They must be treated with respect. For example, the crucifix, Bible, and religious medals are important to Roman Catholics. The prayer rug is significant to the Islamic, who pray five times each day in the direction of their holy city, Mecca. Amulets and special charms are important to the religious beliefs of Native Americans and to some peoples in the Middle East. **Talismans** are engraved stones, rings, or other objects that are used to ward off evil. Copper or silver bracelets and religious medals are important and sacred to some cultures.

If a patient requests a visit from clergy, be sure the request is promptly given to the nurse. When the clergy visits, be sure to provide privacy. It is also important to provide privacy when the patient is engaged in a religious act such as praying. Table 10-5 lists five religious faiths common in the United States and some of their beliefs and religious items. Special religious rituals and practices related to dying, death, and care of the body after death are discussed in Unit 30.

Foods are important in some religions. For example, those of the Orthodox Jewish faith may not be served milk and meat products at the same time. Roman Catholics restrict food intake on specific dates and some Baptists, Muslims, and others are not permitted to drink alcohol. Other food restrictions are discussed in Unit 25.

An understanding of some of the major belief systems will help you be more sensitive to your patient's needs. You can support your patient's spirituality and religious practices by:

- Being a willing listener
- Respecting the patient's belief system
- Never trying to convert the patient to your belief system
- Respecting religious symbols
- Not interrupting during religious rituals
- Reading aloud the patient's favorite passages from religious books such as the Bible, Talmud, Koran, or Book of Mormon
- Providing privacy during prayers and meditation or when clergy visits

TRADITIONS

Traditions are customs and practices followed by members of a culture and passed from generation to generation. Often traditions are related to religious rituals and holiday celebrations. Foods are particularly traditional at holidays. Think about ham at Easter, corned beef and cabbage on St. Patrick's Day, and traditional tacos, tamales, and enchiladas on Cinco de Mayo.

Families carry out traditions from generation to generation. For example, it is a Chinese tradition to have a celebration accompanied by a colorful procession with a dragon to welcome in the Chinese New Year. People all over America watch fireworks to celebrate the Fourth of July. Holidays specific to cultures are celebrated each year.

Many traditions involve the coming to maturity of young people and are related to religious practice. For example, young Jewish boys have a bar mitzvah as they reach puberty. Many Protestant churches present Bibles to children when they are in the third grade of school and are able to read on their own.

Honoring and practicing traditions gives people a sense of stability and continuity. Traditions help to bind the people of a culture closer together.

Nursing assistants have a unique opportunity to learn about other cultures directly from their patients. There are ways to make this process easier for yourself and your patient (see the following guidelines). Always remember that even though a person is part of an identifiable culture, he or she must always be recognized as an individual within the culture.

TABLE 10-5 SOME COMMON BELIEF SYSTEMS (RELIGIOUS)

Religion	Belief in a Deity	Value of Prayer	Belief in Hereafter	Special Practices or Symbols
Protestant	Yes	Important	Yes	Baptism, Holy Communion, cross, Bible
Roman Catholic	Yes	Important	Yes	Baptism, Holy Communion, Anointing the Sick, Reconciliation, Bible, medals, pictures and statues of saints, rosaries, crucifix
Orthodox Judaism	Yes	Important	Yes	Torah, yarmulke (cap), tallith, menorah
Hinduism	Yes (many forms)	Important	Yes	No sacraments
Buddhism	Yes	Important	Yes	No sacraments
Moslems (Islam)	Yes	Important	Yes	Koran, prayer rug

Within the framework of each belief system, there are individual differences in the depth of belief and extent of practice.

GUIDELINES
for

Developing Cultural Sensitivity

- Review your own belief systems.
- Consider how your own culture influences your behavior.
- Always view patients as individuals within a culture.
- Recognize that patients are a combination of heritage, culture, and community.
- Understand that culture influences how people behave and interact with others.
- Remember that personal space needs, eye contact, and ways of communicating are often culturally related.

- Check with the supervisor to learn special ways to deal with patients of different cultural backgrounds.
- Care for religious articles with respect.
- Provide privacy when a spiritual advisor is visiting the patient or the patient is practicing a devotional act.
- Try to learn about the practices, beliefs, and cultural heritage of the people who are most likely to be your patients. A library and the Internet are good sources.
- Ask patients politely about practices that are unfamiliar.
- Attend staff development classes designed to promote cultural sensitivity.

REVIEW

A. Matching.

Match each word with its definition.

1. _____ amulet
2. _____ mores
3. _____ sensitivity
4. _____ standard
5. _____ tradition

a. rules of conduct
b. charms against evil
c. passed from generation to generation
d. awareness and appreciation of
e. customs

B. Completion.

Complete the following sentences by choosing the correct word.

6. Rigid, biased ideas about people are called _____.

   (stereotypes) (characteristics)

7. Classification by shared physical characteristics is based on _____.

   (ethnicity) (race)

8. The way a group views the world, and the group's traditions, are the foundation of a _____.

   (race) (culture)

9. Commonly held opinions, knowledge, and attitudes about life are called _____.

   (standards) (beliefs)

10. Solemn and ceremonial acts that reinforce faith are called _____.

    (rituals) (traditions)

C. Multiple Choice.

Select the one best answer for each question.

11. The cultural language common to most Hispanics is
    a. English.
    b. French.
    c. Spanish.
    d. German.

12. You may expect that a new black immigrant was born in
    a. Egypt.
    b. Haiti.
    c. China.
    d. Poland.

13. The nuclear family is most commonly seen in
    a. African American culture.
    b. Asian culture.
    c. Hispanic culture.
    d. Caucasian culture.

14. Caucasians prefer to stand and speak about
    a. six inches apart.
    b. eighteen inches.
    c. three feet apart.
    d. five feet apart.

15. A Middle Eastern man may greet another man by
    a. nodding.
    b. shaking hands.
    c. kissing on either cheek.
    d. none of the above.

16. Your patient has a prayer rug and prays five times a day. You believe he is from which culture?

    a. Middle Eastern

    b. African American

    c. Asian

    d. Native American

17. Your Asian patient looks down and says little when you speak. This is

    a. rude in his culture.

    b. respectful in his culture.

    c. his way of showing his anger.

    d. his way of showing fear.

18. Your patient makes direct and prolonged eye contact as you speak. He probably is of what culture?

    a. Asian

    b. Native American

    c. Hispanic

    d. Caucasian

19. Your patient speaks only a few words of English. When you speak to him, you should

    a. raise your voice.

    b. speak slowly.

    c. use slang.

    d. look away.

20. Sand painters help diagnose illness in which culture?

    a. Asian

    b. Hispanic

    c. Native American

    d. African American

D. Short Answer.

21. You have a Catholic patient. Briefly explain how you can show sensitivity to her religious beliefs.

22. Name your own culture. List two traditions that are common to your culture.

23. List two ways you can improve your cultural sensitivity to a new patient who has a culture different from your own.

E. Nursing Assistant Challenge.

You have a patient who is a new immigrant from Iran. He is Islamic and 60 years old. Mark the following true or false.

24. T F The Torah is his holy book.

25. T F He will wish to pray once daily.

26. T F He will be the person most likely to make his own medical decisions.

27. T F He probably feels his condition is due to the "Will of Allah."

28. T F He would celebrate Easter and Christmas if he were at home.

Infection and Infection Control

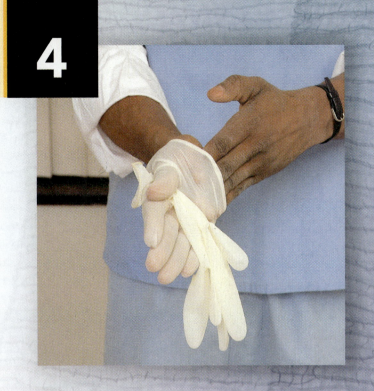

UNIT 11
Infection

UNIT 12
Infection Control

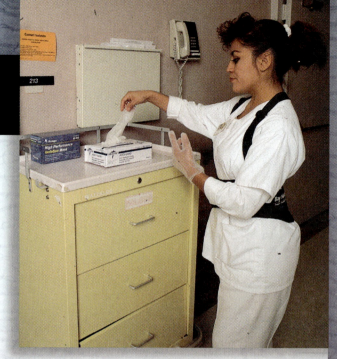

UNIT 11

Infection

See Appendix (page 667) for additional information

As a result of this unit, you will be able to:

- Spell and define terms.
- Identify the most common microbes and describe some of their characteristics.
- Define infectious disease.
- Name five serious infectious diseases.
- Identify the causes of several important infectious diseases.
- List the ways that infectious diseases are spread.
- List the steps of the chain of infection.
- Describe common treatments for infectious disease.
- List natural body defenses against infections.
- Explain why patients are at risk for infections.

VOCABULARY

Learn the meaning and the correct spelling of the following words and phrases:

acquired immune	contamination	incubation	risk factor
deficiency syndrome	culture and sensitivity	infection	seropositive
(AIDS)	diplo-	infectious	source
airborne transmission	droplet transmission	inflammation	spirillum, spirilla
allergy	dysentery	methicillin-resistant	staphylo-
antibiotic	flora	*Staphylococcus aureus*	strepto-
antibody	fomites	microbe	toxin
antigen	fungus, fungi	microorganism	transmission
bacillus, bacilli	hemoptysis	mold	tubercle
bacteremia	hepatitis	nonpathogen	tuberculosis disease
bacterium, bacteria	host	organism	tuberculosis infection
carrier	human	parasite	vaccine
causative agent	immunodeficiency	pathogen	vancomycin-resistant
chain of infection	virus (HIV)	phagocyte	enterococci
coccus, cocci	immune response	portal of entry	vector
colony	immunity	portal of exit	virus
contact transmission	immunization	protozoan, protozoa	yeast
contagious	immunosuppression	reservoir	

INTRODUCTION

Humans are surrounded by a world of tiny **organisms** (living beings). These beings cannot be seen with the naked eye. They make their presence known only by their effect. This is much the same way we become aware of the wind. We cannot see it, but we do see its effect on the trees, which bend and sway.

These organisms can be seen only with a microscope. They are everywhere—in us, on us, and around us. They are:

- On our skin
- In our mouths
- Within our bodies
- In and on the food we eat
- On what we touch or handle

Micro means small. Because these organisms (agents) are so tiny, they are called **microorganisms** or **microbes**. The organisms live in relationship with us and with each other.

Many of these microbes are useful to us. They are called **nonpathogens** because they do not produce disease. They help in the

- Processing of cheese, beer, and yogurt
- Curing of leather
- Baking of bread

Other microbes are not useful. Microbes that cause disease in humans are called **pathogens** or pathogenic organisms. Pathogens grow best:

- At body temperature
- Where light is limited
- Where there is moisture
- Where there is a food supply
- Where oxygen needs can be met

Infections occur when the pathogens invade the body and cause disease.

MICROBES

There are many different types of microbes, many of which are pathogenic to human beings. Microbes are classified as:

- Bacteria
- Viruses
- Fungi
- Protozoa

Bacteria

Bacteria (singular: **bacterium**) are simple one-celled microbes. They are named according to their shapes and arrangement. They cause infections in the skin, respiratory tract, urinary tract, and bloodstream.

Shapes. In the following list, the first term is the singular form of the word. The word in parentheses is the plural form.

- **Coccus** (**cocci**)—round or spherical (Figure 11-1)
- **Bacillus** (**bacilli**)—straight rod (Figure 11-2)
- **Spirillum** (**spirilla**)—spiral, corkscrew, or slightly curved (Figure 11-3)

Arrangements. Bacteria grow in groups called **colonies**. If we look at a small part of a colony under a microscope, we see that the bacteria typically are arranged in pairs, clusters, or chains.

- Single
- Pairs (**diplo-**)
- Chains (**strepto-**)
- Clusters (**staphylo-**)

The shape and group arrangement of bacteria are important factors in their identification. For example, round microorganisms grouped in chains are called streptococci. A very important member of this family is the *Streptococcus hemolyticus.* It causes septic sore throat and rheumatic fever.

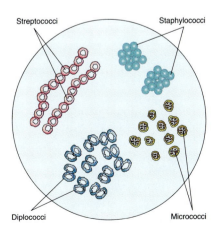

FIGURE 11-1 Forms of cocci

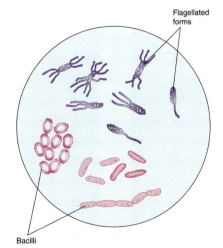

FIGURE 11-2 Forms of bacilli

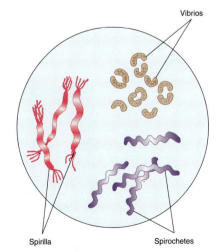

FIGURE 11-3 Spiral forms of bacteria

Round organisms grouped in a cluster are called staphylococci. An example of this family is *Staphylococcus aureus*. Staphylococci cause many infections such as:

- Surgical wound infections
- Abscesses
- Boils
- Toxic shock

Round organisms in pairs are called diplococci. A diplococcus, the *Neisseria gonorrheae* (Figure 11-4) causes gonorrhea.

Fungi

Two groups of **fungi** (singular: **fungus**) are most commonly associated with infection in humans:

- **Yeasts**—single-celled budding forms of a fungus. Yeast can infect areas of the body such as:
  - Mouth/vagina: *Candida albicans*
  - Skin: *Tinea capitis* (ringworm)
  - Feet: *Tinea pedis* (athlete's foot)
- **Molds**—A common mold that can cause infection in the lungs of humans is *Aspergillus*

Yeasts and molds are known as opportunistic parasites. (A **parasite** is an organism that lives in or on another organism without benefiting the host organism.) Under normal conditions, the organisms are harmless. However, when the human immune system is impaired and unable to protect the body, these organisms can invade the body and cause severe infections. For example, a patient with AIDS is very susceptible to fungal infections because the immune system is not working properly.

Viruses

A **virus** is the smallest microbe and has a variety of shapes. Ways viruses are classified include:

- Type of nucleic acid core (DNA or RNA)
- Clinical properties

Common viral infections include:

- Hepatitis (Figure 11-5)
- Herpes
- Acquired immune deficiency syndrome (AIDS)
- Chickenpox

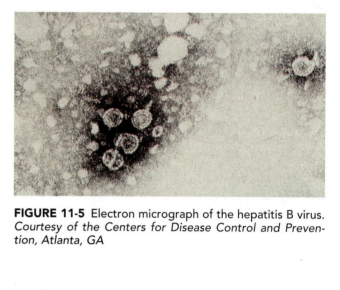

FIGURE 11-5 Electron micrograph of the hepatitis B virus. *Courtesy of the Centers for Disease Control and Prevention, Atlanta, GA*

- Influenza (Figure 11-6)
- Common cold
- Measles
- Mumps

Protozoa

Protozoa (singular: **protozoan**) are simple one-celled organisms that live on living matter (Figure 11-7). These organisms have a true nucleus. They are classified by the way in which they move. For example, some move by whiplike tails, others by hairlike projections. They cause diseases such as:

- Malaria
- Toxoplasmosis
- African sleeping sickness
- Amebiasis

Some signs and symptoms of diseases caused by protozoa include:

- Diarrhea
- **Dysentery** (infection in the lower bowel)
- Inflammation of the brain (encephalitis)

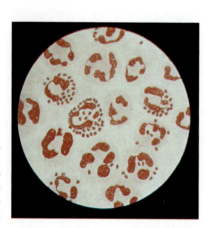

FIGURE 11-4 *Neisseria gonorrheae. Courtesy of the Centers for Disease Control and Prevention, Atlanta, GA*

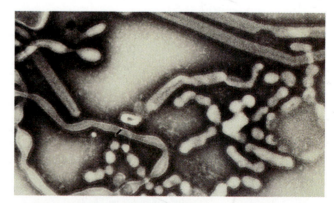

FIGURE 11-6 Electron micrograph of the influenza A virus, early passage. *Courtesy of the Centers for Disease Control and Prevention, Atlanta, GA*

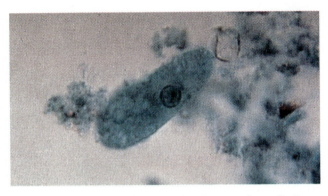

FIGURE 11-7 Intestinal protozoan *Entamoeba coli. Courtesy of the Centers for Disease Control and Prevention, Atlanta, GA*

THE CHAIN OF INFECTION

Infections occur when certain conditions exist. These conditions are called the **chain of infection** (Figure 11-8) and include:

- Causative agent (pathogens) that causes the disease
- Reservoir or source (human body in which the pathogen can live)
- Portal of exit (manner in which the pathogen leaves the body)
- Method or mode of transmission (manner in which the pathogen is carried to another person)
- Portal of entry (manner in which the pathogen enters another person)
- Susceptible host (a person who will become ill from the entry of pathogens into the body)

Pathogens cause disease by entering the body through a portal of entry. They spread disease to others by leaving the body through a portal of exit and being transmitted to another person. They enter that person's body and can again cause disease.

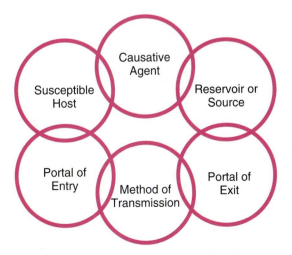

FIGURE 11-8 The chain of infection

Pathogens enter and leave the body through body openings such as:

- Eyes, ears, nose, or mouth
- Breaks in the skin
- Penis, vagina, urinary meatus (bladder opening), or rectum

Causative Agent

The **causative agent** is the microorganism that can produce the disease process in humans. The most common biological agents of infectious disease are:

- Bacteria
- Viruses
- Fungi
- Protozoa

Reservoir

The **reservoir** or **source** is where the pathogens can survive. They may or may not multiply in the reservoir. The four most common reservoirs are:

1. Humans—active cases and carriers
2. Animals
3. Environment
4. **Fomites**—objects that become **contaminated** with infectious material that contains the microbe. Fomites are anything that comes in direct contact with the excretions or secretions of an infected person. This includes:
   - Bedpans and urinals
   - Linens
   - Instruments
   - Containers with specimens for laboratory analysis

In the health care setting, the reservoirs include the:

- Patient
- Health care workers
- Environment
- Equipment

Human Reservoirs. The two major human reservoirs are cases and carriers.

- Cases—people with acute illness including obvious signs and symptoms. An example is a person with chickenpox.
- **Carriers**—those who have and transmit the disease organisms but do not have symptoms and do not display evidence of the disease. Chronic (sustained or intermittent) carriers can spread the disease without being recognized because the illness is not apparent. Another type of carrier is one in whom the organisms are multiplying (**incubating**) before signs and symptoms develop.

Specific diseases can persist in humans for an indefinite period of time, such as salmonella, hepatitis B, AIDS, and typhoid.

Portals of Entry or Exit

Portals of Entry. Organisms enter the body through the following portals of entry:

- Breaks in the skin or mucous membranes—Many organisms that are part of the normal flora, such as staphylococci, enter through breaks in the skin.
- Respiratory tract—Organisms causing the common cold and many childhood communicable diseases (such as mumps and measles) may enter this way.
- Genitourinary tract—Organisms that cause syphilis, AIDS, gonorrhea, and other sexually transmitted diseases enter this way.
- Gastrointestinal tract—Salmonellosis, typhoid fever, and hepatitis A are examples of diseases caused by organisms that enter the digestive tract.
- Circulatory system—Malaria, yellow fever, and meningitis are diseases that can enter the body directly into the blood through the bite of insects.
- Transplacental (mother to fetus) (AIDS and hepatitis B).

Portals of Exit. Infectious organisms leave the reservoir of the host through body secretions (portals of exit), including:

- Excretions of the respiratory tract (sputum) or genital tract (semen or vaginal excretions)
- Draining wounds
- Urine
- Feces
- Blood
- Saliva
- Tears

In infected persons, these products must be considered infectious or capable of transmitting the disease agent.

Transmission of Disease

Transmission (spread) of infectious organisms may happen in one of three ways (Table 11-1):

- **Airborne transmission.** Small particles remain suspended in the air and move with air currents, or become trapped in dust, which is also carried in air currents. The patient breathes in pathogens carried in this manner.
- **Droplet transmission.** Droplets are moist particles from coughing, sneezing, talking, laughing, or singing. Pathogens are transmitted into the air with the droplets. Droplets usually travel only three feet from the source.
- **Contact transmission.** Direct contact occurs with a person who is the source of the pathogens. Indirect contact occurs when a person touches an item contaminated with pathogens, such as soiled linen.

Not all organisms are transmitted in the same way, and some organisms may be transmitted in more than one way.

Host

The person who harbors infectious organisms is called a host. This person does not have enough resistance to the infectious agent. An infection develops in the host when infectious organisms:

- Penetrate the body
- Begin to multiply
- Cause damage to the host

Risk Factors. Specific characteristics about a person make him or her more or less likely to develop an infection. These characteristics are called risk factors and include:

- Number and strength of the infectious organisms
- General health of the individual
- Age, sex, and heredity of the individual
- Condition of the person's immune system

Emotional stress and fatigue also play a role in the progress of an infectious disease.

TABLE 11-1 WAYS IN WHICH MICROBES ARE SPREAD FROM ONE PERSON TO OTHERS

Airborne Transmission
- Pathogens carried by moisture or dust particles in air; can be carried long distances

Droplet Transmission
- Droplet spread within approximately 3 feet (no personal contact) or infected person by:
  - Coughing
  - Sneezing
  - Talking
  - Laughing
  - Singing

Contact Transmission
- Direct contact with infected person:
  - Touching
  - Sexual contact
  - Blood
  - Body fluids (drainage, urine, feces, sputum, saliva, vomitus)

- Indirect contact with infected person:
  - Clothing
  - Dressings
  - Equipment used in care and treatment
  - Bed linens
  - Personal belongings
  - Specimen containers
  - Instruments used in treatment
  - Food
  - Water

See Appendix

Note that pathogens can also be carried by insects and animals (**vectors**) and passed to humans.

TYPES OF INFECTIONS

Infections can be:

- Local (confined to one area)—such as a boil or skin abscess
- Generalized—such as pneumonia (in the lungs)
- Systemic—widespread through the bloodstream (**bacteremia**)

People who have pathogens in their bodies, but do not show signs of disease, are called *carriers*. Carriers can transmit diseases to others. The pathogens in these persons' bodies are not harmful to the carriers, but they may be harmful to other people.

BODY FLORA

Different microbes live on our body surfaces. These microbes are called the normal body **flora**. The flora are not the same in all body areas. For example, the organisms making up the flora of the intestinal tract are different from those of the respiratory tract. Healthy individuals live in harmony with the normal body flora. However, the balance may be disturbed by:

- Pathogenic organisms
- Normal flora organisms that become pathogenic
- Flora from one area that are transferred into a different body area
- Drugs such as antibiotics that upset the normal balance of organisms within a flora, allowing one group to flourish

When the organisms of one normal flora, such as those in the intestinal tract, remain within their normal environment, the body functions properly. However, when microbes from the intestines are transferred into the urinary tract, a serious urinary tract infection can result. Organisms that are nonpathogenic in their own environment may become pathogenic when they enter a different environment.

HOW PATHOGENS AFFECT THE BODY

The potential for infection depends on the risk factors listed previously. Two major factors are the susceptibility of the host and the amount of infectious agent that finds a portal of entry into the host. Even then an infection may not occur unless all elements of the chain of infection are present.

Microbes act in different ways to produce disease in the human body. Some pathogens:

- Attack and destroy the cells they invade. For example, the microscopic protozoan that causes malaria invades the red blood cells and eventually causes them to split. The person experiences chills and fever.
- Produce poisons called **toxins** that harm the body. For example, the tetanus organism produces toxins that travel to and damage the nervous system.

- Cause sensitivity responses called **allergies**. For example, the person may have a runny nose and watery eyes but no rise in temperature. This same response occurs when pollens or dust irritate the respiratory membranes.

BODY DEFENSES

The body has some natural defenses to protect it from infections. There are several natural external defenses. The most important of these is the skin. Intact skin acts as a mechanical barrier against the entry of pathogens. Other defenses include:

- Mucous membranes lining the respiratory, reproductive, gastrointestinal, and urinary tracts. The mucus is sticky and traps foreign materials before they can cause damage.
- Cilia (fine microscopic hairs) lining the respiratory tract propel the mucus and trapped microbes out of the body.
- Coughing and sneezing remove foreign materials from the respiratory tract.
- Hydrochloric acid, a strong chemical that is produced in the stomach, destroys many microbes.
- Eyes are protected by tears that provide a flushing action to remove most microbes that enter the eyes.

The body also has a number of internal defenses against infectious agents, including:

- Fever.
- Special cells in the blood called **phagocytes** that destroy microbes.
- **Inflammation**—a process that brings blood and phagocytes to the area of infection (Figure 11-9). A skin infection, for example, generally becomes swollen, hot, and painful, signs that inflammation is occurring.

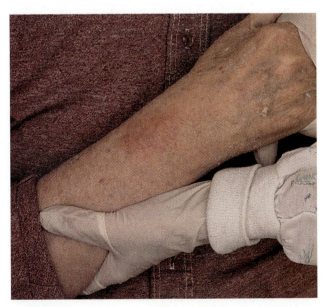

FIGURE 11-9 Redness, swelling, heat, pain, and loss of function are signs of the inflammatory process.

- Temperature—an elevated temperature is believed to increase the body's ability to fight infection.
- Immune response—the body develops protective proteins after having an infectious disease.

IMMUNITY

Immunity is the ability to fight off disease caused by microbes. A pathogenic microbe that enters the body is an antigen. In response to this, the blood develops substances called antibodies. These antibodies provide immunity (resistance) to the disease caused by that particular antigen. For example, if an individual has had antigens in the bloodstream from measles, he or she will form antibodies in the blood that prevent the occurrence of measles a second time.

IMMUNIZATIONS

Artificial defenses called immunizations protect against specific pathogens. Immunization is provided by vaccines. These are artificial or weakened antigens that help the body develop protective antibodies before the need arises. Vaccines are available to prevent most childhood diseases, such as measles, rubella (German measles), meningitis, mumps, polio, diphtheria, chickenpox, whooping cough, and tetanus. Pneumonia vaccine and influenza vaccine are frequently given to elderly people. Health workers who have direct contact with patients are advised to take hepatitis B vaccine. Federal legislation requires that employers provide this vaccine without charge to employees who are considered at risk.

Table 11-2 shows the immunizations for health care providers as recommended by the U.S. Public Health Services Advisory Committee in Immunization Practices.

IMMUNOSUPPRESSION

Immunosuppression occurs when the body's immune system is inadequate and fails to respond to the challenge of infectious disease organisms that it normally would fight successfully. The individual becomes more likely to develop a variety of infections. A number of factors can lead to this condition, including:

- Advanced age
- Frailty
- Drug therapy
- Infection with human immunodeficiency virus (HIV)
- Injury or removal of the spleen
- Radiation therapy

SERIOUS INFECTIONS IN HEALTH CARE FACILITIES

Serious bacterial and viral infections are increasing in health care facilities as well as in the general public. Ill patients, especially those who are elderly or frail, are particularly susceptible to infectious diseases, as are the very young and those with compromised (poorly functioning) immune systems.

BACTERIAL INFECTIONS

Bacteria are often the cause of serious skin, respiratory, urinary, and gastrointestinal infections in patients. If the physician suspects that a patient has a bacterial infection, a culture and sensitivity test may be ordered. This test can be done on urine, drainage from a wound, blood, or other body fluid. The culture tells the physician what type of microbe is causing the infection. The sensitivity tells the physician which antibiotic (antibacterial drug) should be used to treat the infection.

When an antibiotic is prescribed, it is important for the patient to take all the medication prescribed for the stated length of time. If the patient stops taking the antibiotic too soon, some of the microbes may remain and develop a resistance to the antibiotic.

Certain infectious microbes have become resistant to the antibiotics most commonly used against them. This is a serious problem in controlling infections in health care facilities. The antibiotics that are still effective often are more expensive and may have serious side effects compared to the previously preferred antibiotics. It is possible that, in time, these infectious microbes may also become resistant to these antibiotics.

MRSA and VRE

Two groups of organisms have become resistant to two powerful antibiotics, methicillin and vancomycin. These organisms are:

- Methicillin-resistant *Staphylococcus aureus* (MRSA). Staphylococci are normally found on skin and mucous membranes. Figure 11-10 shows *Staphylococcus aureus* organisms.
  See Appendix
- Vancomycin-resistant enterococci (VRE). Enterococci are found in the gastrointestinal tract. They are a major cause of hospital-acquired infections in health care facilities. Most strains are highly resistant to many antibiotics. Newer strains are resistant to vancomycin.

Other Bacterial Pathogens

Serious infections are also caused by the following types of bacteria:

- *Pseudomonas aeruginosa*—this organism is found in water and on other environmental surfaces. It causes urinary tract infections.
- *Escherichia coli*—bacterium commonly found in the intestinal tract, where it is normally nonpathogenic. Outside the intestinal tract, however, it can cause urinary tract infections or infections in pressure ulcers.

Refer to Appendix for additional information.

TABLE 11-2 IMMUNIZATIONS

Vaccine Name	Primary Booster Dose Schedule	Indications	Major Precautions	Special Considerations
Hepatitis B (recombinant vaccine)	Two doses 4 weeks apart. Third dose 5 months after second dosed. No booster necessary.	Health care personnel who may be exposed to blood and body fluids.	Warning: may cause shock in individuals allergic to baker's yeast.	No apparent adverse effects to developing fetuses. Not contraindicated in pregnancy.
Influenza vaccine (inactivated whole or split virus vaccine)	Annual single dose vaccine with current virus strain	Health care personnel who have contact with high-risk residents in long-term care facilities; individuals with high-risk medical conditions.	Warning: may cause shock in individuals with allergy to eggs.	No evidence of maternal or fetal risk when given to pregnant women with underlying medical conditions that cause high risk for serious influenza complications.
Measles (live virus vaccine)	One dose immediately, second dose one month later.	Health care workers born after or in 1957 without documentation of previous vaccine, physician diagnosed measles, or laboratory evidence of immunity. Vaccine should be considered for all workers born before 1957 who have no proof of immunity.	Do not give during pregnancy; immunocompromised state*, history of shock following gelatin ingestion or receipt of neomycin. Do not use if recent recipient of immune globulin.	MMR is the vaccine of choice if the health care worker is also susceptible to rubella and/or mumps. Persons vaccinated between 1963 and 1967, or vaccine of unknown type, should consider being revaccinated.
Mumps (live virus vaccine)	One dose, no booster	Health care workers believed to be susceptible should be vaccinated. Adults born before 1957 can be considered to be immune.	Do not use during pregnancy, immunocompromised state*, history of shock following gelatin ingestion or receipt of neomycin.	MMR is the vaccine of choice if the health care worker is also susceptible to rubella and/or measles.
Rubella (live virus vaccine)	One dose, no booster	Health care personnel who lack documentation or live vaccine on or after their first birthday, or of laboratory evidence of immunity. Adults born before 1957 can be considered immune except women of childbearing age.	Do not use during pregnancy, immunocompromised state*, history of shock following receipt of neomycin.	Risks to fetus if pregnant when vaccinated or women who become pregnant within 3 months of vaccination. MMR is the vaccine of choice if the health care worker is also susceptible to mumps and/or measles.
Varicella zoster (live virus vaccine)	Two doses, 4–8 weeks apart	Health care workers without reliable history of chickenpox or laboratory evidence of immunity.	Do not use during pregnancy, immunocompromised state*, history of shock following gelatin ingestion or receipt of neomycin. Salycilate use should be avoided for 6 weeks after vaccination.	Many individuals without a history of chickenpox are immune. Serologic testing may be cost effective.

*Persons immunocompromised because of immune deficiency diseases, HIV infection (who should primarily not receive BCG, OPV, and yellow fever vaccines), leukemia, lymphoma or generalized malignancy or immunosuppressed as a result or therapy with corticosteroids, alkylating drugs, antimetabolites, or radiation.

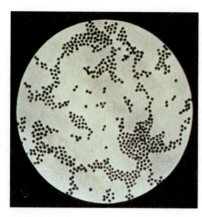

FIGURE 11-10 Methicillin-resistant *Staphylococcus aureus* (MRSA) has developed a resistance to the antibiotic of choice for treating the infection. *Courtesy of the Centers for Disease Control and Prevention, Atlanta, GA*

- Streptococcus A—a bacterium that produces powerful enzymes that destroy tissue and blood cells.
- Salmonella—a group of bacteria that cause mild to life-threatening intestinal infections, including "food poisoning"
- *Mycobacterium tuberculosis*—the bacterium that causes tuberculosis

Tuberculosis

Before the development of antibiotics, tuberculosis was a widespread disease with a high fatality rate. In the 1950s, the use of antibiotics effective against tuberculosis caused the numbers of cases and deaths to drop sharply. Since 1985, the number of people infected with tuberculosis has increased, in part because new strains of *Mycobacterium tuberculosis* are resistant to several antibiotics used to treat tuberculosis. There has also been an increase in the number of people who are at risk for infection, including those who:

- Are HIV positive
- Are infected but fail to take their medication for the full treatment period
- Live in poverty and are malnourished
- Have immigrated to the United States from countries where tuberculosis is still common
- Have inactive tuberculosis and have grown older and experience increased disability

Tuberculosis Infection. Tuberculosis infection occurs when the bacterium that causes the disease enters the body. The lungs are the most common site of infection. The body usually responds to the infection by creating a barrier that prevents the spread of pathogens to other parts of the body. This barrier is called a tubercle. As long as the tubercle remains intact and no other tuberculosis bacteria enter the body, the infection is called inactive or controlled. In this state the person is not contagious (capable of passing the infection to others). If the person is immunocompromised, the tubercle may not form and the person develops active tuberculosis disease.

Tuberculosis Disease. Tuberculosis disease develops if the tubercle breaks down or more tuberculosis bacteria enter the body. The bacteria multiply, tissue damage increases, and the bacteria may spread to other parts of the

body. As the disease progresses, the person will show one or more of the following signs and symptoms:

- Fatigue
- Loss of appetite and weight
- Weakness
- Elevated temperature in the afternoon and evening
- Night sweats
- Spitting up blood (hemoptysis)
- Coughing

The person with tuberculosis in the lungs can spread it to others through droplets in respiratory secretions.

Diagnosis. The presence of tuberculosis bacterium in the body can be shown by:

- A sputum culture—grows the organisms from a specimen of secretions from the person's lungs
- Chest x-rays—show the extent of the disease process in the lungs
- A positive skin test (Mantoux test)—shows the presence of antibodies to the tuberculosis organisms in the body (Figure 11-11)

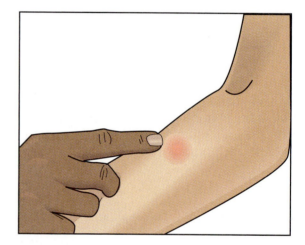
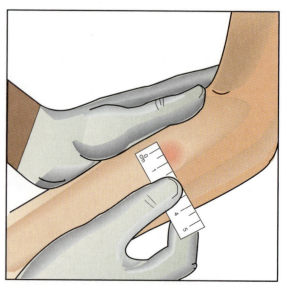

FIGURE 11-11 Positive Mantoux skin test showing an area of redness and swelling 48 hours after the test.

Health care providers in long-term care must undergo a skin test for tuberculosis before employment.

Treatment. A person with tuberculosis is treated with a selected antibiotic or combination of antibiotics. Because many disease organisms have become resistant to specific drugs, a combination of drugs must be used to control them. Once antitubercular drug therapy starts, the patient usually becomes noncontagious (cannot spread the disease organism) within two to three weeks. The therapy, however, continues for six months to two years.

VIRAL INFECTIONS

See Appendix

Several viral infections are described in this section:

- Shingles (herpes zoster)
- Influenza
- Hepatitis
- Acquired immune deficiency syndrome (AIDS)

The viral infection herpes venereum is covered in Unit 43.

Shingles

Shingles (herpes zoster) occurs in people who were infected by the virus that causes chickenpox. Although the person recovered from chickenpox, the organisms did not leave the body. They remained in the body's nervous system in a nonactive state.

Years later, when the person is in a weakened condition, the organisms become active. Painful blister-like lesions develop in the skin along the paths of sensitive nerves. Eventually the lesions heal on their own. However, they contain infectious organisms, so precautions should be used by anyone caring for a person with shingles.

Influenza

Influenza (or flu) is caused by a family of viruses. The infection can lead to serious consequences for elderly or frail people. Each year new types of viruses spread rapidly from person to person by way of respiratory secretions, causing many to become ill. Vaccines offer some protection against influenza viruses and are often given to residents in long-term care.

Someone with the flu may experience:

- Malaise (general unwell feeling)
- Chills
- Fever
- Muscle aches and pains
- Coldlike symptoms

In addition to making the person feel ill, the viruses may lower the patient's resistance to other infectious organisms. These other organisms can cause pneumonia and other life-threatening infections. Medicines may be given to limit the effects of the viruses and antibiotics are given to combat bacterial infections that may develop.

You can help protect the patients in your care by:

- Staying healthy
- Not reporting for duty when you are ill
- Carrying out standard precautions faithfully
- Following the facility's policies regarding special precautions when a patient has a respiratory infection
- Encouraging the patient to drink fluids
- Reporting to the charge nurse when a visitor seems to be ill

Hepatitis

Hepatitis is an inflammation of the liver caused by several viruses, including:

- Hepatitis A virus
- Hepatitis B virus
- Hepatitis C virus

Characteristics of these viruses are:

- Hepatitis A virus (HAV)
  - Most common
  - Transmitted by feces or saliva
  - Vaccine being developed
- Hepatitis B virus (HBV)
  - Most serious
  - Transmitted by blood, sexual secretions, feces, and saliva
  - Vaccine available for protection
- Hepatitis C virus (HCV)
  - 50% of people infected develop chronic hepatitis
  - Transmitted mainly through blood and blood products
  - Treated with alpha interferon

Any infection of the liver is serious because the liver is a vital organ. You can best protect yourself by:

- Using standard precautions (discussed in Unit 12)
- Taking the vaccine, if available
- Practicing safe sex (using condoms)
- Not using illegal drugs
- Giving your full attention to the handling of sharps such as needles or razors

Acquired Immune Deficiency Syndrome (AIDS)

Acquired immune deficiency syndrome (**AIDS**) is a viral disease. It is transmitted primarily through direct contact with the bodily secretions of an infected person. The virus that causes AIDS is the **human immunodeficiency virus** (**HIV**).

The ways in which HIV is transmitted include:

- Blood to blood through:
  - Transfusion of infected blood. Note that federal regulations prohibit the use of untested and unregulated blood in the United States.

— Treatment of hemophilia with clotting factor from infected blood

— Needle sharing among drug users

— Prick from a contaminated needle or sharp

— Unsterile instruments used for procedures such as ear piercing or tattooing

- Unprotected vaginal or anal intercourse when one partner is infected

- Infected mother to infant during:

— Pregnancy

— Birth process

— Nursing

The AIDS Virus. The AIDS virus (HIV):

- Has many variants

- Does not live for long outside the body

- Is affected by common chemicals such as bleach

- Depresses the body's immune system

- Makes the infected person more susceptible to infections

- Makes the infected person more likely to experience complications such as:

— *Pneumocystis carinii* pneumonia—a serious lung infection

— Kaposi's sarcoma—a serious malignancy affecting many body organs

— Brain involvement leading to dementia

— Eye involvement leading to blindness

— Tuberculosis

— Other opportunistic infections

Incubation Period. Not everyone who comes in contact with the HIV virus becomes infected. For those who are infected, there is always a period of time between contact and the start of the signs and symptoms of the infection.

- During this period the virus is in infected cells but is not active. The body does not make antibodies to the virus.

- Most people become **seropositive** or HIV positive (show antibodies to HIV in the bloodstream) approximately three to six months after infection. The person has HIV disease, which may progress to AIDS.

- The asymptomatic period (when no signs and symptoms are present) following infection may last months to years. AIDS does not always develop, but the person is an HIV carrier for life.

Disease Progression. Progression of the disease process is determined by the effect of the viruses on special protective white blood cells known as CD4 cells (T cells). Over time, the number of these protective white blood cells drops. As a result, the immune system of the infected person becomes more suppressed and less able to fight infection. When the number of CD4 cells drops to a critical level (below 200 cells/mm^3), the person is diagnosed with AIDS.

Symptoms of HIV infection, when they do appear, consist of:

- Acute flulike symptoms

- Fever

- Night sweats

- Fatigue

- Swollen lymph nodes

- Sore throat

- Gastrointestinal problems

- Headache

One-fourth to one-half of people exposed to HIV show evidence of disease within 5 to 10 years of antibody development (becoming seropositive).

Testing. Several tests have been developed to confirm the presence of antibodies to HIV (positive for HIV infection), to test the level of viral activity, and to confirm the presence of AIDS.

The test for antibodies is also used to check the national blood supply. When people donate blood, it is tested to be sure that it is free of HIV antibodies, to protect the people who receive blood transfusions and other blood products.

Treatment. No specific treatment is able to cure AIDS at the present time. A combination of drugs currently in use reduces both the symptoms and viral activity.

- No vaccine prevents the infection from developing. However, millions of dollars are being spent on research to develop a vaccine.

- Therapy is directed toward vigorously treating each infection as it appears.

- Nutritional and other forms of preventive therapy are aimed at maintaining a person with AIDS in the best health possible.

- The drug industry continues to develop drugs that slow down the disease process or reinforce the immune system. Patients treated with combinations of drugs show decreased viral loads and improved CD4 counts. Every dose must be taken properly. When patients fail to follow the protocol exactly, the disease state returns quickly and more strongly than before. These drugs, however, do not cure the disease.

- At present there is no evidence that AIDS is transmitted:

— Through kissing, touching, or hugging an HIV-infected person

— By eating at the same table with an infected person

— By using the same toilet seat

— Through insect bites

OTHER IMPORTANT INFECTIONS

Infection Caused by Fungi

Coccidioidomycosis (valley fever) is caused by *Coccidioides immitis*. It occurs primarily as a respiratory infection. It is seldom fatal in otherwise healthy people. In people with

GUIDELINES *for*

Preventing Infections

- Assist patients to maintain adequate fluid intake. This helps prevent urinary tract and respiratory tract infections and keeps the skin healthier.
- Assist patients to maintain adequate nutritional intake. Report to the nurse when patients eat less or refuse food.
- Assist patients to carry out exercise programs established by the nurse or physical therapist. Follow positioning schedules and orders for range-of-motion exercises and ambulation. Exercise improves breathing and circulation.
- Toilet patients who need assistance. This keeps the bladder empty and also assures patients that they will receive help when they need to urinate.
- When cleaning the perineal area of patients, be sure to wipe women from front to back. This prevents contaminating the urethra (bladder opening) with stool or vaginal excretions.
- Perform catheter care as directed. Avoid opening the drainage system.
- Observe patients carefully and report any unusual signs or changes, such as:
  - Changes in frequency of urination or amount of urine voided
  - Complaints of pain or burning on urination
  - Changes in character of urine
  - Coughing or respiratory problems
  - Confusion or disorientation that was not present before or that has increased
  - Drainage or discharge from any body opening or skin wound
  - Changes in skin color
  - Complaints of pain, discomfort, or nausea
  - Elevated temperature
  - Red, swollen areas on body

- Keep patients clean (Figure 11-12).
- Staff members who have an infectious disease should not be on duty. Caring for your own health is vital in preventing illness in patients. Friends and family of residents should be advised not to visit when they do not feel well. If you notice a visitor coughing and sneezing, or otherwise obviously sick, inform your supervisor.
- Follow your facility policies and procedure for prevention of infection and injury. If you identify health risks, take the proper precautions. It is your responsibility to learn and follow these practices. Cooperate with your infection control nurse or department during audits, education, investigation of outbreaks and exposure, and review of infection control practices. Sometimes recommendations to prevent infection change. It is your responsibility to learn new techniques and make changes in the way you practice.

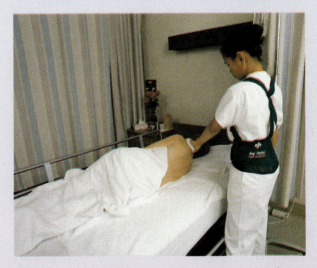

FIGURE 11-12 Maintaining the patient's cleanliness helps prevent infectious disease.

---

immunosuppression, however, the death rate is high. It is treated with antibiotics.

Infection Caused by Protozoa

Two diseases caused by protozoa are becoming more common in the general public and in health facilities. Giardiasis is caused by *Giardia lamblia*, which is found in the water supplies of many communities. It causes severe diarrhea but responds to medication. Cryptosporidiosis is caused by the *Cryptosporidium* protozoa, which is found in the digestive tracts of domestic animals and is transferred by contact. It causes severe diarrhea, especially in immunosuppressed people. There is no specific treatment.

OUTBREAK OF INFECTIOUS DISEASE IN A HEALTH CARE FACILITY

See Appendix

An outbreak of an infection in the facility can be serious for all patients. Unless steps are taken immediately, the infection can spread rapidly. Examples of outbreaks include:

- Influenza
- Gastroenteritis
- Hepatitis
- MRSA
- Scabies (parasites that invade the skin)

Most facilities have an action plan for responding to an outbreak of infection. Nursing assistants will receive instructions from the nurse.

SELF-CARE

You can take steps to stay healthy and free from infections:
- Eat a healthy diet
- Get enough sleep each day
- Keep your body clean
- Live in a clean environment
- Avoid unhealthy habits such as smoking and substance abuse
- Learn how to cope with stress

REVIEW

A. Matching.

Match Column I with Column II.

Column I

1. _____ spiral-shaped bacterium
2. _____ organism that causes ringworm
3. _____ bacteria that grow in pairs
4. _____ organism that causes AIDS
5. _____ bacteria that grow as clusters

Column II

a. staphylococci
b. protozoan
c. diplococci
d. streptococci
e. virus
f. fungus
g. spirillum

B. Word Choice.

Fill in the blanks with the correct word or phrase from the following list.

insects
method of transmission
portal of entry
portal of exit
reservoir

sexual contact
sneezing
susceptible host
water

6. Complete the chain of infection by naming the parts missing from the following figure.

a. _____   c. _____
b. _____   d. _____

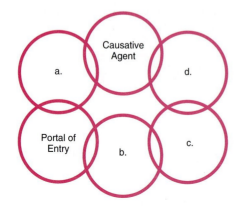

7. An example of transmission by direct contact is _____.

8. An example of transmission by indirect contact is _____.

9. A common vehicle for the transmission of microbes is _____.

10. Vectors, such as animals and _____, also transmit disease organisms.

C. True/False.

Mark the following true or false by circling T or F.

11. T F Normal body flora are the same in each part of the body.

12. T F The rectum is a common portal of exit for some infectious organisms.

13. T F The general health of an individual is an important factor in determining if infectious disease will occur.

14. T F Unbroken skin is a mechanical defense against infection.

15. T F A boil is an example of a generalized infection.

16. T F Allergies are known as sensitivity reactions.

17. T F The term *reservoir* may refer to a human body in which the organisms live.

18. T F An immunizing vaccine causes the body to produce antibodies that protect the person against certain infectious diseases.

19. T F MRSA infections are easy to control.

20. T F Bedpans and urinals can act as fomites.

D. Multiple Choice.

Select the one best answer for each question.

21. White blood cells that multiply and attempt to destroy pathogens are

a. antigens.

b. phagocytes.

c. antibodies.

d. red blood cells.

22. Which of the following is not a natural body defense?

a. Antibiotic

b. Hydrochloric acid in the stomach

c. Hair in the nose

d. Tears

23. Which is an example of a local infection?

a. Pneumonia

b. Septicemia

c. Boil

d. AIDS

24. One patient's visitor is coughing and looks flushed. Your best action is to

a. ask the visitor to leave.

b. put a mask on the visitor.

c. put a mask on the patient.

d. refer the matter to the nurse.

25. You woke up not feeling well this morning. You have an elevated temperature. Your best action is to

a. call in sick.

b. go to work.

c. stay home without notifying the facility.

d. call a friend to go to work for you.

E. Nursing Assistant Challenge.

26. Your patient, Mrs. Wallace, has a cold.

a. What organism is responsible? _____

b. Could Mrs. Wallace be immunized against this condition? _____

c. How is the condition most likely transmitted? _____

27. Mr. Reynolds has a staphylococcal infection in his finger.

a. What class of organisms are staphylococci? _____

b. What shape are these organisms? _____

c. How might Mr. Reynolds have acquired this infection? _____

Infection Control

See Appendix (page 667) for additional information

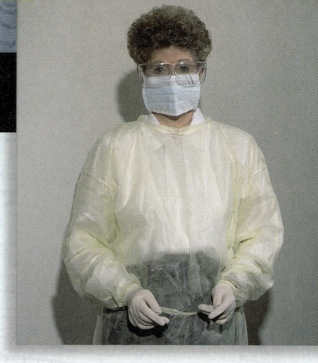

OBJECTIVES

As a result of this unit, you will be able to:

- Define and spell all vocabulary words and terms.
- Explain the principles of medical asepsis.
- Explain the components of standard precautions.
- List the types of personal protective equipment.
- Describe nursing assistant actions related to standard precautions.
- Describe airborne precautions.
- Describe droplet precautions.
- Describe contact precautions.
- Demonstrate the following:
  - Procedure 1 Handwashing
  - Procedure 2 Putting on a Mask
  - Procedure 3 Putting on a Gown
  - Procedure 4 Putting on Gloves

- Procedure 5 Removing Contaminated Gloves
- Procedure 6 Removing Contaminated Gloves, Mask, and Gown
- Procedure 7 Serving a Meal in an Isolation Unit
- Procedure 8 Measuring Vital Signs in an Isolation Unit
- Procedure 9 Transferring Nondisposable Equipment Outside of Isolation Unit
- Procedure 10 Specimen Collection from Patient in an Isolation Unit
- Procedure 11 Caring for Linens in an Isolation Unit
- Procedure 12 Transporting Patient to and from Isolation Unit
- Procedure 13 Opening a Sterile Package

VOCABULARY

Learn the meaning and the correct spelling of the following words and phrases:

airborne precautions	disposable	isolation technique	sharps
airborne transmission	disinfection	isolation unit	standard precautions
asepsis	droplet precautions	medical asepsis	sterile
autoclave	droplet transmission	N95 respirator	sterile field
biohazard	exposure incident	nosocomial infection	sterilization
communicable disease	face shield	occupational exposure	surgical mask
contact precautions	goggles	personal protective	transmission-based
contact transmission	high-efficiency	equipment (PPE)	precautions
contagious disease	particulate air	PFR95 respirator	work practice controls
contaminated	(HEPA) filter mask	potentially infectious	
dirty	isolation	material	

DISEASE PREVENTION

In the last unit you learned what infections are and some of their causes. In this unit, you will be introduced to actions and procedures that can help prevent the transmission (spread) of infection to protect yourself, your coworkers, and those in your care.

MEDICAL ASEPSIS

Asepsis is defined as the absence of disease-producing microorganisms. Two ways of achieving asepsis are by medical aseptic technique and surgical aseptic technique.

Medical asepsis refers to medical practices that reduce the numbers of microorganisms or interrupt transmission from

GUIDELINES *for*

Maintaining Medical Asepsis

To maintain medical asepsis, the nursing assistant should follow these guidelines:

- Wash hands thoroughly and at appropriate times. Protect the skin on the hands by using warm water, drying thoroughly, then applying lotion if needed.
- Treat breaks in the skin immediately by washing thoroughly, cleaning with an antiseptic, and covering. Report any breaks in the skin to your supervisor.
- Use gloves when required.
- Bathe or shower daily. Daily changes of clothing are necessary. Keep your hair clean and away from your face and shoulders. Keep fingernails short and clean. Do not wear rings, other than a plain wedding band.
- Assist patients with their personal hygiene.
- *Never* use one patient's items for another patient.
- Keep patient personal care items in the proper areas.

  In the top two drawers of the patient's bedside stand, place:

  — toothbrush and toothpaste

  — comb and hairbrush

  — denture cup if patient wears dentures

  Items such as a toothbrush, denture cup, wash basin, and emesis basin should always be placed on a different shelf from items such as a bedpan and a urinal.

  In the second drawer or on the shelf of the bedside stand, or in the bathroom, place:

  — emesis basin

  — wash basin

  — soap and soap dish

  Store on the lower shelf:

  — bedpan

  — urinal for male patients

- Disinfect bathtubs and shower chairs after each use according to facility policy.
- Disinfect equipment that is used by more than one health care provider or patient, such as a stethoscope, before and after each use.
- Disinfect personal care equipment, such as bedpans, urinals, and commodes, according to facility policy.
- Be careful when handling bedpans and urinals after use to prevent spills and splashes. Use a cover when transporting.
- Keep food and water supplies clean. Food trays are to remain covered until they reach their destination. Remove food dishes immediately after use. Do not place used trays on a cart until all clean trays have been delivered to patients.
- Do not allow patients to keep puddings or custards from meal trays. Bacteria multiply rapidly in these foods when they are not refrigerated.
- Carry soiled equipment, supplies, and linens away from your uniform so that you do not spread microorganisms from patient to patient. Dispose of items according to facility policy.
- Do not use anything that has touched the floor without recleaning or sterilizing it first. If you are in doubt about whether an item is clean, do not use it. Any personal items that touch the floor should be disinfected before use. The floor is heavily contaminated with pathogens.
- Avoid raising dust.
- Do not shake linens. This scatters contaminated dust and lint. Gather or fold linens inward with the dirtiest area toward the center. Keep soiled linen hampers covered. Keep linens (even if soiled) off the floor.
- Clean from least soiled areas toward the most soiled.
- Keep work areas such as utility rooms clean. Return clean equipment to the proper storage areas after use.

one person to another person or from person to place or object. These practices are often referred to as *medical aseptic technique (clean technique).*

You will hear the terms *clean* and *dirty* applied to equipment and supplies used in the facility. For example, the linen you take from the linen cart is "clean." After it is carried into the patient's room, it is considered "dirty." If it is not used, it cannot be returned to the clean linen cart but must be placed in the laundry hamper. Once linen is in the patient's room, it is exposed to the patient's pathogens. To prevent the spread of these pathogens to other patients, the linen must be laundered. Keeping each patient's equipment and supplies separate from those for other patients is part of medical aseptic technique. Articles that have come into contact with known pathogens or have been exposed to potential pathogens are called **dirty** or **contaminated**. Articles that are free of pathogens are considered clean or uncontaminated.

It is not possible to eliminate all microorganisms from our bodies or the environment. However, microbes can be reduced by always using the essential practices of medical aseptic technique:

- Handwashing
- Using nonsterile gloves when contact with blood, moist body fluids (except sweat), mucous membranes, or non-intact skin is likely
- Cleaning and/or disinfecting equipment

See Appendix

HANDWASHING

Handwashing is the single most important health procedure any individual can perform to prevent the spread of microbes. Handwashing is a vigorous, short rubbing together of all the surfaces of soap-lathered hands. It is followed by rinsing under a stream of running warm water. Warm water is used because it makes a good lather. It is also less damaging to the skin than hot water. In health care facilities, soap is provided in a dispenser. Bar soap is easily contaminated because microbes can grow in the wet soap dish.

When washing your hands, always keep your fingertips pointed down. Never lean against the sink with your uniform or touch the inside of the sink with your hands.

The most important aspect of handwashing is the friction created by rubbing the hands together. This friction mechanically removes microbes from the hands. Routine handwashing with soap, running water, and friction by all health care providers:

- Is the most significant control measure for the prevention of a **nosocomial infection** (infection acquired by a patient while being cared for in a health care facility)
- Is the single most important control measure to break the chain of infection.

The recommended handwashing technique depends on the purpose of the handwashing. Hands can usually be washed effectively in 10 to 15 seconds. More time will be needed, however, if hands are visibly soiled (refer to Procedure 1).

PROCEDURE   1   OBRA

HANDWASHING

1. Check that there is an adequate supply of soap and paper towels. A waste container lined with a plastic bag should be in the area near you.

2. Turn on the faucet with a dry paper towel held between your hand and the faucet (Figure 12-1).

3. Adjust water to a warm temperature. Drop the towel in the waste container. Stand back from the sink so you do not contaminate your uniform. Wet your hands with the fingertips pointed downward (Figure 12-2).

4. Apply soap and lather over your hands and wrists and between fingers. Use friction and interlace your fingers (Figure 12-3). Work lather over every part of your hands and wrists. Clean your fingernails by rubbing them against the palm of the other hand to

force soap under the nails for 10 to 15 seconds (Figure 12-4).

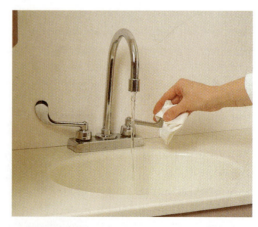

FIGURE 12-1 Use a dry, clean paper towel to turn faucets on and off.

continues

PROCEDURE **1** *continued*

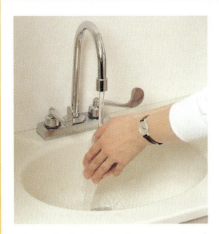

FIGURE 12-2 Point fingertips down while washing hands.

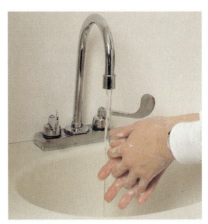

FIGURE 12-3 Interlace the fingers to clean between them.

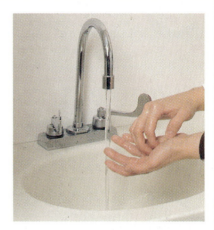

FIGURE 12-4 Rub nails against the palms of the hands to clean under the nails.

5. Rinse hands with your fingertips pointed down. Do not shake water from hands.

6. Dry hands thoroughly with a clean paper towel.

7. Turn off the faucet with another paper towel; drop the towel in the waste container.

8. Apply lotion to your hands.

Handwashing should be done:
- At the beginning of your shift
- After picking up any item from the floor
- Before handling food
- After personal use of the bathroom
- After using a tissue
- After handling a patient's belongings
- After touching any item or environmental surface that is soiled
- Immediately after accidental contact with blood, moist body fluids, mucous membranes, or nonintact skin
- Before and after any contact with your mouth or mucous membranes, such as touching, eating, drinking, smoking, using lip balm, or manipulating contact lenses
- Before and after caring for each patient
- Before applying and after removing gloves
- At the end of your shift before going home

PROTECTING YOURSELF

As you perform your duties, you may contact **potentially infectious material** such as blood or other body fluids that may contain pathogens. This is called **occupational exposure**. Using proper medical asepsis technique and following standard precautions according to your facility policy are the best ways to limit the potential for being infected.

An **exposure incident** means that your eyes, mouth, or nonintact skin had contact with blood or other potentially infec-

tious material. Rinse immediately with clear water. Report this at once to your supervisor and follow facility procedure.

STANDARD PRECAUTIONS

Standard precautions (Figure 12-5) are the infection control actions used for all people receiving care, regardless of their condition or diagnosis. Standard precautions apply to situations in which care providers may contact:

- Blood, body fluids (except sweat), secretions, and excretions
- Mucous membranes
- Nonintact skin

Some examples of secretions and excretions are:
- Respiratory mucus (phlegm)
- Cerebrospinal fluid
- Urine
- Feces
- Vaginal secretions
- Semen
- Vomitus

This means that all health care workers follow specific procedures called **work practice controls** to prevent the spread of infections.

Standard precautions stress handwashing and the use of **personal protective equipment** (**PPE**): gloves, gown, mask, and goggles or face shield.

STANDARD PRECAUTIONS FOR INFECTION CONTROL

Wash Hands (Plain soap)
Wash after touching blood, body fluids, secretions, excretions, and contaminated items. Wash immediately after gloves are removed and between patient contacts. Avoid transfer of microorganisms to other patients or environments.

Wear Gloves
Wear when touching blood, body fluids, secretions, excretions, and contaminated items. Put on clean gloves just before touching mucous membranes and nonintact skin. Change gloves between tasks and procedures on the same patient after contact with material that may contain high concentrations of microorganisms. Remove gloves promptly after use, before touching noncontaminated items and environmental surfaces, and before going to another patient, and wash hands immediately to avoid transfer of microorganisms to other patients or environments.

Wear Mask and Eye Protection or Face Shield
Protect mucous membranes of the eyes, nose and mouth during procedures and patient-care activities that are likely to generate splashes or sprays of blood, body fluids, secretions, or excretions.

Wear Gown
Protect skin and prevent soiling of clothing during procedures that are likely to generate splashes or sprays of blood, body fluids, secretions, or excretions. Remove a soiled gown as promptly as possible and wash hands to avoid transfer of microorganisms to other patients or environments.

Patient-Care Equipment
Handle used patient-care equipment soiled with blood, body fluids, secretions, or excretions in a manner that prevents skin and mucous membrane exposures, contamination of clothing, and transfer of microorganisms to other patients and environments. Ensure that reusable equipment is not used for the care of another patient until it has been appropriately cleaned and reprocessed and single use items are properly discarded.

Environmental Control
Follow hospital procedures for routine care, cleaning, and disinfection of environmental surfaces, beds, bedrails, bedside equipment and other frequently touched surfaces.

Linen
Handle, transport, and process used linen soiled with blood, body fluids, secretions, or excretions in a manner that prevents exposure and contamination of clothing, and avoids transfer of microorganisms to other patients and environments.

Occupational Health and Bloodborne Pathogens
Prevent injuries when using needles, scalpels, and other sharp instruments or devices; when handling sharp instruments after procedures; when cleaning used instruments; and when disposing of used needles.

Never recap used needles using both hands or any other technique that involves directing the point of a needle towards any part of the body; rather, use either a one-handed "scoop" technique or a mechanical device designed for holding the needle sheath.

Do not remove used needles from disposable syringes by hand, and do not bend, break, or otherwise manipulate used needles by hand. Place used disposable syringes and needles, scalpels, blades, and other sharp items in puncture-resistant sharps containers located as close as practical to the area in which the items were used, and place reusable syringes and needles in a puncture-resistant container for transport to the reprocessing area.

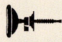

Use resuscitation devices as an alternative to mouth-to-mouth resuscitation.

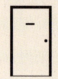

Patient Placement
Use a private room for a patient who contaminates the environment or who does not (or cannot be expected to) assist in maintaining appropriate hygiene or environmental control. Consult Infection Control if a private room is not available.

FIGURE 12-5 Standard precautions. *Courtesy of BREVIS Corporation, Salt Lake City, UT*

See Appendix for additional information

GUIDELINES *for*

Standard Precautions

1. Wash hands in the situations listed under "Handwashing."
2. Wear gloves for any contact with blood, body fluids, mucous membranes, or nonintact skin, such as when:
   — Hands are cut, scratched, or have a rash
   — Cleaning up body fluid spills
   — Cleaning potentially contaminated equipment
3. Gloves are provided in patient rooms on supply carts, or in wall-mounted dispensers.
4. Carry gloves with you so they will always be available as you need them.

5. If you have an allergy to latex gloves, follow your physician's advice. Three possible options are:
   — Change to nonlatex gloves (facilities must supply them because latex allergies are not uncommon).
   — Apply a skin barrier cream to your hands before putting on latex gloves; the cream protects hands against most irritants, including latex.
   — Put on glove liners that prevent direct contact between the skin of the hands and the latex gloves.

continues

GUIDELINES
continued

6. Change gloves:
   — After contacting each patient
   — Before touching noncontaminated articles or environmental surfaces
   — Between tasks with the same patient if there is contact with infectious materials
7. Dispose of gloves according to facility policy.
8. Wear a waterproof gown for procedures likely to produce splashes of blood or other body fluids.
   — Remove soiled gown as soon as possible and dispose of it properly according to facility policy.
   — Wash your hands.
9. Wear a mask and protective eyewear or face shield for procedures likely to produce splashes of blood or other moist body fluids. This is to prevent contact with pathogens by your mucous membranes.
   The surgical mask covers both the nose and

mouth. The mask is used once and discarded. When a mask is required, a new one is put on for each patient receiving care. If the mask becomes wet, a new one must be put on because the mask loses its effectiveness when moist.
10. Goggles or a face shield help protect the mucous membranes of the eyes from splashes or sprays of blood and other body fluids. A surgical mask must be worn with goggles and with a face shield to protect the nose and mouth.
11. When using PPE, you should:
    — Know where to obtain these items in your work area.
    — Always remove the items before leaving the work area, whether the patient's room, an isolation unit, or the utility room.
    — Place these items in the proper container for laundering, decontamination, or disposal, according to facility policy.

GUIDELINES
for

Environmental Procedures

1. Handle all patient care items so that infectious organisms will not be transferred to skin, mucous membranes, clothing, or the environment. Reusable equipment must be cleaned and decontaminated according to facility policy before it can be used with another patient. Dispose of single-use items according to facility policy.
2. Follow facility procedures for routine care and cleaning of environmental surfaces, such as beds, bedside equipment, and other frequently touched surfaces.
3. Dispose of sharps—needles with syringes, razors, and other sharp items—in a puncture-resistant, leakproof container near the point of use (Figure 12-6). The container should be labeled with the biohazard symbol (Figure 12-7) and color-coded red.
4. Do not recap needles or otherwise handle them before disposal.
5. Mouthpieces or resuscitator bags should be available to minimize the need for mouth-to-mouth resuscitation. Remember that you must be trained to use them.
6. Waste and soiled linen should be placed in plastic bags and handled according to facility

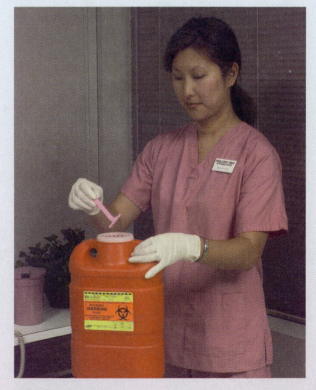

FIGURE 12-6 Sharps must be disposed of carefully in a safety container designed specifically for this use.

continues

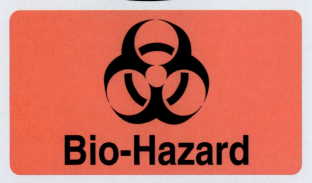

FIGURE 12-7 Containers for contaminated items are identified with the biohazard label. The background is red or orange and the symbol is black.

policy. There are separate containers for regular waste and for biohazardous waste (waste that has contacted blood or body fluids). Containers for biohazardous waste should have the biohazard symbol, or be color-coded in red (Figure 12-8). Learn your facility policy for what is biohazardous waste and follow the guidelines.

7. Wipe up blood spills immediately. Disinfect the floor according to facility policy.
   — Use disposable gloves.
   — For small spills, use 1:10 dilution of bleach or disinfectant required by facility policy.

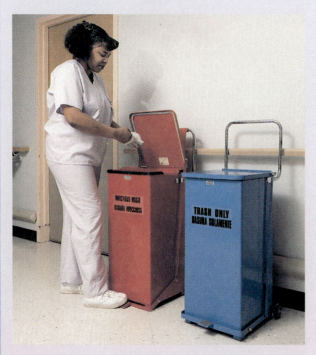

FIGURE 12-8 All potentially infectious materials should be disposed of in the correct waste container.

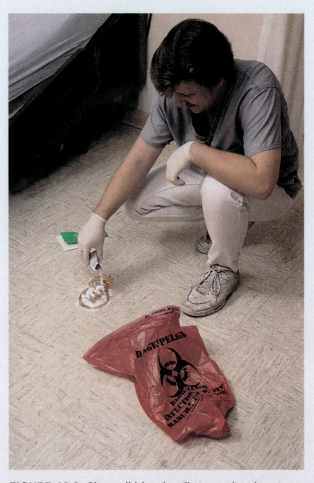

FIGURE 12-9 Clean all blood spills immediately using a 1:10 dilution of bleach or the disinfectant approved by your facility. For larger spills, a blood spill kit can be used. The powder absorbs the blood quickly and can be scooped up for disposal in the biohazard bag.

   — For larger spills, use a commercial blood cleanup kit. This contains an absorbent powder that is sprinkled over the blood to absorb the spill. The blood and powder are then scooped up with the scoop provided in the kit. The material and scoop are placed in a biohazard bag for disposal (Figure 12-9).
   — Use disposable cleaning cloths.
   — Dispose of gloves and cleaning cloths in appropriate infectious waste receptacles.

8. Dispose of body fluids and contaminated articles according to facility policy. This includes the contents of:
   — Urinary drainage bags
   — Bedpans
   — Urinals
   — Emesis basins

continues

GUIDELINES
continued

— Drainage receptacles from tracheal and gastric suction
— Solutions returned from vaginal douches, enemas, and bladder irrigations
— Soiled dressings
— Incontinence pads (Chux®)
— Vaginal pads
— Incontinent briefs

9. Eating, drinking, smoking, applying cosmetics or lip balm, and handling contact lenses are prohibited in work areas where there may be exposure to infectious material.

10. Food and drink should not be kept in refrigerators, freezers, shelves, cabinets, or on countertops or benchtops where they may be exposed to blood or other materials that may be contaminated.

11. Do not pick up potentially contaminated broken glassware with your bare hands. Use a brush and dust pan, tongs, or forceps. Clean and disinfect properly. Discard according to facility policy.

12. Consider laboratory specimens and specimen containers to be potentially infectious materials.

TRANSMISSION-BASED PRECAUTIONS

Standard precautions do not eliminate the need for other isolation precautions. A second set of precautions is used with certain highly transmissible diseases. This second tier of precautions is called **transmission-based precautions**. Transmission-based precautions are designed to interrupt the mode of transmission so that the disease cannot spread to others. Standard precautions are always used in addition to transmission-based precautions.

Diseases may be transferred from one person to another either directly or indirectly. Such diseases are called **communicable** or **contagious diseases**. Some diseases are transmitted more easily than others. Specific precautions must be taken to control their spread.

Communicable diseases may be spread:

● Through upper respiratory secretions by **airborne transmission** and **droplet transmission**

● By **contact transmission** (direct contact or indirect contact) with feces or other body secretions and excretions

● Through draining wounds or infective material such as blood on needles

Each mode of transmission requires special precautions to interrupt the movement of microbes from the infected person to others.

If a disease is transmitted by more than one mode, all methods of transmission must be considered when selecting precautions for a specific patient. Table 12-1 lists transmission-based precautions and common diseases in each category.

Isolation

Isolation means being separated or set apart. The purpose of isolation is to separate the patient with a communicable or contagious disease, to help prevent the spread of the infectious pathogens.

When a patient is in isolation precautions, a private room is used. Two patients with the same disease may share a room.

TABLE 12-1 TRANSMISSION-BASED PRECAUTIONS FOR COMMON DISEASES

Transmission-Based Precautions Category	Disease or Condition
Airborne	Tuberculosis Measles
Airborne and Contact	Chickenpox Widespread shingles
Droplet	German measles Mumps Influenza
Contact	Head or body lice, scabies Impetigo Infected pressure ulcer with heavy drainage

(This practice is called *cohorting*.) For patients in isolation, the proper use of precautions requires extra effort by all care providers, but especially nursing assistants, and is more time-consuming. The fear of infection also makes working with these precautions more stressful for the care providers. Patients in isolation and their families and other visitors also feel stress.

Psychological Aspects of Isolation

The patient in isolation fears both the disease condition that makes the isolation precautions necessary and the practices that must be followed for these precautions to be effective. These include:

● PPE worn by all who enter the isolation unit

● Special procedures for handling waste, specimens, food, linens, and personal effects of the patient

● Restrictions on the patient's movement in the facility

- Procedures to be followed when patient is moved outside of the isolation unit
- Possible restrictions on visiting hours or number of visitors
- Need for visitors to use PPE
- Likelihood that close personal contact, such as kissing of family members, is not permitted

The patient may be afraid of passing the infection to family and friends. If the patient does not understand the infectious process, this fear is increased. If the patient is confused, he or she may be very fearful of the PPE.

Because of the patient's fears and the need for decreased contact with other patients, family, and friends, the patient in isolation requires more emotional support and care. The extra time required to follow the isolation precautions, such as putting on PPE, could easily lessen the time the care providers spend with the patient at a time when emotional attention is most needed. Nursing assistants are mindful of the patient's needs and will plan their schedules to spend the necessary time with a patient in isolation.

Transmission-Based Isolation Precautions

Standard precautions are used with all patients regardless of their condition. When patients are known to have or are suspected of having an infectious disease, isolation precautions are used *in addition to* standard precautions. The isolation precautions used depend on the way in which the infectious pathogens are transmitted. Guidelines from the Centers for Disease Control and Prevention (CDC) indicate the specific precautions and personal protective equipment to be used based on how the disease is transmitted. The three transmission precautions are:

- Airborne precautions
- Droplet precautions
- Contact precautions

Airborne Precautions. Airborne precautions are used for diseases that are transmitted by air currents. The pathogens are small and light and are suspended in the air or on dust particles in the air. They can travel a long distance from the source by natural air currents and through ventilation systems. Tuberculosis is a disease that requires airborne precautions. Figure 12-10 shows the required precautions.

- The patient must be in a private room with negative air pressure. This means that air is drawn into the room and leaves the room through a special exhaust system to the outside. Air from the room does not circulate directly into the facility.
- The door to the room is kept closed.
- All care providers who enter the room must wear a **high-efficiency particulate air** (**HEPA**) **filter mask** (Figure 12-11). The special filters in this mask protect the care provider from the very small disease-causing pathogens. A surgical mask does not provide protection. Each care provider must be fitted with a HEPA filter

AIRBORNE PRECAUTIONS
(in addition to Standard Precautions)
VISITORS: Report to nurse before entering.

Patient Placement
Use **private room** that has:
Monitored negative air pressure,
6 to 12 air changes per hour,
Discharge of air outdoors or HEPA filtration if recirculated.
Keep room door closed and patient in room.

Respiratory Protection
Wear an N95 respirator when entering the room of a patient with known or suspected infectious pulmonary **tuberculosis**.
Susceptible persons should not enter the room of patients known or suspected to have **measles** (rubeola) or **varicella** (chickenpox) if other immune caregivers are available. If susceptible persons must enter, they should wear an **N95 respirator**. (Respirator or surgical mask not required if immune to measles and varicella.)

Patient Transport
Limit transport of patient from room to essential purposes only. Use **surgical mask** on patient during transport.

FIGURE 12-10 Airborne precautions. *Courtesy of BREVIS Corporation, Salt Lake City, UT*

mask. This ensures that air entering the mask comes through the filters only. Follow all facility policies for the use of HEPA filter masks.

The HEPA mask may be disposable or reusable. Men with facial hair cannot wear a HEPA mask because the beard prevents an airtight seal. In this case, a special HEPA-filtered hood can be worn. Other types of masks can be worn in place of a HEPA mask, such as the **PFR95 respirator** (Figure 12-12) and the **N95 respirator** (Figure 12-13). Fit testing of a HEPA mask or respirator is required each time one is put on. Figure 12-14 shows the procedure for fit testing the N95 respirator.

- People who are not immune to measles (rubeola) or chickenpox (varicella) should not enter the room of a patient known or suspected to have either of these infections.
- If transport from the room is necessary, the patient must wear a surgical mask.
- Remember: these precautions are in addition to standard precautions.

Droplet Precautions. Droplet precautions are used for diseases that can be spread by means of large droplets in the air. A person can spread droplets containing infectious pathogens by sneezing, coughing, talking, singing, or laughing. The droplets generally do not travel more than three feet from the source. Influenza is an example of a disease spread by droplets.

Figure 12-15 shows the requirements for droplet precautions.

- If a patient cannot be placed in a private room, then residents requiring the same precautions can be placed together.

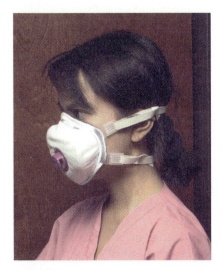

FIGURE 12-11 Different types of HEPA masks

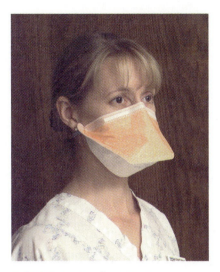

FIGURE 12-12 The PFR95 respirator

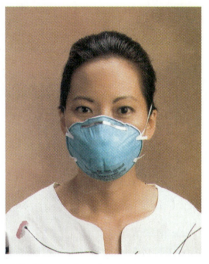

FIGURE 12-13 The N95 respirator. *Courtesy of 3M Health Care, St. Paul, MN*

Donning instructions (to be followed each time product is worn):

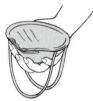

1 Cup the respirator in your hand with the nosepiece at fingertips, allowing the headbands to hang freely below hands.

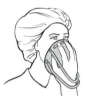

2 Position the respirator under your chin with the nosepiece up.

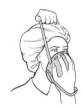

3 Pull the top strap over your head so it rests high on the back of head.

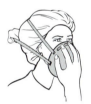

4 Pull the bottom strap over your head and position it around neck below ears.

5 Using two hands, mold the nosepiece to the shape of your nose by pushing inward while moving fingertips down both sides of the nosepiece. Pinching the nosepiece using one hand may result in less effective respirator performance.

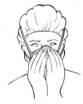

6 FACE FIT CHECK
The respirator seal should be checked before each use. To check fit, place both hands completely over the respirator and exhale. If air leaks around your nose, adjust the nosepiece as described in step 5. If air leaks at respirator edges, adjust the straps back along the sides of your head. Recheck.

NOTE: If you cannot achieve proper fit, do not enter the isolation or treatment area. See your supervisor.

Removal instructions:

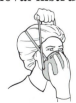

1 Cup the respirator in your hand to maintain position on face. Pull bottom strap over head.

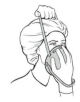

2 Still holding respirator in position, pull top strap over head.

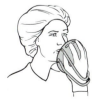

3 Remove respirator from face and discard or store according to your facility's policy.

FIGURE 12-14 The respirator must be fit tested each time you wear it. *Courtesy of 3M Health Care, St. Paul, MN*

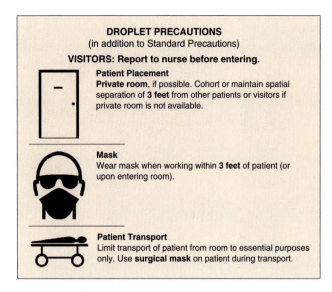

FIGURE 12-15 Droplet precautions. *Courtesy of BREVIS Corporation, Salt Lake City, UT*

- The caregivers should wear surgical masks if they expect to be working within three feet of the resident. The door can be open if the bed is more than three feet from the door.
- If transport from the room is necessary, the patient must wear a surgical mask.
- Remember that these precautions are in addition to standard precautions.

Contact Precautions. Contact precautions are used when the infectious pathogen is spread by direct or indirect contact. *Direct contact* occurs when the caregiver touches a contaminated area on the patient's skin or blood or body fluids containing the infectious pathogen. *Indirect contact* occurs when the caregiver touches items contaminated with the infectious material, such as the patient's personal belongings, equipment or supplies used in the care of the patient, contaminated linens, and so on. Examples of infections requiring contact precautions are scabies, infected pressure ulcers, and gastroenteritis.

Figure 12-16 shows the requirements for contact precautions.

- The patient should be in a private room. If this is not possible, then patients requiring the same type of

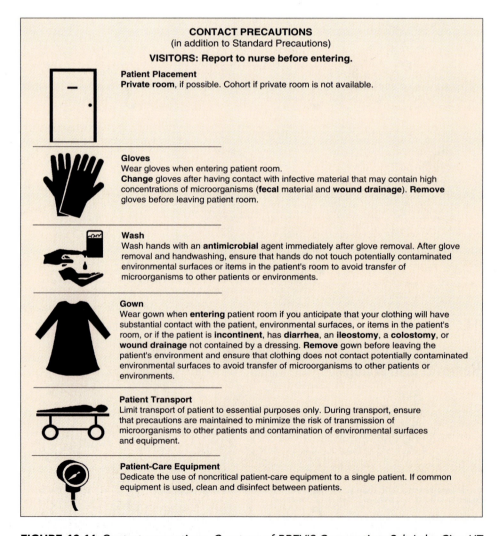

FIGURE 12-16 Contact precautions. *Courtesy of BREVIS Corporation, Salt Lake City, UT*

isolation precautions can be placed in the same room. The door can be open.

- Gloves are put on before the caregiver enters the patient's room. Gloves are changed whenever there is contact with highly contaminated matter in the room. After removing gloves, always wash your hands before putting on a new pair of gloves. After care is completed, remove gloves and wash hands. Use a paper towel to open the door to leave the room and discard the towel in the trash container inside the room.
- Wear a gown when entering the patient's room if your uniform may contact the resident, blood or body fluids, environmental surfaces, or other items in the room. Remove the gown before leaving the room and dispose of it according to facility policy for biohazardous waste. Be careful not to touch environmental surfaces or other items with your uniform as you leave the room.
- Transport the patient from the room only when necessary. Continue precautions to minimize contamination of environmental surfaces, other patients, and health care personnel.
- Disposable equipment and supplies should be used whenever possible. Noncritical, nondisposable equipment should be used for one patient only. If equipment must be used for more than one patient, it must be cleaned and disinfected between patients.
- Remember that these precautions are used in addition to standard precautions.

ISOLATION TECHNIQUE

There are four key points to be remembered at all times for isolation technique:

1. **Isolation technique** is the name given to the method of caring for patients with easily transmitted diseases.
2. It is essential that every person take responsibility and use the proper isolation techniques to prevent the spread of disease to others.
3. All items that come into contact with the patient's excretions, secretions, blood, body fluids, mucous membranes, or nonintact skin are considered contaminated. This potentially infective material must be treated in a special way.
4. Standard precautions are always used in addition to transmission-based precautions.

Isolation Unit

The **isolation unit** may be an area or a private room. Patients with the same disease may share a room. A room with handwashing facilities and an adjoining room with bathing and toilet facilities is best. A private room is indicated for patients who:

- Are highly infectious
- Have poor personal hygiene
- Require special air control procedures within the room

Preparing for Isolation

To prepare a patient room for isolation, do the following:

1. Place a card indicating the type of isolation precaution on the door to the patient's room.
2. Place an isolation cart outside the room, next to the door. Place in it quantities of personal protective equipment as needed:
   - Gowns
   - Masks
   - Gloves
   - Goggles or face shields
   - Plastic bags marked for biohazardous waste
   - Plastic bags for soiled linen
3. Line the wastepaper basket inside the room with a plastic bag labeled or color-coded for infectious waste.
4. Place a laundry hamper in the room and line it with a yellow biohazard laundry bag.
5. At the sink, check the supply of paper towels and soap. Soap should be in a wall dispenser or foot-operated dispenser.

PERSONAL PROTECTIVE EQUIPMENT

Personal protective equipment includes gloves, gown, mask, and goggles or face shield. The following sections describe the correct use of this equipment (see Procedures 2 through 6).

Cover Gown

A gown made of a moisture-resistant material is used when soiling or splashing with blood, body fluids, secretions, or excretions is likely (Figure 12-17). The gown prevents

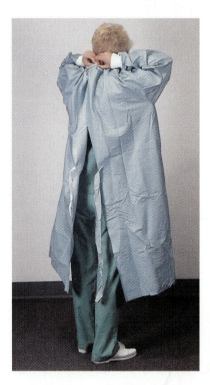

FIGURE 12-17 Put on a gown if your uniform may contact blood or moist body fluids.

contamination of the health care provider's uniform. A gown should be worn only once. Discard gowns according to facility policy after use.

Gloves

The use of gloves prevents the spread of disease. Usually the nursing assistant will wear nonsterile latex or vinyl disposable gloves, but there are also times when other types of gloves are worn. Gloves should be worn for most health care procedures, and they are always worn when contact with blood, body fluids (except sweat), secretions, excretions, mucous membranes, or nonintact skin is expected. You should also wear gloves if you have cuts or open sores on your hands. Gloves are also used during many routine cleaning procedures that the nursing assistant performs. In this case, utility gloves may be worn. The use of gloves does not replace the need for handwashing. Always wash your hands before and after glove use. If you accidentally touch a potentially contaminated environmental surface after removing your gloves, wash your hands again.

Gloves are used for three main purposes:

1. To prevent the nursing assistant from picking up a pathogen from the patient
2. To avoid giving the patient a pathogen that the nursing assistant has picked up on the hands
3. To avoid picking up a pathogen on a patient or the environment and carrying it to another patient on the hands

For gloves to be effective, they must be intact and have no visible cuts, tears, or cracks. They must fit your hands well. Gloves come in different sizes. Select the size that most comfortably fits your hand. If the glove is too large or too small, a measure of protection is lost. Do not wash your hands while wearing gloves. Handwashing damages the pores of the gloves and may allow microbes to enter. If your hands need to be washed, remove the gloves, wash your hands, then reapply new gloves. Table 12-2 lists times when gloves should be changed. Remember to wash your hands every time you remove gloves. Table 12-3 lists common nursing assistant tasks and the correct personal protective equipment to use for each job.

Gloves are for single patient use only. Do not wear them to care for more than one patient. Take care that you do not contaminate environmental surfaces with your gloves. Some facilities use the "one-glove technique" (Figure 12-18). This involves carrying a contaminated item in a gloved hand. The glove on the other hand is removed to open doors, turn on faucets, and touch other environmental surfaces and supplies.

Health care facilities have many different policies regarding how and where gloves are discarded. Many facilities require the staff to discard gloves in sealed or covered containers and not open wastebaskets in the room. Know and follow your facility policy.

TABLE 12-2 SUGGESTED TIMES TO CHANGE GLOVES
Remember to wash your hands before applying and after removing gloves. Never touch environmental surfaces with a contaminated glove.
Change gloves:
• Before giving any patient care
• After giving patient care
• Immediately before touching mucous membranes
• Immediately before touching nonintact skin
• Immediately after touching secretions or excretions
• Immediately after touching blood or body fluids
• After touching equipment or environmental surfaces that are potentially contaminated
• Any time your gloves are torn
• If your gloves become visibly soiled

Face Mask

Surgical masks should be worn when exposure to droplet secretions may occur. The mask should cover the nursing assistant's nose and mouth. For example, a mask would be worn when caring for a patient with influenza who is coughing and releasing droplets containing the flu pathogen into the environment. The mask protects you when you are working within three feet of the patient. It is also used whenever protective eyewear is worn. When a surgical mask is needed, it is:

- Used only once and discarded
- Changed if it becomes moist
- Handled only by the ties
- Never left secured around the neck because it can contaminate the uniform and the environment

Protective Eyewear

A full **face shield** (Figure 12-19), or **goggles** (Figure 12-20), are worn any time splashing of blood, body fluid, secretions, or excretions may occur. The eyewear does not protect the mucous membranes of the nose and mouth, so a surgical mask is always worn with eyewear. A good rule to follow is that a surgical mask may be worn without protective eyewear, but protective eyewear is never worn without a surgical mask. Some masks have a protective eyeshield attached to them. The mask is put on before the protective eyewear. When removing the mask and eyewear, wash your hands, remove the eyewear, then the mask.

TABLE 12-3 PERSONAL PROTECTIVE EQUIPMENT IN COMMON NURSING ASSISTANT TASKS

Note: Use this chart as a general guideline only. Add protective equipment if special circumstances exist. Know and follow your facility policies for using personal protective equipment.

Nursing Assistant Task	Gloves	Gown	Goggles/Face Shield	Surgical Mask
Washing/rinsing utensils in the soiled utility room	Yes	Yes if splashing is likely	Yes if splashing is likely	Yes if splashing is likely
Holding pressure on a bleeding wound	Yes	Yes	Yes	Yes
Wiping the shower chair with disinfectant	Yes	No	No	No
Emptying a catheter bag	Yes	Yes if facility policy	Yes if facility policy	Yes if facility policy
Passing meal trays	No	No	No	No
Passing ice	No	No	No	No
Giving a back rub to a patient with a rash	Yes	No	No	No
Giving special mouth care to an unconscious patient	Yes	Yes if facility policy	Yes if facility policy	Yes if facility policy
Assisting with a dental procedure	Yes	Yes	Yes	Yes
Changing the bed after an incontinent patient has an episode of diarrhea	Yes	Yes	No	No
Taking an oral temperature with a glass thermometer (gloves are not necessary with an electronic thermometer unless this is your facility policy)	Yes	No	No	No
Taking a rectal temperature	Yes	No	No	No
Taking an axillary temperature	No	No	No	No
Taking a blood pressure	No	No	No	No
Assisting an alert patient to brush teeth	Yes	Yes if facility policy	Yes if facility policy	Yes if facility policy
Washing a patient's eyes	Yes	No	No	No
Giving perineal care	Yes	No	No	No
Washing the patient's abdomen when the skin is not broken	No	No	No	No
Washing the patient's arms when skin tears are present	Yes	No	No	No
Brushing a patient's dentures	Yes	No	No	No
Assisting the nurse while he or she suctions an unconscious patient with a tracheostomy	Yes	Yes	Yes	Yes
Turning an incontinent patient who weighs 85 pounds	Yes if linen is soiled	Yes, if your uniform will have substantial contact with the linen	No	No
Shaving a patient with a disposable razor	Yes, because this is a high-risk procedure	No	No	No
Shaving a patient with an electric razor	No	No	No	No
Cleaning the soiled utility room at the end of your shift	Yes	No	No	No

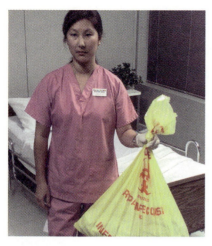

FIGURE 12-18 One-glove technique is used to carry contaminated items.

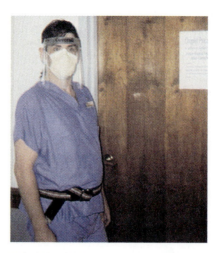

FIGURE 12-19 A surgical mask is always worn with a face shield.

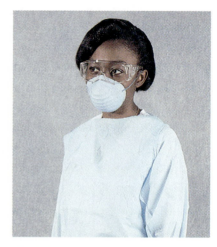

FIGURE 12-20 A surgical mask is always worn with goggles.

Sequence for Applying Personal Protective Equipment

1. Wash hands
2. Mask
3. Gown
4. Goggles or face shield
5. Gloves

Sequence for Removing Personal Protective Equipment

1. Gloves
2. Wash hands
3. Goggles or face shield
4. Mask
5. Gown
6. Wash hands

Equipment

Disposable (used once and discarded) patient care equipment is used by many facilities. It is ideal for patients on isolation precautions. Frequently used equipment remains in the patient's unit. Most articles will not require special handling unless they are contaminated (or likely to be contaminated) with infective material.

Special precautions are not necessary for dishes unless they are visibly contaminated with infective material. An example of this is dishes that have blood, drainage, or secretions on them. Disposable dishes contaminated with infective material can be handled as disposable patient care equipment.

Containment of Contaminated Articles

Contaminated articles leaving the patient's room must be handled so that pathogens will not be spread. It is important that contaminated equipment be bagged, labeled, and disposed of according to the health care facility's policy for the disposal of infectious waste. Used articles are placed in an impenetrable bag (such as plastic) before they are removed from the room or unit of the patient. A single bag may be used if it is waterproof and sturdy enough to confine and contain the article without contaminating the outside of the bag. (Refer to Procedures 7 through 10.)

PROCEDURE **2** OBRA

PUTTING ON A MASK

1. Assemble equipment:
   - mask
2. If gown and gloves are needed, the mask goes on first. (If a face shield is used, it is put on next.)
3. Adjust mask over nose and mouth.

4. Tie top strings of mask first, then bottom strings.
5. Replace mask if it becomes moist during procedures.
6. Do not reuse a mask and do not let the mask hang around your neck.

PROCEDURE **3**

PUTTING ON A GOWN

To be effective, a gown should have long sleeves, be long enough to cover the uniform, and big enough to overlap in the back. Gowns should be waterproof.

1. Assemble equipment:
   - Clean gown
   - Paper towel
2. Remove wristwatch; place it on paper towel.
3. Wash hands.
4. If a mask and goggles or face shield are required, put them on first.
5. After tying on the mask, put on the gown outside the patient's room. Put on gown by slipping arms into sleeves (Figure 12-21A).

6. Slip fingers of both hands under inside neckband and grasp ties in back. Secure neckband (Figure 12-21B).
7. Reach behind and overlap edges of gown. Secure waist ties (Figure 12-21C).
8. Take watch into isolation unit, leaving it on paper towel.
9. Remember when using gowns:
   - A disposable gown is worn only once and then is discarded as infectious waste.
   - A reusable cloth gown is worn only once and then is handled as contaminated linen.
   - Carry out all procedures in the unit at one time, to avoid unnecessary waste of gowns.

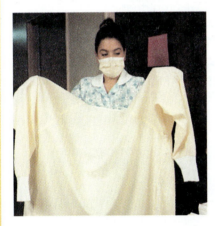

FIGURE 12-21A Putting on the clean cover gown before entering the patient's room. After putting on the mask, put on the gown.

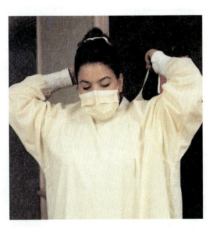

FIGURE 12-21B Slip fingers inside the neckband and tie gown.

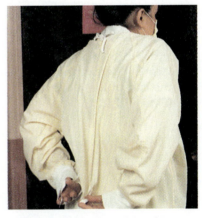

FIGURE 12-21C Reach behind, overlap the edges of the gown so the uniform is completely covered, and tie the waist ties.

PROCEDURE **4**

PUTTING ON GLOVES

1. Assemble equipment:
   - Disposable gloves in correct size
2. Wash hands.
3. If gown is required, put gloves on after gown is put on.

4. Pick up glove by the cuff and place it on the other hand.
5. Repeat with glove for other hand.
6. Interlace fingers to adjust gloves on hands.

continues

PROCEDURE   4   continued

7. Remember when using gloves:
   - Wash hands before and after using gloves.
   - Remove gloves if they tear or become heavily soiled. Wash hands and put on a new pair.
   - Gloves are used whenever there is the possibility of contacting body fluids,

   blood, secretions, or excretions with mucous membranes or nonintact skin.
   - Change gloves between patients and wash hands.
   - Discard gloves immediately after removing, in biohazardous waste receptacle.

PROCEDURE   5

REMOVING CONTAMINATED GLOVES

1. Grasp cuff of one glove on the outside with the fingers of the other hand (Figure 12-22A).

2. Pull cuff of glove down, drawing it over the glove and turning the glove inside out (Figure 12-22B). Pull glove off hand.

3. Hold the glove with the still-gloved hand.

4. Insert fingers of the ungloved hand under the cuff of the glove on the other hand (Figure 12-22C).

5. Pull the glove off inside out, drawing it over the first glove.

6. Drop both gloves together into the biohazardous waste receptacle (Figure 12-22D).

7. Wash hands. Dry with a paper towel and discard towel in proper container. Use a dry towel to turn off water faucet. Discard towel.

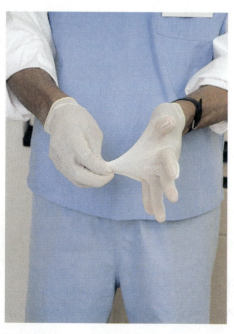

FIGURE 12-22A With fingers of one hand, grasp glove of other hand.

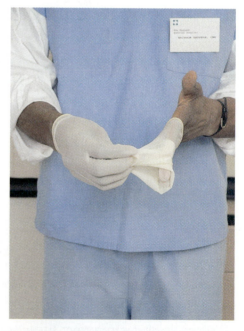

FIGURE 12-22B Pull the glove down over the hand and the fingers and remove it. The glove is inside out with the contaminated side inside.

continues

P R O C E D U R E   5   continued

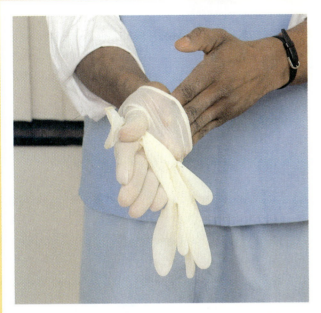

FIGURE 12-22C Hold the glove just removed in the gloved hand. Insert fingers of the ungloved hand inside the cuff of the other glove.

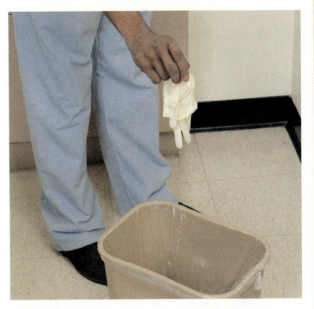

FIGURE 12-22D Pull the glove down over the hand and glove and then pull both gloves off, holding the inside (noncontaminated side of glove). Discard the gloves in the receptacle for contaminated trash.

P R O C E D U R E   6

REMOVING CONTAMINATED GLOVES, MASK, AND GOWN

1. Assemble equipment:

   - Biohazardous waste receptacle for disposable items
   - Waste receptacle for gown if it is not disposable
   - Paper towels

2. Follow Procedure 5 for removing contaminated gloves.

3. Undo waist ties of gown (Figure 12-23A).

4. Turn faucets on with clean paper towel. Discard towel.

5. Wash hands and dry with clean paper towel.

6. Hold clean, dry paper towel to turn off faucet.

7. Remove goggles if used. Dispose of according to facility policy.

8. Remove mask:

   - Undo bottom ties first, then top ties (Figure 12-23B).
   - Holding top ties, dispose of mask in appropriate waste receptacle.

9. Undo neck ties and loosen gown at shoulders (Figure 12-23C).

10. Slip fingers of dominant hand inside cuff of other hand without touching outside of gown (Figure 12-23D).

11. Using gown-covered hand, pull the gown down over the dominant hand (Figure 12-23E) and then off both arms.

continues

PROCEDURE **6** *continued*

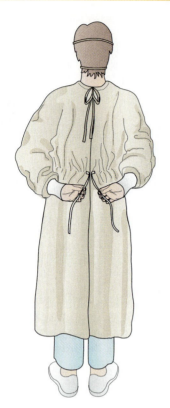

FIGURE 12-23A Remove gloves. Wash hands and then untie waist tie of gown.

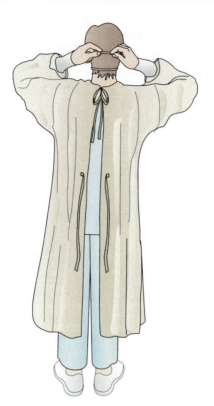

FIGURE 12-23B Remove mask by untying top ties first and then bottom ties. Holding mask by ties, place it in the receptacle for contaminated trash.

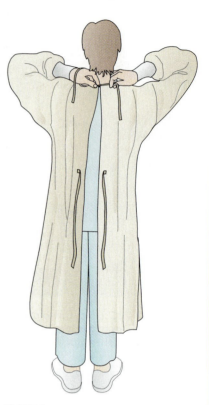

FIGURE 12-23C Untie neck ties of gown.

12. As the gown is removed, fold it away from the body with the contaminated side inward and then roll it up (Figure 12-23F). Dispose of contaminated gown in appropriate receptacle.

13. Wash hands.

14. Remove watch from paper towel. Hold clean side of paper towel and dispose of towel in wastepaper receptacle.

15. Use paper towel to grasp handle to door as you leave patient's room. Discard paper towel in appropriate receptacle before you leave the unit.

continues

PROCEDURE 6 continued

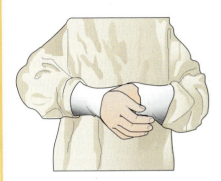

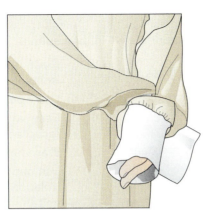

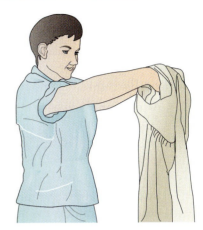

FIGURE 12-23D Slip fingers of one hand inside the cuff of the other hand. Pull gown down over the hand. Do not touch the outside of the gown with either hand.

FIGURE 12-23E Using the gown-covered hand, pull the gown down over the other hand.

FIGURE 12-23F Pull the gown down off the arms, being careful that the hands do not touch the outside of the gown. Hold the gown away from your uniform and roll it up with the contaminated side inside. If gown is disposable, place it in the receptacle for contaminated trash. If gown is not disposable, place it in laundry hamper for contaminated linens.

PROCEDURE 7

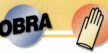

SERVING A MEAL IN AN ISOLATION UNIT

1. Before entering the isolation unit:
   - Wash hands.
   - Obtain the meal tray for the patient. Check the meal card on the tray and check that the correct menu was provided.
   - Ask for the assistance of another member of the team.
   - Place the tray on the isolation cart.
   - Put on PPE as required by the type of isolation precautions used.
2. Enter the isolation room and identify the patient.
3. Explain what you plan to do.
4. Provide privacy.
5. Allow patient to help as much as possible.

6. Raise the bed to comfortable working height.
7. Pick up the meal tray that remains in the room. Make sure the tray is clean.
8. Return to the door and open it. The team member assisting holds the meal tray while you carefully transfer items to the isolation tray.
9. Place isolation meal tray on overbed table. Prepare patient for the meal.
10. Check patient's identification band against the meal tray card.
11. Assist patient with food preparation and feeding as needed.
12. When the patient finishes, note how much food and liquid have been eaten. Uneaten food (except bones) is flushed down the toilet.

continues

PROCEDURE   7   continued

13. All disposable items (bones, dishes, eating utensils, covers, plastic wrap, foil, napkins, cups, cartons) are placed in the appropriate waste receptacle.

14. Reusable dishes may be handled as follows:

    • Use a paper towel to open door to isolation unit.

    • Prop door open with your foot. Transfer dishes to a tray held by another assistant outside the door.

    • Assistant outside the room covers the dishes and returns the tray to the food cart.

Note: CDC no longer requires the use of disposable dishes on transmission-based precautions.

15. Clean isolation meal tray and store in the isolation unit.

16. Carry out all procedure completion actions.

17. Remove PPE and discard in the appropriate receptacle.

18. Wash hands.

19. Use paper towel to open door to leave the isolation unit. Discard towel before leaving unit.

PROCEDURE   8

MEASURING VITAL SIGNS IN AN ISOLATION UNIT

Note: Equipment to measure vital signs in isolation should be dedicated to the patient. (This means that the equipment will remain in the room with the patient.) If the equipment must be shared with other patients, it must be cleaned and disinfected before use with another patient.

1. Before entering the isolation unit:

    • Wash hands.

    • Remove wristwatch and place it on a clean paper towel.

    • Put on PPE as required by the type of transmission-based precautions used.

2. Pick up the paper towel with the watch. Enter the isolation unit.

3. With the watch still on the paper towel, place it where you can see it during the procedures.

4. Identify the patient and explain what you plan to do.

5. Provide privacy.

6. Allow patient to help as much as possible.

7. Raise bed to comfortable working height.

8. Using the equipment dedicated to the patient, measure vital signs.

9. Note the readings so you do not forget them.

10. Clean and store the equipment used according to facility policy.

11. Carry out all procedure completion actions.

12. Remove and discard PPE according to facility policy.

13. Wash hands, dry, and pick up watch.

14. Handling only the clean side of the paper towel, discard it in the appropriate receptacle.

15. Pick up your notes. Use a clean paper towel to open the door and leave the isolation unit. Discard paper towel before you leave the unit.

Soiled linen is a source of pathogens and should be handled with care. (Refer to Procedure 11.) Some facilities place dirty linen in water-soluble bags that melt in the washer. If these bags are used, they must be placed inside a second plastic bag, because the water-soluble bag will begin to melt if it touches wet linen.

• Handle linen as little as possible.

• Fold the dirtiest side inward.

• Do not shake.

• Do not place soiled linen on the floor or tabletop.

• Bag linen before leaving the room.

- Keep soiled linen separate from general linen.
- Transport soiled, wet linen in a leakproof bag.

Transporting the Patient in Isolation

At times a patient in isolation needs to be transported to another area of the health care facility for treatment or testing. Notify the receiving unit of your intention to transport the patient and describe the type of transmission-based precautions being used. If the patient is on airborne or droplet precautions, the patient should wear a surgical mask while out of the isolation room. (HEPA masks are not used on patients.) If the patient is on contact precautions, the infectious area of the skin should be covered while the patient is out of the room. The nursing assistant wears personal protective equipment when picking up and returning the patient to the isolation room, but does not wear the personal protective equipment while transporting the patient in the hallway. (Refer to Procedure 12.)

You may remove your PPE after you have finished all tasks in the patient's room. Follow the instructions in Procedures 5 and 6.

Table 12-4 summarizes some rules for nursing assistants in the practice of infection control. (See page 154.)

PROCEDURE 9

TRANSFERRING NONDISPOSABLE EQUIPMENT OUTSIDE OF ISOLATION UNIT

1. Nondisposable equipment used with a patient in transmission-based precautions may be dedicated to that patient. This means that the equipment remains in the isolation unit and is used only by that patient. Cleaning as required is done in the room by the nursing assistant or the housekeeping staff according to facility policy.

2. If the equipment must be used for other patients, it must be removed from the isolation unit and disinfected or sterilized before use with another patient.

3. Before leaving the isolation unit, clean the equipment with a disinfectant.

4. Place the equipment in a biohazard plastic bag.

5. Follow Procedure 6 for removing contaminated gloves, mask, and gown.

6. Pick up the bag containing the equipment and leave the isolation unit.

7. Once outside the unit, follow facility policy for disinfection or sterilization of the equipment.

8. Some equipment may be terminally (finally and completely) cleaned with disinfectant in the patient's unit when isolation is discontinued.

PROCEDURE 10

SPECIMEN COLLECTION FROM PATIENT IN AN ISOLATION UNIT

1. Outside the isolation unit, assemble equipment:

   - Clean specimen container and cover
   - Paper towel
   - Biohazard bag for specimen container (Figure 12-24)
   - Two completed labels, one for the specimen container and one for the specimen bag

   📝 *Note: The specimen bag may have a preprinted block on the bag that can be completed with the required information. In this case, a second label is not needed.*

2. Place the equipment on the isolation cart while you put on PPE.

3. The biohazard bag for specimen transport remains outside the isolation unit.

continues

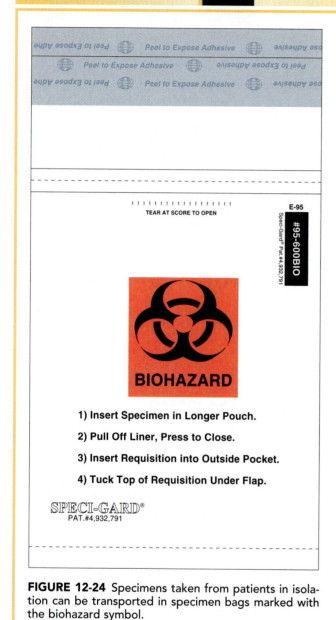

FIGURE 12-24 Specimens taken from patients in isolation can be transported in specimen bags marked with the biohazard symbol.

4. Carry the specimen equipment into the isolation unit. Place container and cover on a paper towel.

5. Identify patient and explain what you plan to do.

6. Provide privacy.

7. Allow patient to help as much as possible.

8. Raise bed to comfortable working height.

9. Place specimen into container without touching the outside of the container.

10. Cover the container and apply label.

11. Clean equipment used to obtain the specimen according to facility policy.

12. Carry out all procedure completion actions.

13. Remove personal protective equipment as described in Procedures 5 and 6.

14. Wash hands.

15. Use a paper towel to pick up specimen container. Use another paper towel to open door to leave isolation unit.

16. Outside the unit, gather the towel in your hands so the edges do not hang loosely. Place the specimen container in the biohazard transport bag, being careful not to allow the paper towel to touch the outside of the transport bag.

17. Discard the paper towels in the appropriate receptacle.

18. Follow facility policy for transporting the specimen.

19. Wash hands.

PROCEDURE 11

OBRA

CARING FOR LINENS IN AN ISOLATION UNIT

1. Assemble linen required and place on chair or stand outside isolation unit.

2. Wash and dry hands.

3. Outside the isolation unit, put on PPE as required by type of transmission precautions.

4. Once inside the isolation unit, place clean linen on a chair.

5. Identify the patient and explain what you plan to do.

6. Provide privacy.

continues

PROCEDURE 11 *continued*

7. Allow patient to help as much as possible.

8. Raise bed to comfortable working height.

9. Remove soiled linen from bed by starting at the edges and working toward the center. Roll the linen toward the center with the soiled side inside.

10. Handle soiled linen as little as possible. Pick up the linen from the bed and hold it away from your uniform and gown (if used).

11. Place soiled linen in a meltaway laundry bag (a bag that dissolves in the wash water in the laundry), or follow facility policy.

12. Place meltaway bag in laundry hamper lined with biohazard plastic bag, or follow facility policy. Bag should be labeled as biohazardous material for laundry.

13. Secure bag and route soiled linen to laundry according to facility policy.

14. If gloves are heavily contaminated from the soiled linens, remove gloves and dispose of in appropriate receptacle. Wash hands, dry, and put on a clean pair of gloves. Then remake patient's bed with the clean linens.

15. Carry out all procedure completion actions. (See Chapter 14.)

PROCEDURE 12

TRANSPORTING PATIENT TO AND FROM ISOLATION UNIT

1. Wash your hands.

2. Assemble equipment:
   - Transport vehicle (wheelchair or stretcher)
   - Clean sheet
   - Mask for patient, if isolation precautions require it

3. Notify department to which patient is to be transported that a patient from an isolation unit is being transported.

4. If the patient is to be transported by stretcher, ask for assistance in moving the patient to the stretcher. Two other care providers will be needed.

5. Cover transport vehicle with clean sheet. Do not let the sheet touch the floor.

6. Wash your hands.

7. Put on PPE as required by type of precautions being used. If other care providers are needed to move the patient onto a stretcher, they also must put on PPE.

8. Wheel transport vehicle into isolation unit.

9. Identify patient. Explain what you plan to do.

10. Provide privacy.

11. Allow patient to help as much as possible.

12. If patient is to be transported by wheelchair, the bed must be in the lowest horizontal position. For transport by stretcher, raise the bed to the same height as the stretcher.

13. Assist the patient into the wheelchair or onto the stretcher.

14. Put mask on patient, if required.

15. Wrap patient in sheet, if required. Make sure sheet does not touch the floor.

16. Remove PPE and wash hands. Open door and take patient out of isolation unit (Figure 12-25).

17. To return patient to isolation unit, place wheelchair or stretcher near wall of room as you put on PPE.

18. Enter the isolation unit, unwrap patient from sheet and remove mask, if used.

19. Assist patient from wheelchair or stretcher (with help of other caregivers) and return to bed.

20. Carry out procedure completion actions.

21. Place sheet in laundry hamper for contaminated linens and discard mask in receptacle for biohazardous trash.

continues

22. Remove PPE and wash your hands.

23. Remove transport vehicle from isolation unit. Follow facility procedure for cleaning and storing vehicle used with patient in isolation.

24. Report completion of procedure: transport of patient in isolation to another department and back to isolation unit.

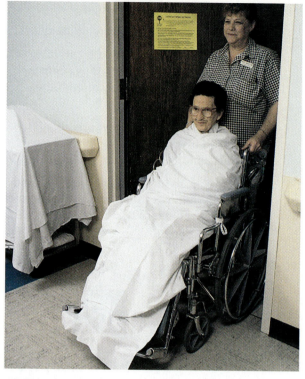

FIGURE 12-25 This patient is leaving her room, where contact precautions are in effect, and is to be transported to another area of the facility.

TABLE 12-4 RULES OF INFECTION CONTROL
Do
• Observe standard precautions and use barrier equipment (PPE) any time contact with blood, body fluids, secretions, excretions, mucous membranes, or nonintact skin is likely. Contact may be with a patient or an environmental surface.
• Clean up dishes immediately after use.
• Damp dust daily and be conscientious about cleaning while you carry out a task.
• Provide a bag for the disposal of used tissues.
• Turn the face to one side so that the assistant and the patient are not breathing directly on each other.
• Cover your nose and mouth when coughing or sneezing.
• Protect the skin on your hands by using warm water, drying thoroughly, and applying lotion if needed.
• Treat breaks in the skin immediately by washing thoroughly, cleaning with an antiseptic, and covering. Report any breaks in the skin to the nurse.
• Disinfect equipment that is used by more than one staff member or patient, such as a stethoscope, before and after each use.
• Gather or fold linen inward, with the dirtiest area toward the center.

continues

TABLE 12-4 *continued*

- Clean reusable equipment immediately after use.
- Handle and dispose of soiled material according to facility policy.
- Practice good personal hygiene.
- Wash your hands frequently.
- Keep clean and dirty items separate in patient rooms and storage areas.
- Bring only needed items into the patient's room.
- Keep soiled linen and trash covered in closed containers.
- Perform procedures in the manner in which you were taught.
- Empty wastebaskets frequently, if this is your responsibility.

Do Not

- Shake bed linens, because any microbes present could be released into the air.
- Allow dirty linen to touch your uniform.
- Eat or share food from a patient's tray.
- Borrow personal care items from another patient or employee.
- Permit the contents of bedpans or urinals to splash when being emptied.
- Report for duty if you have an infectious disease.
- Permit linen to touch the floor, which is always considered dirty.
- Carry clean linen against your uniform or bring more linen than necessary into the patient's room.
- Store lab specimens in the refrigerator with food.

DISINFECTION AND STERILIZATION

Disinfection is the process of eliminating harmful pathogens from equipment and instruments. A chemical called a *disinfectant* is used for this procedure. You may be required to disinfect personal care items such as wash basins, bedpans, and urinals. You may also use disinfectants to clean wheelchairs and other furniture items. Items are usually washed before they are disinfected. The procedure for disinfecting depends on the chemicals used. Follow the directions of your facility for use of disinfectants. Wear disposable gloves and a gown for completing these procedures. You may also need a face shield. Wear PPE that is appropriate to the procedure.

Sterilization removes all microorganisms from an item. This process can be completed in an **autoclave**, which uses steam and pressure to kill organisms. Gas sterilization is also used in some health care facilities. Sterilization procedures are used for all nondisposable equipment that is exposed to potentially infectious materials. Equipment to be sterilized is wrapped in special material. Strips on the packaging material turn a particular color when the package is sterilized (Figure 12-26). Do

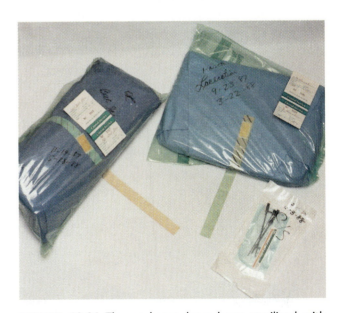

FIGURE 12-26 The packages have been sterilized with steam or gas. The strips below each package show how they look before sterilization. The strips shown on the packages have changed color because they have been sterilized.

not use the package if the strip has not turned the appropriate color. Do not use a sterilized package that has been accidentally opened.

STERILE PROCEDURES

Surgical asepsis is the means by which the environment is kept free of microorganisms, both pathogens and nonpathogens. In procedures where surgical asepsis is used, equipment and supplies must be sterile. In other words, items used in the procedure must go through a sterilization process.

In most facilities, nursing assistants are not expected to carry out procedures requiring sterile techniques. If you are responsible for sterile procedures, you should first be given thorough training. Your responsibilities may include opening sterile packages such as gloves. (See Procedure 13.)

Sterile Field

The term sterile field refers to an area of sterile equipment and materials. When working with a sterile field and sterile equipment, keep the following points in mind:

- The sterile field may be a table covered with a sterilized sheet or a sterile towel placed on an overbed table.
- Only the center of the towel is actually used.
- Equipment is kept two inches in from the edges all around, as an added precaution.
- Never reach for or pass anything that is unsterile over a sterile field. You might drop the unsterile article onto the field or touch the field. Instead, carry the unsterile object around the sterile field or hold it away from the sterile field.
- If there is even a suspicion that anything unsterile has touched any part of the sterile field, the field must be

---

PROCEDURE   13

OPENING A STERILE PACKAGE

1. Wash your hands.

2. Assemble equipment:
   - Sterile package

3. If color code has not changed, or seal does not look intact, do not consider article sterile. *If you have any doubt about sterility, consider item unsterile and inform the nurse.*

4. Touch only outside of package. Only sterile surfaces contact other sterile surfaces. Never reach over a sterile field.

5. Commercially prepared products will be sealed. If package is in poor condition or

discolored, do not consider item sterile. Discard item.

6. Place package with fold side up on a flat, clean surface.

7. Remove tape.

8. Unfold flap farthest away from you by grasping outer surface only between thumb and forefinger (Figure 12-27A).

9. Open right flap with right hand using same technique (Figure 12-27B).

10. Open left flap with left hand using same technique (Figure 12-27C).

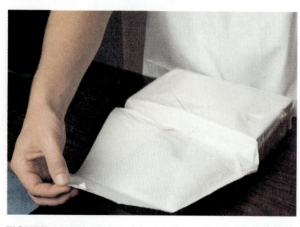

FIGURE 12-27A Open the top flap away from you; handle only the outside.

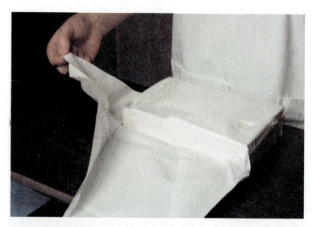

FIGURE 12-27B Open the right side. Do not touch the inside of the folded-over portion.

continues

PROCEDURE 13 continued

11. Open final flap (nearest you) (Figure 12-27D). Touch only the outside of flap. Be careful not to stand too close. Do not allow uniform to

touch flap as it is lifted free. Be sure the flaps are pulled open completely to prevent them from folding back over sterile items.

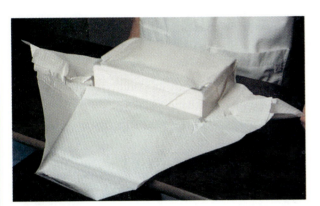

FIGURE 12-27C Open the left side, drawing the left flap to the side.

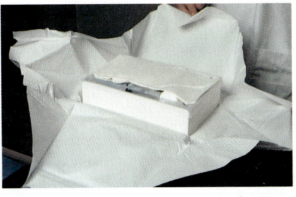

FIGURE 12-27D Without reaching over the sterile field, open the side toward you.

considered contaminated. The entire setup must be discarded.

- Coughing or sneezing while preparing a sterile field or after the field has been set up means contamination of the field.

- Moisture means contamination. If a sterile towel is placed on an unsterile surface, any wetness on the towel means that the towel is contaminated. The towel and anything on the towel must be discarded.

REVIEW

A. True/False.

Mark the following true or false by circling T or F.

1. T F When working in the droplet precautions room, always wear a HEPA mask.

2. T F Surgical masks may be reused.

3. T F It is permitted for two patients in the same room to share equipment.

4. T F Food and drink should not be kept where they may be exposed to contaminated materials.

5. T F When a patient is placed in transmission-based precautions, only licensed nurses are responsible for carrying out proper isolation technique.

6. T F Disposable patient care equipment is preferred when caring for a patient in isolation.

7. T F Droplet precautions do not require the use of a covering gown.

8. T F Handwashing should be done in cold water.

9. T F Always hold fingertips up when rinsing hands during handwashing.

10. T F Handling sterile equipment is a routine procedure for the nursing assistant.

11. T F A mask need not be worn if protective eye equipment is in place.

12. T F Asepsis is the absence of pathogens.

13. T F If an article is "clean," that means it is sterile.

B. Completion.

Complete the statements by choosing the correct word.

14. The single most important health procedure a nursing assistant can carry out is _____.
(wearing gloves) (washing hands)

15. Accidental contact with infectious or potentially infectious materials is known as a/an _____.
(exposure incident) (sepsis mishap)

16. Gloves, gown, masks, goggles, and face masks are part of _____.
(personal protective equipment) (protective hazardous outfits)

17. Small blood spills may be cleaned up by using _____.
(soap and water) (1:10 dilution of bleach)

18. Sharps and needles should be disposed of by placing them in the _____.
(designated container) (wastebasket)

C. Complete the Chart.

In addition to standard precautions, indicate the transmission-based precautions required by each disease condition. Place an x to make your choice.

Disease	Airborne	Droplet	Contact
19. Draining infected pressure ulcer			
20. Tuberculosis			
21. Mumps			
22. Infected surgical wound			
23. Influenza			

D. Multiple Choice.

Select the one best answer for each question.

24. Housing and caring for a person with an infection is known as
a. segregation.
b. isolation.
c. sequestration.
d. separation.

25. To remove PPE after caring for a resident on isolation precautions, you should
a. remove the gown first.
b. remove the gloves first.
c. remove the mask first.
d. remove PPE in any order.

26. If a nursing assistant is sensitive to latex gloves, he or she
a. need not wear gloves.
b. should wear the latex gloves anyway.
c. should ask the supervisor for nonlatex gloves.
d. should put powder in the gloves.

27. The basic foundation of medical asepsis is
a. handwashing.
b. wearing goggles.
c. wearing a mask.
d. wearing a gown.

28. If there is an exposure incident, you should
a. ignore the situation.
b. report it at once to the supervisor.
c. call the doctor.
d. tell other nursing assistants.

E. Nursing Assistant Challenge.

29. Mrs. Minion has just been placed on isolation. Your assignment is to set up the room.
a. What equipment should be assembled and where is each item placed? _____
b. What effect might being placed on isolation have on Mrs. Minion? _____
c. What might you do to make her adjustment easier? _____
d. How might her visitors feel? _____

30. You are reporting on duty. Some of your responsibilities will be handling food trays, making beds, straightening out your patients' overbed tables, and helping to change a patient who is wet with urine. During your shift you will use a facial tissue and visit the rest room.
List six times you will need to wash your hands.
a. _____
b. _____
c. _____
d. _____
e. _____
f. _____

Safety and Mobility

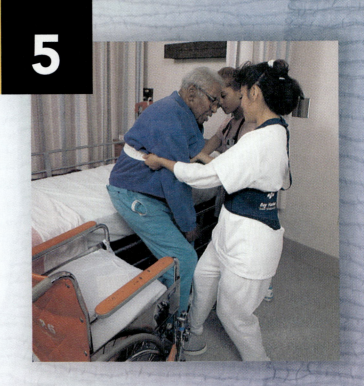

UNIT 13
Environmental and Nursing Assistant Safety

UNIT 14
Patient Safety and Positioning

UNIT 15
The Patient's Mobility: Transfer Skills

UNIT 16
The Patient's Mobility: Ambulation

Environmental and Nursing Assistant Safety

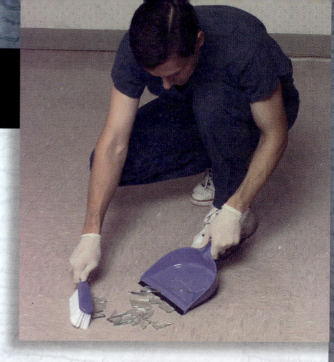

As a result of this unit, you will be able to:

- Spell and define terms.
- Describe the health care facility environment.
- Identify measures to promote environmental safety.
- List situations when equipment must be repaired.
- Describe the elements required for fire.
- List five measures to prevent fire.
- Describe the procedure to follow if a fire occurs.
- Demonstrate the use of a fire extinguisher.
- List techniques for using ergonomics on the job.
- Demonstrate appropriate body mechanics.
- Describe the types of information contained in Material Safety Data Sheets (MSDS).

Learn the meaning and the correct spelling of the following words and phrases:

concurrent cleaning
environmental safety
ergonomics
incident
incident report

Material Safety Data Sheet (MSDS)
Occupational Safety and Health Administration (OSHA)

PASS
private room
RACE
semiprivate room

side rails
ward

INTRODUCTION

The hospital room is the patient's home while he or she is hospitalized (Figure 13-1). The room becomes the patient's world. Cheerful and pleasant surroundings give the patient a better sense of well-being. Consistent attention to safety helps foster feelings of security in this strange environment. *Both* aid in speeding recovery.

The nursing assistant helps keep the patient's unit safe and clean. All health care providers share the task of keeping the entire nursing unit safe and clean.

Environmental safety refers to the condition of an entire facility—patient rooms, hallways, and all departments. The environment includes:

- Temperature (heating and air conditioning)
- Air circulation
- Light
- Cleanliness
- Noise control
- Walls, ceilings, and floors
- Plumbing
- Electricity
- Equipment and furniture

Prevention of injuries to patients, visitors, volunteers, and staff members is of primary concern.

THE PATIENT ENVIRONMENT

In a health care facility, the basic patient unit consists of a/an:

- Hospital bed with rails (Figure 13-2)
- Bedside table
- Chair
- Reading lamp
- Overbed table
- Signal cord

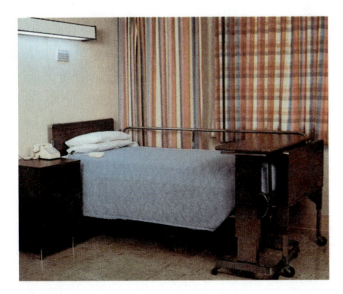

FIGURE 13-1 The patient's unit is his home.

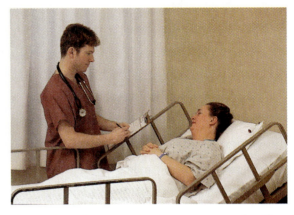

FIGURE 13-2 All hospital beds are equipped with side rails.

This equipment may be located in a single-, double-, or multiple-bed room. A private room contains only one bed. Semiprivate rooms contain two beds. Wards are multiple-bed rooms.

Each room is numbered. The beds are marked by letters or numbers. For example, Room 871 in a large medical center may be a four-unit ward. The beds are labeled A, B, C, D (or 1, 2, 3, 4). The patient in the fourth bed is in Unit 871–D or Unit 871–4.

The equipment from one unit should not be used by other patients. For home care, the same unit elements will be present, but they will be modified. For example, there may not be an adjustable hospital bed or an overbed table.

Hospital Beds

Hospital beds mostly have the same features, but there may be some differences. Hospital beds:

- Differ in the ways in which they operate. Some are controlled electrically (Figure 13-3). Others are operated by the turning of cranks or gatch handles (Figure 13-4).
- May be raised to a high horizontal position. In this position, there is less strain for those giving care. Beds must be returned to the lowest horizontal position when you leave the room.

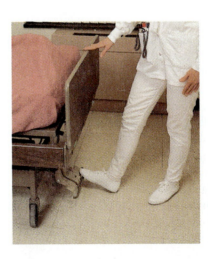

FIGURE 13-3 Bed positions may be changed with electric-powered foot controls.

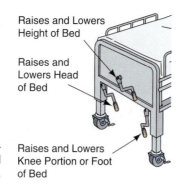

Raises and Lowers
Height of Bed

Raises and
Lowers Head
of Bed

FIGURE 13-4 Nonelec-
tric beds are operated
with gatch handles.

Raises and Lowers
Knee Portion or Foot
of Bed

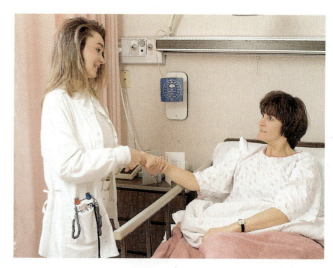

FIGURE 13-5 The overbed light can be adjusted to several
lighting levels.

- Are on wheels, to make it easy to move beds from one place to another. The wheels should always be locked unless the bed is being moved.
- Break in the middle so that the head may be raised.
- Break behind the knees to increase physical comfort for the bedridden patient.

Side rails are attached to the hospital bed. They protect the patient from falling. Side rails:

- Should be checked and attached securely before you leave the patient unless ordered otherwise.
- Should be down only when beds are in the lowest horizontal position or if a release form has been signed by the patient.
- May be raised at night, because patients may become disoriented in dim light and unfamiliar surroundings.
- Should never be used for the attachment of tubes such as IV lines or catheters. Raising and lowering the side rails could put undue stress on such tubes and even pull them out.
- Should never be used for the attachment of restraints.

The use of side rails may upset some patients. Sometimes it may be necessary to reassure the patient that her condition is not becoming worse. The patient should be told that the raising of side rails is hospital policy or is being done as a reminder of a new environment.

- In long-term care facilities the rails may be left down.

Temperature, Air Circulation, and Light

As you adjust and maintain the temperature, light, and ventilation, keep in mind the patient's condition, the patient's personal preference, and the needs of the other patients in the room.

- Best temperature is about 70 degrees. A lower temperature may cause chilling and a higher one may make the patient uncomfortable.
- Movement of air and the temperature may be controlled by opening windows at the top and bottom if air conditioning is not being used. (In some facilities the windows are sealed shut.)
- Patients can be shielded from drafts by screens or curtains.

In most hospitals and health facilities, rooms are automatically air-conditioned. The thermostat may be set from a central location, or set individually in each patient's room.

Lighting comes from several sources. There will be times when less light is desired. At other times, more light will be needed (Figure 13-5). Use as much light as needed to safely carry out your job. Be careful to shield other patients as much as possible.

Patients often find it difficult to sleep if lights are too bright. There should be only enough light at night to enable the staff to work safely.

- Rooms are equipped with lights above each bed. These illuminate a single patient bed.
- There may also be a ceiling light.
- Additional spotlights can be brought from the utility room when needed to provide extra light for delicate procedures.
- The best lighting is indirect; glare causes fatigue.
- Be sure to return extra lights as soon as you are finished, because added clutter in a room is hazardous.
- Be sure to turn ceiling lights off when leaving the room.
- Night lights are often left on for very ill or elderly patients.

Cleanliness and Noise Reduction

You are responsible for the cleanliness, quiet, and order of the patient units to which you are assigned. To contribute to the comfort of the patient:

- Speak quietly.
- Report squeaky wheels on equipment that need to be oiled.
- Avoid banging equipment and trays against other surfaces.
- Keep the area neat as you work. Check its overall appearance before you leave.

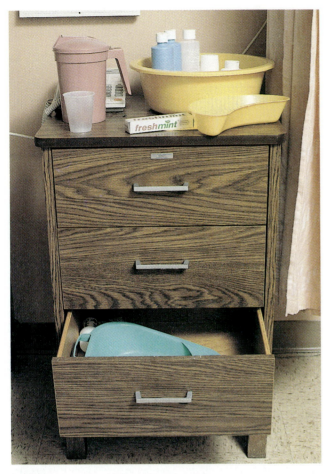

FIGURE 13-6 Standard equipment for personal care is kept in the bedside stand.

- Return equipment to its proper location after completing patient care.
- Do not turn the TV on or up while giving care to patients unless the patient asks you to do so.

You are responsible for keeping the patient supplied with fresh water, ice, disposable drinking cups, tissues, and straws. Make sure that all necessary pieces of equipment, such as the wash basin, emesis basin, bedpan, urinal, soap, and towels, are always available, clean, and in good condition (Figure 13-6). These items should always be stored in the bedside table.

SAFETY MEASURES

Safety is the responsibility of everyone. A safe environment is essential for both the patients and the staff. Safety must be a part of everything you do. This concern extends to the safety of the unit and the entire environment. The number of accidents involving patients and staff can be greatly reduced if simple measures are followed.

When an accident occurs in the health care facility, it is referred to as an **incident**. An incident is any unexpected situation that can cause harm to a patient, employee, or any other person. If you see an incident or are involved in one, you need to report it to your charge nurse. The nurse fills out

an **incident report** (Figure 13-7) after obtaining information from the persons involved. Prevention of incidents depends on employees:

- Knowing their jobs and all policies and procedures related to safety
- Maintaining a safe environment
- Knowing the patients and implementing safety measures to decrease their risk of injury.

Environmental Safety Conditions

Incidents can be prevented by keeping hallways and other walkways free of equipment and clutter. Most facilities require that all equipment that must be in the hall be kept on the same side of the hall. Report these situations promptly:

- Burnt-out light bulbs or light switches that do not work.
- Water leaks from faucets or pipes.
- Faucets or water fountains that do not flow properly.
- Loose or missing floor tiles.
- Windows that do not close tightly or are cracked or broken.
- Temperatures that are too hot or too cold and cannot be controlled within the room. (State licensing agencies have strict regulations regarding environmental temperatures.)
- Loose or missing ceiling tiles or leaks from the ceiling.
- Toilets that do not flush properly.

Equipment and Its Care

The daily or **concurrent cleaning** of equipment is an important part of your job. It contributes to the safety of your patient. The housekeeping department maintains environmental cleanliness. However, spills must be mopped up immediately to avoid falls.

In most health care facilities, equipment is tagged when it needs repair (Figure 13-8). That equipment is not to be used again until the tag is removed. Facility policy differs as to who is responsible for applying and removing the tag. Reporting broken or nonfunctioning equipment is the responsibility of everyone.

You can prevent accidents related to equipment by:

1. Reporting needed repairs promptly. Possible hazards include:
   - lost screws
   - frayed straps
   - loose wheels
   - broken control knobs
   - latches that do not hook
   - side rails that do not fasten correctly
   - faulty brakes on wheelchairs and stretchers
   - frayed electrical cords
2. Reporting call lights (signal cords) immediately if they are not working.

INCIDENT REPORT

Family Name	First Name	M.I.	Room No.	Hosp. No.

Address	City	State	Zip Code	Age	Sex M F

Date of Incident	Time a.m. p.m.	Place	Attending Physician

Status of person involved: Patient _____   Employee _____   Visitor _____   Other _____

Diagnosis: _____

_____

Describe condition before incident: Disoriented ____Senile ___ Sedated ___ Normal ___Other ___

_____

Was height of bed adjustable? Yes ___No ___ Was bed up? Yes ___No ___ Was bed down? Yes ___No ___

Were bedrails ordered? Yes___No ___Were they present? Yes___ No ___Were they up? Yes___No ___

Were they down? Yes ___No ___Other _____

Describe incident entirely, include part of body injured and treatment:

_____

_____

_____

_____

_____

_____

_____

_____

_____

_____

_____

Vital Signs: Temp _____   Pulse _____   Resp _____   Blood Pressure _____

Indicate on diagram location of injury

– over –

FIGURE 13-7 A special report is completed any time an incident occurs.

Was physician called? Yes _____ No _____ Time _____ a.m.
                                                                p.m.

Who responded? _____ Time _____ a.m.
                                                                           p.m.
                Attending physician _____ On-Call physician _____

Statement of physician _____

_____

_____

_____

Was family called? Yes _____ No _____ Time _____ a.m. Who: _____
                                                            p.m.

Give names, addresses and phone numbers of any who witnessed incident _____

_____

_____

_____

A copy of this report will be sent to Patient's physician.

Date of Report _____ Signed _____
                                                    Signature and title of person preparing report

Nursing Office Review of Incident: Date _____ Signed _____

Comments: _____

_____

_____

_____

_____

FIGURE 13-7 *continued*

3. Disposing of equipment in proper containers. Facilities must dispose of "sharps," such as needles and blades, in special containers.

4. Never handling broken bits of glass with your hands. Put on gloves. Large pieces can be picked up with forceps. Broken glass can also be cleaned up using a brush or broom and a dustpan (Figure 13-9).

5. Always knowing what you are handling and the proper method for its disposal.

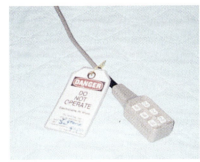

FIGURE 13-8 Equipment that needs repair is tagged.

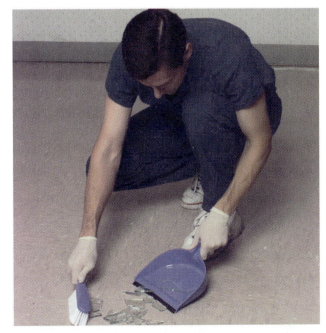

FIGURE 13-9 Sweep up pieces of glass. Wear gloves.

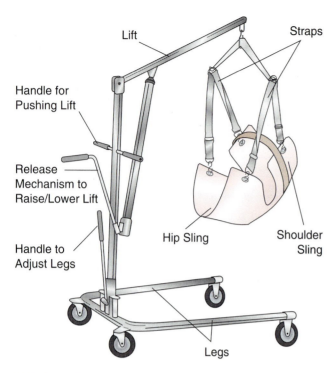

Lift

Straps

Handle for
Pushing Lift

Release
Mechanism to
Raise/Lower Lift

Handle to
Adjust Legs

Hip Sling

Shoulder
Sling

Legs

FIGURE 13-10 Carefully examine the mechanical lift before using it.

6. Inspecting mechanical lifts (Figure 13-10) carefully before using. Check:

   — Handle to make sure legs open and close safely

   — Release mechanism for raising and lowering lift

   — All straps and chains for frayed areas or clasps that do not close correctly

   — Sling to be sure it is the right sling to use with that lift and that there are no frays or tears

   — For hydraulic fluid on the floor—do not use the lift if fluid is present

FIRE SAFETY

It is a scientific fact that if three elements are present in the right proportions (Figure 13-11), there will be a fire. The three elements are heat, fuel, and oxygen.

It is the responsibility of every staff member to know and regularly practice the fire and evacuation plans for the facility.

- Role-play the emergency procedures until you are completely secure. Remember that in any emergency the welfare and safety of the patients are most important.

- Learn the location of escape routes and the location and operation of all fire control equipment (Figure 13-12), such as:
   — Fire alarms
   — Extinguishers
   — Sprinklers
   — Fire doors
   — Fire escapes

- Know and practice fire drill procedures. These are conducted on a regular basis by each facility. Many patients could be injured during a fire because of the confusion and their inability to help themselves.

- Keep alert to all possible fire hazards. Report them immediately to the proper authorities.

Fire Hazards

Some possible fire hazards include:

- Frayed electrical wires
- Overloaded circuits
- Plugs that are not properly grounded
- Accumulated clutter such as papers and rags
- Improper protection during oxygen therapy
- Uncontrolled smoking; most health care facilities prohibit smoking throughout the facility
- Matches left where children or others have unauthorized access to them
- Smoking in rooms where oxygen is in use

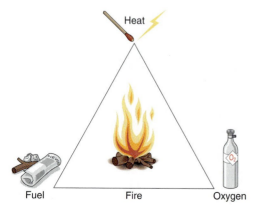

Heat

Fuel

Fire

Oxygen

FIGURE 13-11 The fire triangle—elements needed for combustion (burning).

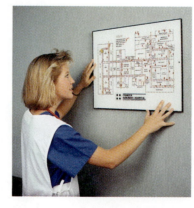

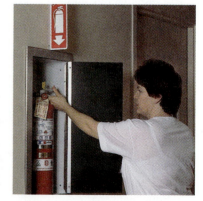

FIGURE 13-12 In the event of fire, all personnel should know the escape plan, where the extinguishers are, and how to use them.

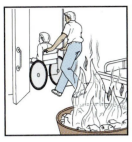
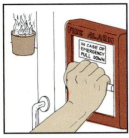
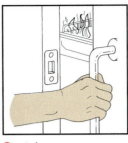
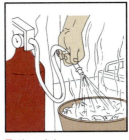
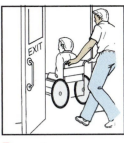

Remove   **A**ctivate   **C**ontain or   **E**xtinguish or   **E**vacuate

FIGURE 13-13 Remember the sequence of critical actions in case of fire.

Fire Prevention

You and every staff member can do a great deal to prevent the disaster of fire. In general:

- Check for frayed electrical wires.
- Do not overload circuits with too many electrical cords.
- Do not use a lightweight electrical cord with heavily powered equipment.
- Use three-prong grounded plugs.
- Do not allow clutter to accumulate in doorways or traffic lanes.
- Empty wastepaper cans in proper receptacles.
- Do not store oily rags or paint rags.
- Report any possible hazards right away.
- Report smoke and/or burning smells.
- Keep all fire exits clear of equipment and debris.
- Know and practice fire drill safety.
- Do not let visitors give cigarettes to patients.

Smoking

Smoking in bed should never be permitted. Smoking should be strictly limited to specific areas, if it is permitted at all. Most health care facilities do not permit smoking by anyone in any area.

This applies to patients, visitors, and staff alike. Ashtrays should be large. The use of matches should be watched. Smoking materials are usually stored at the nurse's station. Patients who do not have smoking privileges should not have smoking materials. If you notice that a patient who is not allowed to smoke has smoking materials, collect the materials and inform the nurse. Some patients may need direct supervision whenever they smoke.

Oxygen Precautions

The use of oxygen presents a specific hazard. When oxygen is in use:

- Never permit smoking, lighted matches, or open flames in the area.
- Do not use flammable liquids such as oils, alcohol, or nail polish.
- Do not use electrical equipment such as radios, hair dryers, electric razors, heating pads, or toys.

- Post a sign indicating that oxygen is in use.
- Use cotton blankets and gowns for the patient.
- Wear cotton uniforms and nonwool sweaters when providing care.
- Be certain there are no cigarettes, matches, or lighters in the room.

In Case of Fire

You must be familiar with the fire policies and procedures for your facility. In case of fire, keep calm. Be sure those in immediate danger are moved to safety. Then sound the alarm according to facility policy. Follow the evacuation plan as you have practiced. The patients may be confused and frightened. Therefore, the staff must be calm and in control. In a fire emergency, remember **RACE** as defined here (Figure 13-13):

- **R** = Remove patients. Move patients to safety. Patients who can walk can be escorted. In some cases, they may be called upon to assist others to escape routes. Patients may need to be moved in their beds out of the danger areas. If a person is unable to walk and the bed cannot be moved, bedsheets may be used as cradles and the patient pulled to safety.
- **A** = Alarm. Sound the alarm. Use the intercom, emergency signal bell, telephone, or fire alarm as directed by facility policy. Give the location and type of fire.
- **C** = Contain fire. Close windows and doors (Figure 13-14) to prevent drafts, which cause the fire to spread more rapidly.
- **E** = Extinguish fire.

Follow the fire emergency plan for your facility:

- Keep calm. Be prepared to follow directions when a person of authority takes charge.

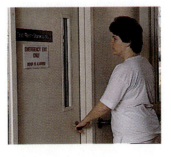

FIGURE 13-14 When closed, fire doors slow the spread of fire.

- Shut off air conditioning and other electrical equipment.
- Shut off oxygen.
- Do not use elevators.

Use of a Fire Extinguisher

If you have been trained in the use of a fire extinguisher, you may use it on small fires.

- Fire extinguishers should be carried upright.
- Remove the safety pin.
- Push the top handle down.
- Direct the hose at the base of the fire.

Remember the letters **PASS**.

    P—PULL the pin

    A—AIM the nozzle at the base of the fire

    S—SQUEEZE the handle

    S—SWEEP back and forth along the base of the fire

OTHER EMERGENCIES

There may be other disasters for which you and your facility must be prepared. Tornadoes, hurricanes, floods, earthquakes, and bomb threats are examples of such disasters. Each facility has its own policies. Be sure you are familiar with them.

In all emergency situations, get patients to safety, follow hospital policy, and keep calm.

NURSING ASSISTANT SAFETY

The work performed by nursing assistants requires a great deal of lifting and moving of patients, objects, and equipment. It is important that you use your body correctly to avoid injury.

Ergonomics

The word **ergonomics** means adapting the environment and using techniques and equipment to prevent injury to the body. If certain risk factors are present, it is more likely that an ergonomic (work-related) problem will occur. These risk factors include:

1. Performing the same motion or motion pattern every few seconds for more than two to four hours at a time.
2. Being in a fixed or awkward posture for more than a total of two to four hours.
3. Using forceful hand exertions for more than two to four hours at a time.
4. Doing heavy lifting, unassisted, for more than one to two hours.

Here are several ergonomic techniques you can use to reduce the risk of having an incident:

1. Use correct body mechanics at all times, both at work and when you are off duty.

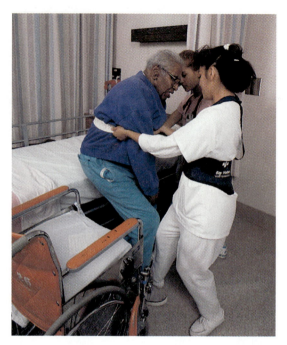

FIGURE 13-15 Many employers require employees to wear back supports.

2. Raise beds to a comfortable working height (remember to lower the beds when you finish your task).
3. Use mechanical lifts when you need to transfer very heavy and/or dependent patients from the bed or back to the bed.
4. Use back supports if your employer requires them. The use of back supports is controversial, but many nursing assistants find them helpful (Figure 13-15).
5. Get another person to help when you need to transfer a patient who cannot bear his own weight fully.
6. Use a cart to move heavy items.

If you follow these eight commandments for lifting, you will greatly decrease the risk of injuring yourself.

1. Plan your lift and test the load (Figure 13-16A).
2. Ask for help (Figure 13-16B).
3. Get a firm footing (Figure 13-16C).
4. Bend your knees (Figure 13-16D).
5. Tighten your abdominal muscles (Figure 13-16E).
6. Lift with your legs (Figure 13-16F).
7. Keep the load close (Figure 13-16G).
8. Keep your back upright (Figure 13-16H).

Warming up before working is another way to maintain a healthy body. The exercises shown in Figures 13-17A through 13-17J can be performed before each work shift. Check with your physician before beginning any exercise program.

Remember that you can avoid many problems if you also:

- Exercise every day.
- Eat a nourishing, well-balanced diet.
- Get adequate sleep.

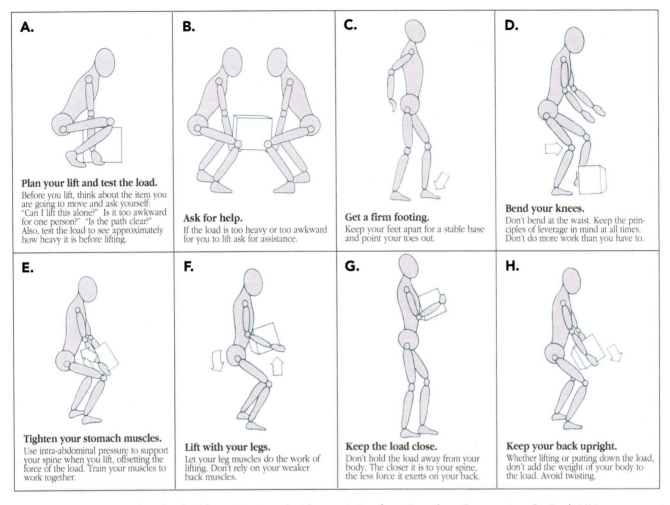

A.

Plan your lift and test the load.
Before you lift, think about the item you are going to move and ask yourself: "Can I lift this alone?" "Is it too awkward for one person?" "Is the path clear?" Also, test the load to see approximately how heavy it is before lifting.

B.

Ask for help.
If the load is too heavy or too awkward for you to lift ask for assistance.

C.

Get a firm footing.
Keep your feet apart for a stable base and point your toes out.

D.

Bend your knees.
Don't bend at the waist. Keep the principles of leverage in mind at all times. Don't do more work than you have to.

E.

Tighten your stomach muscles.
Use intra-abdominal pressure to support your spine when you lift, offsetting the force of the load. Train your muscles to work together.

F.

Lift with your legs.
Let your leg muscles do the work of lifting. Don't rely on your weaker back muscles.

G.

Keep the load close.
Don't hold the load away from your body. The closer it is to your spine, the less force it exerts on your back.

H.

Keep your back upright.
Whether lifting or putting down the load, don't add the weight of your body to the load. Avoid twisting.

FIGURE 13-16A–H Eight rules for lifting. *Reprinted with permission from Ergodyne Corporation, St. Paul, MN*

- Avoid alcohol, cigarettes, drug use, and too much caffeine.
- Wear comfortable shoes with good support.

Hazards in the Work Environment

All health care facilities have hazards in the work environment that can potentially cause injury to employees. Many of these items are chemicals that you may have in your own home (chlorine bleach, for example). On a nursing unit you might find cleaning supplies, disinfectants, and other products that are considered hazardous. Injuries can be prevented if you know what the hazards are and how to protect yourself and others. The Occupational Safety and Health Administration (OSHA) is a section of the Department of Labor under the federal government. OSHA is responsible for employee safety. OSHA requires that all manufacturers of these items supply Material Safety Data Sheets (MSDS) (Figure 13-18) with any hazardous products they sell. The MSDS provide hazard communications that explain:

- what precautions to take in the presence of a hazard (for example, wearing personal protective equipment)

- instructions for safe use of the potentially dangerous substance
- how to clean up and dispose of the hazardous product
- first aid measures to use if exposure occurs

OSHA has also established other rules for a safe environment. Employers are required to inform employees of:

- the location of the MSDS
- the hazards in the work environment and where they are in the building
- the location of information related to the hazards
- how to read and understand chemical labels and hazard signs
- what type of personal protective equipment should be worn while working with these chemicals, and where the personal protective equipment is stored
- how to manage spills and where cleaning equipment is stored

All hazardous products must be kept in their original containers with the original labels intact and legible. Health care facilities must keep all chemicals in locked cupboards.

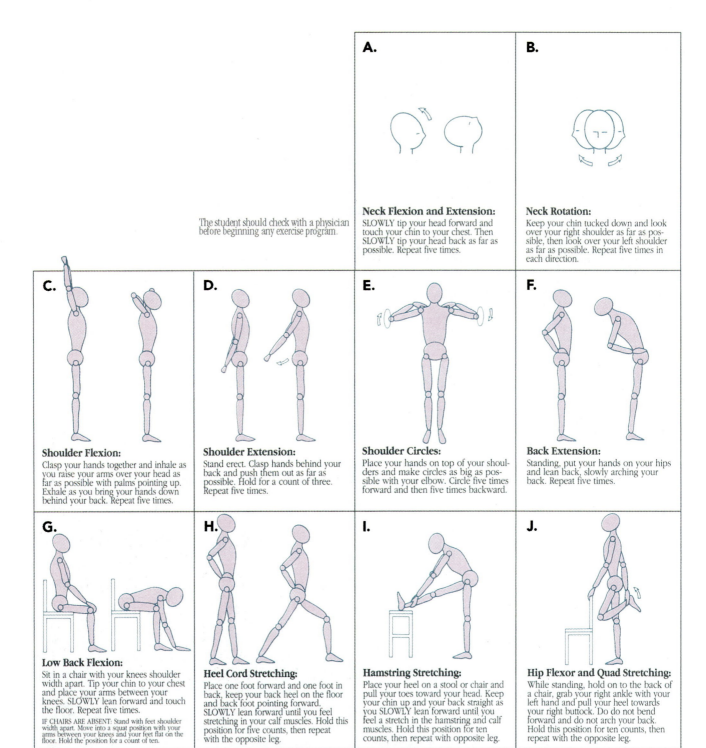

The student should check with a physician before beginning any exercise program.

A.

Neck Flexion and Extension:
SLOWLY tip your head forward and touch your chin to your chest. Then SLOWLY tip your head back as far as possible. Repeat five times.

B.

Neck Rotation:
Keep your chin tucked down and look over your right shoulder as far as possible, then look over your left shoulder as far as possible. Repeat five times in each direction.

C.

Shoulder Flexion:
Clasp your hands together and inhale as you raise your arms over your head as far as possible with palms pointing up. Exhale as you bring your hands down behind your back. Repeat five times.

D.

Shoulder Extension:
Stand erect. Clasp hands behind your back and push them out as far as possible. Hold for a count of three. Repeat five times.

E.

Shoulder Circles:
Place your hands on top of your shoulders and make circles as big as possible with your elbow. Circle five times forward and then five times backward.

F.

Back Extension:
Standing, put your hands on your hips and lean back, slowly arching your back. Repeat five times.

G.

Low Back Flexion:
Sit in a chair with your knees shoulder width apart. Tip your chin to your chest and place your arms between your knees. SLOWLY lean forward and touch the floor. Repeat five times.
IF CHAIRS ARE ABSENT: Stand with feet shoulder width apart. Move into a squat position with your arms between your knees and your feet flat on the floor. Hold the position for a count of ten.

H.

Heel Cord Stretching:
Place one foot forward and one foot in back, keep your back heel on the floor and back foot pointing forward. SLOWLY lean forward until you feel stretching in your calf muscles. Hold this position for five counts, then repeat with the opposite leg.

I.

Hamstring Stretching:
Place your heel on a stool or chair and pull your toes toward your head. Keep your chin up and your back straight as you SLOWLY lean forward until you feel a stretch in the hamstring and calf muscles. Hold this position for ten counts, then repeat with opposite leg.

J.

Hip Flexor and Quad Stretching:
While standing, hold on to the back of a chair, grab your right ankle with your left hand and pull your heel towards your right buttock. Do do not bend forward and do not arch your back. Hold this position for ten counts, then repeat with the opposite leg.

FIGURE 13-17A–J Warming up before work can help prevent injuries. *Reprinted with permission from Ergodyne Corporation, St. Paul, MN*

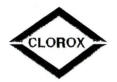

The Clorox Company
7200 Johnson Drive
Pleasanton, California 94588
Tel. (510) 847-6100

Material Safety Data Sheet

I Product:
REGULAR CLOROX BLEACH

Description:
CLEAR, LIGHT YELLOW LIQUID WITH CHLORINE ODOR

Other Designations	Manufacturer	Emergency Telephone No.
Sodium hypochlorite solution Liquid chlorine bleach Clorox Liquid Bleach	The Clorox Company 1221 Broadway Oakland, CA 94612	Notify your Supervisor Rocky Mountain Poison Center (800) 446-1014 For Transportation Emergencies Chemtrec (800) 424-9300

II Health Hazard Data

*Causes substantial but temporary eye injury. May irritate skin. May cause nausea and vomiting if ingested. Exposure to vapor or mist may irritate nose, throat and lungs. The following medical conditions may be aggravated by exposure to high concentrations of vapor or mist; heart conditions or chronic respiratory problems such as asthma, chronic bronchitis or obstructive lung disease. Under normal consumer use conditions the likelihood of any adverse health effects are low.

FIRST AID: EYE CONTACT: Immediately flush eyes with plenty of water. If irritation persists, see a doctor. SKIN CONTACT: Remove contaminated clothing. Wash area with water. INGESTION: Drink a glassful of water and call a physician. INHALATION: If breathing problems develop remove to fresh air.

III Hazardous Ingredients

Ingredients	Concentration	Worker Exposure Limit
Sodium hypochlorite CAS # 7681-52-9	5.25%	not established

None of the ingredients in this product are on the IARC, NTP or OSHA carcinogen list. Occasional clinical reports suggest a low potential for sensitization upon exaggerated exposure to sodium hypochlorite if skin damage (e.g. irritation) occurs during exposure. Routine clinical tests conducted on intact skin with Clorox Liquid Bleach found no sensitization in the test subjects.

IV Special Protection and Precautions

Hygienic Practices: Wear safety glasses. With repeated or prolonged use, wear gloves.

Engineering Controls: Use general ventilation to minimize exposure to vapor or mist.

Work Practices: Avoid eye and skin contact and inhalation of vapor or mist.

Keep out of the reach of children.

V Transportation and Regulatory Data

U.S. DOT Hazard Class: Not restricted

U.S. DOT Proper Shipping Name: Hypochlorite solution with not more than 7% available chlorine. Not Restricted per 49CFR172.101(c)(12)(iv).

Section 313 (Title III Superfund Amendment and Reauthorization Act): As a consumer product, this product is exempt from supplier notification requirements under Section 313 Title III of the Superfund Amendment and Reauthorization Act of 1986 (reference 40 CFR Part 372).

VI Spill or Leak Procedures

Small Spills (<5 gallons)
1) Absorb, containerize, and landfill in accordance with local regulations.
(2) Wash down residual to sanitary sewer.*
Large Spills (>5 gallons)
1) Absorb, containerize, and landfill in accordance with local regulations; wash down residual to sanitary sewer.* - OR - (2) Pump material to waste drum(s) and dispose in accordance with local regulations; wash down residual to sanitary sewer.*

* Contact the sanitary treatment facility in advance to assure ability to process washed-down material.

VII Reactivity Data

Stable under normal use and storage conditions. Strong oxidizing agent. Reacts with other household chemicals such as toilet bowl cleaners, rust removers, vinegar, acids or ammonia containing products to produce hazardous gases, such as chlorine and other chlorinated species. Prolonged contact with metal may cause pitting or discoloration.

VIII Fire and Explosion Data

Not flammable or explosive. In a fire, cool containers to prevent rupture and release of sodium chlorate.

IX Physical Data

Boiling point . . . . 212°F/100°C decomposes)
Specific Gravity ($H_2O=1$) 1.085
Solubility in Water . . . . complete
pH 11.4

©1983, 1991 THE CLOROX COMPANY
DATA SUPPLIED IS FOR USE ONLY IN CONNECTION WITH OCCUPATIONAL SAFETY AND HEALTH

DATE PREPARED 11/92

FIGURE 13-18 Example of a Material Safety Data Sheet (MSDS). *Courtesy of The Clorox Company, Pleasanton, CA*

REVIEW

A. Multiple Choice.

Select the one best answer for each question.

1. The patient's name is Phe Quan. She is in Room 116-D. From this information, you would understand that she is occupying a bed in a
   a. private room.
   b. rehabilitation department.
   c. semiprivate room.
   d. ward.

2. Side rails should be up and secure when
   a. the bed is at the lowest horizontal height (unless you are giving care).
   b. the patient is in bed for the night.
   c. leaving the patient after care unless there is a signed release.
   d. all of these.

3. The best room temperature is approximately
   a. 45°F.
   b. 65°F.
   c. 70°F.
   d. 78°F.

4. Which of the following represents a fire hazard?
   a. Frayed electrical wire
   b. Overloaded circuits
   c. Uncontrolled smoking
   d. All of these

5. Ashtrays should be emptied
   a. into a plastic container.
   b. into a metal container.
   c. into a paper sack.
   d. anywhere—it really doesn't matter.

6. Which of the following contributes to unsafe conditions in the facility?
   a. Equipment sitting in the halls
   b. Chemicals in locked cupboards
   c. Allowing patients to smoke only with supervision
   d. Teaching patients how to use assistive devices such as canes and walkers

7. When oxygen is in use, you should not
   a. use woolen blankets on the patient's bed.
   b. allow smoking in the room.
   c. adjust the liter flow.
   d. all of these.

8. Every staff member should know
   a. the facility fire procedure.
   b. the location of fire extinguishers.

   c. evacuation routes from the unit and building.
   d. all of these.

9. The word that means adapting the environment to prevent body injury is
   a. body mechanics.
   b. incident.
   c. ergonomics.
   d. RACE.

10. One principle of good body mechanics is to
    a. bend from the waist when lifting.
    b. keep your feet close together when lifting.
    c. use the muscles of your arms and legs for lifting.
    d. keep the load as far from your body as possible.

11. Material Safety Data Sheets (MSDS) are required to include information that
    a. explains whether you need personal protective equipment when using the product.
    b. explains first aid measures to use if exposure occurs.
    c. explains how to clean up and dispose of the product.
    d. all of these.

B. Completion.

Choose the correct word from the following list to complete each statement in questions 12–20.

body mechanics	mechanical lift
call light	Material Safety Data
ergonomics	Sheets (MSDS)
hips and knees	OSHA
incident	RACE

12. Using your body correctly while you are working is called _____.

13. Basic rules for lifting include bend from the _____ and not from the waist.

14. An unexpected situation that can cause harm to an employee, a patient, or a visitor is called (a, an) _____.

15. Adapting the environment and using techniques and equipment to prevent body injury is called _____.

16. You should use a _____ when you need to transfer very heavy or dependent patients.

17. All patients must have access to a _____ because it may be the only way they have to summon help.

18. All manufacturers must supply _____ with the hazardous products they sell.

19. The section of the federal government that oversees employee safety is called _____.

20. The acronym used to remember the sequence of critical actions in case of fire is _____.

C. True/False.

Mark the following true or false by circling T or F.

21. T F The bed should be left in lowest horizontal position when the patient is sleeping.

22. T F Some patients may have side rails down so they will not feel confined.

23. T F There should always be enough light to enable the staff to work safely.

24. T F Noise and clutter are very disturbing to most people.

25. T F Needed repairs should be reported immediately.

26. T F The signal cord is the patient's way of letting the staff know that he is in need.

27. T F It is all right to play while at work as long as no one gets hurt.

28. T F You are responsible for knowing and practicing fire drill procedures.

29. T F In case of a fire, follow your own plan of action.

30. T F It is wise to use an elevator during a fire emergency.

D. Nursing Assistant Challenge.

Mary Hernandez is a new nursing assistant at Community Memorial Hospital. She has just completed her CNA course. Consider the information she needs to receive in orientation in order to be a safe and efficient worker.

31. What information does Mary need to learn about the facility to prevent fires and to follow correct procedure in the event of a fire?

32. Mary will need information on equipment she will be working with. What items of equipment is she likely to be using on her job?

33. Discuss everything Mary can do to prevent work-related injuries.

34. What chemicals is she likely to be using?

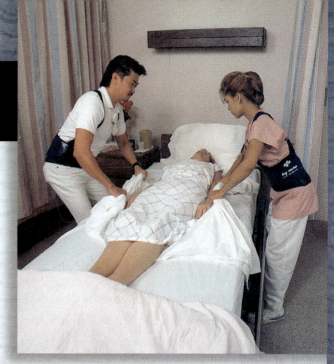

Patient Safety and Positioning

OBJECTIVES

As a result of this unit, you will be able to:

- Spell and define terms.
- List the elements that are common to all procedures.
- Identify patients who are at risk for having incidents.
- List alternatives to the use of physical restraints.
- Describe the guidelines for the use of restraints.
- Demonstrate the correct application of restraints.
- Describe two measures for preventing these types of incidents: accidental poisoning, thermal injuries, skin injuries, and choking.

- Describe correct body alignment for the patient.
- List the purposes of repositioning patients.
- Demonstrate these positions using the correct supportive devices: supine, semisupine, prone, semiprone, lateral, Fowler's, and orthopneic.
- Demonstrate the following procedures:
  - Procedure 14 Turning the Patient Toward You
  - Procedure 15 Turning the Patient Away from You
  - Procedure 16 Moving a Patient to the Head of the Bed
  - Procedure 17 Logrolling the Patient

VOCABULARY

Learn the meaning and the correct spelling of the following words and phrases:

ambulate
aspiration
body alignment
chemical restraint
contracture
draw sheet
Fowler's position

high Fowler's
laceration
lateral
mobility
orthopneic position
orthoses
physical restraint

pressure ulcer
procedure
prone
semi-Fowler's
semiprone
semisupine
Sims' position

spasticity
splint
supine
supportive device
transfer
trochanter roll
turning (moving) sheet

PATIENT SAFETY

In Unit 13, you learned how to maintain a safe environment and how to avoid personal injuries. The prevention of patient injuries is another very important part of your job as a nursing assistant. Patients in health care facilities are at risk for incidents, because they may:

- Have impaired **mobility** (ability to move about) due to an injury, disease, or surgery
- Be receiving medications that affect mental status, balance, and coordination
- Be disoriented because of the change in environment or because of a medical disorder
- Have impaired hearing or impaired vision

Because of these risk factors, most incidents involving patients in any health care setting are falls. Falls may occur because the patient:

- Misjudges the distance from the bed to the floor
- Feels weak or dizzy when trying to get up
- Changes position too rapidly and loses balance when trying to stand up
- Encounters hazards when walking
- Is walking in a poorly lit area

GUIDELINES *for*

Preventing Patient Falls

- Always leave the bed in its lowest horizontal position when you have finished giving care.
- Check to see whether the side rails are to be raised. Make sure they are attached securely.
- Check and adjust protruding objects such as bed wheels or gatch handles.
- Do not block or clutter open areas with supplies and equipment.
- Wipe up spills immediately.
- Encourage patients to use the rails along corridor walls when walking (Figure 14-1).

- Monitor patients for signs of weakness, fatigue, dizziness, and loss of balance.
- Monitor patients for safe practice if they independently:
  - propel their wheelchairs
  - **transfer** (get out of bed)
  - **ambulate** (walk)
- Provide adequate lighting.
- Eliminate noise and other distractions that may increase confusion and create anxiety.
- Avoid leaving patients alone in the tub or shower unless you are given specific permission to do so.
- Check patients' clothing for fit and safety. Loose shoes and laces, long robes, and slacks increase the risk of falling. Patients should wear nonskid shoes when walking and during transfers (Figure 14-2).
- Care for the patient's physical needs promptly. Many incidents occur when patients attempt to get out of bed to go to the bathroom.
- Always use the correct techniques for transferring and walking patients.

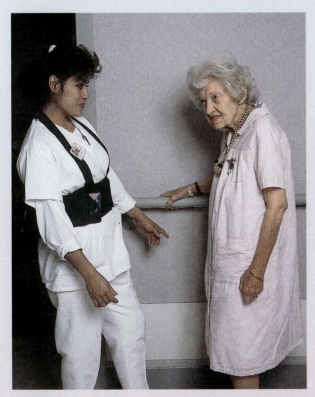

FIGURE 14-1 Encourage patients to use rails along corridor walls when walking.

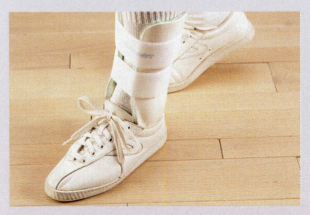

FIGURE 14-2 Patients should wear nonskid shoes for transfers and walking. *Aircast® ankle stirrup is provided by Sammons Preston, Inc., a Bissell® HealthCare Company. Reprinted with permission*

Physical Restraint Informed Consent

Patient's name _____

Method of physical restraint used _____

The reason the physical restraint is needed _____

Times when restraint will be applied _____

Alternatives tried _____

In compliance with federal and state regulations, this facility is committed to the limiting of the use of physical restraints only to situations necessary to maximize a patient's physical, mental and psychological well-being. It is the policy of this facility that, if physical restraints are deemed necessary, the least restrictive method will be applied for shortest amount of time possible.

Physical restraints will only be used by this facility when it has been determined that they are required to treat a patient's medical symptoms or a therapeutic intervention, as ordered by a physician, and based on (1) a documented assessment, by an appropriate health professional of the patient's capabilities; the physical condition or mental treatment which requires the use of physical restraints; the less restrictive measures or therapeutic interventions which have proved ineffective; and the specific physical restraint most effective for the patient's condition; and (2) demonstration by the care planning process that using a physical restraint as a therapeutic intervention will promote the care and services necessary for the patient to attain or maintain the highest practicable physical, mental or psychosocial well-being.

This patient has been assessed regarding his or her need for appropriate physical restraint. He or she will be reassessed at least quarterly or as his or her needs change throughout their stay at this facility. A report will be made each quarter as to the effectiveness of the physical restraint in maximizing the patient's physical, mental or psychosocial well-being. On-going assessments help to further this goal. The duration of consent for the use of this physical restraint is good only until the next annual assessment of the patient's needs, or if there is a need for more restrictive physical restraints. At those times, a new informed consent will be required, if needed.

The benefits of physical restraints include the prevention of injuries to oneself or to others, enhancement of functional abilities, reduced potential for falling, and continued provision of medically necessary procedures. Potential complications associated with physical restraints include incontinence, decreased range of motion, decreased ability to ambulate, symptoms of withdrawal or depression, or reduced social contact. This facility will monitor the use of physical restraints daily and respond to any developing complications to physical restraint use.

By virtue of my signature, I state that I received, read, and had an opportunity to discuss any questions I may have regarding the application of physical restraints in this facility. I give consent for the use of physical restraints when the benefits outweigh the identified risks in accordance with this informed consent. I understand that I can revoke consent for this physical restraint at any time. I further consent to physical restraint reduction as soon as feasible.

_____

(Signature of Patient or Authorized Individual)   (Date)

_____

(Signature of Witness)   (Date)

[   ] Patient unable to sign.

FIGURE 14-3 In long-term care facilities, written consent must be obtained from the patient or family before applying a restraint.

USE OF PHYSICAL RESTRAINTS

In the past, restraints were often used routinely as a preventive measure to avoid falls. Research has shown that side rails and restraints do not necessarily accomplish this purpose. In fact, many falls occur with side rails up and restraints intact. This can result in serious injury and even death. There are two types of restraints: physical restraints and chemical restraints. Chemical restraints are medications that affect the patient's mood and behavior. As a nursing assistant, you will be more concerned with the use of physical restraints. Physical restraints are defined as any technique or device that is attached or next to the patient's body that the patient cannot easily remove and that restricts freedom of movement and normal access to the body. OBRA (1987) clearly states when and how chemical and physical restraints may be used in a long-term care facility. The Residents' Rights state that "residents have the right to be free from physical and chemical restraints." These guidelines are also being implemented in acute care facilities. Physical restraints are to be used only when the life of the patient or other persons is at risk. Before a restraint is used, the staff must:

- Document all patient behavior that indicates a need for a restraint.
- Document all actions that were taken as an alternative to restraints.
- Consult with the patient and the family or legal guardian when alternatives are unsuccessful and obtain their approval and written consent to apply a restraint (Figure 14-3).

Examples of physical restraints include:

- Wrist/arm (Figure 14-4) and ankle/leg restraints
- Vests (Figure 14-5)
- Jackets (Figure 14-6)
- Hand mitts (Figure 14-7)
- Geriatric and cardiac chairs (Figure 14-8)
- Wheelchair safety belts, bars, and tables (Figure 14-9)
- Bed rails (if they meet the definition of a restraint)

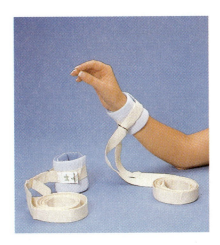

FIGURE 14-4 Wrist restraints may be used to prevent the patient from pulling out an IV.

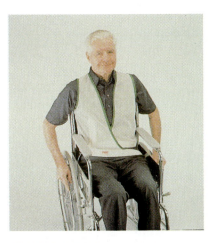

FIGURE 14-5 Vest restraints must always be applied as shown here.

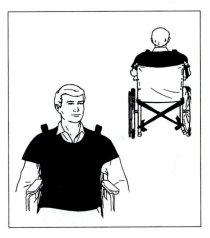

FIGURE 14-6 Jacket restraint. *Courtesy of The J. T. Posey Co., Inc., Arcadia, CA*

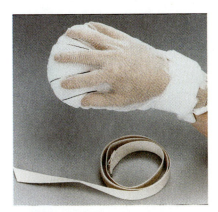

FIGURE 14-7 Hand mitts may be applied to keep the patient from injuring himself.

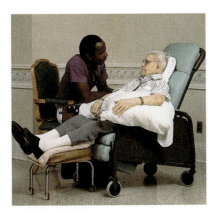

FIGURE 14-8 Geriatric chairs may be considered restraints in some cases.

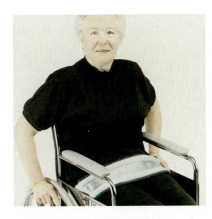

FIGURE 14-9 Wheelchair safety belts, bars, and tables are considered restraints if the patient cannot independently remove them. *Courtesy of The J. T. Posey Co., Inc., Arcadia, CA*

Alternatives to the Use of Restraints

Alternatives to restraints should be tried before restraints are applied. Restraints are used only as a last resort in situations where the patient may harm himself or others. Nursing assistants can take a number of actions to help reduce the need to use restraints.

1. Care for patients' personal needs promptly.
   — Take patients to the bathroom regularly.
   — Provide adequate food and fluids to prevent hunger and thirst.
   — Report signs and symptoms of pain or illness promptly.
   — Follow all instructions for positioning and for assisting patients with exercise.
   — Be sure that patients have their eyeglasses and hearing aids if they need them.
   — Answer call signals promptly.
   — Check patients often to see if they need anything.
   — Provide appropriate exercise and activities.

GUIDELINES *for*

The Use of Restraints

There are a few situations in which a patient may need a restraint, no matter how many alternatives are tried. When restraints are necessary, these guidelines must be followed:

1. A physician's order must be obtained by the nurse before restraints may be used. The order must indicate the type of restraint to use and the reason for its use. Try the least restrictive device first.

2. Use the right type and size of restraint. All restraints must be applied according to manufacturer's directions.
   Check the device before use—do not use if it is frayed, torn, has parts missing, or is soiled. Restraints are put on over clothing, never next to bare skin.

3. Even if the patient does not seem to understand, always explain what you are doing. After application, check the fit of the device. You should be able to slip the width of three fingers between the restraint and the patient's body. The device should never restrict breathing.

4. Tie restraint straps with slip knots for quick release in an emergency.

5. The patient should always have access to the signal light. Check every 15 minutes for the patient's comfort and safety. Make changes as needed.

6. Release the restraint at least every 2 hours for at least 10 minutes to:
   — Check for irritation or poor circulation
   — Change the patient's position
   — Exercise—ambulate the patient or do passive range-of-motion exercises
   — Take the patient to the bathroom
   — Change incontinent patients and cleanse their skin
   — Provide fluid or nourishment
   — Attend to any other needs

Document each of these actions.

7. Maintain good body alignment whether the patient is in bed or a chair.

8. When restraints are used in bed:
   — There must be full side rails on the bed, in the up position
   — The patient should always be positioned in the middle of the mattress
   — Always secure the restraint to the movable part of the bed frame (Figure 14-10)

9. Do not use restraints in moving vehicles or on toilets unless you are sure the device is intended for that use by the manufacturer.

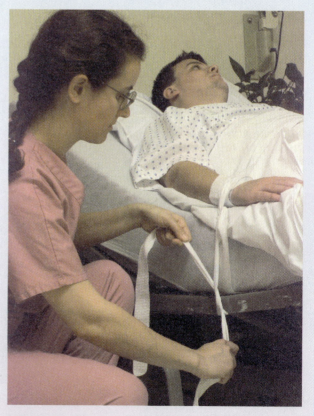

FIGURE 14-10 Always tie restraints to the movable part of the bed frame.

2. Know which patients are at risk for falling. Monitor these patients regularly during your shift.

3. Observe patients who walk and transfer independently. Sometimes falls occur because patients use incorrect and unsafe methods. Report these situations and learn how to teach patients the correct way.

4. Report immediately any physical or mental change that could increase the risk of an incident, such as:
   - Disorientation (patient does not know time, place, or self)
   - Complaints of dizziness
   - Problems with balance and coordination

5. Maintain a safe, quiet, calm, environment.

6. Provide comfortable chairs. Use supportive devices as necessary.

7. A number of security devices are available that are designed to prevent falls and eliminate the need for restraints. These devices include:
   - Special sensors attached to a patient's leg or to a wheelchair. The sensor will set off an alarm if the patient tries to leave the building.
   - Special sensors (a pad) placed in the patient's bed that will set off an alarm if the patient attempts to get out of bed.

PREVENTION OF OTHER INCIDENTS

There are many situations that can result in an incident that can harm the patient. Incidents can be prevented when all staff members are aware of appropriate preventive measures.

Accidental Poisoning

Many common items, such as household chemicals, shaving lotion, plants, and cologne, are poisonous if ingested. Food kept in a bedside table may spoil and also cause illness. Patients who are disoriented may eat or drink any of these items. To prevent accidental poisonings:

- Keep all chemicals and cleaning solutions in locked cupboards.
- Store patients' personal food items in the refrigerator in labeled containers.

Thermal Injuries

Thermal injuries are those caused by heat or cold and result in burns. To prevent thermal injuries:

- Follow procedures accurately when administering warm or cold treatments.
- Check water temperatures before helping a patient into the bathtub or shower. Turn the hot water on last and turn it off first.
- Check food temperatures before feeding patients. Using a microwave oven to reheat food can be dangerous because of the uneven temperatures the oven produces.

- Store smoking materials in a safe place and supervise patients while they smoke. (Most health care facilities do not allow smoking by anyone.)

Skin Injuries

Skin injuries include **lacerations** (cuts or breaks in the skin) and punctures. To prevent these injuries:

- Store knives, scissors, razors, and tools in locked cupboards.
- Store syringes and needles in locked cupboards. These should be disposed of in a sharps container immediately after use.
- Clean up broken glass immediately, as described earlier.

Choking

Aspiration is the accidental entry of food or a foreign object into the trachea (windpipe). This causes choking. Because swallowing becomes less efficient as people age, choking occurs more often in the elderly. Persons who are disoriented or who have impaired consciousness are also at risk. To prevent choking or aspiration:

1. Be aware of patients who have problems with swallowing. Follow all instructions when helping with feeding:
   - Cut food into small pieces.
   - Feed slowly.
   - Offer fluids carefully between solid foods.
   - If the patient has had a stroke, place the food in the unaffected side of the mouth.
   - Use thickeners for liquids if ordered.

2. Place patients upright in good body alignment before meals. Have them remain in this position for at least 30 minutes after eating.

3. At the end of the meal, give oral care to patients who are known to keep food in their mouths. Food may remain in the mouth for several minutes after a meal and be accidentally aspirated if the patient coughs or goes to sleep.

4. Know the procedure to clear an obstructed airway. (See Unit 48.)

INTRODUCTION TO PROCEDURES

Caring for patients' safely means that you must faithfully and carefully carry out specific routines. The normal manner of carrying out a task is called a **procedure**.

As you progress in your studies, you will learn the procedures for many nursing assistant tasks. You have already been introduced to the procedure for washing your hands and using PPE. The procedures that follow give you step-by-step directions for carrying out tasks that involve patients.

Certain things must be done before you carry out patient care procedures. These actions are called *preprocedure* or beginning procedure actions. At the end of each patient care procedure, a standard series of procedure completion actions is also followed.

Beginning Procedure Actions

Steps to be followed at the beginning of each procedure include the following:

- Wash your hands thoroughly (Figure 14-11A).
- Assemble equipment.
- At the patient's room, knock and pause before entering (Figure 14-11B).
- Introduce yourself and identify the patient by checking his or her identification bracelet (Figure 14-11C).

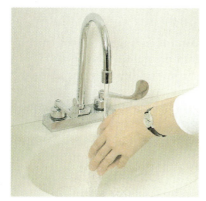

FIGURE 14-11A
Wash your hands.

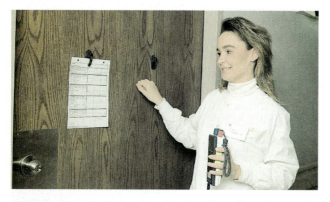

FIGURE 14-11B If the door is closed or the privacy curtains are drawn, knock or speak before entering.

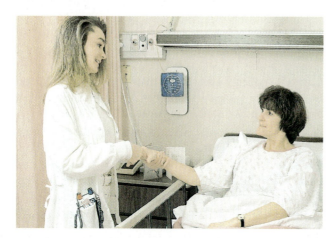

FIGURE 14-11C Identify the patient.

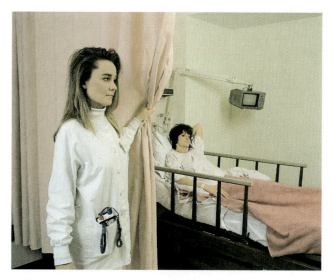

FIGURE 14-11D Draw curtains for privacy.

- Ask visitors to leave the room and inform them where they may wait.
- Provide privacy (Figure 14-11D).
- Explain what will happen and answer questions.
- Allow the patient to assist as much as possible.
- Raise the bed to a comfortable working height.
- Carry out precaution gowning and gloving.
- Use standard precautions when contact with blood, body fluids, mucous membranes, or nonintact skin is likely.

Procedure Completion Actions

Steps to be followed when a procedure is completed include the following:

- Position the patient comfortably.
- Return the bed to the lowest horizontal position.
- Leave signal cord (Figure 14-12A), telephone, and fresh water where the patient can reach them.
- Perform a general safety check of the patient and the environment.
- Open privacy curtains.

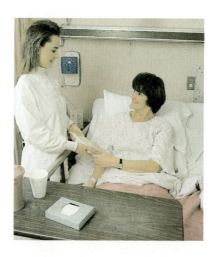

FIGURE 14-12A
Lower the bed and place the signal cord where the patient can reach it.

- Remove and discard personal protective equipment, if used, according to facility policy.
- Care for equipment following facility policy.
- Wash your hands (Figure 14-12B).
- Let visitors know when they may reenter (Figure 14-12C).
- Report completion of task (Figure 14-12D).
- Document action and your observations.

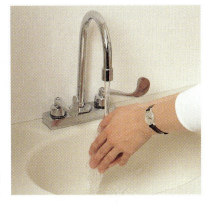

FIGURE 14-12B Wash your hands.

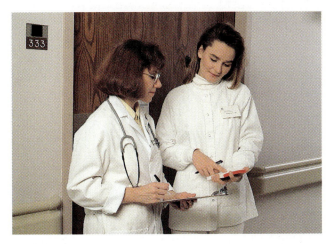

FIGURE 14-12C Let visitors know when they may reenter the patient's room.

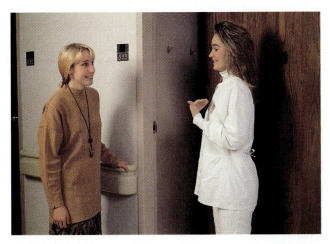

FIGURE 14-12D Report and document your actions and the patient's response.

Note: Where there are open lesions, wet linen, or possible contact with patient body fluids, blood, mucous membranes, or nonintact skin, wear disposable gloves during the procedure. Put on gloves before contact with the patient or linen. Dispose of gloves according to facility policy after they are removed. **ALWAYS APPLY STANDARD PRECAUTIONS**.

So much handwashing may seem unnecessary, because of the short length of time that you are with the patient. Just remember that your hands can transmit germs. Patients already weakened by disease have a much lower resistance to germs.

Because the beginning procedure and procedure completion actions are the same for each patient care procedure, they are not restated in this book as individual steps with each procedure. Rather, a general reference is made to these steps at the beginning and end of each procedure. You must, however, learn and faithfully complete each of these steps for each patient care procedure you perform.

BODY MECHANICS FOR THE PATIENT

Body mechanics for the patient are very similar to those for the health care team. Although the patient probably is not doing any lifting, good posture habits should not be neglected. Good posture for the patient means that moving in bed, getting out of bed, standing, and walking are done safely.

Bed patients sometimes find it hard to stay in a position; they tend to slide toward the foot of the bed when the head of the bed is elevated (Figure 14-13). Patients who are dependent

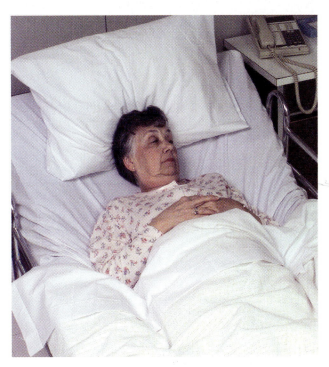

FIGURE 14-13 Patients frequently slide down in bed and are not in proper body alignment.

are not able to change their position. These patients need extra help to gain and maintain proper alignment. Remember to:

- Get help.
- Use turning or lifting sheets.
- Change the patient's position frequently, at least every two hours.

Body Alignment and Positioning

Body alignment means maintaining a person in a position in which the body can properly function. Patients who are weak, have impaired consciousness, are disoriented, or in pain have problems keeping good alignment. Body alignment is maintained by moving, turning, and positioning the patient in a manner that:

- Helps the patient feel more comfortable
- Relieves strain
- Helps the body function more efficiently
- Prevents complications like contractures and pressure ulcers

Complications of Incorrect Positioning

Complications can occur when body alignment is not maintained or when the patient's position is not changed often enough. The two most common complications are pressure ulcers and contractures. **Pressure ulcers** (bedsores) result when unrelieved pressure on a bony prominence interferes with blood flow to the area. Pressure ulcers are dangerous and expensive to treat. (These are discussed in Unit 23.) **Contractures** occur when a joint is allowed to remain in the same position for too long (Figure 14-14). The muscles stiffen and shorten (atrophy), preventing the joint from full movement. The joint becomes fixed in a bent position (position of flexion). Contractures are permanent and can interfere with mobility.

Supportive Devices

Supportive devices are used to maintain proper body alignment and position in the bed or in a chair. Supportive devices include:

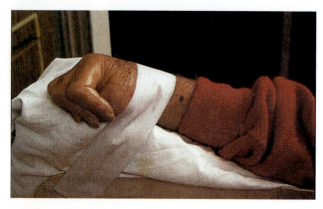

FIGURE 14-14 Contractures occur when a joint is allowed to remain in the same position for too long.

- Pillows and/or folded sheets, bath blankets, or mattress pads to support the trunk and extremities
- Special boots or shoes that are worn in bed to keep the feet in alignment (Figure 14-15A)
- Bed cradles, which prevent pressure on the feet from the bed covers (Figure 14-15B)
- Footboards to maintain foot alignment

A folded pillow placed between the soles of the feet and the foot of the bed, or a pillow resting against the footboard (Figure 14-16), can take the place of a footboard alone. In some cases, a footboard may be harmful. For example, a footboard against the soles of the feet can stimulate **spasticity** (involuntary muscle contraction) in the legs and possibly cause skin breakdown from the rubbing of the feet against the footboard. Special shoes are sometimes worn in bed to maintain the feet in correct alignment. In most cases, ankle contractures can be avoided by doing passive range-of-motion exercises consistently.

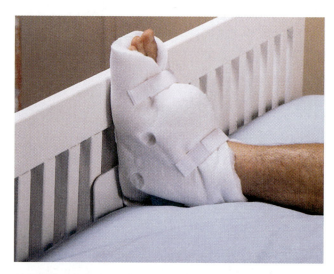

FIGURE 14-15A Special boots will maintain the ankles and feet in alignment. *Bunny boot foot support is provided by Sammons Preston, Inc. a Bissell® HealthCare Company. Reprinted with permission*

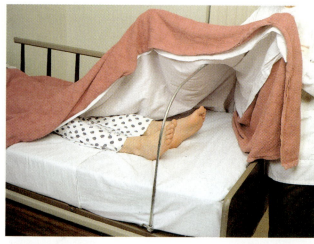

FIGURE 14-15B Bed cradles prevent pressure on the feet from bed covers.

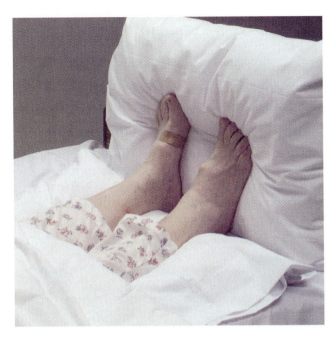

FIGURE 14-16 Footboards or a pillow resting against the footboard may be used to maintain alignment.

There are many other commercially designed products that are used as supportive devices. Remember that a supportive device is also a restraint if it is attached or next to the patient's body, if the patient cannot easily remove it, and if it restricts freedom of movement and normal access to the patient's body.

Basic Body Positions

There are four basic positions, with variations for each one. These are:

- **Prone** (on the abdomen), with a variation of **semiprone**
- **Supine** (on the back), with a variation of **semisupine**
- **Lateral** (on either side), with a variation of **Sims' position**

- **Fowler's position**, with variations of **high Fowler's**, **semi-Fowler's**, and **orthopneic position**

Changing a patient's position involves these steps:

1. Moving the patient into body alignment. You may need to move the patient up in bed or to one side of the bed. If the patient will be positioned on his left side, move him to the right side of the bed. If the patient will be positioned on his right side, move him to the left side of the bed. That way he will not be too close to the edge of the bed after he is turned.
2. Turning the patient onto the back, onto the abdomen, or to the side.
3. Placing the patient's trunk and extremities in proper position and maintaining alignment with the use of supportive devices.

MOVING AND LIFTING PATIENTS

Lifting, moving, and transporting patients is a major responsibility of the nursing assistant. Using proper body mechanics and following safety rules will protect both you and your patients from injury. *Always* ask the nurse whether help is needed to lift or move a patient before proceeding with your assignment. Never be afraid to ask for help. By exercising caution, you are also preventing potentially serious injuries. Always check the care plan to see if there are special positioning instructions.

A **turning sheet** or **draw sheet** (folded large sheet or half sheet) may be placed under a heavy or helpless patient to make moving easier. The sheet must extend from above the shoulders to below the hips to be effective.

Procedures 14 to 17 should be followed when you are lifting or moving patients. As you practice these procedures, keep in mind the 10 basic rules of good body mechanics that were discussed in Unit 13.

PROCEDURE   14

TURNING THE PATIENT TOWARD YOU

1. Carry out each beginning procedure action.
2. Lower the side rail nearest to you. Cross the patient's far leg over the leg that is nearest to you.
3. Cross the far arm over patient's chest. Bend the near arm at the elbow, bringing the hand toward the head of the bed.
4. Place your hand nearest the head of the bed on patient's far shoulder. Place your

other hand on patient's hips on the far side. Brace your thighs against the side of the bed.

5. Roll patient toward you (Figure 14-17A). Do it slowly, gently, and smoothly. Help patient bring the upper leg toward you and bend it comfortably.
6. Put up the side rail. Be sure it is secure.
7. Go to the opposite side of the bed.

continues

PROCEDURE   14   *continued*

8. Place your hands under patient's shoulders and then the hips. Pull toward the center of the bed (Figure 14-17B). This helps patient maintain the side-lying position.

9. Make sure patient's body is properly aligned and safely positioned.

10. A pillow may be placed behind patient's back. Secure it by pushing the near side under patient to form a roll.

11. If patient is unable to move independently, position the arms and legs. Support them with pillows between the shoulders, hands and knees, and ankles to prevent friction and contractures (Figure 14-17C). If patient has an indwelling catheter, make sure the tubing is not between the legs, in order to prevent undue stress on the catheter and to prevent pressure ulcers.

12. Carry out each procedure completion action.

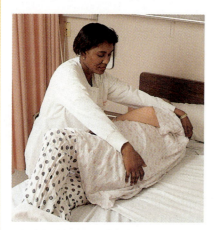
FIGURE 14-17A With your hands on patient's far shoulder and hip, turn patient toward you.

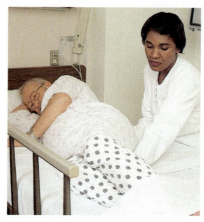
FIGURE 14-17B Keeping your back straight, move patient to center of bed.

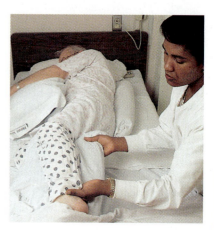
FIGURE 14-17C Make sure patient is in alignment and place pillows to support and maintain position.

PROCEDURE   15

TURNING THE PATIENT AWAY FROM YOU

1. Carry out each beginning procedure action.

2. Lower near side rail. Be sure the side rail on the opposite side of the bed is up and secure.

3. Have patient bend his knees, if able. Cross the arms on the chest.

4. Place your arm nearest the head of the bed under patient's head and shoulders. Place the other hand and forearm under the small of his back. Bend your body at the hips and knees. Keep your back straight. Pull patient toward the edge of the bed.

5. Place your forearms under patient's hips and pull them toward you.

6. Move patient's ankles and knees toward you by placing one hand under the ankles and one under the knees.

7. Cross patient's nearer leg over the other leg at ankles.

8. Roll patient slowly and carefully away from you (Figure 14-18) by placing one hand under patient's shoulder and one hand under the hips.

9. Place your hands under patient's head and shoulders. Draw them back toward the center of the bed.

10. Move patient's hips to the center of the bed, as in step 5.

continues

PROCEDURE 15 *continued*

11. Place a pillow for support behind patient's back.

12. Make sure that patient's body is in a good position. Support the upper leg with a pillow. Place the lower arm in a flexed position. Support the upper arm with a pillow.

13. Replace side rail on near side of the bed. Return bed to the lowest position.

14. Carry out each procedure completion action.

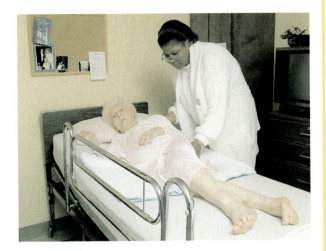

FIGURE 14-18 Roll patient away from you.

PROCEDURE 16

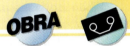

MOVING A PATIENT TO THE HEAD OF THE BED

1. Carry out each beginning procedure action.

2. Ask a coworker to assist from the opposite side of the bed.

3. Lock wheels of bed. Raise bed to comfortable horizontal working height. Lower side rails.

4. Remove pillow. Place it at the head of the bed, on its edge, for safety.

5. Lift top bedding and expose draw sheet. Loosen both sides of the draw sheet.

6. Roll edges close to both sides of the patient's body (Figure 14-19).

7. Face the foot of the bed. Grasp the draw sheet with the hand closest to the foot of the bed.

8. Position your feet 12 inches apart, with the foot that is farthest from the bed edge forward.

9. Place your free hand and arm under patient's neck and shoulders, cradling the head from both sides.

10. Bend your hips slightly.

11. Together, on a count of three, raise the patient's hips and back with the draw sheet, while supporting the head and shoulders.

Move the patient smoothly toward the head of the bed.

12. Replace the pillow under the patient's head.

13. Tighten and tuck in the draw sheet. Adjust top bedding.

14. Carry out each procedure completion action.

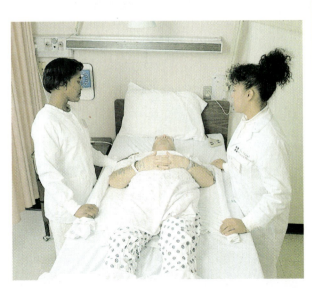

FIGURE 14-19 Using an overhand grasp, roll both edges of the turning (moving) sheet close to the patient's sides.

P R O C E D U R E   17

OBRA

LOGROLLING THE PATIENT

Note: *This procedure is performed when the patient's spinal column must be kept straight, such as following spinal surgery or spinal cord or vertebral column injury. It is a good procedure to use with any dependent patient.*

1. Carry out each beginning procedure action.

2. Get help from another nursing assistant.

3. Raise the bed to waist-high horizontal position. Lock the wheels.

4. Lower the side rail on the side opposite to which patient will be turned. Both assistants should be on the same side of the bed.

5. One assistant places hands under patient's head and shoulders. The second person places hands under patient's hips and legs. Then move the patient as a unit toward you.

6. Place a pillow lengthwise between patient's legs. Fold patient's arm over chest.

7. Raise the side rail. Check for security.

8. Go to the opposite side of the bed and lower the side rail.

9. Turning the patient to side may be done by:

   a. Using a turning sheet that was previously placed under the patient.

   - Reach over patient, grasping and rolling the turning sheet toward patient (Figure 14-20A).
   - One nursing assistant should be positioned beside patient to keep patient's shoulders and hips straight.
   - Second assistant should be positioned to keep patient's thighs and lower legs straight.

   b. If a turning sheet is not in position, the first assistant should position hands on patient's far shoulder and hips.

   - Second assistant positions hands on patient's far thigh and lower leg.

10. At a specified signal, patient is drawn toward both assistants in a single movement, keeping patient's spine, head, and legs in a straight position. If turning sheet is used, grasp sheet and move patient as a unit, onto her side (Figure 14-20B).

11. Place additional pillows behind patient to maintain position. A small pillow or folded bath blanket may be permitted under patient's head and neck. Leave a pillow between patient's legs. Position small pillows or folded towels to support patient's arms.

12. Carry out each procedure completion action.

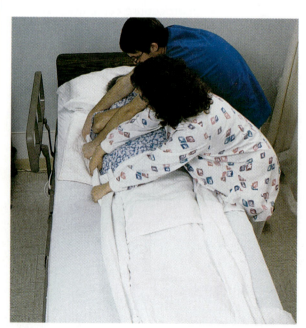

FIGURE 14-20A Roll turning sheet against patient.

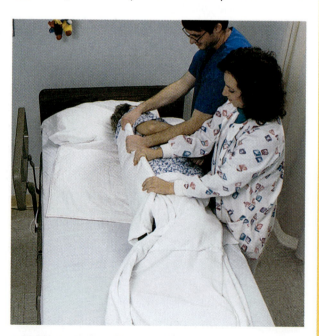

FIGURE 14-20B Pulling together, turn patient to side in one smooth motion.

Positioning the Patient

After you have turned and moved the patient into proper body alignment, you can place pillows and other supportive devices to help the patient maintain the position. Directions are given here for the basic four positions and their variations.

Supine Position (Figure 14-21A).

1. Start with the bed flat and the patient lying on the back. The patient's head should be about two to three inches from the head of the bed.

2. Place a pillow under the patient's head. It should extend about two inches below the patient's shoulders, with the head in the middle of the pillow.

3. Place a trochanter roll along the affected hip or along both hips if the patient has little control over the legs. A trochanter roll is devised by rolling a bath blanket into a shape about 12 inches long. The roll should be just long enough to reach from above the hip to above the knee (Figure 14-21B). The trochanter roll prevents external rotation (Figure 14-21C) of the hip.

4. Place pillows under the legs to reach from above the back of the knee to the ankle so that the ankles and heels do not rub on the sheets.

5. If care plan so indicates, position the footboard or place a folded pillow to support the patient's feet. The ankles should be at 90° angles.

6. Extend the patient's arms and place small pillows to reach from the elbow to below the wrist. The hand should be in alignment with the wrist (Figure 14-21D).

Semisupine Position (Figure 14-22).

Start with the patient in supine position. Roll the patient's trunk and shoulder away from you so that there is a 45° angle between the patient's back and the bed.

1. Place a pillow behind the patient's back for support.

2. Bring the patient's left shoulder forward. Flex the elbow of the left arm and place the lower left arm, palm up, on a pillow.

3. Flex the elbow of the right arm and bring the forearm across the chest with palm down.

4. Extend both legs. Place right leg a little behind left leg. Support right leg with two pillows folded in half that extend from groin to ankle.

Prone Position (Figure 14-23A).

Start with the bed flat and the patient lying on the abdomen with head turned to either side, spine straight and legs extended.

1. Place a small pillow under the head so that it extends to the patient's shoulders and five to six inches beyond the face.

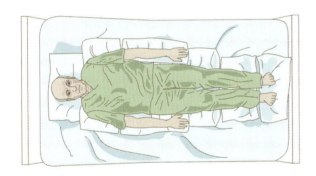

FIGURE 14-21A Supine position

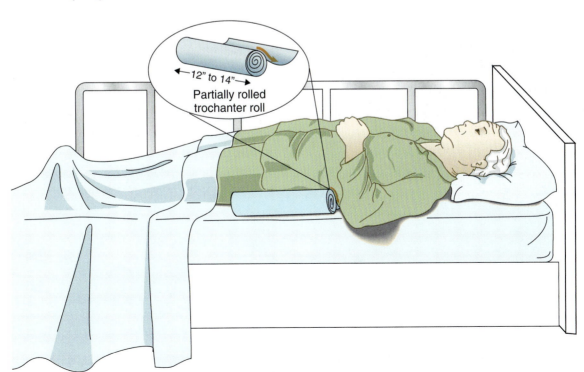

FIGURE 14-21B The trochanter roll should reach from above the hip to just above the knee.

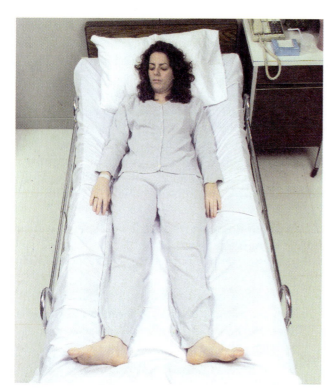

FIGURE 14-21C A correctly placed trochanter roll prevents external rotation of the hip.

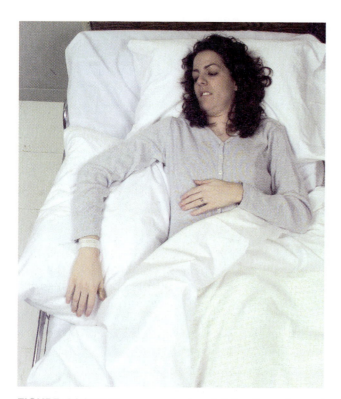

FIGURE 14-21D Proper support maintains the wrist and arm in body alignment.

2. Place a small pillow under the abdomen. This relieves pressure on the back and reduces pressure against a female patient's breasts. An alternate method is to roll a towel and place it under the shoulders.

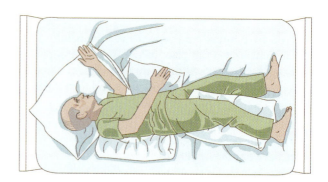

FIGURE 14-22 Semisupine position is a variation of supine.

3. Place a pillow under the arms to reach from the elbow to below the wrists. The shoulders and elbows may be flexed or extended, whichever is more comfortable for the patient (Figure 14-23B).

4. Place a pillow under the lower legs to prevent pressure on the toes. The patient may be moved down in bed before starting the procedure, so that the feet extend over the end of the mattress. This allows the foot to assume a normal standing position (Figure 14-23C).

Semiprone Position (Figure 14-24). This position relieves pressure on the hips. Breathing is easier in this position than in the full prone position. Directions are for the patient lying on the left side.

1. Extend the patient's left arm and tuck it slightly beneath the patient's body.

2. Place a pillow in front of and at right angles to the patient's chest.

3. Flex the patient's right knee and hip. Support with pillows that are parallel to the leg.

4. Grasp the patient's left arm from the back of the patient. Turn the patient onto his chest facing away from you. Gently pull his left arm toward you and push on her hip.

5. Extend the right arm upward and toward the head of the bed. Place it on the head pillow with the fingers and palm against the bed.

6. Flex the upper arm on a pillow.

7. Lift up the sheepskin and place a foam block under the sheepskin above the iliac crest (hipbone).

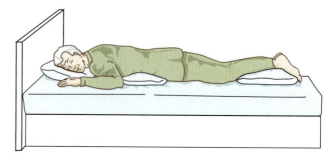

FIGURE 14-23A Prone position

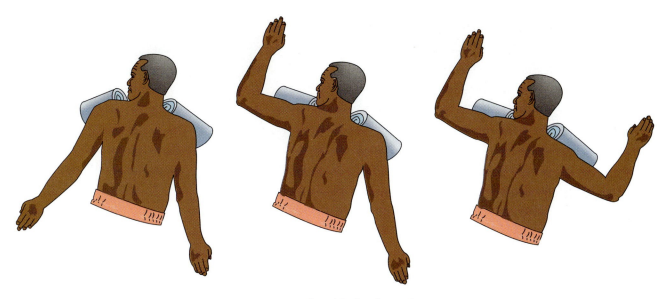

FIGURE 14-23B Position the arms in the way most comfortable for the patient.

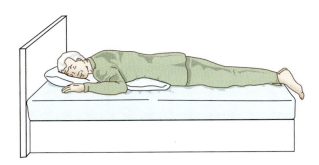

FIGURE 14-23C The patient may be moved down in bed so the feet hang over the end of the mattress.

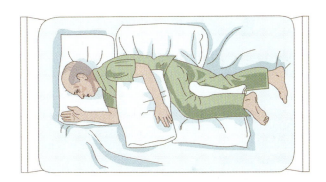

FIGURE 14-25 Right lateral position

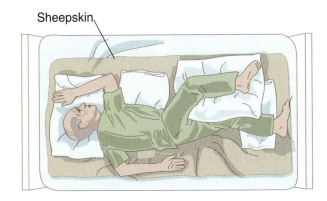

FIGURE 14-24 Semiprone position is a variation of prone.

8. Place another foam block under the sheepskin just below the iliac crest. You should be able to slide your hand between the hip and the bed.

Right Lateral Position (Figure 14-25). Reverse directions for left lateral position.

1. Start with the bed flat and the patient turned to the left side, with spine straight. Remember before turning to move the patient to the right side of the bed.

2. Place a pillow under the head so it extends five to six inches beyond the patient's face and down to the shoulders.

3. Position patient's right arm so shoulder and elbow are flexed and palm of hand is facing up.

4. Place patient's left arm so it is extended or only slightly flexed and rest it on patient's hip or bring it forward and place it on a pillow. The patient's shoulder, elbow, and wrist should be at approximately the same height.

5. Place a pillow between the patient's legs so that it extends from above the knee to below the ankle. The patient's hip, knee, and ankle should be at approximately the same height.

6. A pillow may be placed behind the patient to help maintain the position.

Sims' Position (Figure 14-26). This is a variation of lateral position with the patient on the left side, left leg extended and right leg flexed. This position is often used for rectal examinations and treatments and enemas.

1. Place a pillow under the patient's head as for lateral position.

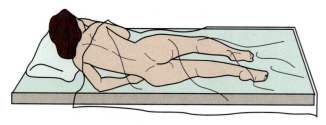

FIGURE 14-26 Sims' position

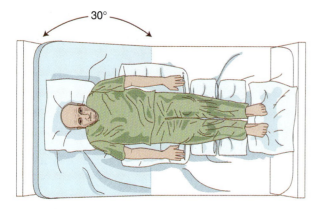

FIGURE 14-27 Fowler's position

2. Start with the bed flat and the patient moved and turned onto the left side.
3. Extend the patient's left arm and position it behind the patient's back.
4. Flex the right arm and bring it forward. Support arm with a pillow.

Fowler's Position. This position, or a variation of it, is used for feeding patients in bed, for certain treatments and procedures, for the patient's comfort while visiting or watching television, and for those who have trouble breathing.

1. Start with the patient on the back, in the middle of the bed and in good alignment. The patient's hips should be at the place where the bed bends when the bed head is rolled up. Place head of bed at 30° (Figure 14-27) for semi-Fowler's, 45° to 60° for Fowler's, and 90° for high Fowler's.
2. Place one or two pillows behind the patient's head to extend four to five inches below the patient's shoulders.
3. Flex elbows and place a pillow under each arm to prevent pull on the shoulders.
4. Place a pillow under each leg to extend from above the knee and to the ankle, to prevent pressure on heels.
5. Place footboard or folded pillow to keep feet in position if necessary.

Orthopneic Position (Figure 14-28). This is a variation of high Fowler's position and is used for patients who have difficulty breathing.

1. The position of the bed remains the same as high Fowler's.

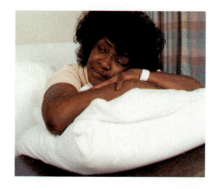

FIGURE 14-28 Orthopneic position

2. Bring the bedside table across the bed and place one or two pillows on top of the table.
3. Have the patient lean forward across the table with her arms on or beside the pillows. Have her rest her head on the pillows.
4. Place another pillow low behind the patient's back for support.

Sitting Position. Patients should be positioned in a comfortable, well-constructed chair, so that the head and spine are erect (Figure 14-29). The back and buttocks should be up against the chair back. The feet should be flat on the floor.

1. Pillows or postural supports may be needed to maintain the position.

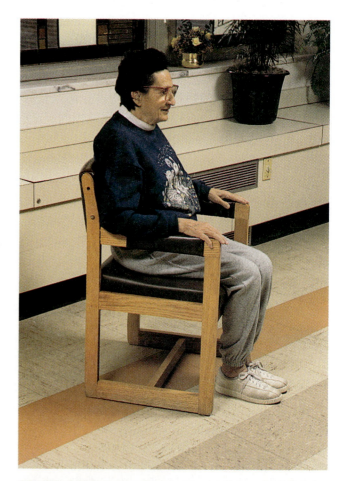

FIGURE 14-29 Body alignment must be maintained for patients sitting in chairs.

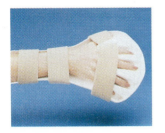
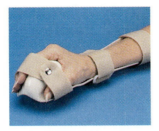
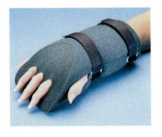
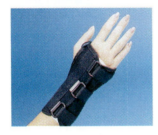

FIGURE 14-30 There are several different types of orthoses (splints) that may be used to maintain alignment of the wrist, hand, and fingers. *Photos provided by Sammons Preston, Inc. a Bissell® HealthCare Company. Reprinted with permission*

2. A small pillow may be folded and placed at the small of the back to add comfort and support.
3. Do not permit the back of the patient's knees to rest against the chair.

Positioning Devices. Several types of devices, called **orthoses**, are used to maintain position of an extremity. The correct use of these devices prevents contracture formation. Orthoses are also called **splints**. Figure 14-30 are examples of orthoses for the upper extremities.

The physician may also order splints or orthoses for the lower extremities. A common type is called the *ankle foot orthosis (AFO)*. The AFO provides support for an unstable ankle and helps reduce extensor spasticity. The AFO is applied to the lower leg before the shoe is put on.

REVIEW

A. Multiple Choice.

Select the one best answer for each question.

1. Patients may be at risk for incidents because they
   a. have impaired mobility.
   b. are receiving medications that affect mental status, balance, and coordination.
   c. are disoriented.
   d. all of these.

2. Patient falls can be prevented by
   a. encouraging the patient to remain in bed.
   b. using restraints when the patient is up.
   c. keeping the side rails up at all times.
   d. caring for the patient's physical needs promptly.

3. Alternatives to restraints include
   a. taking patients to the bathroom regularly.
   b. giving medications to sedate the patient.
   c. playing music throughout the day to distract the patient.
   d. all of these.

4. When restraints are used, they must be released
   a. every two hours.
   b. once each shift.
   c. every hour.
   d. every four hours.

5. When restraints are used on patients in bed,
   a. there must be full side rails on the bed, in the raised position.
   b. the patient should always be positioned in the middle of the bed.
   c. the restraints should be secured to the movable part of the bed frame.
   d. all of these.

6. Injuries caused by heat or cold are called
   a. lacerations.
   b. bruises.
   c. thermal injuries.
   d. aspiration.

7. Choking may be prevented by
   a. giving the patient only fluids.
   b. giving the patient finger foods.
   c. using thickeners for liquids.
   d. all of these.

8. Beginning procedure actions include
   a. handwashing.
   b. assembling equipment.
   c. providing privacy.
   d. all of these.

9. Correct body alignment will
   a. help the patient feel more comfortable.
   b. relieve strain.
   c. help the body function more efficiently.
   d. all of these.

10. Examples of supportive devices include
    a. restraints.
    b. pillows.
    c. side rails.
    d. all of these.

11. Supine position is
    a. lying on the back.
    b. lying on the abdomen.
    c. lying on the side.
    d. sitting in the chair.

12. A position used for patients who have trouble breathing is
    a. orthopneic.
    b. semiprone.
    c. lateral.
    d. supine.

13. Logrolling is a procedure performed for
    a. persons who have had both legs amputated.
    b. ambulatory patients.
    c. all conscious patients.
    d. patients who have had spinal surgery or spinal cord injury.

14. A trochanter roll is used to
    a. maintain the hip in alignment.
    b. maintain the feet in alignment.
    c. support the patient's back.
    d. prevent contractures of the hand.

15. Splints may be used to
    a. maintain position of an extremity.
    b. prevent contracture formation.
    c. provide support for an unstable ankle.
    d. all of these.

B. True/False.

Mark the following true or false by circling T or F.

16. T F Restraints are attached to the side rails for security.

17. T F Restraints may be needed for some patients.

18. T F A physician's order is not necessary before applying restraints.

19. T F The position of bed patients should be changed at least every two hours.

20. T F The left Sims' position is often used for rectal treatments and enemas.

21. T F When turning a patient toward you, cross the patient's near leg over the leg that is farthest from you.

22. T F You must wash your hands before and after completing every nursing assistant task.

23. T F After patient care, the bed should be left in the highest horizontal position.

24. T F Turning sheets make moving heavy patients an easier task.

25. T F You should always explain what you plan to do even if the patient seems not to hear or understand.

C. Matching.

Complete the following by matching Column I with Column II.

Column I

26. _____ Supine
27. _____ Prone
28. _____ Orthopneic
29. _____ Trochanter roll
30. _____ Splint
31. _____ Contracture
32. _____ Supportive devices
33. _____ Physical restraints

Column II

a. prevents external rotation of hip
b. joint deformity caused by shortening of the muscles
c. devices used to maintain patient's position
d. device used to maintain position of an extremity
e. position for patients with difficult breathing
f. lying on the back
g. lying on the abdomen
h. devices that inhibit movement

D. Nursing Assistant Challenge.

Sara Abrams is 76 years old, has Parkinson's disease, and is a resident in a long-term care facility. She is ambulatory, with a shuffling walk, and has tremors of her hands related to the Parkinson's. She is disoriented and frequently walks into other patients' rooms.

34. Discuss safety issues related to Ms. Abrams's condition.

35. Which of the Residents' Rights may be a special issue in this situation?

36. What steps can you take to meet Ms. Abrams's physical needs? Will doing so lower her risk of falling?

37. How can you incorporate exercise into her daily routine?

38. What types of activities might interest Ms. Abrams?

39. Are there are actions that can be taken to avoid restraints and falls?

The Patient's Mobility: Transfer Skills

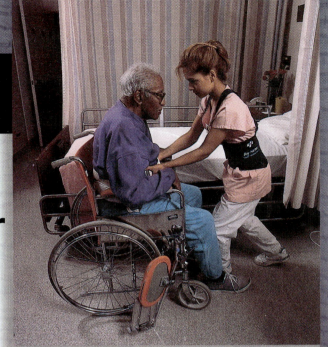

As a result of this unit, you will be able to:

- Spell and define terms.
- List the guidelines for safe transfers.
- Describe the difference between a standing transfer and a sitting transfer.
- Demonstrate correct application of a transfer belt.
- Demonstrate the following procedures:
  - Procedure 18 Applying a Transfer Belt
  - Procedure 19 Transferring the Patient from Bed to Chair—One Assistant
  - Procedure 20 Transferring the Patient from Bed to Chair—Two Assistants
  - Procedure 21 Transferring the Patient from Chair to Bed—One Assistant
  - Procedure 22 Transferring the Patient from Chair to Bed—Two Assistants
  - Procedure 23 Independent Transfer, Standby Assist
  - Procedure 24 Transferring the Patient from Bed to Stretcher
  - Procedure 25 Transferring the Patient from Stretcher to Bed
  - Procedure 26 Transferring the Patient with a Mechanical Lift
  - Procedure 27 Transferring the Patient onto and off the Toilet
  - Procedure 28 Transferring the Patient into and out of the Bathtub
  - Procedure 29 Transferring a Patient into and out of a Car

Learn the meaning and the correct spelling of the following words and phrases:

full weight-bearing	nonweight-bearing	pivot	transfer belt
gait belt	paralysis	sitting transfer	weight-bearing
mechanical lift	partial weight-bearing	standing transfer	

INTRODUCTION

As a nursing assistant, you will work with many patients who have impaired mobility. In the last unit you learned how to move and position patients in bed. In this unit you will learn how to transfer patients (to move them from one place to another). Patients transfer:

- Out of bed into a chair and back to bed from the chair
- Out of bed onto a stretcher and back to bed from the stretcher
- Onto and off of a toilet
- Into and out of a car
- Into and out of a bathtub or shower

Refer to Procedures 19 through 29 later in this unit.

TYPES OF TRANSFERS

There are basically two types of transfers. A standing transfer means the patient stands during the transfer with the help of one or two nursing assistants. A sitting transfer means the patient is sitting throughout the transfer, such as when a mechanical lift is used. A mechanical lift is a piece of equipment that is used to move dependent patients out of bed.

The nurse or the physical therapist determines which method is used to transfer a patient (Figure 15-1). It is

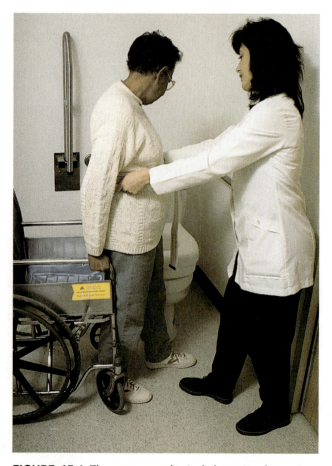

FIGURE 15-1 The nurse or physical therapist determines the method of transfer.

GUIDELINES for

Safe Patient Transfers

Moving dependent patients can result in injury to you or the patient unless all safety measures are followed.

- Know the method of transfer that has been ordered by the nurse or physical therapist.
- Know the patient's capabilities.
- Use correct body mechanics.
- Place the bed in the lowest position before starting the transfer. Make sure the wheels on the bed and the transfer vehicle (wheelchair, stretcher) are locked before the move.
- *Never allow patients to place their hands on your body during a transfer.* This is a dangerous practice. A patient who is disoriented or frightened can cause you to lose your balance. If this happens, the patient can pull you down, possibly injuring both of you.
- *Never place your hands under a patient's arms or shoulders.* This practice can cause the patient severe shoulder injury.
- Use a transfer belt for standing transfers unless it is contraindicated.
- Make sure the patient is wearing shoes with sturdy, nonslip soles and that clothing is not too loose or dragging on the floor.
- Be aware of any tubes, orthoses, or other items that must be dealt with during the transfer.
- Transfer the patient toward his strongest side if possible.
- Allow the patient to see the surface to which he is being transferred. Encourage the patient to keep his head up.
- Stand close to the patient during the transfer.
- If the patient has a weak or paralyzed leg, brace the knee of that leg with your knee or leg. If the patient has a paralyzed arm, be sure it is supported during the transfer to avoid dangling and pulling on the patient's shoulder.
- Always explain to the patient what you are doing and how he can help.
- Give the patient only the assistance that she needs.
- Never have the patient use a footstool unless it is absolutely necessary.

important to follow instructions carefully to avoid injury. The method selected depends on:

1. The patient's physical condition. This takes into consideration:

   — **Paralysis** (inability to move) of any extremity

   — Absence of an extremity due to amputation

   — Recent hip surgery

2. The patient's strength, endurance, and balance. These abilities may be affected by:

   — Respiratory (lung) disease

   — Cardiac (heart) disease

   — Neurological disease, such as multiple sclerosis

   — The ability to stand on one or both legs. This is called **weight-bearing**. For example, a patient may not be able to place full weight on a paralyzed leg. The physician may order the patient to be **non-weight-bearing** or only **partial weight-bearing** if the patient has had hip surgery. A patient who can stand on both legs is called **full weight-bearing**. For a standing transfer, the patient must be able to stand and have at least partial weight bearing on one leg.

3. The patient's mental condition. Can the patient understand and follow the instructions?

4. The patient's size. For example, a very tall or large person who cannot bear full weight would need two assistants or a mechanical lift.

In some situations you may be instructed to take the patient's pulse before and after she gets out of bed. If the patient has been inactive for a long time, the heart muscle may be deconditioned. Checking the pulse when the patient is active provides an evaluation of the heart's condition.

TRANSFER BELTS

A **transfer belt** is a webbed belt 1-1/2 to 2 inches wide and about 54 to 60 inches long. It is an assistive and safety device used to transfer or ambulate patients who need help. (Refer to Procedure 18.) When it is used to assist a patient with ambulation, it is called a **gait belt**. Using a transfer belt avoids the need to grasp the patient around the rib cage or under the shoulders. Either of these methods can cause serious injury. It also allows you to have more control in directing the transfer. A transfer belt is not used to "lift" a patient. If the patient has no ability to bear weight, then another method should be used for transferring.

PROCEDURE **18**

APPLYING A TRANSFER BELT

1. Carry out beginning procedure actions.

2. Assemble equipment:

   - Transfer belt

3. Explain procedure. Tell patient that the belt is a safety device that will be removed as soon as the transfer is completed.

4. Apply the belt over patient's clothing (Figure 15-2A). If patient is undressed and being transferred from wheelchair to tub or shower chair, either leave patient's shirt on or place a towel around patient's waist and then apply the belt over the towel.

5. If patient is going to transfer from bed to chair, the belt may be applied after patient comes to a sitting position on the edge of the bed. If patient has inadequate balance, the belt can be applied while patient is still lying down in bed. You may need to readjust the belt after patient sits up.

6. Keep the belt at patient's waist level. Avoid placing it too high. Make sure the belt is right side out and is not twisted.

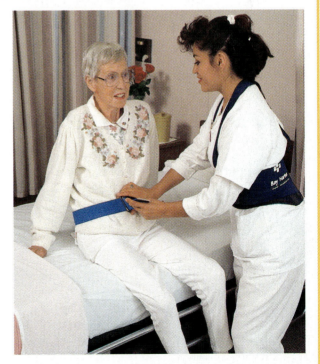

FIGURE 15-2A Always apply a transfer belt over clothing.

continues

P R O C E D U R E   18   c o n t i n u e d

7. Buckle the belt in front by threading belt through teeth side of buckle first and then through both openings (Figure 15-2B). The buckle must be in front.

8. Check female patients to be sure the breasts are not under the belt.

9. The belt should be snug, so that it does not slide up, but not tight (Figure 15-2C).

10. Use an underhand grasp when holding the belt.

11. Do not overuse the belt by pulling patient up with force.

12. The belt may be contraindicated for patients with abdominal, back, or rib injuries or surgery, abdominal pacemakers, advanced heart or lung disease, or abdominal aneurysms.

13. Remove the belt after patient is safely moved.

14. Carry out procedure completion actions.

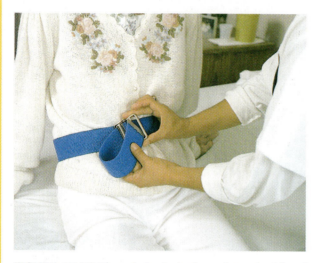

FIGURE 15-2B Thread the belt through teeth side of buckle first.

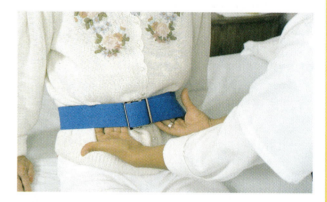

FIGURE 15-2C The belt should be snug but not tight.

P R O C E D U R E   19

TRANSFERRING THE PATIENT FROM BED TO CHAIR— ONE ASSISTANT

1. Carry out beginning procedure actions.

2. Assemble equipment:
   - Transfer belt
   - Chair for patient
   - Bath blanket
   - Robe or clothing
   - Shoes and socks

3. Place chair so patient moves toward his strongest side. Set chair parallel with bed so it faces the foot of the bed on the same side. Lock the wheelchair and raise or remove the foot rests (Figure 15-3A). Cover the chair with a bath blanket, unless patient is fully clothed.

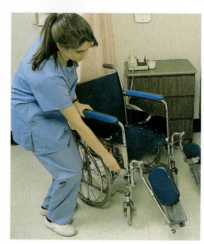

FIGURE 15-3A Lock the wheelchair and lift or remove the footrests before the patient transfers.

continues

4. Lower the bed to the lowest horizontal position and lock the bed wheels.

These instructions are for getting out of the right side (patient's right side) of the bed.

5. Stand against the right side of the bed with the side rail down. Ask patient to slide toward the right side of the bed.

6. Have patient roll over onto his right side, flexing the knees and bending the right arm so it can be used for propping the upper body. Bend the elbow of the left arm so this hand can be used to push off from the bed.

7. Instruct patient to use the elbow of his right arm to raise the upper body and to push with the hand of the right arm so he comes to an upright position (Figure 15-3B).

8. Instruct patient to let his legs slide off the bed at the same time.

9. If assistance is needed, place one arm under patient's shoulders (not his neck) and one arm over and around his knees (Figure 15-3C). Raise patient's upper body at the same time you move his legs off the bed.

10. Give patient time to adjust to sitting up and then apply the transfer belt. Assist patient to put on shoes and socks. (If patient has

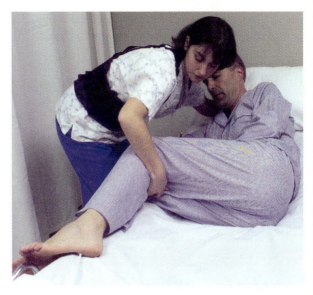

FIGURE 15-3C Place one arm under the patient's shoulders and one arm over and around the patient's knees.

problems with balance, the shoes and socks can be put on while patient is still lying down in bed.)

11. If patient has a weak or paralyzed arm, do not let it hang or dangle during the transfer. Put it in his pocket, or have him cradle it with his strong arm, or carefully tuck his weaker hand in the transfer belt until he is again seated.

12. When patient is ready to transfer:

- Instruct him to move forward or closer to the edge of the mattress, to spread his knees, lean forward from the waist, and place his feet slightly back.

- If one leg is weaker or should not bear weight, have patient place this leg out in front with the strong leg slightly back (Figure 15-3D).

- Remember to spread your feet apart and bend your knees and hips, keeping your back straight.

- Hold belt with underhand grasp, one hand on each side of patient.

- If patient has a weaker leg, press your knee against his knee, or block patient's foot with yours to prevent the weaker leg from sliding out from under him.

- Tell patient on the count of three to use his hands (if able) to press into the

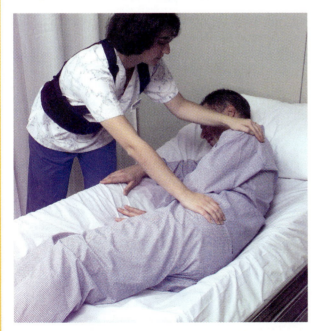

FIGURE 15-3B Instruct the patient to use his hands to come to a sitting position.

continues

mattress, to straighten his elbows and knees and to come to a standing position (Figure 15-3E).

13. If patient cannot walk, have him **pivot** (turn the entire body as one unit) around to the front of the chair until the chair is touching the backs of his legs (Figure 15-3F).

14. Instruct patient to place his hands on the arms of the chair (if able to), to bend his

knees, and to gently lower himself into the chair as you ease him downward (Figure 15-3G). Replace or raise footrests.

15. Position patient comfortably. Place signal light within easy reach.

16. Straighten out bed and prepare it for patient's return.

17. Carry out procedure completion actions.

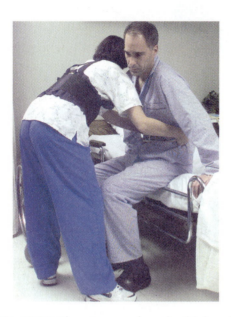

FIGURE 15-3D The stronger leg should be slightly back.

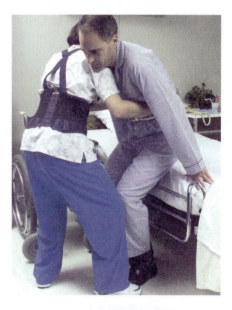

FIGURE 15-3E Tell the patient to straighten his elbows and knees to come to a standing position.

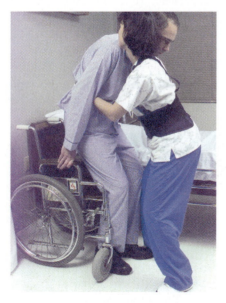

FIGURE 15-3F The patient pivots around to the wheel-chair.

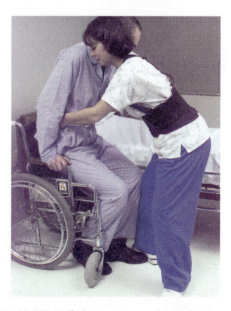

FIGURE 15-3G Tell the patient to bend his knees and lower himself into the chair.

PROCEDURE   **20**

TRANSFERRING THE PATIENT FROM BED TO CHAIR— TWO ASSISTANTS

Two people may be needed to transfer patients who are weak, disoriented, have limited weight-bearing ability, or are very large. Directions are given for transferring toward the patient's right side.

1. Follow steps 1 through 11 in Procedure 19.

2. The nursing assistants stand one on each side of patient, facing patient.

3. Each one places the hand closest to patient through the belt, with an underhand grasp toward the front of patient. The other hand of each assistant grasps the belt toward the back. Coordination of movement is necessary (Figure 15-4A).

4. The nursing assistant closest to the chair (on patient's right side) stands in a position to step or pivot around smoothly to allow patient access to the chair. This person stands with the left leg further back than the right leg.

5. The other nursing assistant uses the left knee to brace patient's weaker left leg. This

assistant's left leg is further back than the right leg.

6. Instruct patient to bend forward and to place the palms of the hands on the edge of the mattress in order to push off.

7. Patient's knees should be spread apart, with both feet back and the stronger foot slightly in back of the weaker foot.

8. The nursing assistants bend their knees and give a broad base of support.

9. On the count of three, patient stands. Allow patient to stand for a moment and bear weight. Tell him to keep his head up. Both nursing assistants help patient pivot by slowly and smoothly pivoting their feet, legs, and hips to their left.

10. To sit, have patient bend forward slightly, bend his knees, and lower onto the chair. At the same time, have patient reach for the arms of the chair with both hands (Figure 15-4B).

11. Complete the procedure as instructed for a one-assistant transfer (Procedure 19).

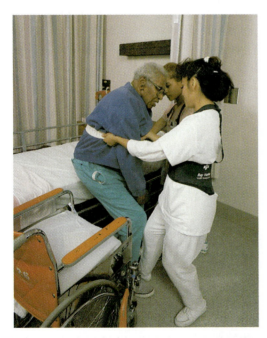

FIGURE 15-4A Coordination of movement is necessary.

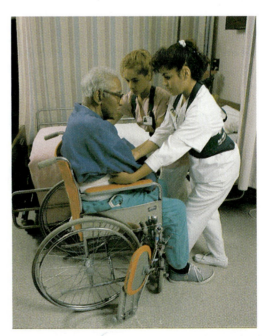

FIGURE 15-4B The patient reaches for the arms of the chair with both hands.

TRANSFERRING THE PATIENT FROM CHAIR TO BED— ONE ASSISTANT

1. Carry out beginning procedure actions.
2. Assemble equipment:
   - Transfer belt
3. Place chair so patient moves toward his strongest side. Set chair parallel with bed so it faces the foot of the bed on the same side.
4. Move the bed to the lowest horizontal position and lock the wheels. Fanfold top covers to foot of bed if necessary and raise the opposite side rail.
5. Lock the wheelchair and raise or remove the footrests.
6. Have patient place both feet flat on the floor.
7. Place transfer belt around patient's waist.
8. Instruct patient to move forward in chair, to bend forward, and to spread his knees apart. Both feet should be back, with the stronger foot slightly in back of the weaker foot. Both of patient's hands should be on the arms of the chair (Figure 15-5).
9. Take hold of the transfer belt with an underhand grasp. Brace patient's weaker leg with your knee or leg, as instructed in Procedure 19. Ask patient to push off the chair on the count of three and to stand up as you provide the necessary assistance.
10. Allow patient to remain standing for a time to stabilize position. Keep your grasp on the transfer belt and continue to brace the weak leg if necessary.
11. To complete the transfer, instruct patient to step or pivot around to stand in front of the

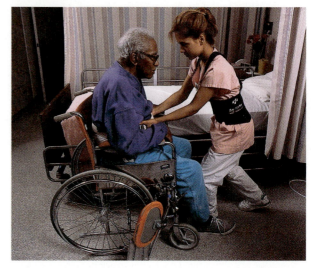

FIGURE 15-5 Both of the patient's hands should be on the arms of the chair.

bed, facing away from it. Tell patient to sit when the edge of the mattress is touching the back of his legs. To sit, have patient bend forward slightly, bend his knees, and lower himself onto the mattress.

12. When patient is safely in bed, remove the transfer belt.
13. Remove patient's slippers and robe. Assist patient to lie down. Position patient as necessary. Draw top bedding over patient. Fold bath blanket and return it to bedside stand. Make sure signal light is within reach.
14. Move the wheelchair out of the way.
15. Perform procedure completion actions.

TRANSFERRING THE PATIENT FROM CHAIR TO BED— TWO ASSISTANTS

Directions are given for moving the patient toward his left side.

1. Follow instructions 1 through 8 in Procedure 21.

2. Each nursing assistant places the hand closest to patient through the belt with an underhand grasp in front of patient; the other hand goes toward the back.

continues

3. The nursing assistant closest to the bed (on patient's left side) stands in a position to step or pivot around smoothly to allow patient access to the bed. This person stands with the right leg further back than the left leg.

4. The other nursing assistant uses the left knee to brace patient's weaker right leg. This person's right leg is further back than the left one (Figure 15-6A).

5. Ask patient to push off the chair on the count of three and to stand up as you provide the necessary assistance.

6. Allow patient to remain standing for a time to stabilize position. Keep your hands on the transfer belt and continue to brace the weak leg if necessary.

7. To complete the transfer, instruct patient to step or pivot around to stand in front of the

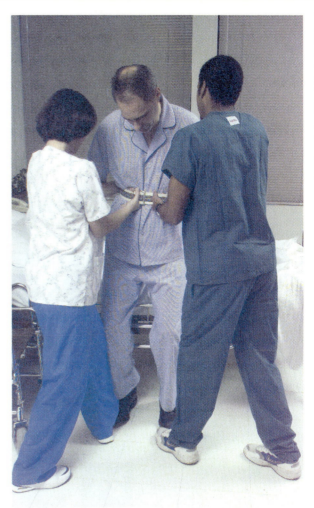

FIGURE 15-6B Tell the patient to bend forward, bend the knee, and lower himself onto the mattress.

bed, facing away from it. Tell the patient to sit when the edge of the mattress is touching the back of his legs. To sit, have patient bend forward slightly, bend his knees, and lower himself onto the mattress (Figure 15-6B).

8. When patient is safely in bed, remove the transfer belt.

9. Remove patient's slippers and robe. Assist patient to lie down and position as necessary. Raise side rails if ordered. Draw top bedding over patient. Fold bath blanket and return to bedside stand. Make sure signal light is within reach.

10. Move the wheelchair out of the way.

11. Perform procedure completion actions.

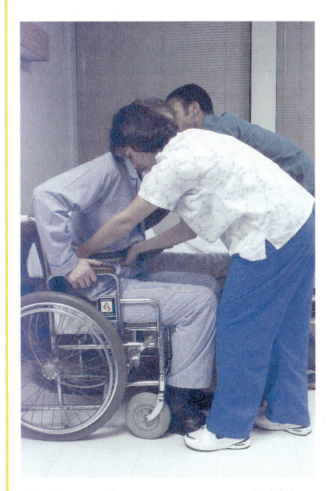

FIGURE 15-6A The nursing assistant uses the left knee to brace the patient's weaker right leg.

PROCEDURE **23**

INDEPENDENT TRANSFER, STANDBY ASSIST

This method is appropriate for the patient who has good balance and strength and can understand instructions. Put a transfer belt on the patient the first time this is attempted.

1. Follow the instructions getting patient to a sitting position on the side of the bed. (See Procedure 19.) For an independent transfer, patient should be able to do this without help.

2. Have patient place the strongest foot slightly in back of the other foot. Patient's knees should be spread slightly apart.

3. Instruct patient to place the palms of the hands at the edge of the bed and to lean slightly forward.

4. Tell patient to press hands into the bed to push off, at the same time the legs straighten, to assume a standing position.

5. Once standing, have patient reach for the far arm of the chair and then step or pivot to stand in front of the chair. Instruct the patient to sit when the edge of the seat is felt against the back of the legs.

6. Perform procedure completion actions.

Reverse these directions when transferring from chair to bed.

STRETCHER TRANSFERS

This procedure is used to move a patient from her room to another room for surgery, treatments, or diagnostic tests. The procedure may be very frightening to the patient. Assure the patient that the procedure is safe.

Note: Procedures 24 and 25 are for moving an unconscious or semiconscious patient. For alert, fully awake patients, two people may be able to perform this procedure with one person against the stretcher and the other person on the opposite side of the bed. Instruct the patient how to help you.

PROCEDURE **24**

TRANSFERRING THE PATIENT FROM BED TO STRETCHER

1. Carry out beginning procedure actions.

2. Assemble equipment:
   - Stretcher
   - Bath blanket

3. You will need three to four people for transferring an unconscious or comatose patient from bed to stretcher.

4. Lock wheels of bed. Raise bed to horizontal position equal to height of stretcher. Lower side rails.

5. Place bath blanket over patient and fanfold top covers to foot of bed, out of the way.

6. Roll turning sheet up against patient on both sides. The sheet should be long enough to support patient's head and shoulders during the move.

7. Position stretcher close to bed. Lock stretcher wheels.

8. Two or three people stand along the open side of the stretcher. The other person stands on the open side of the bed. This assistant may need to get on the bed, on his knees, to avoid overstretching his back.

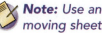 **Note:** *Use an overhand grasp on the moving sheet to avoid wrist strain.*

- Assistant at end of bed grasps moving sheet by placing one hand by patient's legs and other hand by patient's hips.

continues

- Middle assistant grasps moving sheet by placing one hand by patient's hips and other hand by patient's shoulders.
- Assistant at head of bed grasps turning sheet by patient's shoulder and head.
- On the count of three, all persons slide moving sheet from bed to stretcher (Figure 15-7).

9. Center patient on stretcher in good body alignment. Secure stretcher safety belt. Raise side rails of stretcher.

 Note: *Patients on stretchers are not left alone.*

10. Transport patient as directed.

11. Prepare bed for patient's return.

12. Carry out procedure completion actions.

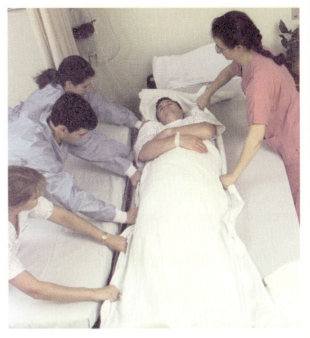

FIGURE 15-7 All persons slide the moving sheet from bed to stretcher.

PROCEDURE 25

TRANSFERRING THE PATIENT FROM STRETCHER TO BED

1. Carry out beginning procedure actions.

2. Assemble equipment:
   - Stretcher
   - Bath blanket (patient should already be covered with one on the stretcher)

3. You will need three to four people for transferring an unconscious or comatose patient from stretcher to bed.

4. Lock wheels of bed. Raise bed to horizontal position equal to height of stretcher. Lower side rails. Fanfold top covers to foot of bed, out of the way.

5. Place bath blanket over patient if necessary.

6. Roll turning sheet up against patient on both sides. The sheet should be long enough to support patient's head and shoulders during the move.

7. Position stretcher close to bed, lock the wheels, and lower the side rails.

8. One person stands along the open side of the stretcher. The other two or three people stand on the open side of the bed. These assistants may need to get on the bed, on their knees, to avoid overstretching their backs.

 Note: *Use an overhand grasp on the moving sheet to avoid wrist strain.*

- Assistant at end of bed grasps moving sheet by placing one hand by patient's legs and other hand by patient's hips.
- Middle assistant grasps moving sheet by placing one hand by patient's hips and other hand by patient's shoulders.

continues

- Assistant at head of bed grasps turning sheet by patient's shoulder and head.
- On the count of three, all persons slide moving sheet from stretcher to bed (Figure 15-8).

9. Center patient on bed in good body alignment. Position patient properly. Raise side rails of bed if ordered.

10. Carry out procedure completion actions.

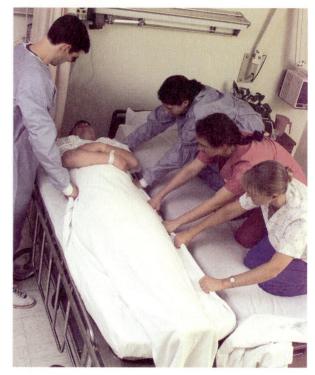

FIGURE 15-8 All persons help slide the moving sheet from stretcher to bed.

PROCEDURE 26

TRANSFERRING THE PATIENT WITH A MECHANICAL LIFT

This procedure is used for heavy residents who have little or no weight-bearing ability.

 Note: Check slings, chains, and straps for frayed areas or clasps that do not close properly. Check the hydraulic lift and the leg spreader to make sure they are both working. Do not use if there is oil on the floor or if equipment is defective. Report need for repair and obtain safe equipment.

1. Carry out beginning procedure actions.

2. Assemble equipment:

- Mechanical lift
- Sling
- Chair

Note: Two people should carry out these procedures to ensure patient safety.

3. Place wheelchair or other chair parallel to foot of bed, facing the head. Lock wheelchair.

4. Elevate bed to comfortable working height. Lock wheels of bed. Lower nearest side rail. Roll patient toward you.

5. Position sling beneath patient's body behind shoulder, thighs, and buttocks. Be sure sling is smooth (Figure 15-9A).

6. Roll patient back onto sling and position properly (Figure 15-9B). If sling has inserts for metal bars, insert them now.

continues

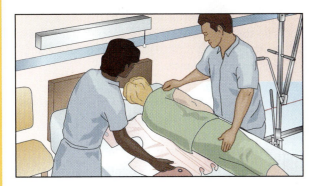

FIGURE 15-9A Position sling under patient.

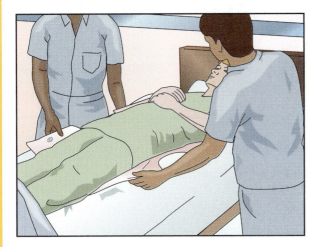

FIGURE 15-9B Roll patient back onto sling.

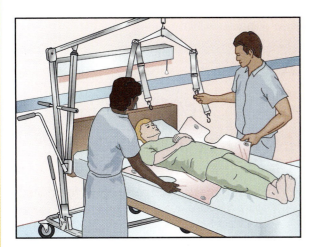

FIGURE 15-9C Position lift frame over bed.

7. Position lift frame over bed with base legs in maximum open position, and lock lift legs (Figure 15-9C).

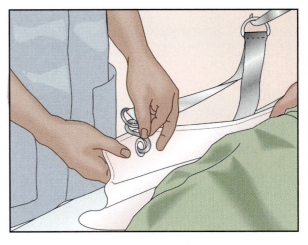

FIGURE 15-9D Attach straps or chains to sling.

8. Attach suspension straps or chains to sling (Figure 15-9D). Check fasteners for security.

📝 *Note: Be sure that the right end of the strap or chain is hooked to the right place on the sling. Always hook straps or chains from inside to outside.*

9. Position patient's crossed arms inside straps.

10. Secure straps or chains if necessary.

11. One assistant operates the lift and the other assistant guides the movement of patient. Talk to patient while slowly lifting him free of the bed.

12. Guide lift away from bed.

13. Position patient and lift over the chair or wheelchair (Figure 15-9E). Make sure that wheels of wheelchair are locked.

14. Slowly lower patient into chair or wheelchair. Pay attention to position of patient's feet and hands.

15. Unhook suspension straps or chains and remove lift.

📝 *Note: Directions are reversed for moving patient from chair to bed.*

16. If patient is in chair, the sling can remain underneath patient so it is in position for transfer back to bed. If sling has metal bars, remove these and make sure sling is smooth and wrinkle-free. Make sure signal light is within reach.

continues

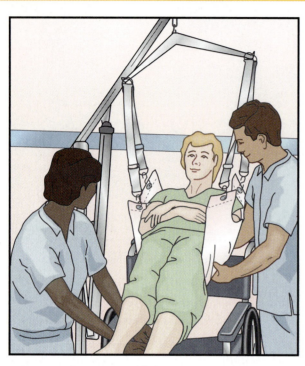

FIGURE 15-9E Position lift frame over chair.

17. If patient has returned to bed, remove sling. Pull top covers up and position patient. Raise both side rails if necessary. Make sure signal light is within reach.

📝 **Note:** *The method for raising and lowering the lift and for moving the base legs varies for different types of equipment. Read manufacturer's directions and practice using equipment before using it with patients.*

18. Carry out procedure completion actions.

TOILET TRANSFERS

The bladder is emptied much more efficiently if patients can use the toilet or commode rather than a urinal or bedpan. To use the toilet, the patient must possess transfer skills. Unless the patient has full weight bearing on both legs and good balance, a wall rail is needed for support while transferring. (Refer to Procedure 27.) Towel racks are not safe for this purpose. Male patients may find it easier and safer to sit rather than stand while urinating.

PROCEDURE **27**

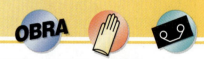

TRANSFERRING THE PATIENT ONTO AND OFF THE TOILET

1. Carry out beginning procedure actions.
2. Assemble equipment:
   - Toilet tissue
   - Transfer belt
   - Disposable gloves
   - Commode if toilet is not available
3. Position the wheelchair at a right angle to the toilet or commode to face the wall rail.

Lock the wheels. Raise or remove footrests (Figure 15-10A).

4. Place transfer belt around patient's waist. Use an underhand grasp with one hand toward patient's back and the other hand toward patient's front.

5. Tell patient to lean forward slightly, to place the strongest foot slightly behind the other

continues

PROCEDURE **27** *continued*

foot, to bring himself to a standing position by pushing off from the wheelchair, and to grasp the wall rail with both hands (Figure 15-10B).

6. Have patient pivot or step around until he feels the toilet against the back of his legs.

7. Slide the pants and underwear down over patient's knees. You may need to keep one hand in the transfer belt and use the other hand to manipulate patient's clothing (Figure 15-10C).

8. Assist patient to a sitting position on the toilet and allow him time to eliminate.

9. When patient is finished, put on the disposable gloves. Instruct patient to stand and to reach for the wall rail. Use the toilet tissue to clean patient if he was unable to do this himself. If the patient is steady, remove and dispose of your gloves. Then pull the patient's pants or underwear up.

10. If the sink is close enough, patient can pivot or step to the sink to wash his hands before sitting down in the wheelchair. Otherwise, unlock wheelchair, replace footrests, and move the wheelchair to the sink so this step can be completed while patient is seated.

11. Wash your hands.

12. Assist patient to leave the bathroom. Make sure he is comfortable and has a signal light within reach.

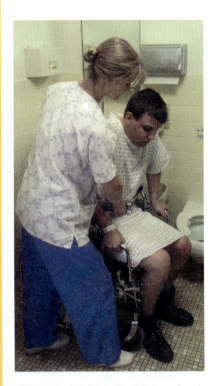

FIGURE 15-10A Position wheelchair at right angle to toilet or commode.

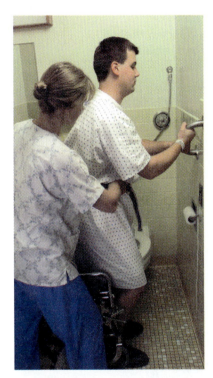

FIGURE 15-10B Tell the patient to grasp the wall rail with both hands.

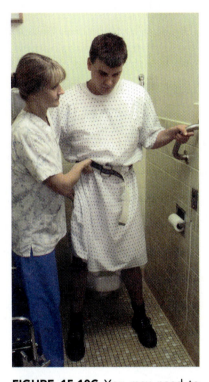

FIGURE 15-10C You may need to keep one hand in the transfer belt as you manipulate the patient's clothing.

TUB TRANSFERS

In the institutional setting, a shower with chair or tub with hydraulic lift is available. If the patient is at home, a tub chair, rail on the wall beside the tub, and slip-proof mats in the tub are needed for safety. Add water to the tub after the patient has safely transferred, with cold water turned on first and off last. A hand-held shower attached to the faucet of the tub is safer and easier for self-bathing.

PROCEDURE **28** OBRA

TRANSFERRING THE PATIENT INTO AND OUT OF THE BATHTUB

1. Carry out beginning procedure actions.

2. Assemble equipment:
   - Towels and washcloths
   - Soap
   - Hand-held shower if available
   - Tub chair
   - Slip-proof bath mats for floor and tub
   - Disposable gloves if necessary
   - Sturdy straight chair if necessary

   Note: If patient's wheelchair has a removable arm or side, remove it and place the wheelchair at the foot of the tub, facing the faucets.

3. Place a sturdy chair beside the tub facing the faucets if wheelchair arm is not removable. (Use this in place of wheelchair.)

4. Have patient transfer from the wheelchair to chair and then into the tub and onto tub chair. Make sure the tub chair is even with the other chair.

5. Once patient is seated in the chair beside the tub, instruct the patient to place the leg closest to the tub into the tub. If this is the weaker leg, the strong arm can be used to

lift the leg over the side of the tub (Figure 15-11A).

6. Tell the patient to use the strongest arm to reach for the wall rail. Sliding across onto the tub chair, have the patient bring the other leg over the side of the tub (Figure 15-11B).

   Note: For this procedure, it is safer to have the weaker side toward the tub, if possible; that way the strong arm can be brought around to the wall rail.

7. Proceed with bath, giving the assistance that is needed or allowing patient privacy to complete bath, if possible. Stay within hearing distance.

8. When patient is ready to get out of the tub, her strong side will be next to the outer chair. This allows her to get her strong leg out of the tub and to use the strong arm to move herself onto the chair. She then uses the strong arm to move her weaker leg out of the tub.

9. Assist patient to dry and dress if necessary.

10. Perform procedure completion actions.

11. Disinfect tub and tub chair.

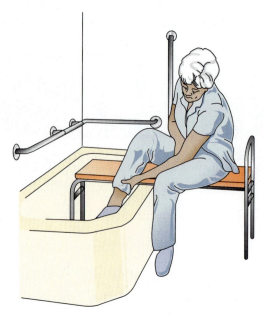

FIGURE 15-11A The patient can use the stronger arm to lift the weak leg over the side of the tub.

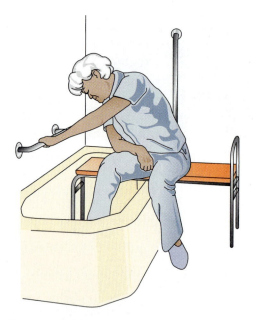

FIGURE 15-11B The patient brings the stronger leg over the side of the tub.

CAR TRANSFERS

You may need to assist a patient to transfer into a car when she is discharged from the facility. If you are working in the patient's home, you may need to be able to help the patient into and out of the car. A two-door car makes the transfer easier because the door is wider and gives more room for moving in and out of the car. With either a two-door or four-door car, the patient should always transfer onto the front seat. The front door is usually wider and opens wider.

PROCEDURE 29

TRANSFERRING A PATIENT INTO AND OUT OF A CAR

1. Carry out beginning procedure actions.

2. Assemble equipment:
   - Car
   - Wheelchair
   - Transfer belt

3. Place the wheelchair at a 45° angle to the car, with brakes set. Put transfer belt on patient if necessary (Figure 15-12A). Have patient come to a standing position in the usual manner.

4. If transferring to the stronger side, the dashboard and car door can be used for support (Figure 15-12B). If moving toward the weaker side, instruct patient to use the strong arm and the door with the window open for support. Another person should hold the door for stability.

5. Tell patient to pivot or step around so the side of the car seat is touching the back of the legs. After she sits down, have patient raise one leg at a time into the car to face forward (Figure 15-12C). Assist with seat belt.

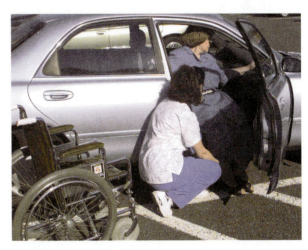

FIGURE 15-12B The dashboard and car door can be used for support.

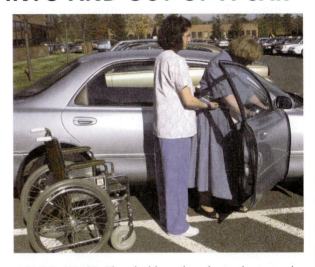

FIGURE 15-12C The patient raises one leg at a time into the car.

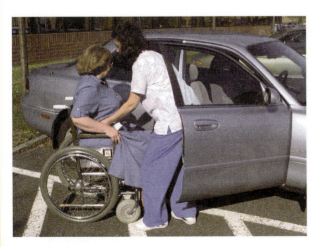

FIGURE 15-12A With the gait belt on, prepare to assist the patient to come to a standing position.

6. To get out of the car, reverse the procedure. Car seats are usually lower than other sitting surfaces and the patient may need help in getting to a standing position.

7. Carry out procedure completion actions.

REVIEW

A. Multiple Choice.

Select the one best answer for each question.

1. The method used for transferring a patient depends on the patient's
   a. size.
   b. physical condition.
   c. strength, endurance, balance.
   d. all of these.

2. A transfer belt should never be used on patients who
   a. have an abdominal aneurysm.
   b. need assistance in transferring.
   c. are tall.
   d. all of these.

3. During a transfer, the patient should never
   a. be allowed to help in the move.
   b. place his hands on your body.
   c. wear shoes.
   d. be allowed to stand.

4. When transferring a patient, you should never place your hands under a patient's arms because
   a. the patient may not want you to stand so close.
   b. the patient cannot see where he is going.
   c. the patient's bones are fragile.
   d. the patient may be ticklish.

5. Using a mechanical lift requires that
   a. there always be two persons to do the procedure.
   b. the patient be able to assist in the move.
   c. the patient be mentally alert.
   d. all of these.

B. True/False.

Mark the following true or false by circling T or F.

6. T F During a transfer, the patient should place his or her hands on the nursing assistant's shoulders.

7. T F A transfer belt should always be used for standing transfers unless contraindicated.

8. T F Always transfer toward the patient's strongest side.

9. T F During a transfer, the nursing assistant should place his or her hands around the patient's trunk.

10. T F During a transfer, always explain to the patient how he or she can help.

11. T F Towel bars are not safe to use as grab bars.

12. T F Before using a mechanical lift, always check the slings and straps for frayed areas.

13. T F One person can safely transfer an unconscious patient from a stretcher to a bed.

14. T F When transferring a patient from a bed to a stretcher, raise the bed to the same horizontal height as the stretcher.

15. T F The unconscious patient should be secured with a safety belt during transport.

C. Nursing Assistant Challenge.

You are assigned to Mrs. McNeely, who is scheduled for surgery. She is alert and able to follow your directions. You know that when she returns from surgery she will be semiconscious from the medications and anesthesia. Consider the differences in procedures when she goes to surgery and when she returns to her room.

16. What instructions will you give Mrs. McNeely when she transfers from her bed to the surgical stretcher?

17. What will you need to do to transfer her back to bed after the surgery?

The Patient's Mobility: Ambulation

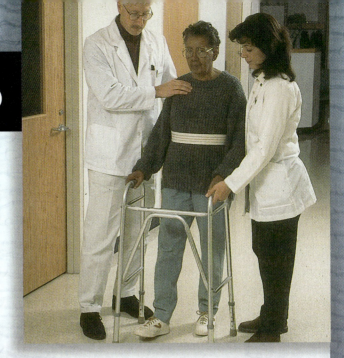

OBJECTIVES

As a result of this unit, you will be able to:

- Spell and define terms.
- Describe the purpose of assistive devices used in ambulation.
- List safety measures for using assistive devices.
- Describe safety measures for using a wheelchair.
- Describe nursing assistant actions for
  — Ambulating a patient using a gait belt.

  — Propelling a patient in a wheelchair.
  — Positioning a patient in a wheelchair.
- Demonstrate the following procedures:
  — Procedure 30 Assisting the Patient to Walk with a Cane and Three-Point Gait
  — Procedure 31 Assisting the Patient to Walk with a Walker and Three-Point Gait
  — Procedure 32 Assisting the Falling Patient

VOCABULARY

Learn the meaning and the correct spelling of the following words and phrases:

ambulate	gait	orthopedic	prosthesis
assistive device	gait training		

AMBULATION

The term **ambulate** means to walk. Some patients may not be able to walk because of a disease or injury. Patients who cannot walk may be able to self-propel their wheelchairs to increase their independence.

The term **gait** refers to the way in which a person walks. Many disorders can affect a person's gait, such as:

- A stroke—one side of the body is paralyzed (hemiplegia).
- Multiple sclerosis—one or both legs are weakened and balance may be disturbed.
- Huntington's disease—the patient has involuntary movements that disturb balance.
- Parkinson's disease—the patient has stiffness and slowness of movements, causing shuffling.
- Arthritis—pain and stiffness of joints.
- Amputation—the patient has a **prosthesis** (artificial limb).
- **Orthopedic** (bones and muscles) surgery.

Evaluation for Ambulation

Before initiating an ambulation program, the nurse or physical therapist (Figure 16-1) will evaluate the patient's:

- Tolerance to movement in bed
- Ability to participate in active (as opposed to passive) exercise
- Ability to safely transfer with minimal assistance
- Ability to stand and bear weight
- Strength, endurance, and balance

- Mental state, to determine if the patient can follow directions
- Ability to walk alone (will the assistance of a person or equipment be needed)

Normal Gait Pattern

There are two phases to a normal gait (walking). The leg is on the floor during the first phase and the leg is brought forward during the second phase. Walking begins with the ankle in *dorsiflexion* (toes pulled toward shin) and the heel striking the floor first (Figure 16-2), rolling onto the ball of the foot. The patient must be able to stand straight on this leg while bringing the other leg forward. The arms normally swing slightly during walking. Each arm moves in the same direction as the opposite leg. To walk safely, the patient must have adequate joint motion in the hips and knees and strength in the muscles of the hips, buttocks, and legs. The physical therapist may work with the patient on exercises to promote movement and strength before the patient starts walking.

Gait Training

The physical therapist may work with the patient on **gait training** (teaching the patient to walk). The physical therapist will teach the patient how to:

- Walk correctly
- Walk on different surfaces, such as linoleum floors, carpet, grass, gravel, etc.
- Go up and down stairs (Figure 16-3)
- Get in and out of a chair
- Use an assistive device if one is ordered

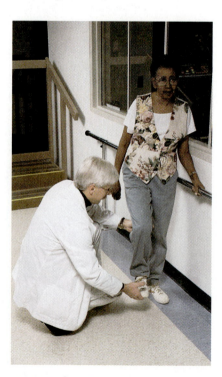

FIGURE 16-1 The physical therapist evaluates the patient's ability to ambulate.

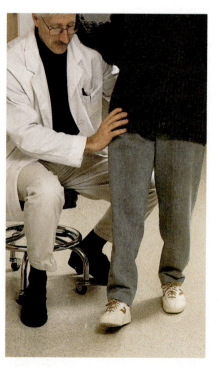

FIGURE 16-2 Walking begins with the ankle in dorsiflexion and the heel striking the floor first.

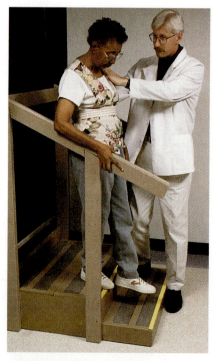

FIGURE 16-3 The physical therapist teaches the patient how to use the stairs.

ASSISTIVE DEVICES

An **assistive device** is often prescribed. These devices include:

- Crutches
- Canes
- Walkers

An assistive device can help compensate for problems the patient has with walking. A walker or crutches may be ordered if the patient has only partial weight bearing on one leg. Canes are usually ordered for persons who have problems with balance. There are several types of crutches, canes, and walkers. Each device is selected according to the needs of the patient and the cause of the problem. The nurse or physical therapist will adjust the device to fit the patient. The gait

---

GUIDELINES *for*

Safe Ambulation

- Encourage independent patients to use the hand rail when walking.
- Always stand on the patient's affected side when walking with her.
- Always use a gait belt (transfer belt) if the patient needs assistance with ambulation. Grasp the belt in the back with an underhand grip (Figure 16-4). Place your other hand on the patient's shoulder if balance is unsteady.
- Make sure the patient is wearing sturdy shoes with nonslip soles and that laces are tied. Clothing should not be too loose or drag on the floor.
- Check floor for clutter or puddles that could cause a fall.
- If you are unsure of the patient's endurance or balance, ask another nursing assistant to follow behind you with the wheelchair. If the patient becomes weak, dizzy, or tired, she can sit in the wheelchair.
- Check rubber tips on bottoms of canes, crutches, and walkers and the rubber handgrips (Figure 16-5). These should be replaced if the ridges are cracked, loose, or worn down. If the ridges are filled with debris, use alcohol and cotton swabs to clean them. Replace the handgrip if it is loose or cracked.
- Check screws, nuts, and bolts for tightness. Do not use any device that appears unsafe. Report the problem to the appropriate person.

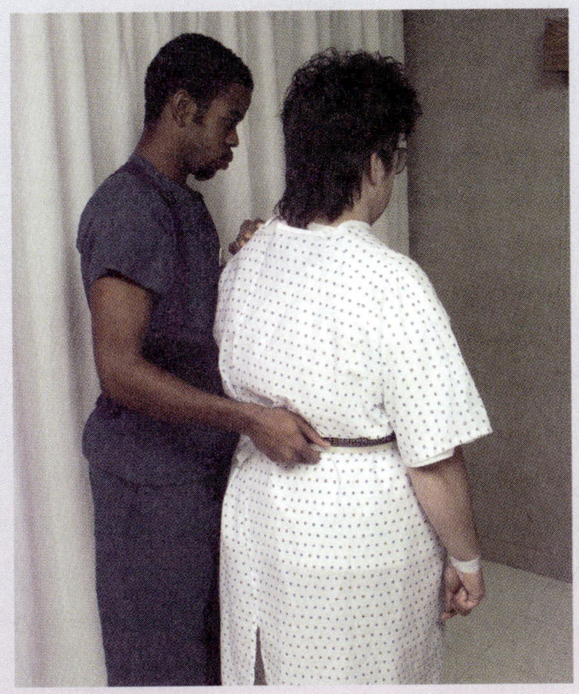

FIGURE 16-4 Grasp the gait belt in back with an underhand grip.

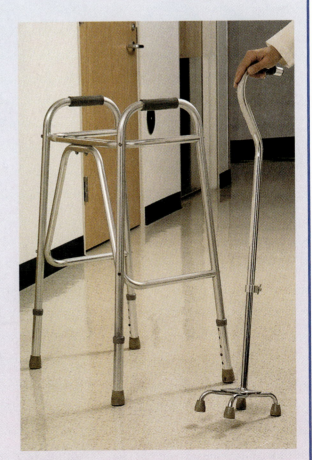

FIGURE 16-5 Check the rubber tips and handgrips.

used with the device is determined by the patient's abilities, the cause of the impairment, and the type of assistive device being used. The nurse or physical therapist will select the appropriate gait. You should know the gaits that have been chosen. When you walk with the patient, you can then help make sure the patient is using the device correctly.

Use of Crutches

Standard crutches (Figure 16-6) are seldom recommended for older adults. They can be cumbersome to handle and require considerable balance and two strong arms. Metal forearm or Canadian crutches may be used by patients who have weakness of both legs. The cuff of the crutch encloses the forearm so the patient can release that hand without dropping the crutch (Figure 16-7).

Forearm crutches with platforms permit weight bearing on the forearms, providing stability. During use, the elbows are in a constant 90° angle to the shoulder (Figure 16-8). The patient may need assistance in attaching the arm straps of the platforms. If you care for patients with crutches, you will be taught the gaits the patients are to use.

Use of Canes

Quad canes and tripod canes provide a wide base of support. Pyramid canes are four-pronged devices with a broad base, and are narrower at the top. Single-prong canes with T-handles or J-handles have straight handles with a handgrip and are easier to hold than half-circle handled canes. For proper fit, the elbow is flexed 30° when the hands are on the handgrip, and the patient's wrist is even with the hip joint. Canes are recommended for aiding balance rather than for providing support. (Refer to Procedure 30.) The cane is always held by the arm on the *strong* side of the body. The patient will be taught to use either a two-point gait or a three-point gait with a cane.

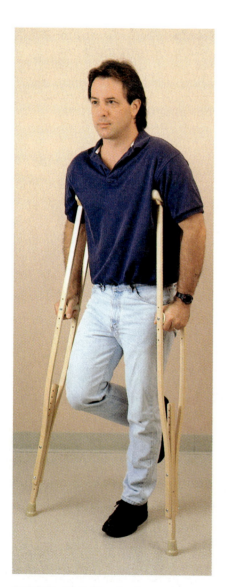

FIGURE 16-6 Standard crutches are not usually appropriate for elderly patients.

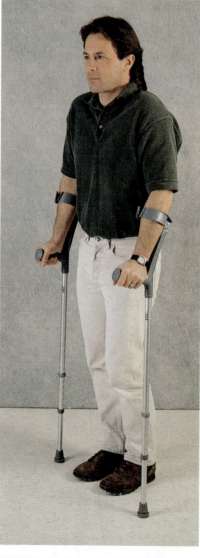

FIGURE 16-7 Forearm crutches can be released to free the hand without dropping the crutch.

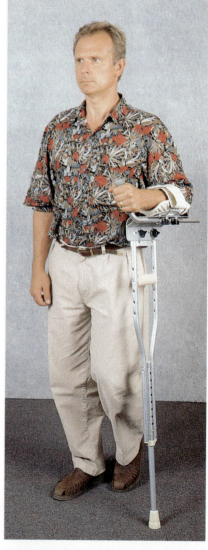

FIGURE 16-8 Forearm crutches with platforms permit weight bearing on the forearms to provide stability.

PROCEDURE **30**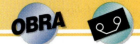

ASSISTING THE PATIENT TO WALK WITH A CANE AND THREE-POINT GAIT

1. Carry out beginning procedure actions.

2. Assemble equipment:
   - Cane as ordered
   - Gait belt

3. Make sure patient has on sturdy shoes with nonslip soles. Check clothing to be sure it does not hang down over shoes.

4. Place bed in lowest horizontal position. Assist patient to sit on edge of bed. Place gait belt on patient and assist patient to standing position. Stand on patient's affected side. Place your closest hand in the gait belt, using an underhand grip.

5. Instruct patient to hold the cane on her stronger side, with the tip about four inches to the side of the stronger foot. Her weight should be distributed evenly between her feet and the cane (Figure 16-9A).

6. Tell patient to shift her body weight to the strong leg and advance the cane about four inches so she is supporting her weight on the strong leg and the cane. Move the weak leg forward so it is even with the cane (Figure 16-9B).

7. Patient then shifts her weight to the weak leg and the cane, moving the strong leg forward, ahead of the cane. This pattern is repeated while patient is walking.

8. Note patient's endurance, balance, and strength while walking. Stop immediately if patient has trouble and help her to the closest chair. Call the nurse.

9. Assist patient to sit in the chair or to lie down in bed. Remove gait belt. Store cane in appropriate area.

10. Document number of feet patient ambulated and her tolerance to the procedure.

11. Carry out procedure completion actions.

FIGURE 16-9A The patient holds the cane on the strong side of the body. The patient's weight should be distributed evenly between her feet and the cane before starting to walk.

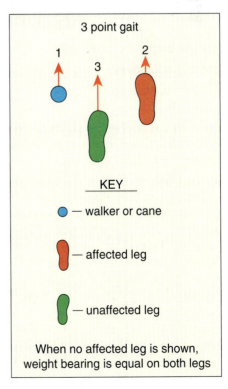

FIGURE 16-9B Three-point gait

Two-Point Gait with Cane. The steps for this procedure are as follows:

1. Follow steps 1 through 5 in Procedure 30.
2. Tell the patient to move the cane and weaker leg forward at the same time, while his weight is on the stronger leg (Figure 16-10).
3. He then shifts his weight to the weak leg and cane, and moves the stronger leg forward.
4. This pattern is repeated while the patient is walking.
5. Repeat steps 8 through 11 in Procedure 30.

Use of Walkers

Walkers also come in a variety of styles. Walkers are recommended for individuals who have general weakness of both legs, partial weight bearing on one leg, or mild balance problems. The patient needs strength in both arms to pick up the walker. The walker should be wide enough to allow the patient to walk into it. For proper fit, the elbow is flexed 30° when the hands are on the handgrip, and the top of the walker reaches the hip joint. Most walkers are adjustable. The nurse or physical therapist will make any necessary changes. There are many additional features available from most manufacturers.

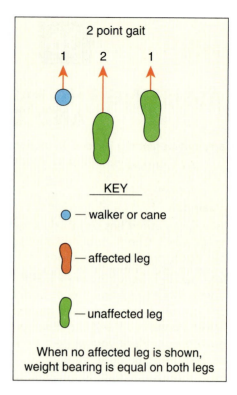

2 point gait

KEY

● — walker or cane

— affected leg

— unaffected leg

When no affected leg is shown, weight bearing is equal on both legs

FIGURE 16-10 Two-point gait

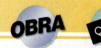

PROCEDURE   31

OBRA

ASSISTING THE PATIENT TO WALK WITH A WALKER AND THREE-POINT GAIT

1. Carry out beginning procedure actions.
2. Assemble equipment:
   - Walker as ordered
   - Gait belt
3. Make sure patient has on sturdy shoes with nonslip soles. Check clothing to be sure it does not hang down over shoes.
4. Place gait belt on patient and assist patient to standing position. Place walker in front of patient and have her grasp the walker with both hands. Stand on patient's affected side. Place your closest hand in the gait belt, using an underhand grip (Figure 16-11).

📝 *Note: The walker is not a transfer device and should not be used by patient to come to a standing position. Patient grasps the walker after she is standing. To sit, patient releases her grip on the walker while still standing, and then places her hands on the arms of the chair before sitting.*

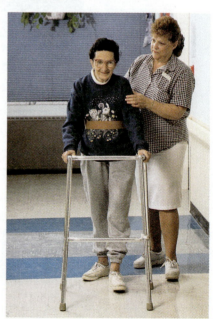

FIGURE 16-11 Stand on the patient's affected side while she grasps the walker with both hands.

continues

PROCEDURE 31 *continued*

5. Instruct patient to stand with her weight evenly distributed between the walker and both legs, with the walker in front of her.

6. Have patient shift her weight to the strong leg as she lifts and moves the walker six to eight inches ahead. All four legs of the walker should strike the floor at the same time.

7. Patient then brings her weak foot forward into the walker.

8. Now have her bring her strong foot forward even with the weak foot.

9. This process is repeated while the patient is walking.

10. Note the patient's endurance, balance, and strength while walking. Stop immediately if the patient has trouble and help her to the closest chair. Call the nurse.

11. Assist patient to sit in the chair or to lie down in bed. Remove gait belt. Store walker in appropriate area.

12. Document number of feet patient ambulated and her tolerance to the procedure.

13. Carry out procedure completion actions.

Two-Point Gait with Walker. The steps for this procedure are as follows:

1. Complete steps 1 through 5 in Procedure 31.
2. Have the patient shift his weight to the strong leg as he lifts and moves the walker and the weak leg six to eight inches ahead.
3. Now have him shift his weight to the weaker leg and the walker (with most of the weight on the walker).
4. He then moves his strong leg six to eight inches ahead.
5. This process is repeated while the patient is walking.
6. Note the patient's endurance, balance, and strength while walking. Stop immediately if the patient has trouble and help him to the closest chair. Call the nurse.
7. Assist patient to sit in the chair or to lie down in bed. Remove gait belt. Store cane in appropriate area.
8. Document number of feet patient ambulated and his tolerance to the procedure.
9. Carry out procedure completion actions.

THE FALLING PATIENT

If a patient starts to fall, you must protect both yourself and the patient. If the patient has started to fall, do not try to hold

PROCEDURE 32

ASSISTING THE FALLING PATIENT

1. Keep your back straight, bend from the hips and knees, and maintain a broad base of support as you assist the falling patient. Maintain your grasp on the transfer belt.

2. Ease the patient to the floor, protecting her head.

3. As you ease the patient to the floor, bend your knees and go down with the patient (Figure 16-12).

4. Call for help.

5. Assist in returning the patient to bed or chair.

6. Carry out each procedure completion action.

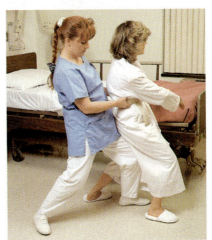

FIGURE 16-12 Ease the falling patient to the floor; bend your knees and go down with the patient.

her upright. This will strain your back and may injure the patient. *If a patient does fall, call the nurse to assess the patient for injuries before she is moved.*

USE OF WHEELCHAIRS

Many individuals who are unable to ambulate are able to gain some independence with the use of a wheelchair. A wheelchair should fit the person using it. Correct fit and body alignment will prevent contractures (Figure 16-13). If the chair fits correctly, there will be:

- About four inches between the top of the back upholstery and the patient's axillae.
- Armrests that support the arms without pushing the shoulders up or forcing them to hang.
- Two to three inches clearance between the front edge of the seat and the back of the patient's knee.
- Enough space between the patient's hip and the chair to slide your hand between the patient's hips on each side and the side of the wheelchair; the right amount of space avoids internal or external rotation of hips.
- Two inches between the bottom of the footrests and the floor.

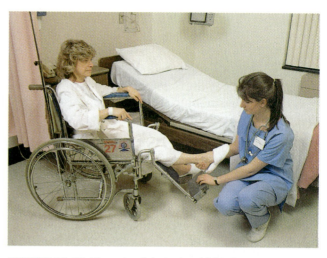

FIGURE 16-13 The wheelchair should fit the patient.

- 90° angles between the feet and the legs, whether they are on the footrests or on the floor (when the footrests have been removed).

If the wheelchair does not fit the patient, check with the nurse or physical therapist to see how you can use pads or other devices to adapt the chair to the patient.

GUIDELINES *for*

Wheelchair Safety

- Check wheelchair to see that brakes are working and wheels are securely attached. If the patient needs footrests, make sure they are in place. Replace arm of wheelchair if it was removed during transfer.
- Place the casters in forward position for balance and stability. To do this, go forward and then back up so the casters swing to the forward position.
- Keep the wheelchair locked when not moving.
- Apply brakes and lift footrests out of the way when the patient is getting in or out of the wheelchair.
- Instruct the patient not to try to pick up an object off the floor. If there is satisfactory trunk stability and balance, the patient may be taught to do so, but instruct the patient to:
  — avoid shifting weight in the direction of the reach
  — not move forward in the seat
  — not reach down between the knees
  The safest method is to position the chair alongside the object with casters in forward position, lock the chair, and reach only as far as the arm will extend.
- Check the patient's body alignment while in the wheelchair and reposition the patient when necessary.

- Prevent bath blankets, lap robes, or clothing from getting caught in wheels.
- Observe the patient's affected arm. A paralyzed arm may fall over the side of the wheelchair and become caught in the wheel.
- Guide the wheelchair from behind, grasping both handgrips (Figure 16-14).
- Always back into doorways and elevators when transporting a patient by wheelchair (Figure 16-15).

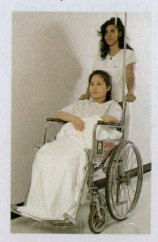
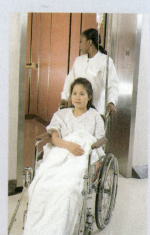

FIGURE 16-14 Guide the wheelchair from behind, grasping both handgrips.

FIGURE 16-15 Always back into doorways and elevators when transporting a patient in a wheelchair.

POSITIONING THE DEPENDENT PATIENT IN A WHEELCHAIR

The dependent person may slide down in the wheelchair, requiring assistance to regain body alignment. Several procedures can be used to correct the dependent patient's position in the wheelchair.

1. Stand in front of the patient; make sure that the feet are in alignment and the arms are on the armrests. Help patient lean forward and push with the hands and legs as you push against the patient's knees (Figure 16-16).

2. For an alternate method, place a soft towel or small sheet under the patient's buttocks and use this as a pull sheet to move the patient up in the chair. This requires two people (Figure 16-17).

3. This method also requires two people. Place the transfer belt around the patient's waist. One assistant stands in back of the wheelchair and grasps the transfer belt with one hand on each side of the patient. The other one stands in front of the patient and places her hands and arms under the patient's knees. On the count of three, this assistant supports the lower extremities while the other one moves the patient back in the chair (Figure 16-18). This is not recommended for a heavy patient.

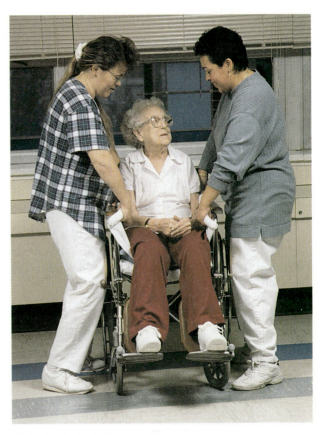

FIGURE 16-17 A draw (pull) sheet may be used to correct the patient's body alignment.

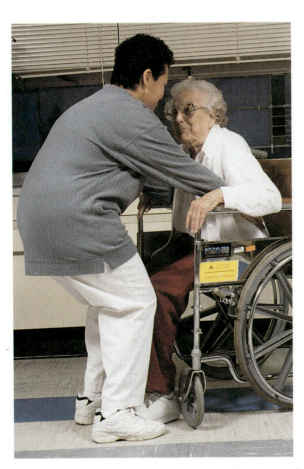

FIGURE 16-16 Push against the patient's knees as she pushes with her hands and legs.

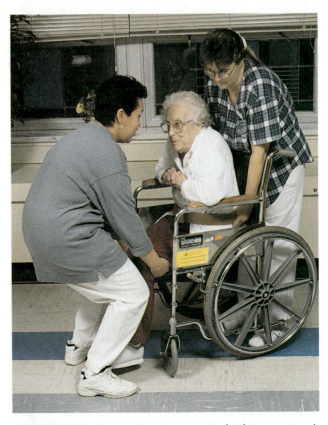

FIGURE 16-18 One assistant supports the lower extremities while the other one uses the transfer belt to move the patient back in the chair.

4. This method also requires two people. Stand in back of the wheelchair and have another assistant in front of the patient. Both assistants work with knees and hips bent and backs straight. Lean forward with your head over the patient's shoulder. Instruct the patient to fold the arms. Place your arms around the patient's trunk. Grasp the patient's right wrist with your left hand and grasp the patient's left wrist with your right hand. The other assistant encircles the patient's knees with hands and arms. On the count of three, both assistants lift and move the patient up (Figure 16-19).

5. One person can do this procedure. The patient needs to be oriented and able to follow directions. Stand in front of the patient. Flex your knees and hips and keep your back straight. Position your feet, one on each side of the patient's feet. Brace your knees against the patient's knees. Have the patient lean forward. Lean forward over the patient's right shoulder with the patient's head under your right arm. Encircle your arms around the patient's trunk. The patient's arms are folded together (Figure 16-20). Rock the patient forward and on the count of three, when the patient's weight is over the legs, push against the patient's knees to move back in the chair.

If the patient can bear weight, it is easier and more beneficial to assist the patient to stand and then sit back down, getting

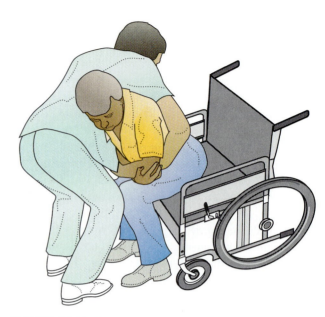

FIGURE 16-20 Put your arms around the patient's trunk.

the hips to the back of the chair. Wedge cushions placed in the wheelchair will prevent the patient from sliding forward.

WHEELCHAIR ACTIVITY

Pressure over the buttocks is dramatically increased when the patient is sitting. Teach the patient (and provide assistance if necessary) to periodically relieve the pressure by shifting

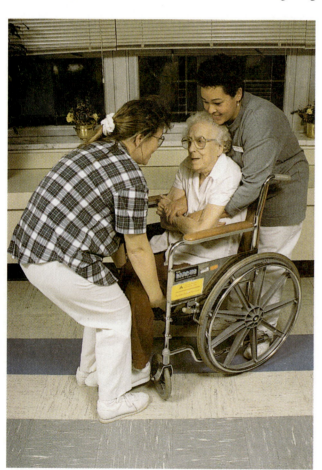

FIGURE 16-19 One assistant encircles the patient's knees with her hands and arms.

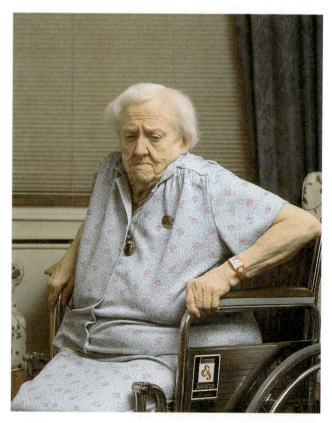

FIGURE 16-21 Wheelchair push-ups can relieve pressure on the buttocks.

weight every 15 minutes. *Be sure wheelchair is locked before beginning any of the following activities involving the patient's movement in the chair.*

Wheelchair Push-ups

1. Teach the patient to place one hand on each armrest, keeping both elbows bent.
2. Then have patient lean forward slightly, pushing on the armrests and straightening the elbows while lifting the buttocks off the seat of the wheelchair. Have patient hold this position to the count of five if possible (Figure 16-21).

Leaning

If the patient cannot do push-ups, teach her to place the hands on the armrests or thighs and lean forward slightly, and then to each side to relieve pressure on the buttocks (Figure 16-22). Monitor the patient with balance problems to avoid falling out of the chair.

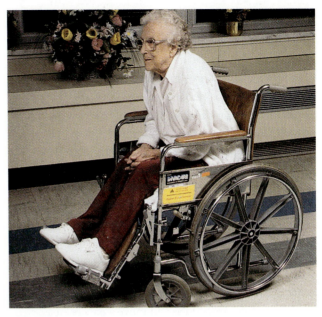

FIGURE 16-22 The patient can lean forward slightly to relieve pressure.

REVIEW

A. Multiple Choice.

Select the one best answer for each question.

1. When ambulating a patient with a weak right side, you should stand
   a. in back of the patient.
   b. on the patient's right side.
   c. on the patient's left side.
   d. in front of the patient.

2. You should hold the gait belt with
   a. an overhand grasp in back of the patient.
   b. an underhand grasp in back of the patient.
   c. one hand on each side of the patient.
   d. one hand in front of the patient.

3. Before helping a patient to walk with a cane or walker, you should check the
   a. handgrips and rubber tips.
   b. screws and bolts for tightness.
   c. height of the cane or wheelchair.
   d. all of these.

4. The cane is always held on the
   a. patient's weaker side.
   b. patient's stronger side.
   c. either side.

5. When using a two-point gait with a cane, the patient will

   a. place the strong foot forward, then the cane, then the weaker foot.
   b. place the strong foot and cane forward at the same time and then the weaker foot.
   c. place the weaker foot and cane forward at the same time and then the stronger foot.
   d. place the weaker foot forward, then the stronger foot, and then the cane.

6. If a patient starts to fall, you should
   a. try to hold the patient upright to prevent a fall.
   b. let go of the patient immediately to avoid back strain.
   c. ease the patient to the floor.
   d. leave the patient and go for help.

7. When using a walker, the walker is set down so that
   a. the front legs strike the floor first and then the back legs.
   b. the back legs strike the floor first and then the front legs.
   c. all four legs strike the floor at the same time.
   d. how the walker is set down depends on the patient's problem.

8. When transporting a patient in a wheelchair, always
   a. stay to the right in corridors.
   b. guide the wheelchair from the front going down ramps.

c. push the patient into an elevator frontwards.

d. all of these.

9. Conditions that can affect a patient's gait include

   a. diseases such as Parkinson's disease.

   b. using a prosthesis.

   c. orthopedic surgery.

   d. all of these.

10. Assistive devices are usually selected by the

    a. nursing assistant.

    b. physician.

    c. physical therapist.

    d. family.

B. True/False.

Mark the following true or false by circling T or F.

11. T F Always back in as you move a patient in a wheelchair into an elevator.

12. T F When transporting a patient in a wheelchair, always walk on the left of the corridor.

13. T F A wheelchair should always be locked unless the patient is being moved.

14. T F A cane is held in the patient's weaker hand.

15. T F When using a walker, the front two tips of the walker should strike the floor first and then the back two tips should strike the floor.

16. T F When assisting a patient to ambulate, you need to use a gait belt only if the patient is using an assistive device.

17. T F To relieve pressure on the buttocks, the patient should be taught how to do wheelchair push-ups or how to lean to relieve the pressure.

18. T F To pick an article up off the floor, the patient should lean forward and reach down between the knees.

19. T F A cane is used for patients who are unable to bear weight on one leg.

20. T F The patient needs to be able to use both hands to manipulate a walker.

C. Nursing Assistant Challenge.

Mr. Santozi is 76 years old and has had right hip surgery. His physician does not want him to bear full weight on the affected leg. He uses a walker to assist his ambulation. He has been taught to use a three-point gait. When you help him out of bed, he reaches for the walker to help pull himself up from the bed. As you watch him walk down the hall, you note that he is setting the walker down by the front legs first and then the back legs. When he walks, he pushes the walker and his strong leg ahead at the same time. What errors is Mr. Santozi making and how can you help him?

Measuring and Recording Vital Signs, Height, and Weight

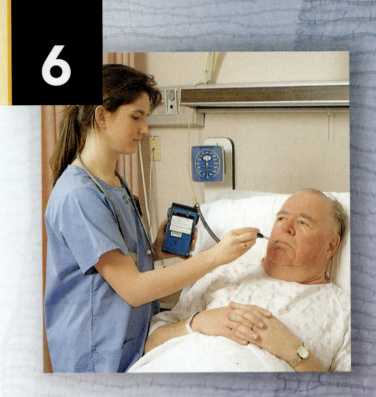

UNIT 17
Body Temperature

UNIT 18
Pulse and Respiration

UNIT 19
Blood Pressure

UNIT 20
Measuring Height and Weight

Body Temperature

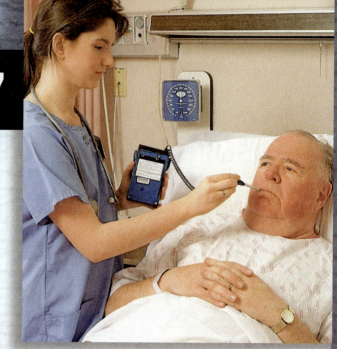

INTRODUCTION

Measurement of body temperature is a common nursing assistant task. Body temperature is one of the vital (living) signs. The patient's other vital signs include the pulse, respiration, and blood pressure. Although they are not part of the vital signs, the height and weight of the patient are other values commonly measured.

Specific equipment is used to determine or measure these values. They must be accurately measured because they tell us a great deal about the patient's condition. Do not tell the patient the results. This is not your responsibility. Tell the patient you will ask the nurse to discuss the results with him. Although they are usually determined as a combined procedure, each vital sign is discussed in a separate unit. Measuring height and weight are discussed in Unit 20.

Many facilities use electronic equipment that automatically registers the four vital signs simultaneously.

TEMPERATURE VALUES

Temperature values may be expressed in either of two scales. They are the:

- Fahrenheit scale, which is indicated by an *F*.
- Celsius scale (centigrade scale), which is indicated by a *C*.

A small ° before either capital letter indicates degrees or levels of temperature.

A formula can be used to convert temperature readings from Celsius to Fahrenheit and from Fahrenheit to Celsius. See Table 17-1 for some important equivalents. Figure 17-1 compares the markings of the Fahrenheit and Celsius thermometers.

DEFINITION OF BODY TEMPERATURE

Temperature is the measurement of body heat. It is the balance between heat produced and heat lost.

Body temperature is:

- Fairly constant. There is a daily variation of 1 to 3°F. Body temperature is lowest in the morning. It is higher in the afternoon and evening.

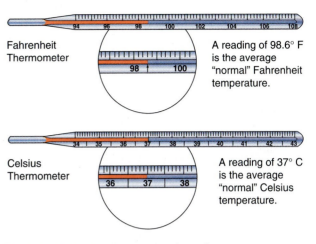

FIGURE 17-1 Fahrenheit and Celsius thermometers

- Lower the closer to the body surface it is measured. The temperature at the center of the body (body core) is much higher than the temperature at the surface of the body.
- Different in the same person when determined from different body areas (Table 17-2). It is important to know the "normal" temperature for an individual, because the normal may vary from person to person.
- Less stable in children. Table 17-3 shows average temperatures in infants and children.
- Affected by
  — illness
  — external temperature/environment

TABLE 17-1 COMPARISON OF FAHRENHEIT AND CELSIUS TEMPERATURE SCALES

	Celsius (C)	Fahrenheit (F)
Freezing	0°	32°
Body temperature	37°	98.6°
Pasteurization	63°	145°
Boiling	100°	212°
Sterilizing (Autoclave)	121°	250°

TABLE 17-2 TEMPERATURE VARIATIONS IN THE SAME PERSON

	Oral	Axillary	Rectal
Average Temperature	98.6°F	97.6°F	99.6°F
Range	97.6–99.6°F (36.5–37.5°C)	96.6–98.6°F (36–37°C)	98.6–100.6°F (37–38.1°C)

TABLE 17-3 AVERAGE TEMPERATURES IN INFANTS AND CHILDREN

Age	Temperature
3 months	99.4°F
6 months	99.5°F
1 year	99.7°F
3 years	99.0°F
5 years	98.6°F
9 years	98.0°F

— medication
— age
— infection
— time of day
— exercise
— emotions
— pregnancy
— menstrual cycle
— crying
— hydration

Excessive body temperature puts stress on vital body organs.

TEMPERATURE CONTROL

Activities to control and regulate body temperature are managed by special cells in the brain.

- Heat is produced by chemical reactions (**metabolism**) in the body core and muscular contractions. For this reason, rectal temperature is highest.
- Blood carries the heat to the skin (**body shell**). The heat is lost from the skin to the outside.
- Heat loss is largely controlled by regulating the amount of blood reaching the skin and through perspiration.
- Average oral temperature range is 96.8°F (36°C) to 100.4°F (38°C). Average temperature is 98.6°F (37°C).

MEASURING BODY TEMPERATURE

There are four body areas in which temperature is usually measured. They are:

- mouth (oral)—most common
- ear (aural)—takes the least amount of time
- rectal—most accurate of commonly used sites (mouth, rectal, axillary); rectal temperature registers 1°F higher than oral
- axillary or groin—least accurate. (This method is used only when the patient's condition does not permit the use of oral, aural, or rectal sites.) An axillary or groin temperature registers 1°F (or 0.6°C) lower than oral temperature.

The patient's condition determines which is the best site for measuring the temperature. The site used most often is the mouth. It is not, however, always the best or safest site to use. In some situations, it would be wiser to use the rectal site.

For example, if the patient is a child or irrational, a glass thermometer in the mouth could result in injury. Patients with respiratory problems, those who breathe through the mouth, or those who are very weak or unconscious may not be able to keep the oral thermometer in their mouths for a long enough time to ensure an accurate recording. In these situations, the best choice is the aural site because the care provider holds the tympanic thermometer in the ear. The reading registers within seconds, so the tympanic ther-

mometer is a good choice for restless patients as well. If the tympanic thermometer is not available, the rectal site might be used. Use a rectal thermometer inserted in the anus for the proper time. Be sure to hold the rectal thermometer in place to avoid possible injury.

CLINICAL THERMOMETERS

A patient's temperature is determined by using a **clinical thermometer**. There are several types of clinical thermometers.

The Glass Clinical Thermometer

The glass clinical thermometer is a slender glass tube containing mercury; the mercury expands when exposed to heat and moves up or down the tube. Three types of glass clinical thermometers are in general use (Figure 17-2). They are the oral, security, and rectal thermometers. They differ mainly in the size and shape of the bulb. The bulb is the end that is inserted into the patient. When only the security or stubby type is in use, the rectal thermometers are marked with a red dot at the end of the stem.

Electronic Thermometer

The **electronic thermometer** (Figure 17-3) is used in many hospitals. One unit can serve many patients because the nursing assistant simply changes the disposable sheath that fits over the probe.

- The electronic thermometer is battery-operated. It registers the temperature on the viewing screen in a few seconds.
- The portion called the **probe** is inserted into the patient.
- The probes are colored red for rectal use and blue for oral use.
- The probe is covered by a plastic sheath before use. The plastic sheath stays on during use. It is discarded after use.

Digital Thermometer

Digital thermometers are hand-held and have a probe that is inserted into the patient's mouth or rectum (Figure 17-4). Sheaths are used to cover the oral or rectal probe before use

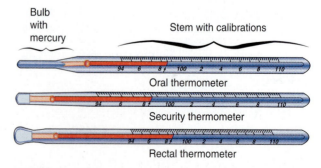

FIGURE 17-2 Clinical thermometers (from top to bottom): oral, security, rectal

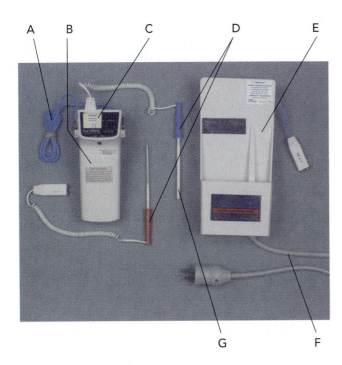

FIGURE 17-3 An electronic thermometer. The temperature is registered in large, easy-to-read numerals. The disposable protective sheath is placed over the probe tip. The probe is then inserted in the patient's mouth in the usual manner. (A) Plastic cord goes around nursing assistant's neck (B) Thermometer (C) Box of disposable probe covers (D) Probe (Blue = oral Red = rectal) (E) Charging unit (F) Probe cord (G) Disposable probe cover

and are discarded after use. The unit is battery-operated. After the sheath-covered probe is inserted, the temperature can be read within 20 to 60 seconds. The temperature is shown as a digital (number) display. The unit is stored in a battery charger between uses.

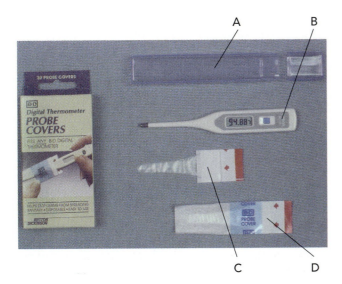

FIGURE 17-4 Digital thermometer (A) Carrying case (B) Digital thermometer (C) Probe cover less backing (D) Probe cover with backing

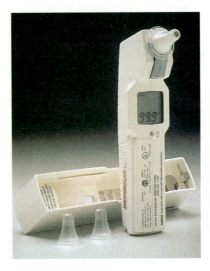

FIGURE 17-5 Cordless, hand-held tympanic thermometer that measures the temperature of the tympanic membrane in the ear. The window on the handset indicates the digital temperature reading. *Courtesy of Thermoscan® Inc., San Diego, CA*

Disposable Oral Thermometers

Plastic or paper thermometers are used in some facilities. They are used once and discarded. They have dots on them. The dots change color from brown to blue, according to the patient's temperature.

Tympanic Thermometer

The **tympanic thermometer** is an instrument that measures the temperature from blood vessels in the tympanic membrane (ear drum) in the ear (Figure 17-5). The temperature reading obtained is close to the core body temperature. To obtain an accurate reading, the probe must be placed solidly into the ear canal. The instrument has a built-in converter that provides the equivalent temperature in rectal or oral values (in both the Fahrenheit and Celsius systems). The type of temperature reading (mode) is selected by the user. The disposable speculum is inserted into the ear canal, gently sealing the canal. The instrument is activated, usually by pressing a button, and within a few seconds it registers the temperature of the blood flowing through the vessels in the eardrum.

Using the Glass Thermometer

The glass thermometer is a long, cylindrical, calibrated tube that contains a column of mercury (Figure 17-6).

● Starting with 94°F (34°C), each long line indicates a one-degree elevation in temperature.

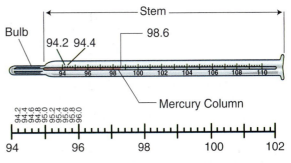

FIGURE 17-6 Reading a thermometer. This thermometer reads 98.6°F. Most Fahrenheit thermometers have an arrow indicating 98.6°.

- Only every other degree is marked with a number.
- In between each long line are four shorter lines.
- Each shorter line equals two-tenths (2/10 or 0.2) of 1 degree.

Mercury (the solid color line shown in Figure 17-6) in the bulb of the thermometer rises in the hollow center of the stem as heat is registered. To read the thermometer:

- Hold it at eye level.
- Find the solid column of mercury.
- Look along the sharper edge between the numbers and lines.
- Read at the point at which the mercury ends.
- If it falls between two lines, read it to the closest line.

Some glass thermometers come individually pre-packaged for patient use. The patient receives it as part of the admission package.

GUIDELINES for

Using an Oral or Rectal Thermometer

Oral Thermometer
1. Do not use if the patient is:
   — uncooperative
   — restless
   — unconscious
   — chilled
   — confused or disoriented
   — coughing
   — an infant or child
   — unable to breathe through the nose
   — has had oral surgery
   — irrational
   — very weak
   — receiving oxygen (except nasal prongs)
   — on seizure precautions
2. An oral temperature reading could be false on denture wearers.
3. To measure an oral temperature accurately, wait 15 minutes after patients have been smoking, eating, or drinking.

Rectal Thermometer
1. Do not use if the patient has:
   — diarrhea
   — fecal impaction
   — combative behavior
   — rectal bleeding
   — hemorrhoids
   — had rectal surgery or rectal or colonic disease
   — a colostomy
2. Always hold a rectal thermometer with probe in place the entire time.

GUIDELINES for

The Safe Use of a Glass Thermometer

- Wear disposable gloves when measuring oral and rectal temperatures.
- Check glass thermometers for chips.
- Shake mercury down before use. Shake away from the patient and hard objects.
- Do not leave the patient alone with a thermometer in place.
- Allow glass thermometer to register for at least 3 minutes for oral temperature, 3 to 5 minutes for rectal temperature, and 10 minutes for axillary temperature.
- Hold rectal and axillary thermometers in place.
- When using a rectal thermometer, lubricate the bulb end of the thermometer before inserting it into the rectum.
- After removing the thermometer and before reading it, wipe the thermometer from end to tip with an alcohol wipe or cotton ball.
- Do not touch bulb end that has been in patient's mouth (oral thermometer) or anus (rectal thermometer).

Using the Electronic Thermometer

Battery-operated electronic thermometers are commonly used. The temperature registers in large numbers on the screen. The probe is placed into the patient. The probe stem is colored blue for oral or axillary use and red for rectal use. A new, disposable probe cover is used for each patient. Following use, the cover is discarded. The temperature registers in about 30 seconds.

The Tympanic Thermometer

Many facilities use tympanic thermometers. The temperature is taken by measuring the heat that is given off by the tympanic membrane (in the ear). This method has several advantages:

- Tympanic thermometers are accurate and easy to use.
- The temperature registers in a few seconds. Because of this, taking the temperature of an agitated patient is safer and faster.
- Temperatures that cannot be taken orally can be taken by the tympanic method, eliminating the need to take rectal or axillary temperatures.
- The tympanic thermometer allows you to select a core, oral, or rectal mode. This means the reading will correlate with the mode selected. Choose the mode according to your facility's policy.
- Wait for 15 minutes to take the temperature if the patient has been outdoors or if the patient has been lying on the ear you will use.

PROCEDURE 33

MEASURING AN ORAL TEMPERATURE (GLASS THERMOMETER)

1. Carry out each beginning procedure action.

2. Assemble the following equipment on a tray:
   - gloves (standard precautions)
   - container with clean thermometers
   - container for used thermometers
   - cotton balls
   - container for soiled tissues
   - container with tissues
   - pad and pencil
   - watch with second hand

3. Have patient rest in a comfortable position in bed or chair. Put on gloves.

4. Remove thermometer from container by holding stem end. Rinse thermometer with cold water and wipe with tissue from stem to mercury bulb end if thermometer has been in disinfectant. Check to be sure the thermometer is intact. Read the mercury column. It should register below 96°F. If necessary, shake it down. (To shake down (Figure 17-7A), move away from table and other hard objects. Grasp the stem tightly between your thumb and fingers. Shake down with downward motion.) If used in your facility, place in disposable plastic cover sheath.

5. Ask patient if he or she has had any liquids to drink or has smoked within the last 15 minutes. Wait 15 minutes before taking oral temperature if the answer is yes.

6. Insert bulb end of thermometer under patient's tongue, toward side of mouth (Figure 17-7B). Tell patient to hold thermometer gently with lips closed for 3 minutes.

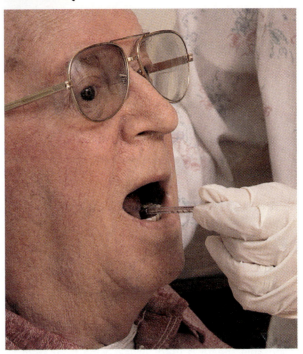

FIGURE 17-7B The bulb end of the thermometer is inserted under the tongue, left 3 minutes, then removed.

7. Remove thermometer, holding by stem. Wipe from stem end toward bulb end (Figure 17-7C).

8. Discard tissue in proper container.

9. Read thermometer and record temperature on pad (Figure 17-7D).

10. Place thermometer in container for used thermometers. If thermometer is to be reused for this patient:
    - Wash it twice in cold water and soap with two separate cotton balls, wiping from stem to bulb.
    - Rinse and dry it.
    - Return it to the individual disinfectant-filled holder.
    - Remove gloves and discard according to facility policy.

11. Carry out each procedure completion action.

12. Report any unusual variations to the nurse at once.

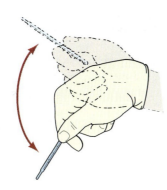

FIGURE 17-7A
Shake mercury down in column by holding the thermometer by the stem and snapping the wrist. Check the reading. Repeat until the reading is below 96°F.

continues

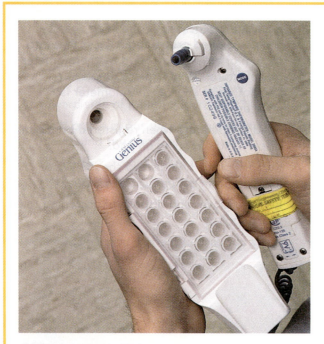

FIGURE 17-14A Check the lens of the tympanic thermometer to make sure it is clean and intact.

contact with blood or body fluids, open lesions, or wet linens.

7. Position the patient so you have access to the ear you will be using.

8. Gently pull the ear pinna back and up (Figure 17-14B). This straightens the ear canal so the thermometer can be placed for an accurate reading.

9. Place the probe in the patient's ear, aiming it toward the tympanic membrane. Insert the probe until it seals the ear canal (Figure 17-14C). Do not apply pressure.

10. Press the activation button (Figure 17-14D). Leave the thermometer in the ear for the time recommended by the manufacturer.

11. When you have a reading, remove the probe from the resident's ear and dispose of the cover. See Table 17-4 for normal ranges of tympanic temperatures by age group.

12. Carry out each procedure completion action.

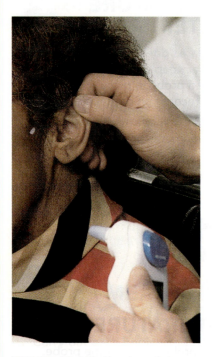

FIGURE 17-14B Gently pull the ear pinna back and up.

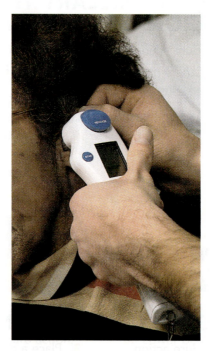

FIGURE 17-14C Place the probe in the patient's ear, aiming it toward the tympanic membrane. Insert the probe until it seals the ear canal.

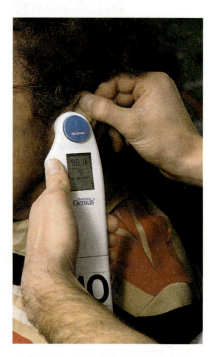

FIGURE 17-14D Press the activation button and leave the thermometer in the ear for the time recommended by the manufacturer.

continues

PROCEDURE **40** *continued*

TABLE 17-4 NORMAL RANGES FOR TYMANIC TEMPERATURES

Years of Age	Fahrenheit	Celsius
0–2	97.5–100.4°F	36.4–38.0°C
3–10	97.0–100.0°F	36.1–37.8°C
11–65	96.6–99.7°F	35.9–37.6°C
>65	96.4–99.5°F	35.8–37.5°C

Cleaning Glass Thermometers

Glass thermometers are reusable. Therefore, they must be cleaned and disinfected between uses. If each patient has an individual thermometer kept in solution at the bedside, you must clean and disinfect it after each use. If a general supply of thermometers is used to determine routine temperature, they too must be disinfected before reuse.

Each used thermometer must be carefully washed with soapy, cold, running water to remove saliva or other body secretions. It must be rinsed to remove the soap and then carefully dried before disinfecting.

PROCEDURE **41**

CLEANING GLASS THERMOMETERS

1. Wash your hands.
2. Assemble equipment:
   - tray
   - towel
   - label
   - washcloth
   - soiled thermometers in container of soapy water
   - container for clean thermometers
   - liquid soap
   - container of cotton balls
   - disinfectant, according to facility policy
   - disposable gloves, according to facility policy
3. Take tray of equipment to utility room.
4. Place towel on sink side.
5. Wash and dry container and cover for clean thermometers. Place on towel with cover top up.
6. Place gauze in bottom of container.
7. Clean sink with cleanser. Then place washcloth in bottom of sink and fill sink 1/3 full with cool water. This is in case you drop a thermometer; it is less likely to break. Put on gloves.
8. Slowly turn on cold water faucet.
9. Moisten a sponge/cotton ball and apply soap.
10. Pick up one thermometer at a time, holding by the stem.
    a. Using a circular motion, cleanse the thermometer from stem to bulb.
    b. Discard cotton ball.
    c. Carefully rinse the thermometer.
    d. Using a circular motion and a dry cotton ball for each, dry each thermometer.
    e. Check thermometers for chips and shake down to 96°F (21°C) or below

continues

PROCEDURE **41** *continued*

before placing in clean container (Figure 17-15A).

f. Fill container half full with disinfectant (Figure 17-15B).

g. Empty water from dirty container.

11. Shut off faucet. Squeeze out washcloth and put into laundry. Shut basin drain and add hot water and soap.

12. Wash, rinse, and dry dirty thermometer container.

13. Remove gloves and discard according to facility policy.

14. Add disinfectant, if necessary, so that each thermometer is completely covered by it.

15. Place cover on container. Place label with date, time, and your initials on container. Remember that disinfectants take time to be effective.

16. Place washcloth and towel in laundry. Dispose of used sponges or cotton balls in trash.

17. Leave area neat and tidy.

18. After disinfecting:

a. Remove label. Remove thermometers.

b. Empty disinfectant.

c. Wash and dry container.

d. Place 4 × 4 folded sponge on the bottom of the container.

19. Rinse and dry thermometers.

20. Place dry, clean thermometers on sponge in container and cover (Figure 17-15C).

21. Store per facility policy in clean area.

22. Wash your hands and report completion of task to the nurse.

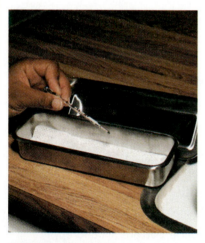

FIGURE 17-15A Place in a clean container that has folded gauze on the bottom to prevent breakage of thermometers.

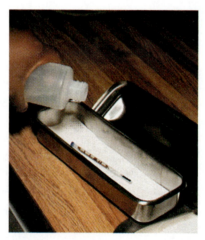

FIGURE 17-15B Add disinfectant solution, being sure to cover entire thermometer.

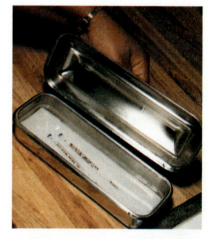

FIGURE 17-15C Allow thermometers to soak the required time. Then remove and rinse well before storing in a clean, dry container.

Remember that glass breaks very easily, so be careful when washing and drying the thermometer. Check each one for chips before putting it into disinfectant and before placing the thermometer in the patient.

Documentation

In many facilities, temperatures are recorded on a temperature clipboard. They are then transferred to the individual patient charts. Changes in readings may be **flagged** (specially noted) by placing a circle around the reading or a star beside it. Make sure to report any changes from previous temperature readings directly to the nurse. Your accurate observations, reporting, and documentation contribute to the nurses' evaluation and assessment of the patient.

REVIEW

A. True/False.

Mark the following true or false by circling T or F.

1. T F When charting an axillary temperature, always print *AX* after the reading.

2. T F Readings taken with a plastic thermometer may not be entirely accurate.

3. T F Temperature is the measurement of body heat.

4. T F The most common method of measuring the temperature of a cooperative adult is by mouth.

5. T F To measure a rectal temperature, the patient is best positioned on her back.

6. T F 96.8°F is an average oral temperature.

7. T F Only temperature variations of more than 5°F should be reported to the nurse.

8. T F Clinical thermometers can be identified by the shapes of their bulbs.

9. T F The probe of an electronic thermometer is covered with a red sheath for rectal use.

10. T F The axillary temperature of a patient will register approximately one degree higher than his oral temperature.

11. T F The tympanic temperature reading is the most accurate.

12. T F A freezing temperature registered in Celsius readings would be 32°.

13. T F It would be unsafe to use glass oral thermometers with children.

14. T F If safely placed, rectal thermometers need not be held.

15. T F Wait five minutes after the patient has taken hot liquids to measure an oral temperature.

16. T F When washing used glass thermometers, always wash them in hot, soapy water.

17. T F Always wipe the axillary area before placing a thermometer.

18. T F When using an electronic thermometer, you should not allow your fingers to touch the probe sheath.

19. T F All rectal thermometers should be lubricated before insertion.

20. T F The oral thermometer should remain in place one minute.

21. T F The mercury column in a glass oral thermometer should register below 96°F at the beginning of the procedure.

22. T F There may be times when a temperature has to be measured in the groin area.

23. T F Each long line on the stem of a clinical thermometer indicates an increase of 2 degrees of temperature.

24. T F Each short line on the stem of the clinical thermometer indicates a 0.2-degree increase in temperature.

25. T F Measuring the temperature in the groin area gives the most accurate indication of body temperature.

B. Completion.

Complete the statements by choosing the correct words from the following list.

Fahrenheit	less
higher	temperature
pulse	tympanic

26. Vital signs include _____ , _____ , respiration, and blood pressure.

27. A normal temperature reading of 98.6° would be in the _____ scale.

28. A _____ thermometer is used to measure the temperature in the ear.

29. A three-month-old child might be expected to have a slightly _____ temperature normally than a child who is nine years old.

30. Temperature is _____ stable in children than in adults.

C. Nursing Assistant Challenge.

31. Mrs. LeJune is having difficulty breathing and is very restless. The nurse instructs you to measure her temperature. What type of thermometer would you choose if all were available?

   a. Glass oral thermometer

   b. Glass rectal thermometer

   c. Electronic oral thermometer

   d. Tympanic thermometer

32. You are about to measure a rectal temperature with a glass thermometer. You find a small chip in the glass. What should you do?

   a. Use the thermometer, because it is just a small chip.

   b. Throw the thermometer in the wastepaper basket.

   c. Break the thermometer in half so no one else will use it.

   d. Replace with another thermometer.

33. You are assigned to measure your patient's rectal temperature using a glass thermometer. How long should you hold the thermometer in place?

   a. 3 minutes

   b. 10 minutes

   c. 15 minutes

   d. 20 minutes

U N I T **18**

Pulse and Respiration

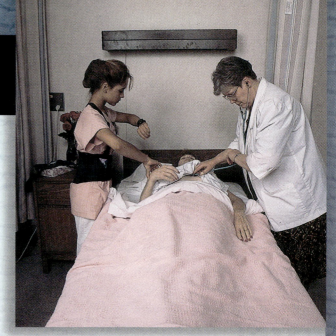

INTRODUCTION

The pulse and respiration of the patient are usually counted during the same procedure. Because breathing is partly under voluntary control, a person is able to stop or alter breathing temporarily for a short period. For example, when a patient realizes that her breathing is being watched and counted, she alters her breathing pattern without meaning to do so. To avoid this, the respirations are counted immediately following the pulse count without telling the patient. The patient's hand is kept in the same position, and your fingers remain upon the pulse so that you seem to still be taking the pulse.

THE PULSE

The **pulse** is:

- The pressure of the blood felt against the wall of an artery as the heart alternately contracts (beats) and relaxes (rests).
- More easily felt in arteries that come fairly close to the skin and can be gently pressed against a bone.
- The same in all arteries throughout the body.
- An indication of how the cardiovascular system is meeting the body's needs.

Radial Pulse

The **radial pulse** is the most commonly measured pulse. It is measured at the radial artery in the wrist. Figure 18-1 shows areas of the body where other large blood vessels come close enough to the surface to be sites for counting the pulse. Conscious patients can be checked at the radial artery. (See Procedure 42.) Unconscious patients should be checked at the carotid artery or apically (over the heart).

Pulse measurement includes determining the:

1. Rate or speed
   a. **Bradycardia**—an unusually slow pulse
   b. **Tachycardia**—an unusually fast pulse
2. Character
   a. **Rhythm**—regularity
   b. Volume or fullness

Report:

- Pulse rates over 100 beats per minute (bpm) (tachycardia)
- Pulse rates under 60 bpm (bradycardia)
- Irregularities in character (rhythm and volume)

Pulse rates can be affected by:

- Illness
- Emotions
- Age
- Exercise
- Elevated temperature
- Sex

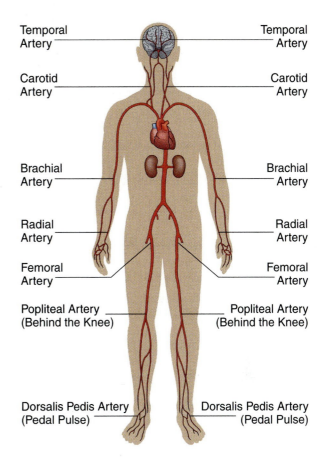

FIGURE 18-1 Common pulse sites of the body

- Position
- Physical training
- Lowered temperature
- Drugs

Table 18-1 shows average pulse rates.

The Apical Pulse

An **apical pulse** is measured by counting the heart contractions. The stethoscope is placed over the apex (tip) of the heart. Listen for the heart sounds that indicate closing of the valves. These sounds occur as the heart pumps blood into the

TABLE 18-1 AVERAGE PULSE RATES	
Patient	**Beats per Minute**
Adult men	60–70
Adult women	65–80
Children over 7 years	75–100
Preschoolers	80–110
Infants	120–160

COUNTING THE RADIAL PULSE

1. Carry out each beginning procedure action.

2. Place patient in a comfortable position. The palm of the hand should be down and the arm should rest on a flat surface.

3. Locate the pulse on the thumb side of the wrist with the tips of your first three fingers (Figure 18-2). Do not use your thumb—it contains a pulse that may be confused with the patient's pulse.

4. When the pulse is felt, exert slight pressure. Use second hand of watch and count for one minute. It is the practice in some hospitals to count for one-half minute and multiply by two and to record the rate for one minute. A one-minute count is preferred and must be done if the pulse is irregular.

5. Carry out procedure completion actions.

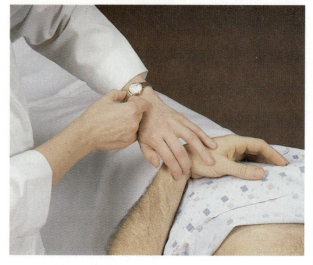

FIGURE 18-2 Locate the pulse on the thumb side of the wrist with the tips of your first three fingers.

---

arteries. The sounds should occur at the same rate as the pulse that is felt as an expansion of the radial artery. The apex of the heart is found:

- On the left side of the front of the chest
- Between the fifth and sixth ribs
- Just below the left nipple
- In women, under the left breast

Listen carefully for two sounds: lub dub. The louder sound (lub) corresponds to the contraction of the ventricles pushing the blood forward through the arteries, and the closing of the valves to prevent the backflow of blood. This is the sound to be counted. The softer sound (dub) corresponds to the relaxation of the ventricles as they fill with blood before the next contraction and the closing of the semilunar valves to prevent backflow from the arteries.

Apical-Radial Pulse Rate

The apical and radial pulse rate is a comparison of the apical rate and the radial rate. Usually they are the same.

Sometimes the contraction of the heart is so weak that it fails to send enough blood to the arteries to expand them. When this happens, no pulse is felt. In this case, the number of loud sounds do not correspond with the number of pulses felt in the radial artery.

The difference between the apical pulse (the loud sounds heard over the heart) and the radial pulse (the expansion felt over the radial pulse) is called a **pulse deficit**. Two people

measure the heart rate and the radial pulse at the same time. (See Procedure 43.) The nurse measures the apical pulse while the second person counts the radial pulse for 1 minute. The rates are then compared.

Apical pulse rates are checked:

- Whenever a pulse deficit exists or is suspected.
- Before the registered nurse administers drugs that alter the heart rate or rhythm.
- In children whose rapid rates might be difficult to count at the radial artery.
- For one full minute.
- On any child 12 months of age or younger.
- Whenever you are uncertain of the accuracy of the radial pulse or it is irregular.

Pulse deficits are found in some forms of heart disease.

RESPIRATION

The main function of **respiration** is to supply the cells in the body with oxygen and to rid the body of excess carbon dioxide. When respirations are inefficient, there is less oxygen in the blood available for body needs. In addition, carbon dioxide is released less efficiently. The skin takes on a bluish or dusky color and the patient develops a condition known as **cyanosis**.

There are two parts to each respiration: one **inspiration** (inhalation) followed by one **expiration** (exhalation).

PROCEDURE **43**

COUNTING THE APICAL-RADIAL PULSE

1. Carry out each beginning procedure action.
2. Clean stethoscope earpieces and bell with disinfectant.
3. Place stethoscope earpieces in your ears.
4. Place the stethoscope diaphragm or bell over the apex of the patient's heart. If it is cold, warm the diaphragm with hands before placing it on patient's chest.
5. Listen carefully for the heartbeat.
6. Count the louder sounding beats for one minute.
7. Check radial pulse for one minute. The best way to obtain these numbers is to have the nurse count the apical pulse while you take the radial pulse (Figure 18-3).
8. Note results on a pad for comparison.
9. Clean earpieces and bell of stethoscope with disinfectant.
10. Carry out each procedure completion action.

    Example: Apical pulse = 108
    Radial pulse = 82
    Pulse deficit = 26 (108 − 82 = 26)

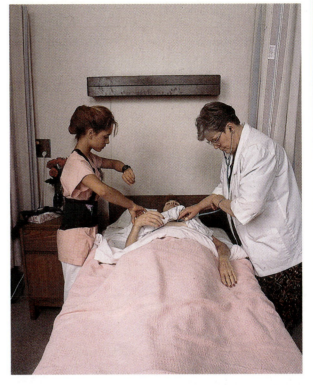

FIGURE 18-3 The nurse takes the apical pulse while the nursing assistant takes the radial pulse.

Special terms describe different breathing patterns:
- Normal—regular, 16 to 20 breaths per minute
- **Tachypnea**—rapid, shallow breathing
- **Dyspnea**—difficult or labored breathing
- Shallow—breaths that only partially fill the lungs
- **Apnea**—a period of no respirations
- **Cheyne-Stokes respirations**—a period of dyspnea followed by periods of apnea
- **Stertorous**—Snoring-like respirations
- **Rales** (gurgles)—moist respirations. At times, fluid (mucus) will collect in the air passages. This causes a bubbling type of respiration. Rales are common in the dying patient.
- Wheezing—difficult breathing accompanied by a whistling or sighing sound due to narrowing of bronchioles (as in asthma) or an increase of mucus in bronchi.

Respirations should be checked for:
- **Rate**—number of respirations per minute
- Rhythm—regularity
- **Symmetry**—ability of the chest to expand equally as air enters each lung

- **Volume**—depth of respiration
- Character—terms used to describe the character of respirations include:
  - Regular
  - Irregular
  - Shallow
  - Deep
  - Labored (difficult)

The rate of respiration is determined by counting the rise or fall of the chest for one minute, using a watch equipped with a second hand. (See Procedure 44.)

- The average rate for adults is 16 to 20 respirations per minute.
- If the rate is more than 25 per minute, it is said to be **accelerated**. Accelerated respiration should be reported.
- If the rate is less than 12 per minute, it is too slow. It should be reported.

Remember that, if possible, respirations should be counted without the patient's knowing that you are doing so; the rate and volume may change if the patient knows they are being

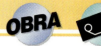

PROCEDURE   44

COUNTING RESPIRATIONS

1. When the pulse rate has been counted, you may leave your fingers on the radial pulse and start counting the number of times the chest rises and falls during one minute (Figure 18-4).

2. Note depth and regularity of respirations.

3. Record the time, rate, depth, and regularity of respirations.

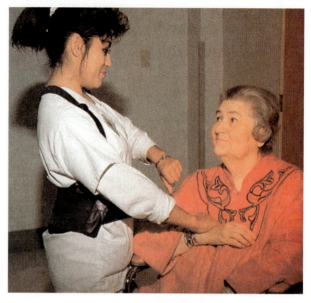

FIGURE 18-4 Continue to rest the back of the hand against the chest wall while counting the respirations.

counted. You might count respirations before or after counting the radial pulse. Continue pressing on the pulse area while counting.

The factors affecting respiratory rates include:

- Illness
- Emotions
- Elevated temperature
- Sex
- Age
- Exercise
- Position
- Drugs

Temperature, pulse, and respiration (TPR) rates and character are recorded in a notebook and then transferred to the patient's chart (Figure 18-5).

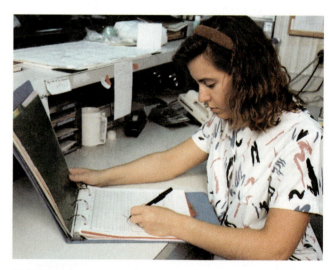

FIGURE 18-5 TPR readings are recorded on the patient's record.

REVIEW

A. True/False.

Mark the following true or false by circling T or F.

1. T F A pulse deficit results when there is a difference between the apical and radial pulses.

2. T F The pulse is the pressure of blood against the arterial wall.

3. T F Cheyne-Stokes respirations are deep and regular.

4. T F Pulses differ when counted at different pulse sites.

5. T F The pulse rate of an infant is 110 to 130 bpm.

6. T F An apical pulse should be counted in children.

7. T F The most often used pulse site is the carotid artery.

8. T F The respiratory system rids the body of excess carbon dioxide.

9. T F Mucus in the air passages causes rales.

10. T F A pulse is best counted using the thumb placed over the artery.

B. Matching.

Choose the correct word from Column II to match the words and phrases in Column I.

Column I	Column II
11. ____ Snoring types of respiration	a. accelerated
12. ____ Bluish discoloration to the skin	b. apnea
13. ____ Regularity	c. bradycardia
14. ____ Periods of no respiration	d. cyanosis
15. ____ Difficult breathing	e. dyspnea
16. ____ Rapid respirations	f. rate
17. ____ Increased or speeded up	g. rhythm
18. ____ Expiration	h. stertorous
19. ____ Speed	i. tachypnea
20. ____ Slow pulse	j. inspiration
	k. exhalation

C. Nursing Assistant Challenge.

21. Mrs. Morgan has a heart condition that makes her heart rate irregular and faster than normal. Her respirations are difficult or rapid, labored, and moist. She receives a medication that profoundly alters her heart action. Your orders are to assist in determining the pulse deficit. Answer the statements using the terms in the following list.

    apical   rales
    dyspnea   tachycardia
    radial   tachypnea

    a. The faster heart rate is described as _____.
    b. The difficult respirations can be charted as _____.
    c. Moist respirations are best described as _____.
    d. Rapid respirations are also called _____.
    e. Which pulse rate will you count? _____.
    f. Which pulse rate will a second person count? _____.

22. List two reasons why a radial-apical pulse rate would be ordered.

    a. _____
    b. _____

Blood Pressure

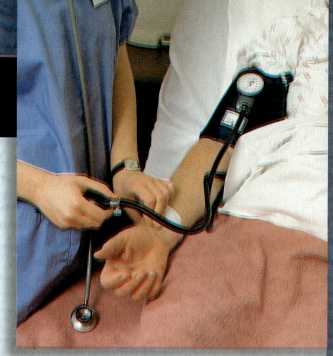

As a result of this unit, you will be able to:
- Spell and define terms.
- Describe the factors that influence blood pressure.
- Identify the range of normal blood pressure values.
- Identify the causes of inaccurate blood pressure readings.
- Select the proper size blood pressure cuff.
- List precautions associated with use of the sphygmomanometer.
- Demonstrate the following procedure:
  - Procedure 45 Taking Blood Pressure

Learn the meaning and the correct spelling of the following words and phrases:

aneroid gauge	diastole	hypertension	stethoscope
auscultatory gap	diastolic pressure	hypotension	stimulant
blood pressure	elasticity	pulse pressure	systole
brachial artery	fasting	sphygmomanometer	systolic pressure
depressant			

INTRODUCTION

Blood pressure is the fourth vital sign. It is the measure of the force of the blood against the walls of the arteries. Blood pressure depends on the:

- Volume (amount of blood in the circulatory system).
- Force of the heartbeat.
- Condition of the arteries. Arteries that have lost their **elasticity** (stretch) give more resistance. The pressure is greater in these arteries.
- Distance from the heart. Blood pressure in the legs is lower than in the arms.

Pressure varies with contraction (**systole**) and relaxation (**diastole**) of the ventricles of the heart.

- Systolic blood pressure reading indicates the period when the pressure within the arteries is the greatest, during contraction of the ventricles.
- Diastolic reading indicates the lowest point of pressure between ventricular contractions.

Blood pressure is elevated by:

- Sex of the patient (males slightly higher than females before menopause)
- Exercise
- Eating
- **Stimulants** (substances that speed up body functions)
- Emotional stress, such as anger, fear, or sexual activity
- Disease conditions, such as arteriosclerosis (hardening of the arteries), elevated cholesterol, or diabetes mellitus
- Hereditary factors
- Pain
- Obesity
- Age
- Condition of blood vessels
- Some drugs

Blood pressure is lowered by:

- **Fasting** (not eating)
- Rest
- **Depressants** (drugs that slow down body functions)
- Weight loss
- Emotions (such as grief)
- Abnormal conditions such as hemorrhage (loss of blood) or shock
- Some drugs, such as antihypertensives (drugs that lower blood pressure in persons who have hypertension)
- Diuretics (drugs that lower the volume of body fluids)

The factors affecting blood pressure are:

- Age
- Sleep
- Weight
- Emotion
- Heredity
- Sex
- Viscosity of blood
- Condition of blood vessels

EQUIPMENT

The **sphygmomanometer** (blood pressure measuring apparatus) consists of:

- A cuff (different sizes are available) that fits around the patient's arm. There is a rubber bladder inside the cuff. A pressure control button is attached to the cuff. It is important to use the proper size cuff when measuring blood pressure. Cuffs that are too wide or too narrow will give inaccurate readings (Figure 19-1). The width of the cuff should measure approximately 80 percent of the diameter of the patient's arm.
- Two tubes. One tube is connected to the pressure control bulb and to the bladder inside the cuff. The other tube is connected to the pressure gauge.
- A pressure gauge, which may be a round **aneroid gauge** dial or a column of mercury (Figure 19-2). Both are marked with numbers.

The **stethoscope** (Figure 19-3) magnifies sounds. It consists of:

- A bell or diaphragm.
- Tubing that carries sounds to the listener.
- Ear pieces that direct the sounds into the listener's ears. The ear pieces and diaphragm must be cleaned with antiseptic before and after each use to prevent transmission of disease.

Electronic sphygmomanometers with attached cuffs are used in some facilities. These units do not require a stethoscope but automatically register the readings on a digital display. Check with your nurse for specific operating instructions.

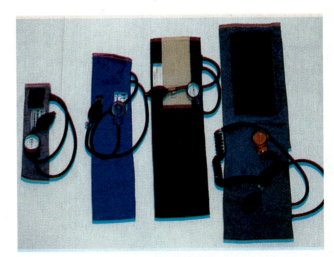

FIGURE 19-1 The cuff must be sized properly (to fit the specific patient) to obtain accurate readings.

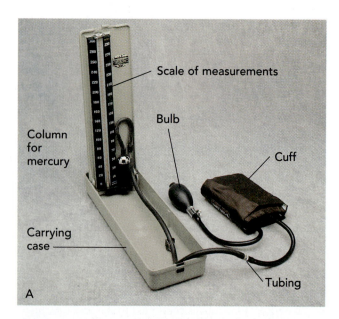

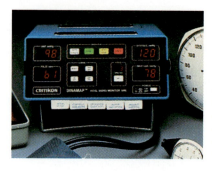

FIGURE 19-4 All vital signs may be checked with a single instrument. *Courtesy of Critikon, Inc.*

Some facilities use an instrument that measures pulse rate, temperature, and blood pressure (Figure 19-4).

MEASURING THE BLOOD PRESSURE

Blood pressure is usually measured in the upper arm over the brachial artery. Blood pressure readings taken anywhere else must be ordered by a doctor.

1. The cuff is smoothly applied directly over the **brachial artery** (1 inch above the antecubital area).
2. The stethoscope bell is placed over the brachial artery.
3. Pressure is then increased by inflating the rubber bladder in the cuff to stop the flow of blood through the artery.
4. The pressure is slowly released and the sounds of heart valves closing can be heard. The sounds correspond to pressure changes in the blood.
5. The blood pressure is measured:
   a. At its highest point as the **systolic pressure**. This will be the first regular sound you will hear. This is the sound of the bicuspid and tricuspid valves shutting.
   b. At its lowest point as the **diastolic pressure**. This will be the change or last sound you will hear. This is the sound of the semilunar valves shutting.
   c. The difference between systolic and diastolic pressure is called **pulse pressure**. The pulse pressure gives important information about the health of the arteries. The average pulse pressure in a healthy adult is about 40 millimeters (mm) of mercury (Hg) (range 30–50 mm Hg). However, factors in both health and disease can alter the pulse pressure. An increase in blood volume or heart rate or a decrease in the ability of the arteries to expand may result in an increased pulse pressure.
6. Blood pressure readings are recorded as an improper fraction; e.g., systolic/diastolic or 130/92. This means the systolic pressure is 130 and the diastolic pressure is 92.
7. Blood pressure values:
   a. Average resting adult brachial artery pressure is between 90 and 140 millimeters of mercury (mm Hg) systolic and between 60 and 90 millimeters of mercury (mm Hg) diastolic.

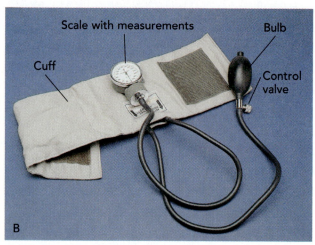

FIGURE 19-2 A. Mercury gravity sphygmomanometer B. Dial (aneroid) sphygmomanometer

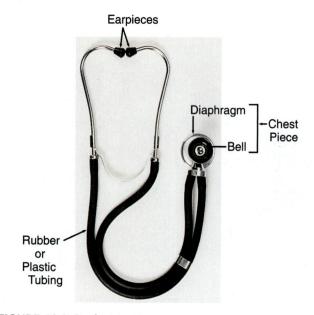

FIGURE 19-3 Stethoscope

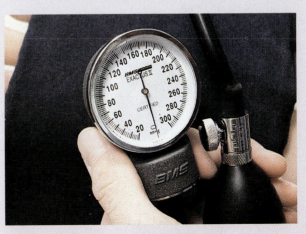

GUIDELINES
for

Preparing to Measure Blood Pressure

Before using the stethoscope:

1. Clean the ear pieces with an alcohol wipe (Figure 19-5) and clean the bell with a different alcohol wipe.
2. Point the ear pieces forward when inserting them in your ears.
3. Use the bell portion of the stethoscope (Figure 19-6).
4. Be sure the bell portion is open so you will hear the beats.

Before using a sphygmomanometer:

1. If using a mercury manometer—if the mercury moves up the column very slowly (Figure 19-7), it may have oxidized. Report this to the nurse and use another sphygmomanometer.

2. If using an aneroid manometer—make sure the needle is on zero before inflating the cuff (Figure 19-8). If it is not, report this to the nurse and use another sphygmomanometer.

Generally:

Turn off radio and television when taking blood pressure. Ask the patient not to talk. Do not take blood pressure on an arm that:

- Has an intravenous feeding or other device inserted
- Is being treated for burns, fractures, or other injuries

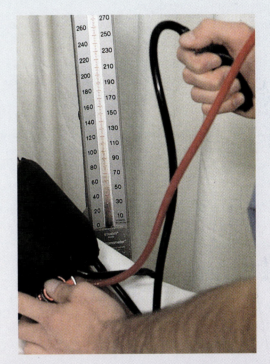

FIGURE 19-7 Do not use the sphygmomanometer if the mercury moves up the column very slowly.

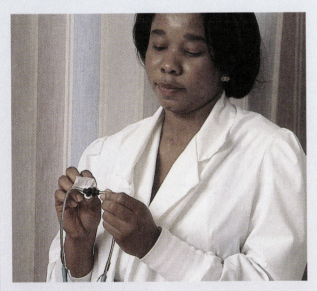

FIGURE 19-5 Carefully clean ear pieces of the stethoscope before use.

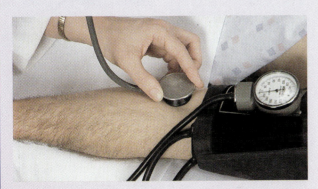

FIGURE 19-6 Use the bell portion of the stethoscope when taking a blood pressure.

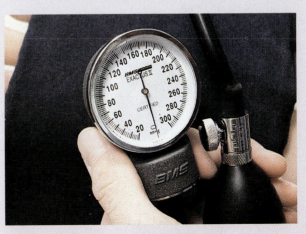

FIGURE 19-8 Make sure the needle is on zero before inflating the cuff of an aneroid manometer.

b. **Hypertension** (high blood pressure) is when values are greater than 140 mm Hg systolic and 90 mm Hg diastolic.

c. **Hypotension** (low blood pressure) is when values are less than 100 mm Hg systolic and 70 mm Hg diastolic. Excessive hypotension can lead to shock.

d. For either hypertension or hypotension, unusual or changed readings must be recorded and reported. (See Procedure 45.)

Inaccurate Blood Pressure Readings

Causes of inaccurate blood pressure readings include:

- Use of a wrong size cuff
- An improperly wrapped cuff
- Incorrect positioning of arm
- Not using the same arm for all readings
- Not having the gauge at eye level
- Deflating the cuff too slowly
- Mistaking an **auscultatory gap** (sound fadeout for 10 to 15 mm Hg which then begins again) as the diastolic pressure

Caution: Do not attempt to measure blood pressure using an arm that is the site of an intravenous infusion, paralyzed, injured, the site of an A-V shunt, or if edema is present.

HOW TO READ THE GAUGE

The gauges are marked with a series of lines. The large lines are at increments of 10 millimeters of mercury pressure. The shorter lines are at 2-mm intervals. For example, the first small line above 80 mm is 82 mm. The first small line below 80 mm is 78 mm (Figure 19-9).

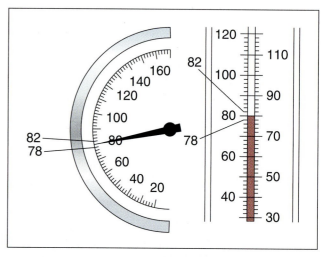

FIGURE 19-9 The aneroid gauge (left) and the mercury gravity gauge (right). Take reading at the closest line.

PROCEDURE 45 OBRA

TAKING BLOOD PRESSURE

1. Carry out each beginning procedure action.
2. Assemble equipment:
   - sphygmomanometer with appropriate size cuff
   - stethoscope
   - alcohol wipes
3. Remove patient's arm from sleeve or roll sleeve 5 inches above elbow; it should not be tight or binding.
4. Locate the brachial artery with your fingers (Figure 19-10).
5. Place patient's arm palm upward, supported on bed or table at heart level.
6. Wrap the cuff smoothly and snugly around arm. Center the bladder over the brachial artery. The bottom of the cuff should be 1 inch above the antecubital space (inner elbow) (Figure 19-11).

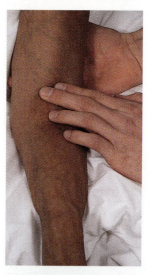

FIGURE 19-10 Locate the brachial artery with your fingers.

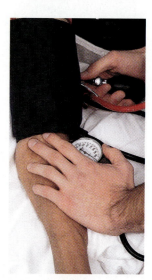

FIGURE 19-11 The bottom of the cuff should be 1 inch above the antecubital space (inner elbow).

continues

7. Place the bulb in your dominant hand and feel for the radial pulse with the fingers of your other hand (Figure 19-12). To find out how high to pump the cuff:

- Rapidly inflate the cuff until you no longer feel the radial pulse.
- Add 30 mm to that reading. (If you no longer feel the pulse when the mercury or needle reaches 130, add 30 mm for a reading of 160.)

8. Quickly and steadily deflate the cuff. Wait 15 to 30 seconds.

9. Place the stethoscope over the brachial artery (Figure 19-13).

10. Reinflate the cuff quickly and steadily to the level you calculated (in the example in step 7, to 160) (Figure 19-14).

11. Release the air at an even pace, about 2 to 3 mm per second. Keep your eyes on the needle or the mercury.

12. Listen for the onset of at least two consecutive beats. Note where the needle is on the sphygmomanometer when you hear the sound. (Do not stop deflating the cuff.) This is your systolic reading.

13. Continue deflating the cuff. The last sound you hear is the diastolic reading. Continue to deflate and to listen for 10 to 20 mm more to make sure you have the correct diastolic reading.

14. Record the reading (blood pressure is always recorded in even numbers with the systolic on top and the diastolic on the bottom, e.g., 128/82). Indicate the arm used and the position of the patient (sitting, lying down, or standing).

15. If you are not sure of the reading and need to retake the blood pressure, wait 1 to 2 minutes before repeating the procedure.

16. Clean the ear pieces of the stethoscope with alcohol wipes. If the tubing has contacted the patient or his linen, wipe it as well.

17. Return equipment to appropriate area.

18. Carry out each procedure completion action.

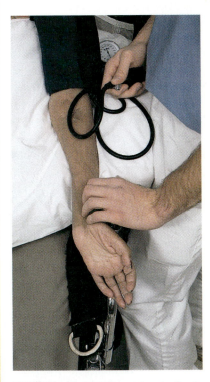

FIGURE 19-12 Place the bulb in your dominant hand and feel for the radial pulse with the fingers of your other hand.

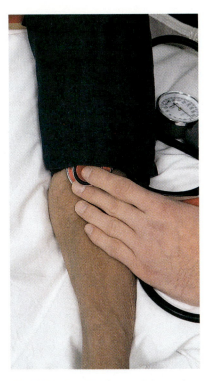

FIGURE 19-13 Place the stethoscope over the brachial artery.

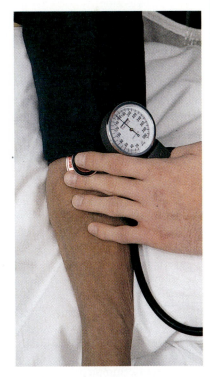

FIGURE 19-14 Reinflate the cuff quickly and steadily to the level you calculated.

To properly read the mercury gauge:
- It should be at eye level.
- It should not be tilted.
- The reading should be taken at the top of the column of mercury. It should not be taken at the "hump" in the middle of the mercury when you hear the first sound.

To properly read the aneroid gauge, observe the gauge at eye level. Do not read it at an angle.

Following completion of the blood pressure measurement, you will record and report the following:
- If you were unable to hear the reading.
- If blood pressure is higher than in previous reading.
- If blood pressure is lower than in previous reading.
- If site of reading was other than brachial artery.

REVIEW

A. True/False.

Mark the following true or false by circling T or F.

1. T F The volume of blood in the circulatory system is a factor in the blood pressure.
2. T F Exercise decreases blood pressure.
3. T F To accurately measure blood pressure, you will need both a sphygmomanometer and a stethoscope.
4. T F Blood pressures taken over arteries closer to the heart will be lower than those taken over arteries farther from the heart.
5. T F A blood pressure below 100/70 would signal hypotension.
6. T F The large lines on the blood pressure gauge are in increments of 20 mm of Hg pressure.
7. T F Depressant drugs elevate the blood pressure.
8. T F Using a blood pressure cuff of the wrong size will give an inaccurate reading.
9. T F When measuring a blood pressure, always keep the gauge at eye level.
10. T F Stethoscope ear pieces should be cleaned both before and after use.

B. Matching.

Choose the correct word from Column II to match each phrase in Column I.

Column I

11. _____ high blood pressure
12. _____ lowest blood pressure reading
13. _____ stretch
14. _____ most common artery used to determine blood pressure
15. _____ blood pressure apparatus

Column II

a. brachial
b. diastolic
c. stethoscope
d. femoral
e. sphygmomanometer
f. hypotension
g. hypertension
h. elasticity
i. systolic

C. Completion.

Complete the statements by choosing the correct word.

16. The closing of the heart valves is heard as the _____ sounds.
    (diastolic) (systolic)
17. High blood pressure is known as _____.
    (hypotension) (hypertension)
18. Blood pressure is lowered when weight is _____.
    (gained) (lost)
19. Blood pressure is raised by _____.
    (rest) (exercise)
20. The ear pieces of the stethoscope should be pointed _____ as they are placed in the ears.
    (forward) (backward)

D. Nursing Assistant Challenge.

You are assigned to take Mr. King's blood pressure at 12 noon. He is a very heavy man with an IV inserted in his left arm. His blood pressure was 180/140 at 8 AM. Answer the following questions:

21. What effect will his size have on your selection of cuff? _____
22. On which arm will you apply the cuff? _____
23. Will you report your findings? _____
24. Why? _____

UNIT 20

Measuring Height and Weight

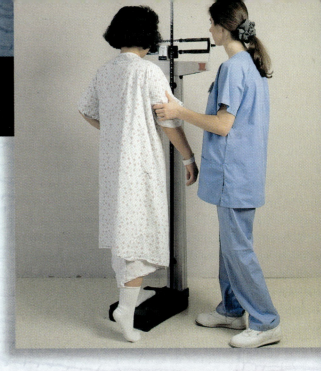

OBJECTIVES

As a result of this unit, you will be able to:

- Spell and define terms.
- Describe the proper use of an overbed scale.
- Demonstrate the following procedures:
  - Procedure 46 Weighing and Measuring the Patient Using an Upright Scale

  - Procedure 47 Weighing the Patient on a Chair Scale
  - Procedure 48 Measuring Weight with an Electronic Wheelchair Scale
  - Procedure 49 Measuring and Weighing the Patient in Bed

VOCABULARY

Learn the meaning and the correct spelling of the following words and phrases:

balance bar	centimeter (cm)	kilogram (kg)
baseline	increment	pound (lb)

WEIGHT AND HEIGHT MEASUREMENTS

Changes in weight are frequently used as an indicator of the patient's condition.

- A baseline (original) measurement of height and weight is usually obtained on admission.
- Weights are frequently measured when patients are given drugs (diuretics) to increase their urine output.
- Weight is an indicator of the patient's nutritional status.
- Measurements of weight and height must be accurately made and recorded according to facility policy because medications may be ordered according to the patient's size.
- Height measurements may be recorded in feet (') and inches ('') or in centimeters (cm).
- Weight measurements may be recorded in pounds (lb) or kilograms (kg).

Note: Some facilities use the metric system, so you may be recording weight in kilograms. If your facility uses this measurement system, the scales will be calibrated for the metric system. You will not be required to convert measurements from the inch and pound system to the metric system.

- The upright scale is used for ambulatory patients who can stand unattended on the platform (Figure 20-1).
- A mechanical lift with scale can be used to weigh patients who cannot stand or sit in a wheelchair (Figure 20-2).

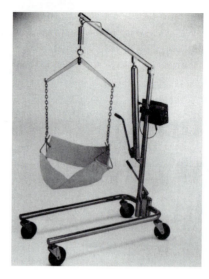

FIGURE 20-2 The scale with the mechanical lift is used when patients are not ambulatory or are too heavy or difficult to move. *Photo courtesy of Health o meter®*

- Sling scales can be used to weigh patients whose conditions do not permit the use of a mechanical lift/scale (Figure 20-3).
- Chair scales are used to weigh patients in wheelchairs (Figure 20-4).

(See Procedures 46 to 49.)

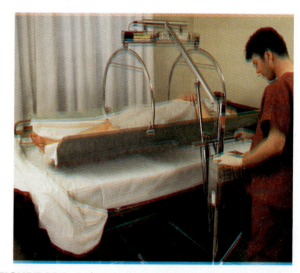

FIGURE 20-3 A sling scale is used to weigh patients in bed who cannot stand on the upright scale and cannot sit up in a wheelchair.

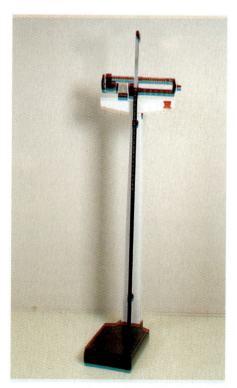

FIGURE 20-1 An upright scale is used only for patients who can stand unattended on the platform.

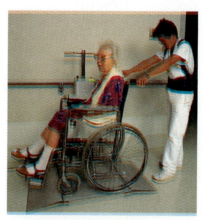

FIGURE 20-4 Electronic chair scales are used for residents who cannot stand on an upright scale.

GUIDELINES for

Obtaining Accurate Weight and Height Measurements

To obtain an accurate weight measurement, you must:

- Always balance the scale before using.
- Have patient empty bladder.
- Weigh the patient at the same time of day each time.
- Have the patient wear the same type of garments each time.
- Use the same method and the same scale each time, if possible.

You must learn to read the scale correctly. There are two bars on the upright scale (see Figure 20-1). The **balance bar** should hang free to start.

- The lower bar indicates weights in 50-pound **increments** (amounts).

- The upper bar indicates one-quarter-pound increments (Figure 20-5).
- The even-numbered pounds are marked with numbers.
- The long line between each number indicates the odd-numbered pounds.
- Each small line indicates one-quarter pound, or 4 ounces.

The two figures are added and recorded as the person's total weight. The sum is recorded according to facility policy in either pounds or kilograms. For example:

Large weight = 100 pounds
Small weight = +22 pounds
Total = 122 pounds

- Height is measured with the ruler attached to an upright scale or with a tape measure when the patient is in bed.

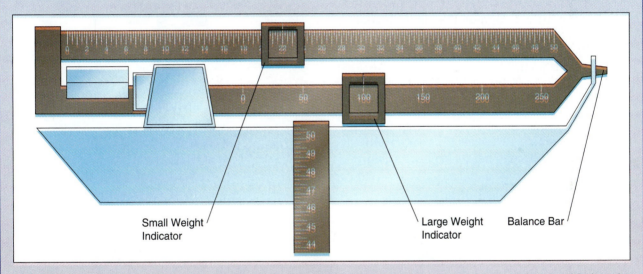

Small Weight Indicator   Large Weight Indicator   Balance Bar

FIGURE 20-5 The upper bar indicates smaller pound weights. The weight shown on the lower bar is added to the weight shown on the upper bar.

PROCEDURE 46

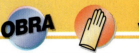

WEIGHING AND MEASURING THE PATIENT USING AN UPRIGHT SCALE

1. Carry out each beginning procedure action.

Note: Use disposable gloves if there may be contact with open lesions, wet linens, or body fluids.

2. Check notes or chart for previous weight as documented. Then escort patient to the scales.

3. Place a paper towel on the platform of the scale.

continues

PROCEDURE   46   continued

4. Be sure the weights are to the extreme left and the balance bar (bar with weight markings) hangs free.

5. Assist patient to remove shoes and step up onto the scale platform, facing the balance bar. The balance bar will rise to the top of the bar guide. Patient should not hold the bar or other parts of the scale.

6. Move the large weight to the right to the closest estimated patient weight.

7. Move the small weight to the right until the balance bar hangs freely halfway between the upper and lower bar guides.

8. Add the two figures and record the total as the patient's weight in pounds or kilograms, according to the type of scale used.

9. Assist patient to turn on the platform until facing away from the balance bar. Raise the height bar until it is level with the top of the patient's head.

10. The reading is made at the movable point of the ruler (Figure 20-6).

11. Note the number of inches indicated. Record this information in inches (″), feet (′) and inches (″), or centimeters (cm) according to

the type of scale. The height shown in Figure 20-6 is 62 inches. This may be recorded as 62 inches or 5 feet 2 inches (62 ÷ 12 = 5 feet 2 inches). Record value on your note pad.

12. Assist patient off the platform. Help patient to put on shoes, if necessary, and return to the room.

13. Carry out each procedure completion action.

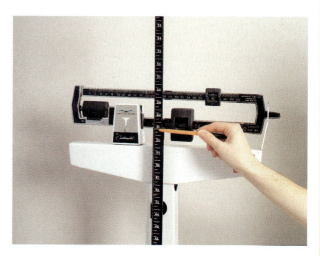

FIGURE 20-6 The patient's height is read at the movable point of the ruler.

PROCEDURE   47

WEIGHING THE PATIENT ON A CHAIR SCALE

1. Carry out each beginning procedure action.

2. Assemble equipment:
   - chair scale

3. Take patient in wheelchair to chair scale.

4. Apply transfer belt to patient and assist in a pivot transfer to chair on scale. Instruct

patient to sit down when the chair is felt against the back of the legs. Be sure patient's feet are on footrest of scale.

5. Walk behind the scale to obtain the reading.

6. Transfer patient back to wheelchair.

7. Carry out each procedure completion action.

MEASURING WEIGHT WITH AN ELECTRONIC WHEELCHAIR SCALE

1. Carry out each beginning procedure action.

2. Assemble equipment:
   - wheelchair scale

3. Determine empty weight of wheelchair by weighing it on the scale.

4. Take wheelchair to patient's room. Help patient into the wheelchair and take patient to the electronic wheelchair scale.

5. Open metal ramp sides on scale to rest on floor. This allows wheelchair access to scale.

6. Press "on" button; scale zeroes automatically (Figure 20-7).

7. Roll wheelchair with patient onto platform of scale. Lock wheels of wheelchair.

8. Digital readout will show weight.

9. Record weight of patient and wheelchair. Subtract wheelchair weight to obtain patient weight.

10. Unlock wheels of wheelchair. Roll wheelchair with patient off scale.

11. Fold scale ramps back into place.

12. Carry out each procedure completion action.

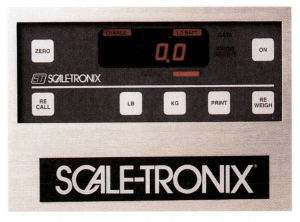

FIGURE 20-7 Press "on" button to zero scale automatically. *Courtesy of Scale-Tronix, White Plains, NY*

MEASURING AND WEIGHING THE PATIENT IN BED

1. Carry out each beginning procedure action.

2. Obtain assistance from coworker.

3. Assemble equipment:
   - overbed scale
   - tape measure
   - pencil

4. Check scale sling and straps for frayed areas or straps that do not close properly.

5. Lower side rail on your side. Make sure side rail is up on other side.

6. Fanfold top linen to foot of bed.

7. Position patient flat on back with arms and legs straight and body in good alignment.

8. Make a small pencil mark at the top of patient's head on the sheet.

9. Make a second pencil mark even with the feet (Figure 20-8).

10. Using the tape measure, measure the distance between the two pencil marks.

11. Note this on a pad with patient's height in feet and inches.

12. Remove the scale sling from suspension straps and position half under the patient.
    - Turn patient away from you.
    - Place the sling, folded lengthwise, under patient.
    - Return patient to recumbent position and place sling so that patient rests securely within it.
    - Attach sling to suspension straps. Check to be sure attachments are secure.

continues

PROCEDURE **49** *continued*

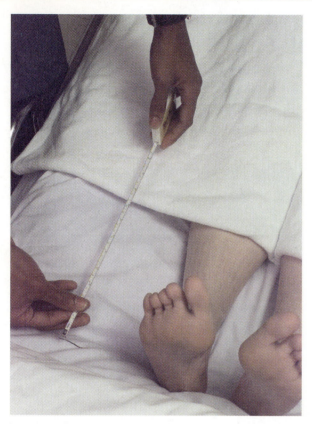

FIGURE 20-8 Measuring the height of the patient in bed. Measure from the pencil line at the bottom of the feet to the pencil line at the top of the head.

13. Position lift frame over bed with base legs in maximum open position and lock.

14. Elevate head of bed and bring patient to sitting position.

15. Attach suspension straps to frame. Position patient's arms inside straps.

16. Slowly raise sling so patient's body is free from bed. Be reassuring.

17. Guide the lift away from the bed so that no part of patient touches the bed.

18. Balance scale according to manufacturer's instructions.

19. Take and note reading.

20. Reposition sling over center of bed.

21. Release knob slowly, lowering patient to bed.

22. Remove sling by reversing the process in step 12.

23. Assist patient to comfortable position.

24. Move overbed scale out of the way.

25. Replace top bed linen over patient. Raise side rail and lower bed to lowest horizontal height.

26. Carry out each procedure completion action.

REVIEW

A. True/False.

Mark the following true or false by circling T or F.

1. T F The lower bar on the scale indicates pounds in increments of 25.

2. T F Always check the overbed scale for needed repairs before use.

3. T F To obtain a proper reading, the scale balance bar must hang freely.

4. T F The scale used most often to weigh ambulatory patients in care facilities is the upright scale.

5. T F A patient who cannot get out of bed cannot be measured.

6. T F When using an overbed scale, the patient's body must be free of the bed.

7. T F To measure a patient confined to bed, first help her assume the left Sims' position.

B. Short Answer.

Choose the correct word from the following list to complete each statement in questions 8–12.

ambulatory	inches
centimeters	kilograms
forward	pounds

8. Weights may be measured in _____.

9. Height measurements may be recorded in feet and _____ or in _____.

10. The upright scale is used to weigh _____ patients.

11. A scale that is calibrated for the metric system will express weights in _____.

12. When a patient is measured on an upright scale, he should face _____.

C. Nursing Assistant Challenge.

Mrs. Haughn is in bed recovering from a stroke. She is unable to walk or stand. She is receiving diuretics. Her doctor wants to order some new medication that is given according to the patient's size. You are assigned to weigh and measure the height of this patient. Answer each of the following by selecting the correct answer.

13. The best way to weigh this patient is with
   a. an upright scale.
   b. an overbed scale.
   c. a wheelchair scale.

14. The best way to measure this patient is
   a. with a height bar.
   b. with a tape measure.
   c. to ask the patient.

15. One reason the physician might have asked for the patient's weight is because the patient
   a. is receiving diuretics.
   b. has had a stroke.
   c. cannot stand.

16. The patient measures 63 inches. This may be expressed as
   a. 5 feet 6 inches.
   b. 5 feet 8 inches.
   c. 5 feet 3 inches.

SECTION 7

Patient Care and Comfort Measures

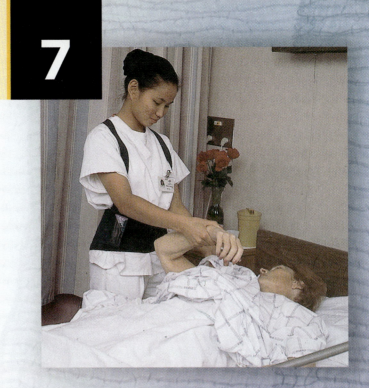

UNIT 21
Admission, Transfer, and Discharge

UNIT 22
Bedmaking

UNIT 23
Patient Bathing

UNIT 24
General Comfort Measures

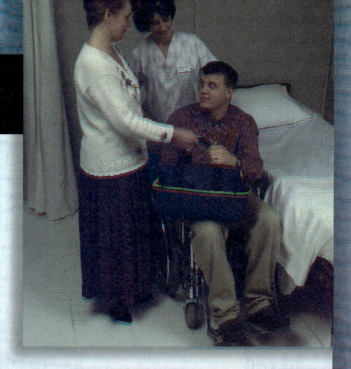

U N I T 21

Admission, Transfer, and Discharge

OBJECTIVES

As a result of this unit, you will be able to:

- Spell and define terms.
- List the ways the nursing assistant can help in the processes of admission, transfer, and discharge.
- Demonstrate the following procedures:
  - Procedure 50 Admitting the Patient
  - Procedure 51 Transferring the Patient
  - Procedure 52 Discharging the Patient

VOCABULARY

Learn the meaning and the correct spelling of the following words and phrases:

admission	diagnosis-related groups	discharge
baseline assessment	(DRGs)	transfer

INTRODUCTION

The nurse is responsible for overseeing and carrying out hospital procedures and physician's orders regarding all admissions, transfers, and discharges. You will usually help the nurse by carrying out the routine procedures associated with these activities.

A nursing assistant, a volunteer, or someone from the admissions office accompanies the patient to the unit. Someone must always escort the patient to the unit. Someone must always escort the patient from the unit during transfer or discharge.

You can do much to make these activities easier for the patient, family, and the other staff members by:

- Having equipment and materials prepared for the activity.
- Being very observant during each activity.
- Documenting observations carefully and accurately. These make a valuable contribution to the nurse's initial **baseline assessment** of the patient's condition.
- Reporting observations directly to the nurse.
- Giving attention to the details of each procedure.
- Being aware of the emotional stress these activities cause patients and their families.
- Being courteous to everyone (Figure 21-1).

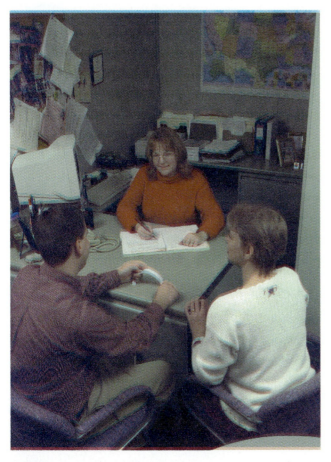

FIGURE 21-1 Be courteous to the patient and family. Remember, they are anxious and concerned.

ADMISSION

When a person enters a health care facility for treatment of an illness or injury, the **admission** process usually causes concern to the patient, family, and friends. The first impression created is very important. You will be one of the first staff members to see the patient, so it is important that you be courteous, confident, and efficient. (See Procedure 50.)

When a patient is ready for admission, ask the nurse if:

- The patient requires a gurney or wheelchair to reach the unit
- Any special equipment such as oxygen or a fracture bed is needed
- There are any special instructions, such as withholding fluids or foods

Introduce yourself and observe the patient carefully. Listen for complaints as you escort and assist the patient to the room and to bed. Initial observations are very important. They become the basis of comparison for future observations.

If it is necessary to ask visitors to leave, do so in a kindly and polite manner. They will be most anxious to remain and see the patient settled and comfortable (Figure 21-2), so

- Show them where they may wait.
- Let them know about how long they will have to wait.
- Tell them where they can get refreshments.
- Answer questions they may have about where to find a chapel and telephones, and visiting hours.
- After you have completed your part of the admission procedure, locate visitors and let them know they may return to the patient's room.

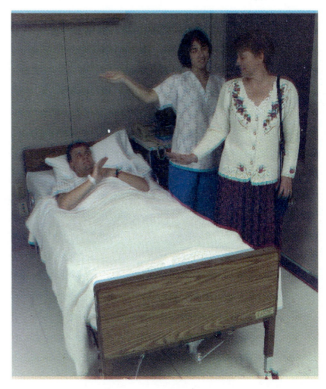

FIGURE 21-2 Explain where visitors can wait in comfort.

TRANSFER

It may be necessary for the patient to be moved to another unit (Figure 21-6, see page 267). Preparations for the **transfer** will be handled by the nurse, but you may be asked to assist. (See Procedure 51.)

The transfer may be the patient's own preference, or because a change in the patient's condition requires a different type of care. The patient may or may not fully understand the reasons for the transfer. Be positive and supportive in your attitude. Recognize that the patient may be feeling very anxious. It would be helpful to know what the patient has been told about the reasons for the transfer. You may learn this from the nurse and by carefully listening to what your patient says.

All details must be taken care of according to facility policy. Following facility policy ensures that there is no interruption of health care services. Some facilities have transportation services for transferring patients.

After the new unit has been notified and prepared for the move, you will:

- Tell the patient what you are doing.
- Gather all the patient's belongings together. Explain to the patient what you are doing.

- Get the patient's medicines, charts, and other personal data from the nurse.
- Assist in the physical transfer.
- Give the records and medication directly to the nurse on the new unit.

 Caution: Never leave the patient, the records, or medications unattended.

- Make sure the patient is comfortable in the new environment before you return to your own unit.

DISCHARGE

In recent years, the cost of health care has increased steadily. A government program known as **diagnosis-related groups (DRGs)** was introduced to control hospital costs. Hospitals are paid a specific amount of money for the care of an individual who has a particular condition or disease that is covered by a DRG.

If the hospital can provide the needed care and discharge the patient early, the hospital saves money and may keep the difference between the actual expenses and the DRG allotted payment. If the patient requires a longer hospital stay than is stated by the DRGs and the costs are higher, the hospital

---

PROCEDURE 50

ADMITTING THE PATIENT

1. Wash hands.
2. Assemble equipment:
   - equipment for urine specimen collection
   - equipment for taking temperature
   - pad and pencil
   - patient's chart or worksheet
   - stethoscope
   - admission kit
     - water pitcher
     - glass
     - liquid soap
     - washcloth
     - towel
     - basin
     - lotion
     - mouthwash
   - scale
   - blood pressure cuff and manometer
   - watch with second hand
   - disposable gloves (if urine specimen is required)

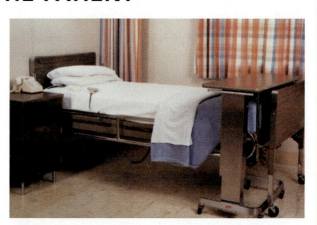

FIGURE 21-3 An open bed lets patients know that they are expected and welcome.

3. Prepare the unit for patient by:
   a. Making sure that all necessary equipment and furniture are in their proper places and in good working order.
   b. Checking the unit for adequate lighting.

continues

PROCEDURE 50 continued

c. Loosening the top linen at the foot of the bed.

d. Opening the bed (Figure 21-3).

4. Identify patient both by asking the name and checking the identification bracelet.

   a. Introduce yourself.

   b. Take patient and family to the unit.

   c. Do not appear to rush patient.

   d. Be courteous and helpful to patient and family.

5. Ask patient to be seated.

   a. Ask the family to go to the lounge or lobby while patient is being admitted.

   b. Introduce patient to the other patients in the room, unless it is a private room.

   c. As permitted, explain what will happen in the next hour.

6. Screen the unit to provide privacy (Figure 21-4).

7. Help patient to undress and put on a hospital gown or night clothes from home. Care for clothing according to facility policy.

8. Check patient's vital signs, weight, and height.

9. Help patient get into bed. Adjust side rails as needed.

10. If patient is wearing any jewelry or has valuables:

    a. Make a list of them and ask patient to sign it. This protects the facility and the patient.

    b. Ask the relatives also to sign the list and take the valuables home, or

    c. After checking and signing, give them to the nurse to put in the hospital safe.

11. Tell patient if a urine specimen is necessary.

    a. Put on gloves and assist patient as necessary.

    b. Allow patient to use the bathroom, if ambulatory, or offer the bedpan or urinal.

12. Pour patient's specimen from the bedpan into the specimen bottle. Put on the cap. Remove gloves and dispose of according to facility policy. Be sure to label the specimen correctly (Unit 42).

13. An admission form is usually completed at this time (Figure 21-5). Vital information includes:

    • observations
    • vital signs (TPR, BP, height, weight)
    • known allergies
    • medications being taken
    • food preferences and dislikes

14. If admission is to a long-term care facility, name labels must be added to belongings.

15. Orient patient to the unit by explaining:

    • visiting hours
    • how to use the telephone and/or television
    • how to use the call light system for assistance
    • standard hospital regulations
    • television rental procedures, if available
    • any questions about facility routines
    • when meals and refreshments are provided

16. Carry out each procedure completion action.

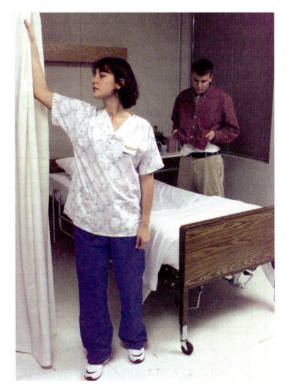

FIGURE 21-4 Provide privacy by closing the curtain while the patient undresses.

continues

The patient should be spared any fatigue or unnecessary delay when being routinely discharged. (See Procedure 52.) You can help if you:

- Check with the nurse to make sure that the physician has written an order for discharge before preparing the patient.
- Gather all the patient's belongings and assist in packing, if necessary. Patients who are well enough usually prefer to assemble their own things. You will need to do this activity completely for other patients.
- Carefully check the closet and bedside table. Disposable

equipment is often sent home with the patient. If this is the policy in your facility, be sure that the equipment is clean.

- Check with the nurse for any medications or other treatment-related equipment that should be sent home with the patient.
- Verify that the patient has received discharge instructions from the nurse, physician, or discharge coordinator.
- Never allow a patient to leave the health care facility unassisted. The patient is the staff's responsibility until he has left the building.

PROCEDURE **52**

DISCHARGING THE PATIENT

1. Check to be sure the physician has ordered the patient to be discharged. If the discharge order has not been written, check with the supervisor before proceeding.

2. Carry out each beginning procedure action.

3. Assemble equipment
   - wheelchair
   - cart to transport items

4. Help patient to dress, if necessary.

5. Collect patient's personal belongings. Help patient check them against the admission list.

   a. Pack, if necessary.

   b. Check valuables against list according to facility policy.

   c. Make sure that all of patient's belongings have been removed from the closet and bedside stand.

   d. Check to see if medications or other equipment are to go home with patient.

   e. Verify that patient has received discharge instructions from the nurse, physician, or discharge coordinator.

6. Tell patient or a member of the family how

to collect valuables from the facility safe, if valuables were put there.

7. Help patient into wheelchair.

8. Take patient to the discharge entrance of the facility.

   a. Help patient to transfer safely into the vehicle.

   b. Be gracious as you say goodbye.

9. Return wheelchair.

10. Return to patient unit.

    a. Strip bed. Dispose of linen according to facility policy.

    b. Clean and replace equipment used in care of patient, according to facility policy.

11. Wash your hands.

12. Record discharge in accordance with facility policy. Include:
    - time
    - method of transport
    - patient's reaction
    - signature

13. Report completion of task to nurse.

REVIEW

A. True/False.

Mark the following true or false by circling T or F.

1. T F When transferring a patient, it is all right to leave the patient unattended and return immediately to your own unit.

2. T F Use all precautions related to safe transport when admitting or discharging a patient.

3. T F You do not need to waste time introducing a new patient to others, because facility stays are very short anyway.

4. T F It is all right to allow patients simply to leave a health care facility.

5. T F After discharge, the patient's unit is stripped, cleaned, and restocked.

6. T F The patient's unit should be prepared as soon as you are notified that there will be an admission.

7. T F During a transfer, the patient's medications remain on the original unit.

8. T F Measuring the patient's height and weight is part of the admission procedure.

9. T F The discharge order is written by the physician.

10. T F You should observe the patient carefully during the admission procedure.

B. Multiple Choice.

Select the one best answer for each question.

11. The assistant can do much to help facilitate the admission procedure by
    a. preparing equipment after the patient arrives on the unit.
    b. letting the nurse make all the observations.
    c. giving attention to the details of the procedure.
    d. recognizing that admission to the facility causes more anxiety to the staff than to the patient.

12. When dealing with the newly admitted patient's family, you should
    a. treat them with courtesy and consideration.
    b. send them home.

c. let the nurse deal with them.
d. allow them to stay at the patient's bedside at all times.

13. Part of the admission procedure includes
    a. securing a stool specimen.
    b. obtaining a sputum specimen.
    c. working in a hurried manner so the patient knows you are efficient.
    d. measuring vital signs.

14. Valuables that accompany the patient to her unit should be
    a. taken away.
    b. listed and signed for.
    c. left in the bedside stand.
    d. tucked under the pillow for safety.

15. When a patient is transferred, you should include his
    a. personal belongings.
    b. chart.
    c. medications.
    d. all of these.

C. Nursing Assistant Challenge.

Mrs. Leon is being admitted because her emphysema is making it very difficult for her to breathe. She is accompanied by her husband and both are obviously nervous. The next morning, her condition worsens. She is moved to the intensive respiratory care unit. Answer the following questions yes or no.

_____ 16. The anxiety of the patient and family is not natural.

_____ 17. You should answer questions about facility routines during admission.

_____ 18. When taking vital signs, you should use an oral thermometer.

_____ 19. When Mrs. Leon is transferred, take all of her personal articles with her.

_____ 20. One way to prepare the unit for admission might include checking for the need for oxygen.

Bedmaking

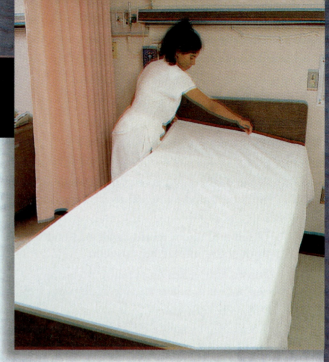

INTRODUCTION

The room, especially the bed, is the patient's home while hospitalized. A well-made bed offers both comfort and safety. It is an extremely important contribution to the well-being of the patient.

OPERATION AND USES OF BEDS IN HEALTH CARE FACILITIES

The types of beds and the methods used to operate them may vary in different health care facilities, but the basic principles of bedmaking are the same. The most common beds are the:

- **gatch bed**—a stationary bed about 26 inches high. Modern facilities are equipped with beds that can be raised to the desired height for bedside nursing or lowered to 13 inches to accommodate the out-of-bed patient. The position of the head and knee areas of the bed can be adjusted for comfort. This operation may be done manually by turning the cranks.
- **electric bed**—a bed similar to the gatch bed, in that it can be raised or lowered and the knee and head areas can be adjusted. It is operated electrically (Figure 22-1). You will be using this bed most often in a large facility.
- **CircOlectric® bed**—a special bed frame placed within a circular frame (Figure 22-2). This bed is operated electrically. The circular frame can be rotated. The patient is secured on the inner frame before the bed is moved. The entire inner frame is rotated forward. This allows for position change without any stress on the patient. After rotating, the patient is on the abdomen.
- **Stryker frame** or spinal bed—a turning frame that serves the same purpose as the CircOlectric® but is oper-

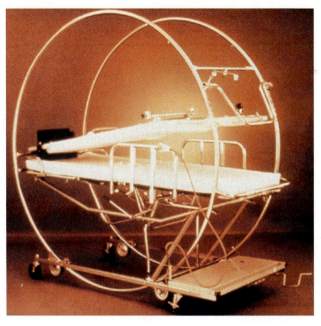

FIGURE 22-2 CircOlectric® bed. *Photo courtesy of Stryker Corporation, Kalamazoo, MI*

ated manually. Once the patient is secured by placement of the upper frame, a crank is used to turn the entire frame and the patient. After turning, the patient is on the abdomen. The patient lies on the frame until turned once more (Figure 22-3).

Patients with severe burns or spinal injuries are examples of patients who are often placed on special beds like the CircOlectric® or Stryker frame, for safety. These beds allow patients to be repositioned with minimal handling of their bodies.

This procedure is frightening for many patients. Reassure the patient that he is secure and that turning will proceed without incident. In most facilities, a licensed nurse must be present during turning.

Other types of beds are available for the treatment of patients with multiple or advanced pressure ulcers, flaps, grafts, burns, and intractable pain. For example, one special unit that supports the patient's body evenly is filled with a sand-

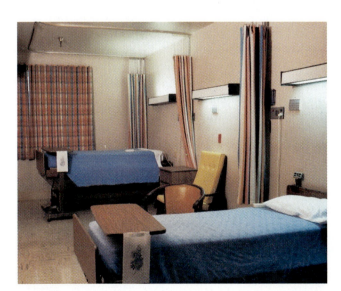

FIGURE 22-1 A typical hospital bed that can be adjusted for height and position. Note that the bed by the window has been raised.

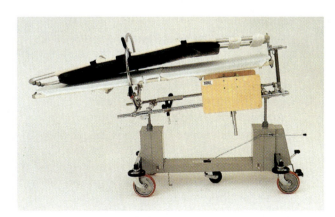

FIGURE 22-3 Turning frame or spinal bed. *Photo courtesy of Stryker Corporation, Kalamazoo, MI*

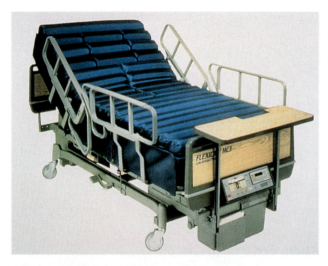

FIGURE 22-4 Alternating air pressure mattress overlay. Alternating air pressure in the mattress cells changes pressure points against the resident's skin and gently massages the skin. *Courtesy of Hill-Rom, Charleston, SC*

like material. Warm, dry air circulates through the material to maintain an even temperature and support the body evenly. An alternating-pressure mattress automatically inflates one section of the mattress at a time, thereby reducing prolonged pressure on any particular part of the body (Figure 22-4).

Correct operation of any bed or equipment is important for patient safety. Always seek help and instruction from the nurse or another health care professional when using any specialized beds. Never try to operate any bed or equipment with a patient in it without first practicing and gaining security and skill in the procedures.

BEDMAKING

Bed linen is always changed when soiled. It is routinely changed:

- daily in the acute care facility.
- two or three times a week in long-term care facilities.

GUIDELINES *for*

Handling Linens and Making the Bed

Handling Linens

1. Wash hands and use gloves as required; other personal protective equipment may be required.
2. Laundry hampers placed in the hallway should be at least two rooms away from clean linen carts.
3. The clean linen cart is always covered; replace covers after removing required linen.
4. Take only the linens you need into the patient's room.
5. Linens that touch the floor are considered dirty and are placed in the laundry hamper; they are not used.
6. Avoid contact between the linens and your uniform (for both clean and soiled linens).
7. Unused linen is never returned to the clean linen cart; it is placed in the laundry hamper.
8. As soiled linen is removed from the bed, keep the soiled areas on the inside and fold or roll the linen toward the center.
9. Never shake soiled bed linens, because microbes will be released into the air.
10. Soiled linen is never placed on environmental surfaces in the room, such as overbed table, chair, or floor; soiled linens are placed in the

appropriate laundry hamper (follow facility policy).
11. Fill laundry hampers no more than two-thirds full.
12. Many facilities do not permit laundry hampers or barrels to be taken into the patient's room. Soiled linen may be placed in a plastic bag or a pillowcase in the room. Make a cuff at the top of the bag or open end of the pillowcase and place the cuff over the back of the chair. When the bag or case is two-thirds full, secure the top and place it in the hamper in the hallway.
13. Laundry hampers or barrels are returned to the utility room after use, or as directed by facility policy.

Making the Bed

1. Use proper body mechanics at all times to prevent back injury.
2. Work on one side of the bed at a time to complete removal of soiled linen and placement of clean linen.
3. Make sure the bottom sheet and draw sheet (if used) are smooth and unwrinkled (wrinkles in bed linens can lead to skin breakdown, especially for patients who must remain in bed).
4. Follow the care plan for positioning the head and foot of the bed, the number of pillows to be used, and the use of pillows for positioning.

Residents in long-term care may prefer to use their own pillows, blankets, and spreads.

Closed Bed

The **closed bed** is made following the discharge of the patient and after the unit is cleaned (terminal cleaning). It remains closed until a new patient is to be admitted. Details are important. The same procedure is followed when making an unoccupied bed, but the bed is opened as a final step when a patient is to occupy it shortly. (Refer to Procedure 53.)

The Unoccupied Bed

Beds are often made while patients are up in a shower or chair. Follow the procedure for making a closed bed but then

---

PROCEDURE 53

MAKING A CLOSED BED

1. Wash your hands and assemble equipment:
   - 2 pillowcases
   - pillow
   - spread
   - blankets, as needed
   - 2 large sheets (90" × 108") (substitute one fitted sheet, if used)
   - cotton draw sheet or half sheet
   - plastic or rubber draw sheet (if used in facility)
   - Mattress pad and cover, if mattress is not plastic-treated

   Note: Mattresses that are treated with plastic do not require a moisture-proof sheet or cotton half sheet (draw sheet). In selected cases, the half sheet is used as a lifter to assist in moving the patient. It is sometimes used simply to keep the bottom sheet clean. Some facilities use fitted bottom sheets. If this is so, use a fitted sheet in place of one of the large sheets.

2. Elevate the bed to a comfortable working height in the horizontal position. Lock bed wheels so the bed will not roll. Place chair at the side of the bed.

3. Arrange linen on chair in order in which it is to be used.

4. Position mattress to the head of the bed by grasping mattress handles (or the edge of the mattress, if no handles are present).

5. If used, place mattress cover on mattress. Adjust it smoothly for corners. You will work entirely from one side of the bed until that side is completed. Then go to the other side of the bed. This conserves time and energy.

6. Place mattress pad even with the top of the mattress and unfold.

7. Place on the bed and unfold the bottom sheet, right side up, wide hem at the top. The small hem should be brought to the foot of the mattress (Figure 22-5). The center fold should be at the center of the bed. If a fitted bottom sheet is used, fit it smoothly around one corner (Figures 22-6A and B).

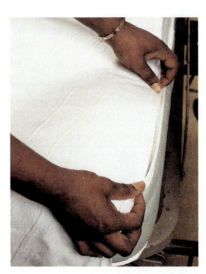

FIGURE 22-5 Place flat bottom sheet even with end of mattress at foot of bed.

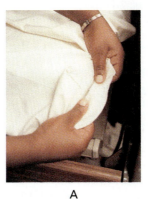
A

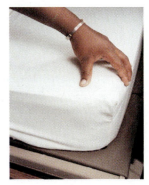
B

FIGURE 22-6A AND B If a fitted bottom sheet is used, fit it properly and smoothly around the corner.

continues

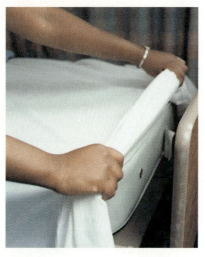

FIGURE 22-7A Gather about 12 to 18 inches of top sheet at bottom of bed.

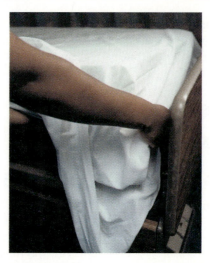

FIGURE 22-7B Face foot of bed and lift mattress with near hand.

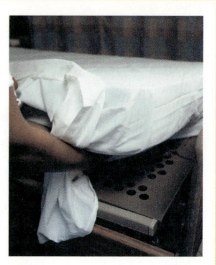

FIGURE 22-7C Bring sheet with opposite hand smoothly over end of mattress.

8. Tuck 12 to 18 inches of sheet smoothly over the top of the mattress (Figures 22-7A to 7C).

9. Make a **mitered corner** (Figure 22-8). The square corner, preferred by some facilities, is made in a way similar to the mitered corner.

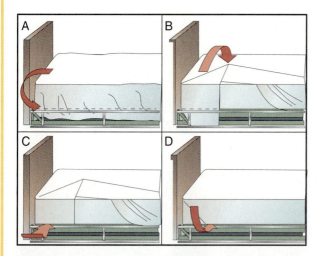

FIGURE 22-8 Making a mitered corner. A. The sheet is hanging loose at the side of the bed. B. Pick up the sheet about 12 inches from the head of the bed to form a triangle. Pull back toward the bed to smooth out the sheet and lay triangle on bed. C. Tuck in sheet at head of bed. D. Pick up triangle and place other hand at edge of bed near head to hold edge of sheet in place. Bring triangle over edge of mattress and tuck smoothly under mattress. Tuck in the rest of the sheet along the side of the mattress. Make sure sheet is smooth.

10. Tuck in the sheet on one side, keeping the sheet straight. Work from the head to the foot of the bed. If using a fitted sheet, adjust it over the head and bottom ends of the mattress.

11. If used, place the plastic draw sheet and half sheet with upper edge about 14 inches from the head of the mattress and tuck under one side. Be sure that the half sheet covers the plastic sheet. It should cover the area from above the patient's shoulders to below the hips.

12. Unfold and place the top sheet on the bed, wrong side up, top hem even with the upper edge of the mattress and the center fold in the center of the bed.

13. Spread the blanket over the top sheet and foot of mattress. Keep blanket centered.

14. Tuck top sheet and blanket under mattress at the foot of the bed as far as the center only. Make a **box (square) corner** (Figures 22-9A to 9C).

15. Place spread with top hem even with head of mattress. Unfold to foot of bed.

16. Tuck spread under mattress at the foot of the bed and make a mitered corner. Sometimes the spread may be placed directly on top of the sheet. Rather than tucking the sheet, blanket, and/or spread under the end of the mattress separately

continues

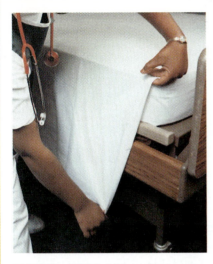

FIGURE 22-9A Make the square (box) corner following the steps shown in Figures 22-8A–C. Then, holding corner with left hand, grasp bottom of sheet and pull it straight down until fold is even with edge of mattress.

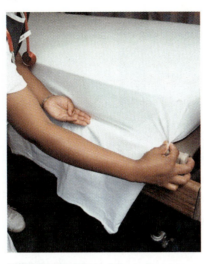

FIGURE 22-9B Holding the square corner in place, tuck remaining sheet under mattress.

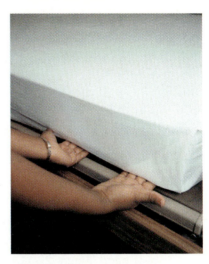

FIGURE 22-9C Finished square corner should look like this.

and forming separate corners, all of the covers may be tucked under at the same time and one corner formed (Figures 22-10A to 10E).

17. Go to other side of the bed. Fanfold the top covers to the center of the bed so you can work with the lower sheets and pad.

18. Tuck bottom sheet under head of mattress and make a mitered corner. Working from top to bottom, smooth out all wrinkles and tighten these sheets as much as possible to provide comfort. (Adjust fitted bottom sheet smoothly and securely around mattress corners.)

19. Grasp protective draw sheet (if used) and cotton draw sheet in the center. Tuck these sheets under the mattress.

20. Tuck in top sheet and blanket at foot of bed and make a mitered corner.

21. Fold top sheet back over blanket, making an 8-inch cuff.

22. Tuck in spread at foot of bed and make a mitered corner. Bring top of spread to head of mattress.

23. Insert pillow into pillowcase:

    a. Place hands in the clean case, freeing the corners.

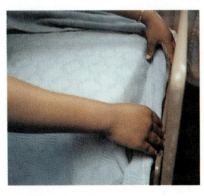

FIGURE 22-10A Gather top sheet and spread together and smooth evenly over end of mattress.

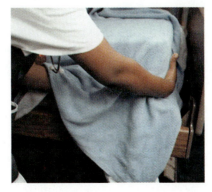

FIGURE 22-10B Tuck sheet and spread under mattress together.

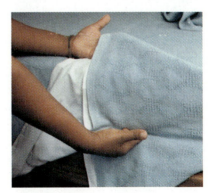

FIGURE 22-10C Continue as with the procedure for a mitered corner.

continues

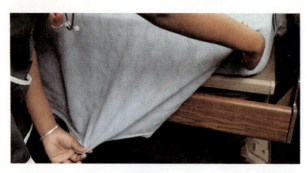

FIGURE 22-10D Slide finger to the end to make a smooth edge.

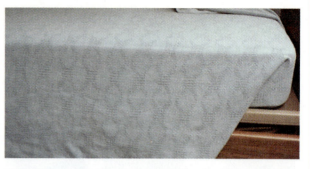

FIGURE 22-10E The completed top bedding. The procedure is repeated on the opposite side of the bed.

b. Grasp the center of the end seam with hand outside the case and turn case back over hand (Figure 22-11A).

c. Grasp the pillow through the case at the center of one end. Pull case over pillow with free hand (Figures 22-11B and 22-11C). (Do not allow pillow to touch uniform.)

d. Adjust the corners of the pillow to fit in the corners of the case.

24. Place pillow at head of bed with open end away from the door.

25. Lower bed to lowest horizontal position.

26. Arrange room as follows:

a. Replace bedside table parallel to bed. Place chair in assigned location.

b. Place overbed table over the foot of the bed opposite the chair.

c. Place signal cord within easy reach of patient.

d. Leave side rails down.

e. Check for possible hazards, such as crank handles out of place.

27. Leave unit neat and tidy.

28. Wash your hands.

29. Report completion of task to the supervisor.

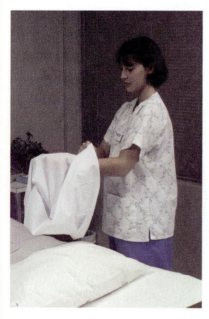

FIGURE 22-11A Grasp the pillowcase at the seam and fold it over your hand.

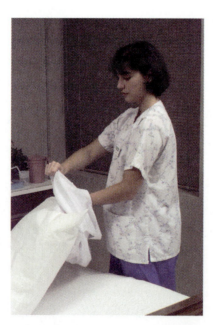

FIGURE 22-11B Grasp the pillow with your pillowcase-covered hand. At all times, hold the pillow and pillowcase away from your uniform.

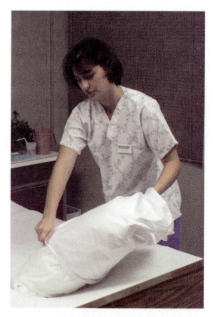

FIGURE 22-11C Unfold the pillowcase over the pillow.

fanfold the top bedding halfway down. This "opens" the bed and makes it easier for the person to get into it.

The Open Bed

The **open bed** is like a sign saying "welcome" to the new patient (Figure 22-12). It indicates that the patient's arrival has been made known to the assistant. It also shows that the unit has been prepared. In long-term care facilities, the bed is not opened unless the resident is going to bed soon. (See Procedure 54.)

The Occupied Bed

Unless the patient is permitted out of bed by physician's order, the bed is made with the patient in it. (See Procedure

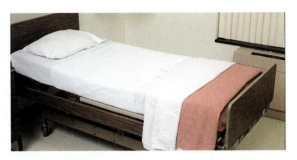

FIGURE 22-12 The closed bed is opened by drawing the bedding to the foot of the bed and fanfolding.

55.) Bedmaking usually follows the bed bath, while the patient is covered with a bath blanket. It may, however, be done any time it would add to the comfort of the patient.

PROCEDURE 54

OPENING THE CLOSED BED

1. Wash your hands.
2. Check assignment for bed location.
3. Raise bed to comfortable working height in the horizontal position. Move overbed table to one side.
4. Lock bed wheels.
5. Loosen top bedding.
6. Facing head of bed, grasp top sheet and spread and fanfold to foot of bed.
7. Return bed to lowest horizontal position. Place overbed table over foot of bed.
8. Place call bell under pillow or within each reach.
9. Leave unit neat and tidy.
10. Wash your hands.
11. Report completion of task to the nurse.

PROCEDURE 55

MAKING AN OCCUPIED BED

1. Carry out each beginning procedure action.
2. Assemble the equipment needed:
   - disposable gloves (if linens are soiled with blood, body fluids, secretions, or excretions)
   - cotton draw sheet or turning sheet for selected patients
   - 2 large flat sheets (or one large flat sheet and one fitted bottom sheet)
   - 2 pillowcases
   - laundry hamper
3. Place bedside chair at the foot of the bed.
4. Arrange clean linen on chair in the order in which it is to be used.
5. Bed should be flat with wheels locked unless otherwise indicated. Raise to working horizontal height. Lower side rail on your side of bed.

continues

PROCEDURE   55   *continued*

6. If bed linens are soiled with blood or other body fluids, wash hands and put on disposable gloves.

7. Loosen the bedclothes on your side by lifting the edge of the mattress with one hand and drawing bedclothes out with the other. Never shake the linen. This spreads germs.

8. Put side rail up and go to opposite side of bed.

9. Adjust mattress to head of bed (Figure 22-13). Get help, if possible.

10. Remove top covers except for top sheet, one at a time. Fold to bottom. Pick up in center. Place over the back of chair if they are to be reused.

📝 *Note: Carefully check each piece of linen for foreign articles (such as patient care equipment, eyeglasses, dentures, items of food, or eating utensils). Remove any such items.*

11. Place the clean sheet or bath blanket over top sheet. Have patient hold the top edge of the clean sheet if she is able. If patient is unable to help, tuck the sheet beneath patient's shoulder.

12. Slide the soiled sheet out, from top to bottom. Put it in hamper.

13. Ask patient to move to the side of the bed toward you. Assist if necessary. Move one pillow with patient and remove the other pillow. Pull up the side rail. (Alternatively, you may ask patient to turn toward the opposite side of the bed, holding onto the raised side rail. You would then fanfold the sheet, as in step 15, but there would be no need to go to the other side of the bed.)

14. Go to the other side of the bed. Fanfold the soiled cotton draw sheet, if used, and bottom sheet close to the patient (Figure 22-14).

15. Straighten mattress pad. If bottom sheet is to be changed, place a clean sheet on the bed so that the narrow hem comes to the edge of the mattress at the foot. The seamed side of the hem is toward the bed. The lengthwise center fold of the sheet is at the center of the bed. Fanfold opposite side of sheet close to patient.

16. Tuck top of sheet under the head of the mattress.

17. Make a mitered corner.

18. Tuck side of sheet under mattress, working toward the foot of the bed.

19. Position fresh draw sheet, if used. Tuck it under the mattress.

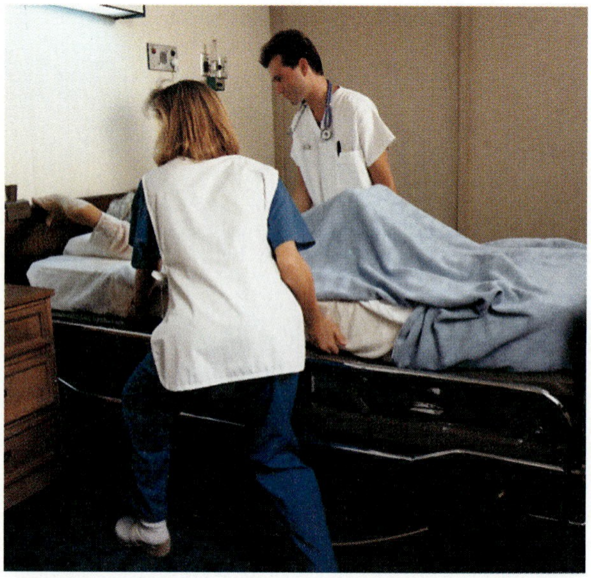

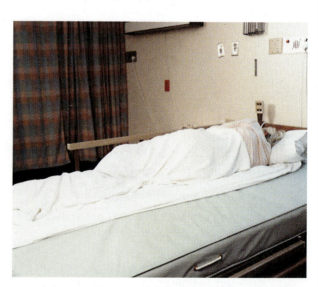

FIGURE 22-13 The patient grasps head of bed and pushes in with heels while two nursing assistants pull mattress to head of the bed.

FIGURE 22-14 Fanfold soiled bottom sheet to center of bed as close to patient as possible. Note that bottom linen is flat and patient is positioned to far side of bed.

continues

PROCEDURE 55 continued

20. Ask or assist patient to roll toward you, over the fanfolded linen. Move the pillow with patient.

21. Raise side rails. Test for security.

22. Go to the other side of the bed. Lower side rail. Remove the soiled linen by rolling the edges inward. *Keep soiled linen away from your uniform.* Placed soiled linen in hamper.

23. Remove gloves, if worn, and discard according to facility policy.

24. Wash your hands.

25. Pull the clean bottom sheet into place. Tuck it under the mattress at the head of the bed. Make a mitered corner.

26. Pull gently to eliminate wrinkles. Then tuck

the side of the sheet under the mattress, working from top to bottom.

27. Pull the draw sheet smoothly into place. Tuck firmly under the mattress.

28. Place the top sheet over the patient. Remove the bath blanket.

29. Complete the bed as an unoccupied bed. To reduce pressure on toes, grasp the top bedding over the toes and pull straight up. Some patients prefer not to have the blanket and top sheet or spread tucked in.

30. Assist the patient to turn on his or her back. Place a clean pillowcase on the pillow not being used. Replace pillow. Change other pillowcase.

31. Carry out each procedure completion action.

Surgical Bed

The surgical bed provides a safe, warm environment to receive the postsurgical patient. It must be made in such a way that movement from gurney to bed is made with maximum safety and minimum effort. For this reason, the bed should be left open and at stretcher height. (See Procedure 56.)

All equipment needed to monitor vital signs and to supervise recovery should be in place and ready for use. You should also keep alert for the patient's return so you can help in the safe transfer from stretcher to bed.

Modern surgical techniques have shortened the time many patients stay in an acute care facility after surgery. Patients are often admitted on the morning of surgery to special units, have the surgery performed, return to these same units immediately after surgery, and are discharged the same day to recuperate at home. These units are called ambulatory, short-term, or day care units. To prepare a postsurgical bed in one of these units:

- Tighten the bottom linen.
- Fanfold top linen to the side or foot of bed.
- Raise bed to gurney height and lock wheels.
- Place equipment to check vital signs, emesis basin, and tissues by recovery bed.

PROCEDURE 56

MAKING THE SURGICAL BED

1. Wash your hands.

2. Check assignment for unit location.

3. Assemble the following equipment:
   - disposable gloves (if linens are soiled with blood or body fluids)
   - articles for basic bed
   - one extra draw sheet
   - bath blanket for warmth
   - one protective (rubber or plastic) draw sheet (if used in facility)
   - roll of one-inch gauze bandage

4. Lock bed.

5. Apply gloves if linen is wet or soiled with blood or body fluids.

continues

PROCEDURE 56 *continued*

6. Strip and discard used linen.

7. Remove gloves and discard according to facility policy.

8. Wash your hands.

9. Make bottom foundation bed (steps 1–11 in Procedure 53). Repeat on opposite side of bed.

10. Place protective draw sheet over head of mattress sheet. Cover with cotton draw sheet. Miter corners and tuck in on sides.

11. Place top sheet, blanket, and spread in usual manner. Do not tuck in.

12. Fold linen back at foot of bed even with edge of mattress.

13. Fanfold upper covers and top sheet to far side of bed (Figure 22-15).

14. Tie waterproof pillow to head of bed with gauze bandaging or place according to facility policy.

15. Arrange bed so there is adequate room to position stretcher next to it. Leave bed locked and at same height as stretcher.

16. Check unit for obvious hazards.

17. Leave the room neat and tidy.

18. Wash your hands.

19. Report completion of task to nurse.

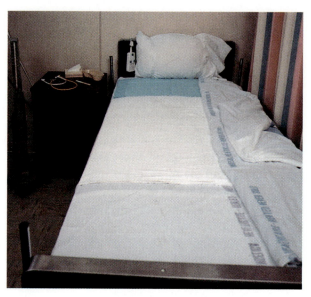

FIGURE 22-15 The bed is prepared for a patient returning from surgery by fanfolding covers to far side of bed and placing bed at stretcher height.

REVIEW

A. True/False.

Mark the following true or false by circling T or F.

1. T F The patient is most comfortable in a closed bed.

2. T F The Stryker frame is used to turn patients easily.

3. T F You should not attempt to operate a bed until you have been thoroughly supervised.

4. T F The closed bed is made after terminal cleaning is finished.

5. T F Bottom bed linen can be loosely tucked as long as there are no wrinkles when you have finished.

6. T F A mitered corner is tucked in, forming a triangle.

7. T F Shaking linen as you change the bed spreads germs.

8. T F The open bed is like a sign saying "welcome."

9. T F Before making an occupied bed, adjust the mattress to the head of the bed.

10. T F The side rail opposite you must be up as you make an occupied bed.

B. Multiple Choice.

Select the one best answer for each question.

11. Loosening the top bedding at the foot of the bed is done
    a. to improve the appearance of the bed.
    b. in unoccupied beds.
    c. as folds in the bottom sheet.
    d. to reduce pressure on the toes.

12. When making an unoccupied bed, make the
    a. entire bottom first.
    b. far side of the bottom and top first.
    c. near side of the entire bed first.
    d. far side of the bottom first.

13. Before making an unoccupied bed,
   a. elevate it to a comfortable working height.
   b. keep the bed at the lowest horizontal height.
   c. raise the head portion.
   d. raise the bed to the highest horizontal height.

14. Before making any bed, always
   a. raise side rails.
   b. lower the bed to the lowest horizontal height.
   c. lock the bed wheels.
   d. raise the bed to its highest horizontal height.

15. Sheets should be smoothly tucked in over the head of the mattress
   a. 5 to 7 inches.
   b. 12 to 18 inches.
   c. 20 to 24 inches.
   d. any amount as long as the job is done quickly.

16. If a draw sheet or lift sheet is used, it should be placed so that it covers the area under the patient's
   a. head and shoulders.
   b. heels and lower legs.
   c. buttocks only.
   d. shoulders and buttocks.

17. When placing the case on the pillow,
   a. tuck it under your chin.
   b. lay the pillow on the bed.

   c. pull the case over while grasping the pillow with the opposite hand.
   d. lay the pillow on the bedside stand.

18. When opening a closed bed,
   a. fanfold top bedding to the foot.
   b. loosen all top bedding.
   c. leave the bed at its highest horizontal height.
   d. raise the head of the bed.

19. The top bedding in a surgical bed is
   a. untucked and draped.
   b. tucked in on two sides.
   c. untucked and fanfolded.
   d. made with toepleats.

20. A common element to all bedmaking is
   a. fanfolding the linen.
   b. leaving the unit neat and tidy.
   c. leaving the bed at its highest horizontal height.
   d. using the same linen and equipment.

C. Nursing Assistant Challenge.

21. You are assigned to make a closed bed. You have washed your hands and assembled the following equipment: pillow, blanket, spread, mattress pad, and mattress cover. What else will you need?

GUIDELINES
for

Patient Bathing

- Wear disposable gloves if there may be contact with open lesions or body fluids.
- Make sure the shower or tub is cleaned before and after each use (Figure 23-2).
- Check that all safety aids, such as handrails, shower chairs, tub seats/benches, and hydraulic lifts are in good repair and proper working order.
- Protect patients from fatigue by transporting patients to and from the tub room and carrying out the bathing procedure as efficiently as possible.
- Make sure the patient's body is covered during transport.
- If a patient falls in the tub or shower room or feels faint during bathing, do not leave him alone. Signal for help, using the emergency call button in the bathroom. Do not lock the bathroom door.
- Use good body mechanics to protect yourself and the patient.
- Nonskid strips placed in the tub and on the floor of the shower prevent slipping.
- Handrails secured to the walls help prevent falls as the patient transfers into and out of the tub.
- The patient should be assisted in all transfer activity related to the bath. Be sure to have enough help.
- The use of a shower chair will prevent patient stress and fatigue but it must be secured so it does not move as the patient transfers into and out of it.
- Never leave the patient alone in the tub or shower.
- A call signal in the bathing area is used to call for emergency help.
- Wipe up all water spilled on the floor immediately, to prevent falls.

- The room should be comfortably warm (about 70°F) and free from drafts, to prevent chilling the patient.
- Cotton bath blankets should be used to cover the patient during a bed bath. They may also be used for added warmth following the tub bath or shower.
- The temperature of the water for shower, tub bath, or bed bath should be maintained at about 105°F. Use a bath thermometer to check the temperature of the water.
- Observe the patient's skin for any changes or irregularities. Note any reddened areas. Do not disturb or injure warts or moles. Report anything unusual.

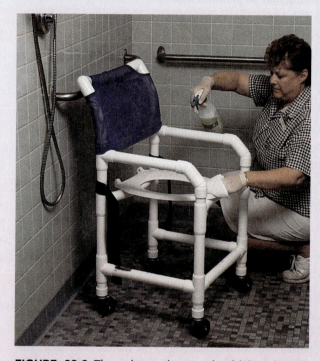

FIGURE 23-2 The tub or shower should be cleaned before and after each use, including handrails that the patient may touch, a shower chair if used, and floor.

PROCEDURE   57

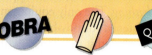

ASSISTING WITH THE TUB BATH OR SHOWER

1. Carry out each beginning procedure action.
2. Assemble equipment needed:
   - disposable gloves
   - liquid soap
   - washcloth
   - 2–3 bath towels

continues

PROCEDURE 57 *continued*

- bath blanket
- bath lotion
- deodorant
- chair or stool beside shower or tub
- bath or shower chair, as needed
- patient's gown, robe, and slippers
- bath mat

3. Take the supplies to the bathroom. Prepare bathroom for patient. Make sure tub is clean.

4. Fill tub half full of water at 105°F or adjust shower flow. If a bath thermometer is available, check the water temperature. If a bath thermometer is not available, test the water with your wrist or elbow. The water should feel comfortably warm.

5. Help patient put on robe and slippers. Escort patient to bathroom. Cover patient with a bath blanket when going to or from the bath or shower.

6. Help patient to undress. Give patient a towel to wrap around the waist.

7. Position shower chair in tub or shower, if needed (Figure 23-3).

8. Assist patient into the tub or shower. For patient's safety, the bottom of the tub and the shower floor are covered with a nonskid surface.

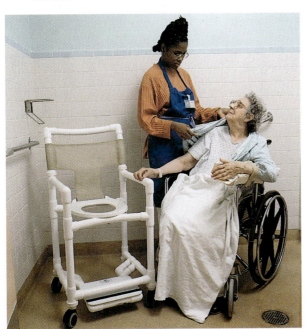

FIGURE 23-3 The shower chair allows the patient to bathe in safety. Always disinfect it after each use.

9. Put on disposable gloves if patient has open skin lesions.

10. Wash patient's back.
    - Observe the skin for signs of redness or breaks. See Unit 35 for information on caring for pressure sores or other skin lesions.

11. Patient may be left alone to wash the **genitalia** (external reproductive organs).
    - If patient is not able to wash the genitalia, then you will also perform this part of the bath. Apply disposable gloves before bathing the genital area.
    - Remove gloves, if worn, and discard according to facility policy.
    - Wash your hands.

12. If patient shows any signs of weakness:
    - Get help. Use the call button.
    - Remove the plug and let the water drain.
    - Turn off the shower.
    - Allow patient to rest until feeling better before making any attempt to assist patient out of the tub or shower.
    - Keep patient covered with a bath blanket to avoid chilling.

13. If patient wants a shampoo and you have permission to do so:
    - Ask patient to hold washcloth over eyes.
    - Pour small amount of water on hair (enough to wet hair thoroughly).
    - Use a small amount of shampoo to lather hair.
    - Massage scalp gently.
    - Rinse hair with warm water.
    - Repeat lathering, massaging, and rinsing, if necessary.
    - Towel hair dry.

14. Hold the bath blanket around patient as he or she steps out of the tub. Patient may choose to remove wet towel under bath blanket.

15. Assist patient to dry, apply deodorant, dress, and return to the unit.

16. Return supplies to patient's unit.

17. Put on gloves and clean bathtub and disinfect. Remove gloves and discard according to facility policy. Wash your hands.

18. Carry out each procedure completion action.

PROCEDURE   **58**

BED BATH

📝 **Note:** *Disposable gloves should be worn if the patient has draining wounds, nonintact skin, or if contact with blood, body fluids, or mucous membranes is likely.*

1. Carry out each beginning procedure action.

2. Assemble equipment needed:

   - disposable gloves
   - bed linen
   - bath blanket
   - laundry bag or hamper
   - bath basin
   - bath thermometer
   - soap and soap dish, or liquid soap
   - washcloth
   - face towel
   - 2 bath towels
   - hospital gown/patient's night clothes
   - lotion
   - equipment for oral hygiene
   - nail brush, emery board, and orangewood stick (if available)
   - deodorant
   - brush and comb
   - bedpan and cover or urinal
   - paper towel or protector

3. Close the windows and door to prevent chilling patient.

4. Close privacy curtain.

5. Put clean towels and linen on chair in order of use (Figure 23-4). Place laundry hamper nearby.

6. Offer bedpan or urinal. If patient wants to use the bedpan or urinal, put on gloves. Empty and clean bedpan or urinal before proceeding with bath. Remove gloves and discard according to facility policy. Wash your hands.

7. Put on disposable gloves.

8. Lower the back of the bed and the side rails, if permitted, on the side where you are working.

9. Loosen top bedclothes. Remove and fold blanket and spread and place over back of chair.

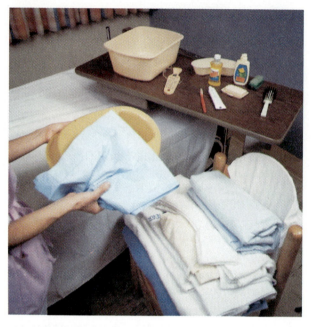

FIGURE 23-4 Assemble equipment. Place bed linens on chair next to bed and remaining items (except bedpan) on overbed table. If used, bedpan or urinal will be removed from bedside stand, used, cleaned immediately, and returned to stand.

10. Place bath blanket over top sheet (Figure 23-5) and remove sheet by sliding it out from under the bath blanket. Place in laundry hamper.

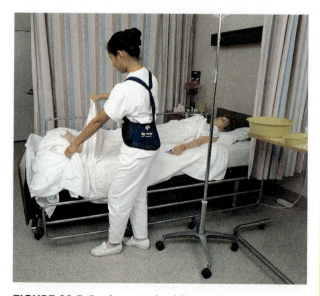

FIGURE 23-5 Replace top bedding with a bath blanket.

continues

PROCEDURE 58 *continued*

11. Leave one pillow under patient's head. Place other pillow on chair.

12. Remove patient's night wear and place in laundry hamper (assuming patient has no IV).

    a. Loosen gown from neck.

    b. Slip gown down arms.

    c. Make sure patient is covered by bath blanket (Figure 23-6).

    Note: This procedure is to be used only when the IV is NOT run through an electric pump. When a pump is used, the patient may wear a gown that snaps at the shoulder. In this case, the gown can be removed without touching the IV bag or tubing. If the patient is wearing a nonsnap gown, call the nurse if the gown is to be changed. Never disconnect the tubing from the pump.

    d. For a patient wearing a regular gown (nonsnap):

       (1) Remove gown from the arm without the IV and bring gown across patient's chest to other arm.

       (2) Place clean gown over patient's chest to avoid exposure.

       (3) On the arm with the IV, gather material of gown in one hand so there

is no pull or pressure in the line (Figure 23-7A) and slowly draw gown over tips of fingers.

       (4) With free hand, lift IV free of standard and slip gown over bag of fluid (Figure 23-7B), removing gown from patient's body. **Never allow the bag of fluid to be lower than patient's arm.**

       (5) Take sleeve of clean gown and slip it over the bag of fluid, over the tubing, and up the patient's arm.

       (6) Replace bag of fluid on IV standard.

       (7) Remove soiled gown and place at end of bed. Finish putting clean gown on patient's other arm. Secure neck ties.

       (8) Place soiled gown in laundry hamper.

       (9) Make sure IV is dripping at required rate and that tubing is not kinked or twisted.

    e. If patient has a weak or paralyzed arm, always undress patient in the following manner:

       (1) Untie the gown and remove the back sides of the gown from underneath patient.

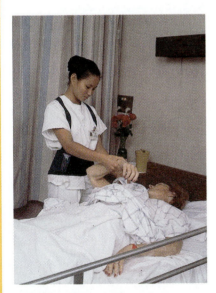

FIGURE 23-6 Keeping patient covered with bath blanket, remove patient's gown.

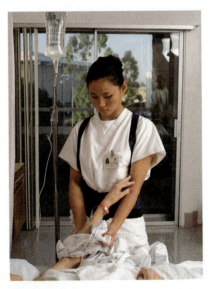

FIGURE 23-7A Gather material of gown in one hand so there is no pull or pressure on the IV line. Slowly draw gown over tips of fingers

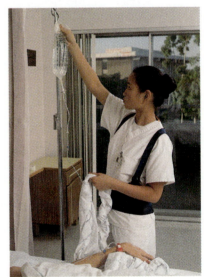

FIGURE 23-7B With free hand, lift IV free of standard and slip gown over bag of fluid.

continues

PROCEDURE **58** *continued*

(2) Remove the gown from the stronger arm first.

(3) Bring the gown across patient's chest and slide the gown down over the weak arm.

(4) Gently lift patient's weak arm to finish removing the gown over patient's hand.

(5) Reverse the procedure to put a clean gown on patient by putting the gown over the weaker arm first.

13. Fill bath basin two-thirds full with water at 105°F. Use a bath thermometer, if available, to be sure of the proper temperature.

14. Assist patient to move to the side of the bed nearest you.

15. Fold face towel over upper edge of bath blanket to keep it dry. Put on gloves.

16. Form a mitt by folding washcloth around hand (Figure 23-8 shows a mitt being made on a gloved hand).

    a. Wet washcloth.

    b. Wash eyes, using separate corners of cloth for each eye.

    c. Wipe from inside to outside corner.

    d. Do not use soap near eyes.

    e. After you have washed the eyes, remove gloves and discard according to facility policy.

    f. Do not use soap on face unless patient requests it.

17. Rinse washcloth and apply soap if patient desires. Squeeze out excess water. Do not leave soap in water.

18. Wash and rinse patient's face (Figure 23-9), ears, and neck well. Use towel to dry.

19. Expose patient's far arm. Protect bed with bath towel placed underneath arm (Figure 23-10).

    a. Wash, rinse, and pat dry arm and hand.

    b. Be sure **axilla** (armpit) is clean and dry.

    c. Repeat for other arm.

    d. Apply deodorant if patient requests it.

20. Care for hands and nails as necessary. Check with the nurse first to see if there are any special instructions.

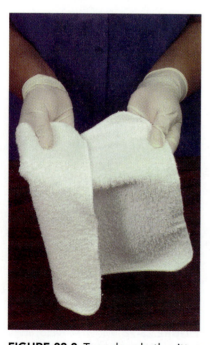 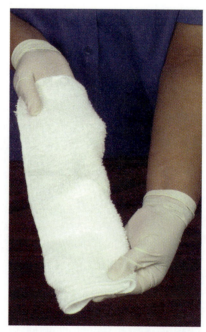 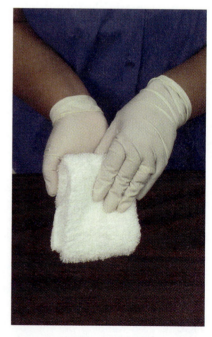

FIGURE 23-8 To make a bath mitt over a gloved hand, wrap the washcloth around one hand. Then bring the free end over palm and tuck in the end. Thumb is free to hold washcloth in place. (If gloves are not required, make the bath mitt in the same manner over the ungloved hand.)

continues

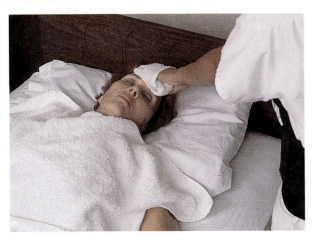

FIGURE 23-9 Wash face carefully, doing eyes separately. Do not use soap on washcloth when cleaning around eyes.

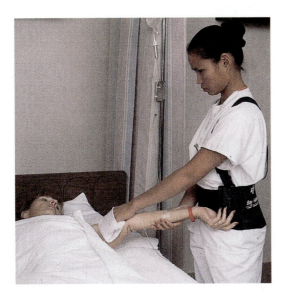

FIGURE 23-10 Place towel under patient's arm and support arm as you wash it.

  a. Place hands in basin of water. Wash each hand carefully. Rinse and dry. Push **cuticle** (base of fingernails) gently with towel while wiping the fingers. Be sure to dry between fingers.

  b. Clean under nails with orangewood stick. Shape with emery board. Be careful not to file nails too close. Do not cut nails if patient is diabetic. Inform the nurse if attention is needed.

21. Discard used bath water and refill basin two-thirds full with water at 105°F.

22. Put bath towel over patient's chest. Then fold blanket to waist. Under towel:

  a. Wash, rinse, and pat dry chest (Figure 23-11).

  b. Rinse and dry folds under breasts of female patient carefully to avoid irritating the skin.

23. Fold bath blanket down to **pubic** area (location of external genitalia). Wash, rinse, and pat dry abdomen. Fold bath blanket up to cover abdomen and chest. Slide towel out from under bath blanket.

24. Ask patient to flex far knee, if possible. Fold bath blanket up to expose thigh, leg, and foot. Protect bed with bath towel.

  a. Put bath basin on towel.

  b. Place patient's foot in basin (Figure 23-12).

  c. Wash and rinse leg and foot.

  d. When moving leg, support leg properly.

25. Lift leg and move basin to the other side of the bed. Dry leg and foot. Dry well between toes.

26. Repeat for other leg and foot. Take basin from bed before drying leg and foot.

27. Care for toenails as necessary. Check with the nurse for any special instructions. Apply lotion to feet of patient with dry skin.

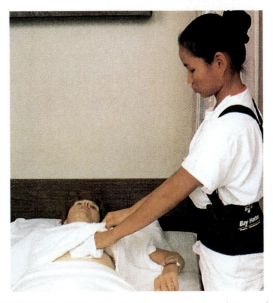

FIGURE 23-11 Lift towel with one hand and use other hand to wash underneath.

continues

PROCEDURE **58** *continued*

- Do not attempt to cut thickened nails.
- File nails straight across.
- Do not round edges.
- Do not push back the cuticle, because it is easily injured and infected.
- If patient is diabetic, inform nurse if toenail care is required.

28. Change water and check for correct temperature with bath thermometer. It may be necessary to change water before this point in the patient's bath if it becomes cold or too soapy.

29. Help patient to turn on side away from you. Help her to move toward the center of the bed. Place bath towel lengthwise next to patient's back.
    - Wash, rinse, and dry neck, back, and buttocks (Figure 23-13).
    - Use long, firm strokes when washing back.

30. A back rub is usually given at this time (see Unit 24).

31. Help patient to turn on back.

32. Place a towel under the buttocks and upper legs. Change water in basin and check for correct temperature. Place washcloth, soap, basin, and bath towel within convenient reach of the patient. Have patient complete bath by washing genitalia. Assist the patient, if necessary. You must take the responsibility for the procedure if the patient has difficulty. Many times patients are reluctant to

acknowledge the need for help. If assisting a patient, always put on disposable gloves.
- For a female patient, wash from front to back, drying carefully.
- For a male patient, carefully wash and dry penis, scrotum, and groin area. If the patient is not circumcised, gently push foreskin back and carefully wash and dry penis. Then gently pull foreskin down to original position.

33. Remove gloves and discard according to facility policy.

34. Carry out range-of-motion exercises as ordered. (See Unit 38 for procedures.)

35. Cover pillow with towel. Comb or brush hair. Oral hygiene is usually given at this time (see Unit 24).

36. Discard towels and washcloth in laundry hamper.

37. Provide clean gown.

38. Clean and replace equipment according to facility policy.

39. Put clean washcloth and towels in bedside stand or hang according to facility policy.

40. Change the bed linen, following the procedure for making an occupied bed. Replace and discard soiled linen in laundry hamper.

41. Remove and discard disposable gloves according to facility policy. Wash your hands.

42. Raise side rails if required.

43. Carry out each procedure completion action.

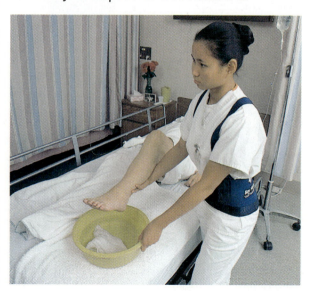

FIGURE 23-12 Support leg and place foot in basin.

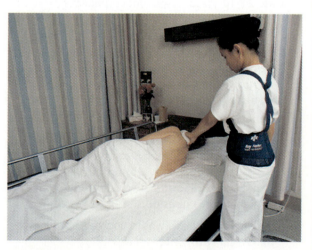

FIGURE 23-13 Change water and wash patient's back.

PROCEDURE **59**

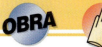

PARTIAL BATH

1. Carry out each beginning procedure action.

2. Assemble equipment needed:
   - disposable gloves
   - bed linen
   - bath blanket
   - bath thermometer
   - soap and soap dish or liquid soap
   - washcloth
   - face towel
   - bath towel
   - gown and robe
   - laundry bag or hamper
   - bath basin
   - lotion
   - equipment for oral hygiene
   - Nail brush, emery board, and orangewood stick
   - brush, comb, and deodorant
   - bedpan or urinal and cover
   - paper towels or protector

   📝 *Note: A package of pre-moistened washcloths can be substituted for the basin of water, soap, washcloth, and towel if the facility has approved the use of the basinless bath. The nursing assistant or the patient (condition permitting) can use the pre-moistened washcloths to perform a sponge bath.*

3. Close windows and door and turn off fans to prevent chilling patient.

4. Put towels and linen on chair in order of use. Make sure laundry hamper is available.

5. Put on disposable gloves.

6. Offer bedpan or urinal (see Unit 24). Empty and clean before proceeding with bath. Remove gloves and discard according to facility policy. Wash hands and put on pair of new gloves.

7. Elevate head rest, if permitted, to comfortable position.

8. Loosen top bedclothes. Remove and fold blanket and spread and place over back of chair. Place bath blanket over top sheet. Remove top sheet by sliding it out from under the bath blanket.

9. Leave one pillow under patient's head. Place other pillow on chair.

10. Assist patient to remove gown. Place it in laundry hamper. Make sure patient is covered with bath blanket.

11. Place paper towels or bed protector on overbed table.

12. Fill bath basin two-thirds full with water at 105°F. Place basin on overbed table.

13. Push overbed table comfortably close to patient.

14. Place towels, washcloth, and soap on overbed table within easy reach.

15. Instruct patient to wash as much as she is able and that you will return to complete the bath.

16. Place call bell within easy reach. Ask patient to signal when ready.

17. Remove gloves and discard according to facility policy. Wash hands and leave unit.

18. Wash hands and return to unit when patient signals. Put on a new pair of gloves.

19. Change the bath water. Complete bathing those areas the patient could not reach. Make sure the face, hands, axillae, buttocks, back, and genitals are washed and dried.

20. Remove gloves and discard according to facility policy.

21. Wash your hands.

22. Give a back rub with lotion.

23. Assist the patient in applying deodorant and a fresh gown.

24. Cover pillow with towel. Comb or brush hair. Assist with oral hygiene, if needed (see Unit 24).

25. Clean and replace equipment according to facility policy.

26. Put clean washcloth and towels in stand or hang according to facility policy.

27. Change the bed linen, following the procedure for making an occupied bed. Put soiled linen in laundry hamper.

28. Carry out each procedure completion action.

Perineal Care

The **perineum** is the area between the legs. In females, it is the area between the vagina and the anus. In males, it is the area between the scrotum and the anus.

Perineal care may be performed as part of general bathing or as a separate procedure, as needed. **Perineal care** means to wash the area including the genitals and anus (see Procedures 60 and 61). Always wear gloves and use standard precautions when caring for the perineal area.

PROCEDURE **60**

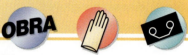

FEMALE PERINEAL CARE

1. Carry out each beginning procedure action.

2. Assemble equipment:
   - disposable gloves
   - bath blanket or top sheet
   - bedpan and cover
   - liquid soap
   - basin
   - bath thermometer
   - bed protector
   - washcloth and towel

3. Lower side rail on side where you will be working. Be sure opposite side rail is up and secure.

4. Remove bedspread and blanket. Fold and place on back of chair.

5. Patient is to be on her back. Cover patient with bath blanket and fanfold sheet to foot of bed.

6. Put on disposable gloves. Fill basin with water at 105°F.

7. Ask patient to raise hips while you place bed protector underneath patient.

8. Offer bedpan to patient.
   a. If used and patient is on intake and output, record amount.
   b. Empty and clean the bedpan before continuing with the procedure.
   c. Remove gloves and discard according to facility policy.
   d. Wash hands and put on a new pair of gloves.

9. Position bath blanket so that only the area between the legs is exposed.

10. Ask patient to separate her legs and flex knees.

📝 **Note:** *If patient is unable to spread legs and flex knees, turn the patient on her side with legs flexed. This position provides easy access to the perineal area.*

11. Wet washcloth, make mitt, and apply a small amount of liquid soap.

📝 **Note:** *Heavy soap application may be difficult to rinse off completely. Soap residue is irritating.*

12. Use one gloved hand to stabilize and separate the vulva (Figure 23-14). With the other gloved hand, proceed as follows.
   a. Bring soaped washcloth in one downward stroke along the far side of outer labia to perineum.
   b. Rinse washcloth, remake mitt, and rinse area just cleaned.
   c. Repeat steps a and b, washing and rinsing inner far labia.
   d. Repeat steps a and b, washing and rinsing inner near labia.
   e. With gloved hands, separate labia. Clean and rinse inner part of vulva to perineum.
   f. Dry washed area with towel.

13. Turn patient away from you. Flex upper leg slightly if permitted.

14. Make a mitt, wet, and apply soap lightly.

15. Expose anal area. Wash area, stroking from perineum to coccyx (front to back) (Figure 23-15).

16. Rinse well in the same manner.

17. Dry carefully.

18. Return patient to back.

19. Remove and dispose of bed protector according to facility policy.

20. Cover patient with sheet or bath blanket.

continues

PROCEDURE **60** *continued*

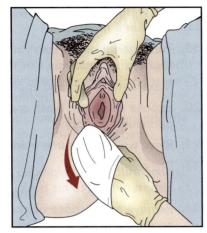

FIGURE 23-14
Spread the vulva with one hand. With the washcloth in the other hand, start at the front and stroke downward along the outer labia.

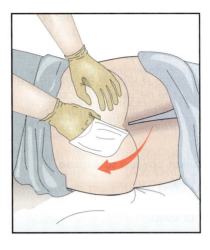

FIGURE 23-15
With one hand, lift up on the buttocks to expose the rectal area. Wipe from the perineum back toward the anus.

21. Remove and dispose of gloves according to facility policy. Wash hands.

22. Remove, fold, and store bath blanket according to facility policy.

23. Replace top covers, tuck under mattress, and make mitered corners. (Patient may prefer that the top covers not be tucked in.)

24. Put up side rail.

25. Put on gloves. Empty water, clean equipment, and dispose of or store, according to facility policy.

26. Remove gloves and discard according to facility policy. Wash hands.

27. Carry out each procedure completion action.

PROCEDURE **61**

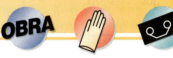

MALE PERINEAL CARE

1. Carry out each beginning procedure action.

2. Assemble equipment:
   - disposable gloves
   - bath blanket
   - bath thermometer
   - urinal and cover or bedpan and cover
   - soap, washcloth, and towel
   - plastic bag
   - bed protector or bath towel
   - ordered solution (if other than water)
   - basin

3. Fill basin with warm water at approximately 105°F.

4. Lower side rail on side where you will be working.

5. Fanfold blanket and spread to foot of bed. Remove, fold, and place on back of chair.

6. Cover patient with bath blanket and fanfold sheet to foot of bed.

7. Place bed protector under patient's buttocks.

8. Put on disposable gloves.

9. Offer bedpan or urinal.

   a. If used and patient is on intake and output, record amount.

   b. Empty and clean the bedpan or urinal before continuing with the procedure.

   c. Remove gloves and discard according to facility policy.

continues

PROCEDURE   63   continued

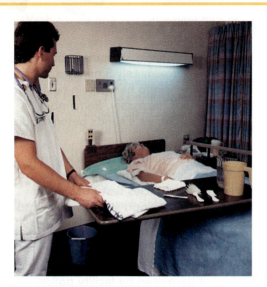

FIGURE 23-18A Assemble equipment.

3. Place large, empty basin on floor under spout of shampoo tray.

4. Arrange on bedside stand within easy reach (Figure 23-18A).

   - Large pitcher of water (105°F)
   - Washcloth
   - 2 bath towels
   - Shampoo
   - Small pitcher of water (105°F)

5. Replace top bedding with bath blanket.

6. Ask patient to move to side of bed nearest you. Assist as needed.

7. Replace pillowcase with waterproof covering.

8. Cover head of bed with bed protector. Be sure it goes well under the shoulders.

9. Loosen neck ties of gown.

10. Place towel under patient's head and shoulders. Brush hair free of tangles, working snarls out carefully.

11. Bring towel down around patient's neck and shoulders and pin. Position pillow under shoulders so that head is tilted slightly backward.

12. Raise bed to high horizontal position.

13. Raise patient's head and position shampoo tray (Figure 23-18B) so that drain is over the edge of the bed directly above the basin.

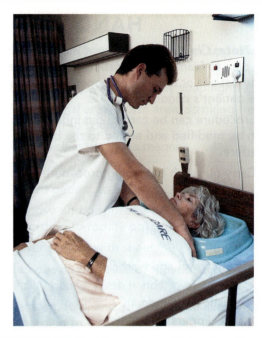

FIGURE 23-18B Position patient with head on shampoo tray. Protect patient with a towel and bed with a protector.

14. Give patient washcloth to cover eyes (Figure 23-18C).

15. Recheck temperature of water in the basin.

16. Using the small pitcher (Figure 23-18D), pour a small amount of water over hair until thoroughly wet. Use one hand to help direct the flow away from the face and ears.

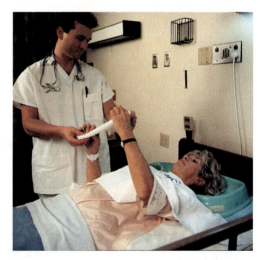

FIGURE 23-18C Give patient folded washcloth to protect her eyes.

continues

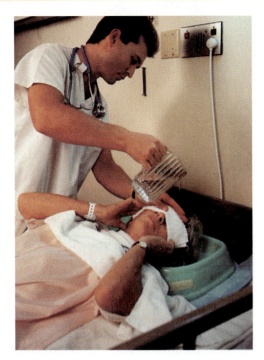

FIGURE 23-18D Use warm water to wet hair.

17. Apply a small amount of shampoo, working up a lather (Figure 23-18E). Work from scalp to hair ends.

18. Massage scalp with tips of fingers. Do not use fingernails.

19. Rinse thoroughly, pouring from hairline to hair tips. Direct flow into drain. Use water from pitcher if needed, but be sure to check temperature of water before use.

20. Repeat lathering and rinsing (steps 16–19).

21. Lift patient's head. Remove tray and bed protector. Adjust pillow and slip a dry bath towel underneath head.

22. Place tray on basin. Wrap hair in towel. Be sure to dry face, neck, and ears as needed.

23. Dry hair with towel. If available and not otherwise contraindicated, a portable hair dryer may be used to complete the drying process. Brushing the hair as you blow dry

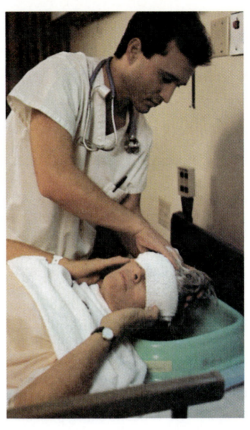

FIGURE 23-18E Apply shampoo and work into a lather.

helps the hair to dry. Be sure to keep the dryer moving and not too close to the hair.

24. Comb hair appropriately. Remove protective pillow cover. Replace with cloth cover.

25. Lower height of bed to comfortable working position.

26. Replace bedding and remove bath blanket.

27. Help patient assume a comfortable position. Lower bed to lowest horizontal position. Leave call bell within reach.

28. Allow patient to rest undisturbed. Length of procedure may tire patient.

29. Empty water from collection basin.

30. Carry out each procedure completion action.

DRESSING A PATIENT

Patients in hospitals generally wear hospital gowns because they are in bed most of the time. However, some patients may prefer to wear their own nightgowns or pajamas and will need assistance in dressing. You may also need to assist patients to dress when they are discharged from the hospital. It is usually easier to help people dress while they are still in bed. (See Procedure 64.)

GUIDELINES
for

Dressing and Undressing Patients

The patient who requires help in dressing may wish to sit in a chair with clothing placed nearby. You can help by:

- Allowing the patient to choose the clothing to be put on.
- Encouraging the patient to participate in the dressing or undressing procedure as much as he or she is able.

- Being prepared to assist with shoes and stockings even for patients who can do much themselves. Bending over to adjust shoes and stockings can result in dizziness and loss of balance.
- Removing clothing from unaffected or strongest side first if the patient has difficulty moving one side or is paralyzed.
- Putting clothing on the affected or weakest side first if the patient has difficulty moving one side or is paralyzed.

PROCEDURE 64

DRESSING AND UNDRESSING PATIENT

1. Carry out each beginning procedure action.

2. Select appropriate clothing and arrange in order of application. Encourage patient to participate in selection.

3. Cover patient with bath blanket and fanfold top bedclothes to foot of bed.

4. Elevate head of bed to sitting position.

5. Assist patient to comfortable sitting position.

6. Remove night clothing, keeping patient covered with bath blanket. Remove from strong side first and then from weaker side. Place in laundry hamper or fold to be taken home.

7. If the patient wears a bra, slip straps over patient's hands (weak side first), move straps up arms, and position on shoulders. Adjust breasts in cups of bra. Then hook bra in back (assist patient to lean forward so bra can be fastened).

8. For an undershirt, or any garment that slips on over the head:

   a. Gather undershirt and place it over the patient's head (Figure 23-19A).

   b. Grasp patient's hand and guide it through the arm hole by reaching into the arm hole from the outside.

   c. Repeat procedure with opposite arm.

   d. Assist patient to lean forward, and adjust undershirt so it is smooth over upper body.

9. Alternate procedure for slipover garments:

   📝 **Note:** *Garment must be large enough or made of stretchy fabric for this procedure.*

   a. Place garment front side down on patient's lap with bottom opening facing the resident.

   b. Put patient's hands into bottom of garment and, one at a time, into the sleeve holes.

   c. Pull the sleeves up as far as possible on patient's arms and pull hands through at wrist if it is a long-sleeved garment. The garment should now be high on the patient's chest.

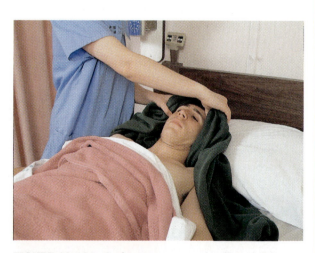

FIGURE 23-19A Gather garment and pull over patient's head.

continues

PROCEDURE **64** *continued*

d. Gather up the back of the garment with your hand and slip the garment over patient's head.

e. Smooth the garment down and position it comfortably about patient's body. Adjust sleeves and shoulders as needed.

10. Shirts or dresses that fasten in the front:

a. Insert your hand through sleeve of garment and grasp patient's hand, drawing sleeve over your hand and patient's.

b. Adjust sleeve at shoulder.

c. Assist patient to sit forward. Arrange clothing across back.

d. Gather sleeve on opposite side by slipping your hand in from the outside.

e. Grasp patient's wrist and pull sleeve of garment over your hand and patient's hand. Draw upward and adjust at shoulder.

f. Button, zip, or snap garment.

11. Underwear or slacks:

a. Facing foot of bed, gather patient's underwear from waist to leg hole.

b. Slip underwear over one foot at a time (Figure 23-19B). Pull underwear up legs as high as possible.

c. Assist patient to raise buttocks and draw garment over buttocks and up to waist. If patient cannot raise buttocks, assist

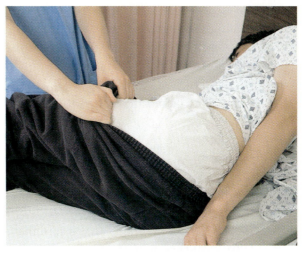

FIGURE 23-19C Have patient roll onto strong side first and pull up pants over hip. Then have patient roll to the other side and pull up pants. Adjust garment for comfort.

patient to roll first to one side as you pull up the garment and then the other side (Figure 23-19C). Adjust garment until it is comfortable.

d. Fasten garment if required.

12. Socks or knee-high (or thigh-high) stockings:

a. Roll sock or stocking with heel in back and place over toes (Figure 23-19D).

b. Draw sock up over foot and adjust until smooth. Pull stockings smoothly up to knee or thigh.

c. Repeat for other foot.

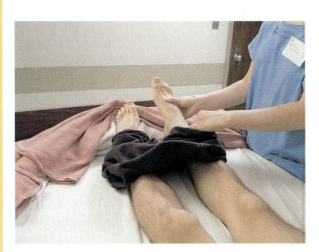

FIGURE 23-19B Slip pants over patient's feet and lower legs.

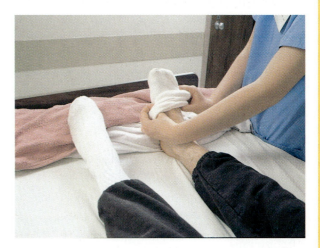

FIGURE 23-19D Adjust socks (or stockings) smoothly over toes.

continues

PROCEDURE 64 continued

13. Pantyhose:

    a. Gather pantyhose and adjust over toes and feet. Draw up legs as high as possible.

    b. Draw over hips as described in step 11c. Adjust until comfortable at waist.

14. Shoes:

    a. Slip shoe on, using shoe horn if necessary. Open laces of shoes completely so foot can easily slip into shoe (Figure 23-19E).

    b. Be sure shoe is fastened securely (Velcro tabs or ties). If the shoes tie, be sure that ends of shoelaces do not drag on the floor. The shoes should be fastened tight enough to prevent them from slipping off the resident's feet but not so tight that circulation is impaired.

    c. Shoes should have rubber soles for better

traction. Leather soles slide easily on tile and linoleum floors.

15. To undress, reverse order of steps.

16. Carry out each procedure completion action.

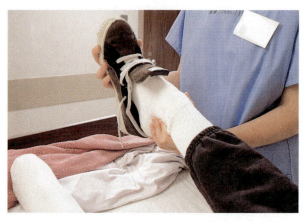

FIGURE 23-19E Laces of shoes are opened completely so that the foot can easily slip into the shoe.

REVIEW

A. True/False.

Mark the following true or false by circling T or F.

1. T F The nursing assistant should carefully observe the patient during the bath procedure.

2. T F Perineal care is given with the patient positioned on a bedpan.

3. T F Range-of-motion exercises are often performed after the bath procedure begins.

4. T F The bath can be omitted if the patient is receiving an IV.

5. T F During the bed bath, only the part being bathed should be exposed.

6. T F Patients should be encouraged to use handrails when getting in and out of the bathtub.

7. T F Stress may be placed on drainage tubes as long as they are not disconnected.

8. T F Because soap is used during the bathing procedure, the tub need not be cleaned between patient uses.

9. T F The bathing procedure can provide the patient with mild exercise.

10. T F Disposable gloves should be worn if the patient has draining wounds.

B. Matching.

Match the words in Column II with the statements in Column I.

Column I	Column II
11. _____ External reproductive organs	**a.** axillae
	b. midriff
12. _____ Area at base of nails	**c.** genitalia
13. _____ Area under the arms	**d.** cuticle
	e. shampoo

C. Multiple Choice.

Select the one best answer for each question.

14. The room temperature during the bath procedure should be about

    a. 62°F.

    b. 68°F.

    c. 70°F.

    d. 78°F.

15. Patients needing special care during the bath period are those who
    a. have drainage tubing.
    b. are receiving an IV.
    c. are receiving oxygen.
    d. all of these.

16. Bath water temperature should be approximately
    a. 105°F.
    b. 90°F.
    c. 100°F.
    d. 115°F.

17. When giving hand and nail care, the hands should be soaked approximately
    a. 1 hour.
    b. 1/2 hour.
    c. 20 minutes.
    d. 5 minutes.

18. When a patient takes a bath, the bathroom door should
    a. not be locked.
    b. be left wide open for easier access.
    c. be locked for privacy.
    d. be left partially open.

D. Nursing Assistant Challenge.

Mr. Rodriguez is taking a shower before going home. He had bowel surgery four days ago. Answer the following about his care by selecting the correct word.

19. The person responsible for the cleanliness of the shower is the _____
    (patient) (nursing assistant)

20. The patient _____ be assisted into and out of the shower.
    (should not) (should)

21. You can protect the patient from fatigue by _____ to the shower.
    (walking slowly) (transporting him by wheelchair)

22. If Mr. Rodriguez feels faint during his shower, you should turn the water _____.
    (to cold) (off)

23. To prevent chilling when Mr. Rodriguez felt weak, you should _____.
    (turn on the warm water) (wrap in a bath blanket)

General Comfort Measures

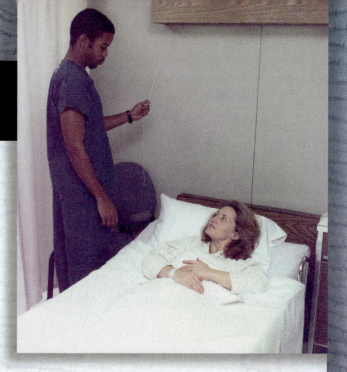

As a result of this unit, you will be able to:

- Spell and define terms.
- Discuss the reasons for early morning and bedtime care.
- Identify patients who require frequent oral hygiene.
- List the purposes of oral hygiene.
- Explain nursing assistant responsibilities for a patient's dentures.
- State the purpose of backrubs.
- Describe safety precautions when shaving a patient.
- Describe the importance of hair care.
- Explain the use of comfort devices.
- Demonstrate the following procedures:

- Procedure 65 Assisting with Routine Oral Hygiene
- Procedure 66 Assisting with Special Oral Hygiene
- Procedure 67 Assisting Patient to Floss and Brush Teeth
- Procedure 68 Caring for Dentures
- Procedure 69 Backrub
- Procedure 70 Shaving a Male Patient
- Procedure 71 Daily Hair Care
- Procedure 72 Giving and Receiving the Bedpan
- Procedure 73 Giving and Receiving the Urinal
- Procedure 74 Assisting with Use of the Bedside Commode

Learn the meaning and the correct spelling of the following words:

AM care	dentures	foot drop	PM care
bridging	feces	halitosis	trochanter roll
caries	footboard	oral hygiene	

INTRODUCTION

There is much that you can do for your patients that will add to their general comfort and feeling of well-being. This includes:

- Providing AM and PM care
- Caring for oral hygiene
- Giving backrubs
- Brushing hair
- Shaving
- Using pillows and special equipment to maintain comfortable positions

AM CARE AND PM CARE

Early morning (AM) care prepares the patient for a day of activities and PM care prepares the patient for a night of rest. Each provides an opportunity for the patient to meet elimination needs and to be refreshed. The nursing assistant has an opportunity to closely observe the patient's condition and to interrelate supportively with the patient.

Early Morning (AM) Care

Early morning or **AM care** helps to set the tone for the entire day. If the patient is refreshed and comfortable before eating breakfast, the day is off to a good start. The nursing assistant provides AM care by:

- Awakening the patient gently—never abruptly—by placing a hand on the patient's arm and saying the patient's name (Figure 24-1).
- Awakening the patient before breakfast.
- Giving the patient the opportunity to use the bathroom, if permitted, or to use the bedpan or urinal.
- Helping the patient to wash hands and face.

The patient is not awakened early if he or she is:

- Going to surgery
- Having tests that prohibit eating

Bedtime (PM Care)

The care given to the patient just before bedtime is similar to that given in the early morning. Bedtime care is called **PM care** (or HS care). The nursing assistant gives PM care:

- In a quiet, unrushed manner that will help prepare the patient for sleep (Figure 24-2)
- Before medication for sleep is given by the nurse

Other routine procedures that may be carried out during AM and PM care include:

- Measuring vital signs
- Giving a backrub
- Providing mouth and hair care
- Giving the patient the opportunity to use the bathroom, if permitted, or to use the bedpan or urinal.

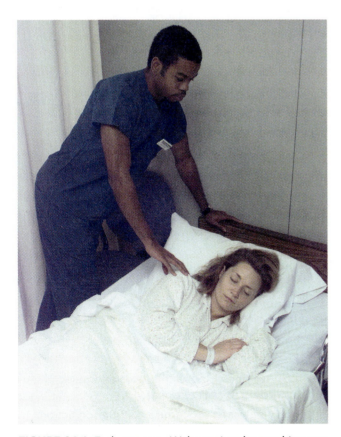

FIGURE 24-1 Early AM care. Wake patient by touching arm gently and saying patient's name.

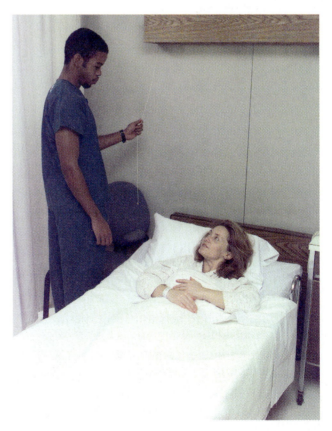

FIGURE 24-2 When you are sure patient is settled and comfortable, turn off light.

ORAL HYGIENE

Oral hygiene is the care of the mouth and teeth. (Refer to Procedures 65 to 67.)

- Routine oral hygiene (including brushing and flossing the teeth) should be performed at least three times a day.
- Patients should be encouraged to do as much as possible for themselves.
- *Special oral hygiene* is the cleansing of the mouth of the helpless patient using commercially prepared lemon and glycerine Toothettes® and other preparations.

Patients requiring more frequent oral hygiene include those who are:

- unconscious
- vomiting
- experiencing a high temperature
- receiving certain medications
- dehydrated
- breathing through the mouth
- receiving oxygen
- dying

Proper cleansing of the teeth and mouth helps

- prevent tooth decay (caries)
- eliminate bad breath (halitosis)
- contribute to the patient's comfort

PROCEDURE **65**

ASSISTING WITH ROUTINE ORAL HYGIENE

1. Carry out each beginning procedure action.
2. Assemble equipment:
   - disposable gloves and face mask
   - toothbrush
   - toothpaste
   - dental floss
   - mouthwash solution in cup
   - emesis basin
   - bath towel
   - drinking tube
   - tissues
   - cup of fresh water
   - plastic bag
   - bed protector
3. Raise back of bed so that patient may sit up, if condition permits.
4. Lower side rails and position overbed table across patient's lap.
5. Cover table with protector and place equipment on table.
6. Place bath towel over patient's gown and bedcovers.
7. Be prepared to help as patient brushes and flosses teeth.
8. Pour water over toothbrush and put toothpaste on brush.
9. Put on disposable gloves and face mask.
10. Brush teeth as follows (Figure 24-3):

    a. Insert toothbrush into the mouth with bristles pointing downward.
    b. Turn toothbrush with bristles toward teeth.
    c. Brush all tooth surfaces with a back-and-forth motion.

11. Give patient water in cup to rinse mouth. Use straw, if necessary. Turn the patient's head to one side with emesis basin near chin for return of fluid.
12. Repeat steps 10 and 11 as necessary.
13. To floss the patient's teeth:

    a. Select a piece of dental floss about twelve inches long. Wrap end of dental floss around middle fingers, leaving the center area free (Figure 24-4).
    b. Ask patient to open her mouth. Gently insert floss between each tooth down to, but not into, the gum line.
    c. Ask patient to rinse mouth using emesis basin.

14. Offer patient mouthwash. Dilute mouthwash, if desired by patient.
15. Remove basin. Wipe patient's mouth and chin with tissue. Discard tissue in paper bag.
16. Remove towel.
17. Rinse toothbrush with water.
18. Remove and dispose of gloves and mask according to facility policy.
19. Carry out each procedure completion action.

continues

PROCEDURE **65** *continued*

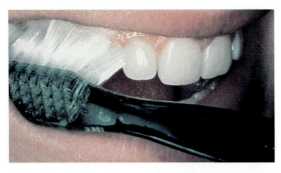

A. Place the head of the toothbrush beside the teeth, with the bristle tips at a 45-degree angle against the gumline. Move the brush back and forth in short (half-a-tooth-wide) strokes several times, using a gentle "scrubbing" motion. Brush the outer surfaces of each tooth, upper and lower, keeping the bristles angled against the gumline.

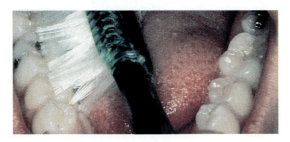

B. Use the same method on the inside surfaces of all the teeth, still using short back-and-forth strokes.

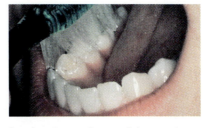

C. Scrub the chewing surfaces of the teeth.

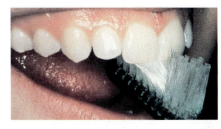

D. To clean the inside surfaces of the front teeth, tilt the brush vertically and make several gentle up-and-down strokes with the "toe" (the front part) of the brush.

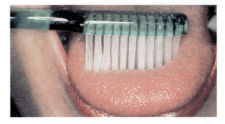

E. Brushing the patient's tongue will help freshen breath and clean the mouth by removing bacteria.

FIGURE 24-3 Brush teeth in the direction they grow and across the chewing surfaces. *Toothbrushing photos and descriptions compliments of the American Dental Association*

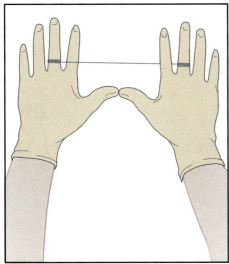
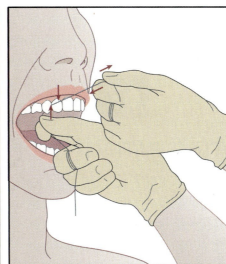

FIGURE 24-4 Floss is wrapped around the middle fingers (*left*). The proper method of using the floss to clean between the teeth (*right*).

PROCEDURE 66

ASSISTING WITH SPECIAL ORAL HYGIENE

Note: *Special oral hygiene is provided when the patient cannot participate actively in such care.*

1. Carry out each beginning procedure action.

2. Assemble equipment:
   - disposable gloves
   - Toothettes® or lemon and glycerine applicators
   - emesis basin
   - bath towel
   - plastic bag
   - pre-moistened applicators
   - tissues
   - tongue depressor
   - water-based lubricant for lips

3. Put on gloves.

4. Cover pillow with towel and turn patient's head to one side and slightly forward so any excess fluid will not run down throat. Place emesis basin under patient's chin.

5. Gently pull down on chin to open mouth or open mouth gently with tongue depressor.

6. Using moistened Toothettes®, wipe gums, teeth, tongue, and inside of mouth (Figure 24-5).

7. Discard used applicators in plastic bag.

8. Using clean applicators, apply lubricant to patient's lips. Place used applicators in plastic bag.

9. Clean and replace equipment.

10. Remove and dispose of gloves properly. Wash hands.

11. Carry out each procedure completion action.

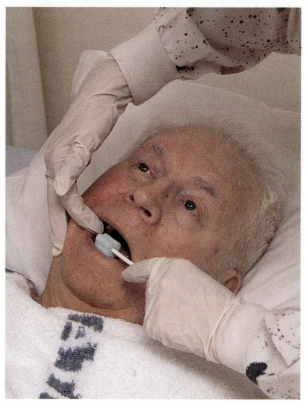

FIGURE 24-5 Using pre-moistened applicators, wipe gums, teeth, and tongue.

PROCEDURE 67

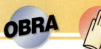

ASSISTING PATIENT TO FLOSS AND BRUSH TEETH

1. Carry out each beginning procedure action.

2. Assemble equipment:
   - disposable gloves
   - emesis basin
   - toothbrush
   - toothpaste
   - dental floss
   - glass of cool water
   - mouthwash (if permitted)
   - hand towel
   - bed protector

3. Elevate the head of the bed. Help patient into a comfortable position.

continues

PROCEDURE **67** *continued*

4. Lower side rails and position overbed table across patient's lap.

5. Cover table with plastic protector.

6. Place emesis basin and glass of water on overbed table.

7. Place towel across patient's chest.

8. Be prepared to help as patient flosses and brushes teeth. Remind patient to clean tongue and gums. Apply gloves and use standard precautions if you will be assisting with the procedure.

9. After patient has flossed and brushed his teeth:

   a. Push overbed table to the foot of the bed.

   b. Remove the emesis basin, clean it, and replace it according to facility policy.

   c. Remove the towel and discard with the soiled linen.

   d. Remove gloves and discard according to facility policy. Wash hands.

10. Carry out each procedure completion action.

DENTURES

Some patients have full sets of dentures. Other patients have partial plates that are removable, but attach by small metal clips to existing teeth. Partial plates should be given the same care as full dentures. Dentures are artificial teeth that are removable. They must be cleaned. The patient may feel embarrassed about wearing dentures and may dislike being seen after the dentures have been removed. Therefore, always provide privacy when dentures are to be removed and cleaned. (See Procedure 68.)

Denture Care

Denture care includes the following:
- Cleaning dentures daily under cool running water.
- Handling dentures carefully to prevent damage.

- Storing dentures in a safe place when out of the patient's mouth, such as in the drawer of the bedside stand in a container labeled with the patient's name (Figure 24-6).
- Cleaning and checking the patient's mouth for signs of irritation.
- Checking the patient's lips for cracking and dryness.
- Applying cream, petroleum jelly, or glycerin to lips for excessive dryness.

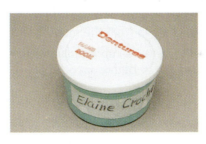

FIGURE 24-6 Dentures are stored in a denture cup labeled with the patient's name.

PROCEDURE **68**

CARING FOR DENTURES

1. Carry out each beginning procedure action.

2. Assemble equipment:
   - disposable gloves
   - tissues
   - emesis basin
   - tongue depressor
   - brush
   - toothpaste or tooth powder
   - mouthwash, if permitted
   - gauze squares
   - applicators
   - denture cup

3. Apply disposable gloves.

4. Allow patient to clean dentures if he or she is able to do so. If patient cannot, give tissue to patient and ask him or her to remove dentures. Assist if necessary.

   a. To remove upper dentures, grasp dentures firmly, ease downward and then forward, and remove from the mouth (Figure 24-7).

continues

PROCEDURE **68** *continued*

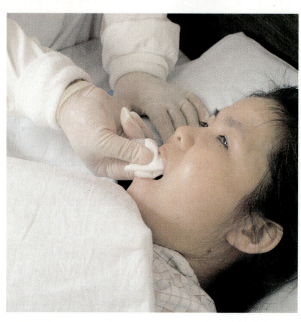

FIGURE 24-7 Firmly grasp upper dentures and ease down and forward to remove.

b. To remove lower dentures, grasp dentures firmly, ease upward and then forward, and remove from the mouth.

5. Place dentures in denture cup padded with gauze squares. Take to bathroom or utility room.

6. Place a paper towel or washcloth in the bottom of the basin to protect the dentures (Figure 24-8). Add a small amount of cool water.

7. Dentures may be soaked in a solution with a cleansing tablet before brushing, if desired.

8. Put toothpaste or tooth powder on brush. Hold dentures and brush until all surfaces are clean.

9. Rinse dentures thoroughly under cool or warm running water. Never use hot water. Rinse denture cup.

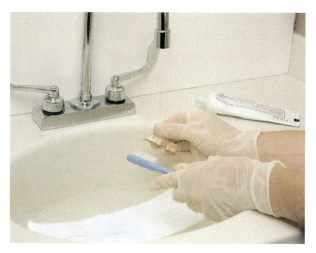

FIGURE 24-8 Brush dentures until all surfaces are clean.

10. Place fresh gauze squares in denture cup with clean, cool water unless instructed otherwise.

11. Place dentures in cup and take them to bedside.

12. Assist patient to rinse mouth with mouthwash, if permitted. Otherwise, use water. Hold mouth open gently with wooden tongue depressor. Clean gums and tongue with applicators moistened with mouthwash or use foam Toothettes.®

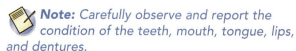 **Note:** *Carefully observe and report the condition of the teeth, mouth, tongue, lips, and dentures.*

13. Use tissue or gauze to hand wet dentures to patient. Insert if necessary, upper denture first.

14. Clean and replace equipment according to facility policy.

15. Remove and dispose of gloves according to facility policy.

16. Carry out each procedure completion action.

BACKRUBS

When properly given, backrubs can be:
- stimulating to the patient's circulation.
- a major aid in preventing skin breakdown (*decubiti*).
- soothing.
- refreshing.

Keep your nails short to prevent injuring the patient. The backrub procedure provides a good opportunity for you to observe the condition of the patient's skin. (See Procedure 69.) Report all observations to the nurse. Look for:
- Reddened areas that do not blanch (whiten) when pressed
- Raw areas of skin

- Condition of skin over bony prominences

Unless contraindicated, the backrub is given:

- routinely as part of the bed bath or partial bath.
- following use of the bedpan.
- when changing the position of the helpless patient.
- at bedtime.
- when it could be a comfort to the patient.

Long, smooth strokes are relaxing. Short, circular strokes tend to be more stimulating.

The backrub is given with warmed lotion.

PROCEDURE   69

BACKRUB

1. Carry out each beginning procedure action.

2. Assemble equipment:
   - disposable gloves
   - basin of water (105°F)
   - bath towel
   - soap and lotion

3. Put up far side rail.

4. Place lotion in basin of water to warm (Figure 24-9).

5. Put on disposable gloves if patient has open lesions.

6. Turn the patient on his or her side with back toward you.

7. Expose and wash back; dry carefully. This step is not necessary if the backrub is given after a bath.

8. Pour a small amount of lotion into one hand.

9. Apply to skin and rub with gentle but firm strokes. Give special attention to all bony prominences (Figure 24-10).

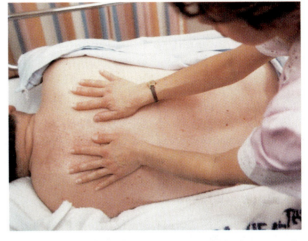

FIGURE 24-10 Use long, smooth strokes as you apply the lotion.

10. Begin at base of spine:
    - With long, soothing strokes, rub up the center of back, around the shoulders, and down sides of back and buttocks (Figure 24-11, *left*).

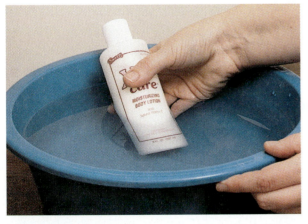

FIGURE 24-9 Before the backrub, the bottle of lotion can be placed in a basin of warm water for several minutes. That way the lotion will not be cold when applied to the patient's back.

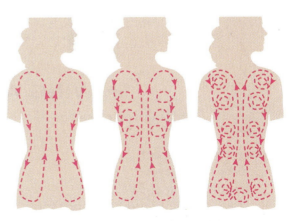

FIGURE 24-11 Strokes to be used during the back rub: soothing strokes (*left*), circular movement (*middle*), passive movement (*right*).

continues

PROCEDURE 69 *continued*

- Repeat previous step four times, using long, soothing upward strokes and circular motion on downstroke (Figure 24-11, *middle*).
- Repeat, but on downward stroke rub in small circular motions with palm of hand. Include areas over coccyx (over base of spine) (Figure 24-11, *right*).
- Repeat long, soothing strokes on muscles for 3 to 5 minutes (Figure 24-11, *left*).

- Dry area well.
- If redness on pressure areas is noted, report to nurse. Straighten and tighten bottom sheet and draw sheet.
11. Change patient's gown if needed.
12. Remove gloves if used. Discard according to facility policy and wash hands.
13. Replace equipment.
14. Carry out each procedure completion action.

DAILY SHAVING

Daily shaving is part of the routine self-care of most men. It should not be neglected in a care facility. When patients are unable to shave themselves and a barber is not available, it is your responsibility. (See Procedure 70.)

Older women have an increase in the growth and coarseness of hairs on the chin and upper lip. Many women find this distressing. Tweezers can be used to remove some of the hairs, but a more permanent method is to have the hairs removed professionally with an electric needle. Some women may require a shave. In some facilities nursing assistants are not permitted to shave women patients. Be sure to check the policy of your facility.

GUIDELINES *for*

Safety in Shaving

- Use the patient's own shaving equipment if possible. For safety, use an electric razor or rotary razor.
- If the patient is receiving anticoagulants, a special procedure may be required. For

example, an electric razor provides the greatest safety. Check with the nurse for the proper procedure.
- If oxygen is being given, it may be possible to discontinue it during this procedure. Consult the nurse and follow hospital policy.

PROCEDURE 70

SHAVING A MALE PATIENT

1. Carry out each beginning procedure action.

2. Assemble equipment:
   - disposable gloves
   - electric shaver or safety razor
   - shaving lather or preshave lotion for electric razor
   - basin of water (105°F)
   - face towels
   - mirror
   - washcloth
   - aftershave lotion

3. Raise the head of the bed. Place equipment on overbed table.

4. Put on gloves.

5. Place one face towel across patient's chest and one under head.

continues

P R O C E D U R E **70** *continued*

6. Moisten face and apply lather (or preshave lotion).

7. Starting in front of ear:
   a. Hold skin taut and bring razor down over cheek toward chin (Figure 24-12).
   b. Repeat until lather on cheek is removed and area has been shaved. Rinse frequently.
   c. Repeat on other cheek.
   d. Use firm short strokes. Shave in direction of hair growth.
   e. Rinse razor frequently.

8. Lather neck area and stroke up toward the chin. Rinse and repeat until all lather is removed.

9. Wash face and neck and dry thoroughly.

10. Apply aftershave lotion if desired.

11. If the skin is nicked, apply pressure directly over the area and then apply an antiseptic and bandage. Report incident to nurse.

12. Clean and replace equipment. Dispose of razor according to facility policy. Remove head of electric razor. Use razor brush to remove clippings. Store razor according to facility policy.

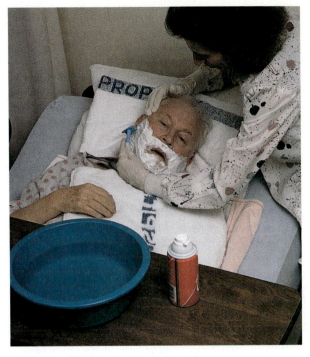

FIGURE 24-12 Shaving is part of the daily routine for most men.

13. Remove and dispose of gloves according to facility policy.

14. Carry out each procedure completion action.

DAILY HAIR CARE

Daily care of the hair, for both male and female patients, is usually performed after the patient's bed bath. (See Procedure 71.)

The hair should be combed and brushed each morning. Tangles can be loosened by sectioning the hair with a comb or brush, working with one section at a time. Grasp the hair near the scalp to reduce pulling (Figure 24-13). Start combing or brushing tangles out starting at the ends and working toward the scalp. Braiding long hair after brushing can help reduce tangles. Tangles can be reduced in wiry, dry hair by using conditioner and keeping the hair short or in braids.

Brushing the hair:

- stimulates circulation of the scalp.
- refreshes the patient.
- removes dust and lint.
- helps to keep the hair shiny and attractive.

If additional care is needed, a fluid dry cleaner to shampoo the hair is available. It leaves the hair soft and manageable and the hairstyle intact. This procedure is so simple that it is

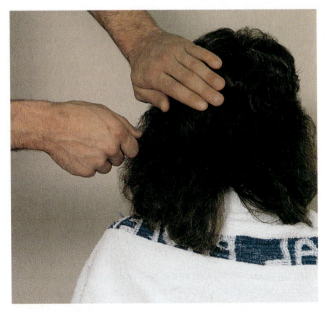

FIGURE 24-13 To remove tangles from long hair, divide the hair into sections. Work with one section at a time. Hold hair near the scalp to reduce pulling and start combing at the end of the hair, working toward the scalp.

PROCEDURE 71

DAILY HAIR CARE

1. Carry out each beginning procedure action.

2. Assemble equipment:
   - towel
   - comb and brush

3. Ask patient to move to the side of the bed nearest you; or patient may sit in chair if permitted. If patient is sitting up, put a towel around her shoulders.

4. Cover pillow with towel.

5. Part or section hair and comb with one hand between scalp and end of hair.

6. Brush carefully and thoroughly.

7. Have resident turn so hair on back of head may be combed and brushed. If hair is tangled, work section by section to unsnarl hair, beginning near ends and working toward scalp.

8. Complete brushing and arrange attractively. Braid long hair to prevent repeated snarling.

9. Clean and replace equipment according to facility policy.

10. Carry out each procedure completion action.

---

often used instead of the regular shampoo for patients who must remain in bed.

Sometimes, however, a shampoo may be advisable for the patient in bed. Approval for the procedure must be obtained from the doctor. Bed shampoos should be given every two weeks when the patient is bedbound for an extended period. (See Unit 23, Procedure 63.)

The following procedure assumes that the patient is a female. Hair care for a male is very similar, however, so the procedure can easily be adapted.

COMFORT DEVICES

The physician, nurse, or physical therapist orders comfort devices such as bed cradles, footboards, and pillows. They are designed to relieve pressure on specific areas or to help maintain body position.

Bed Cradle

A bed cradle (Figure 24-14) prevents the weight of the bedclothes from falling on some part of the body. It can be used therapeutically or as a comfort device. It is used:

- over fractured limbs.
- when there are burns.
- to prevent skin lesions.

Coverings that maintain some degree of warmth within the cradle may also be needed to keep the patient comfortable.

Care must be taken to position the limb within the cradle. It may be necessary to pad the cradle edges.

Footboard or Footrest

The footboard or footrest is a device placed between the mattress and bed to keep the feet at right angles to the legs

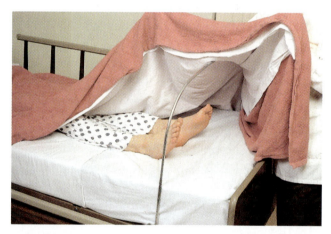

FIGURE 24-14 A bed cradle keeps the sheet and blanket from putting pressure on the feet.

(natural standing position). A footboard is always padded. It is used to prevent foot drop. In foot drop, the muscle in the calf of the leg tends to tighten, causing the toes to point downward. Foot drop may happen when the patient must remain in bed over a long period of time. Even a brief period in bed is sufficient to cause a degree of foot drop that makes walking difficult when the patient does get out of bed.

If a footboard is not available, a pillow folded lengthwise may be placed against the foot of the bed to serve the same purpose.

Pillows

Pillows can be used as comfort devices and to maintain alignment when properly arranged. For directions on properly altering the patient's positions, refer to Unit 14.

A trochanter roll or support can be made as follows:

1. Fold a bath blanket lengthwise in thirds.

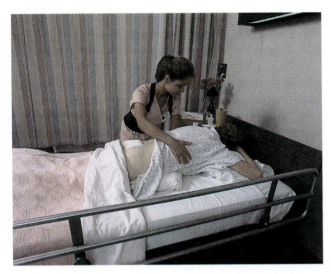

FIGURE 24-15 The patient is positioned on her abdomen and pillows are used to form a bridge, preventing pressure on her breasts.

2. Position patient in center of folded bath blanket. Blanket should extend from mid-thigh to above the waist.

3. Roll each side of the blanket under and toward the patient until the blanket roll is firmly against the patient. Then tuck roll inward toward bed and patient to maintain patient's position.

Pillows are also used to relieve pressure in such a way that spaces are left to relieve pressure on specific areas (Figure 24-15). This technique is called **bridging**.

ELIMINATION NEEDS

Regular, periodic elimination of body wastes is essential for maintaining health. Patients who are confined to bed must rely on you to help them with this physical task. (See Procedures 72 to 74.) You should know that:

- The patient must regularly empty the bladder by urinating (voiding).

- A urinal (duct or bottle) is used by male patients when they need to urinate. A bedpan is used by female patients to void when they are confined to bed.
- A regular bowel movement (which is the discharge of solid waste from the body) is also important to a patient's health.
- The solid waste produced by the patient is called **feces** or *stool*.
- Both male and female patients use a bedpan for solid waste elimination when confined to bed.
- Many patients are somewhat sensitive about using a bedpan or urinal.
- Personal hygiene is exceedingly important in carrying out these procedures properly.
- Bedpans are very uncomfortable.

Four important points must be kept in mind. You must:

1. Wear disposable gloves.
2. Wash your hands immediately before and after the procedure. This will help prevent the transmission of any disease to others and to yourself.
3. Provide privacy for the patient. Obtain the proper bedpan according to patient needs.
4. As soon as possible, answer the light indicating that the patient is finished.

One-Glove Technique

Some facilities require health care providers to use the one-glove technique when removing bedpans, urinals, and other contaminated items. Gloves are worn on both hands when the contaminated item is removed. The bedpan or contaminated item is covered if it is to be carried to the bathroom or into the hallway. A glove is then removed from one hand. Do not put the glove on an environmental surface. The gloved hand carries the glove that you removed and the contaminated item. The ungloved hand is used to open doors and turn on faucets. By using this method, you avoid contaminating the environment with your gloves.

P R O C E D U R E **72**

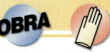

GIVING AND RECEIVING THE BEDPAN

1. Carry out each beginning procedure action.
2. Assemble equipment:
   - disposable gloves
   - bedpan and cover
   - basin
   - washcloth
   - paper towels/protector
   - toilet tissue
   - soap
   - towel
3. Lower the head of the bed, if necessary.
4. Put on gloves.

continues

PROCEDURE   72   continued

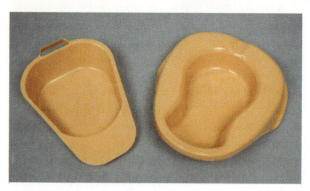

FIGURE 24-16 Orthopedic bedpan (*left*) and regular bedpan (*right*)

5. Take the bedpan and tissue from the bedside stand.

   - Place protector on chair. Place bedpan (Figure 24-16) on it.
   - Never place a bedpan on the side stand or overbed table.
   - Put the remainder of the articles on the bedside table.

6. Place bedpan cover at the foot of the bed.

   - The bedpan may be warmed by running warm water into it and then emptying and drying it.
   - Plastic bedpans may be comfortable without warming.

   Note: *Never carry or allow a used bedpan to sit uncovered. If a bedpan cover is not available, cover the bedpan with a towel, pillowcase, or paper towels.*

7. Fold top bedcovers back at a right angle. Raise patient's gown. If patient is thin or has a pressure sore, consult the nurse for the appropriate action. The nursing care plan may have specific instructions for such cases. For example, it may be necessary to pad the bedpan with a folded towel or to take some other action.

8. Ask patient to flex knees and rest weight on heels, if able.

9. Help patient to raise buttocks by:

   - Putting one hand under the small of patient's back and lifting gently and slowly with that hand.
   - With the other hand, place the bedpan under patient's hips.

   - If patient is unable to raise the buttocks, two assistants may be needed to lift patient.
   - The pan may also be placed by rolling patient to one side, positioning the bedpan against the buttocks, and rolling the patient back on it (Figure 24-17). Check to be sure bedpan is positioned properly.
   - Alternatively, if a trapeze is in place over the bed, place the bedpan under patient as patient lifts self using the trapeze (Figure 24-18).
   - Patient's buttocks should rest on the rounded shelf of the regular bedpan.
   - The narrow end should face the foot of the bed.

10. Replace top bedcovers. Raise the head of the bed to a comfortable height. Remove gloves and dispose of properly.

11. Make sure the toilet paper and signal cord are within easy reach of patient. Leave patient alone unless contraindicated in the nursing care plan.

12. Wash your hands.

   Note: *If a specimen is to be taken, instruct patient that toilet tissue is not to be placed in the bedpan. In this case, the nursing assistant will clean patient and provide perineal care.*

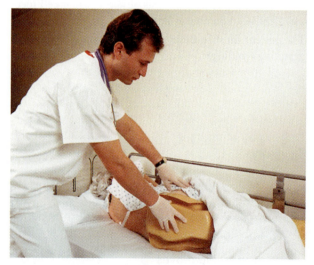

FIGURE 24-17 Roll patient away from you while supporting patient with one hand on patient's hip and arm. Place bedpan with the other hand. Then roll patient back onto the bedpan.

continues

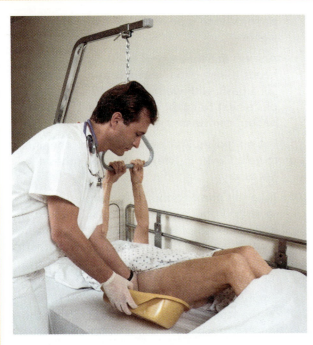

FIGURE 24-18 The patient assists by lifting with the trapeze as the nursing assistant places the bedpan under the patient. Note that the nursing assistant supports the patient's back with his hand.

13. Watch for patient's signal.

14. Answer patient's call signal immediately. Wash hands and put on disposable gloves. Fill the basin with warm water (105°F) and place next to soap, washcloth, and towel on overbed table.

15. Remove bedpan from under patient.

   - Ask patient to flex knees and rest weight on heels. Place one hand under the small of the back and lift gently to help raise the buttocks off bedpan. Take the bedpan with the other hand. Cover it and place it on the chair.

   - If patient is unable to raise the buttocks, two assistants may be needed to lift. Otherwise, roll patient off the pan to the side and remove the pan. Lift and move carefully. Hold the pan firmly with one hand.

   - Many patients have difficulty cleaning adequately after using the bedpan. You may need to clean and dry patient yourself.

16. Assist patient to a clean area of the bed, if necessary. Provide perineal care.

   - Discard tissue in bedpan unless specimen is to be collected.

   - Cover bedpan again.

   - Cleanse patient with warm water and soap, if necessary.

17. Replace bedclothes, changing linen or protective pads as necessary.

18. Encourage patient to wash hands and freshen up after the procedure.

19. Take the bedpan to the bathroom or utility room and observe contents. Measure, if required.

20. Empty bedpan.

21. Turn on faucet, using a paper towel in the hand. Rinse bedpan with cold water and disinfectant. Rinse, dry, and return bedpan to storage in patient's bedside stand.

22. Remove gloves and dispose of them properly. Wash hands.

23. Carry out each procedure completion action.

PROCEDURE **73**

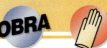

GIVING AND RECEIVING THE URINAL

1. Carry out each beginning procedure action.

2. Assemble equipment:
   - urinal (Figure 24-19)
   - basin
   - soap
   - washcloth
   - towel
   - disposable gloves

continues

PROCEDURE **73** *continued*

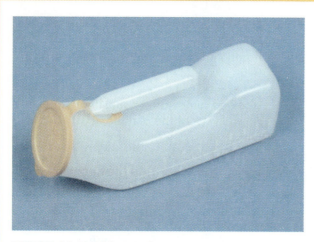

FIGURE 24-19 Male urinal

3. Put on gloves. Lift the top bedcovers and place the urinal under the covers so patient may grasp the handle. Instruct patient to place his penis in the urinal opening. If he cannot do this, you must position the urinal and ensure that the penis is placed in the opening.

4. Remove gloves and dispose of them properly. Wash hands. Make sure the signal cord is within easy reach of patient. Leave patient alone if possible. Watch for his signal.

5. Answer patient's signal immediately. Wash hands. Use a paper towel to turn on faucet. Fill a basin with warm water (105°F), and place next to soap, washcloth, and towel so patient can wash and dry hands.

6. Put on gloves. Ask patient to hand the urinal to you. Cover it. Rearrange bedclothes if necessary.

7. Take the urinal to the bathroom or utility room and observe the contents. Measure, if required. Do not empty urinal if anything unusual (such as blood) is observed. Rather, save the contents of the urinal for the nurse's inspection.

8. Empty the urinal. Use a paper towel to turn on the faucet and another towel to turn the faucet off. Rinse with cold water and clean with warm soapy water. Rinse, dry, and cover urinal. Remove gloves and dispose of them properly. Wash hands.

9. Place urinal inside patient's bedside table. Clean and replace other articles.

10. Carry out each procedure completion action.

PROCEDURE **74**

ASSISTING WITH USE OF THE BEDSIDE COMMODE

1. Carry out each beginning procedure action.

2. Assemble equipment:
   - disposable gloves
   - portable commode
   - toilet tissue
   - basin
   - washcloth
   - soap
   - towel

3. Position commode beside bed, facing head. Lock wheels and open lid. Be sure receptacle is in place under seat.

4. If bed and side rails are elevated, lower side rail nearest you and lower bed to lowest horizontal position. Lock bed wheels.

5. Put on gloves.

6. Assist patient to sitting position. Swing patient's legs over edge of bed.

7. Assist patient to put on robe. Put slippers on patient. Assist patient to stand. If needed, use a transfer belt.

8. Support patient with hands on either side of the chest. Remember to use proper body mechanics. Pivot patient to the right and lower to commode.

continues

PROCEDURE 74 continued

9. Leave call bell and tissue within reach.

10. Remove gloves and discard according to facility policy.

11. When patient signals, return promptly. Wash hands and put on gloves. Fill basin with water at 105°F. Bring basin to bedside along with soap, towel, and washcloth.

12. Assist patient to stand.

13. Cleanse anus or perineum if patient is unable to help self.

14. Allow patient to wash and dry hands. Remove gloves and dispose of according to facility policy. Wash hands.

15. Assist patient to return to bed. Adjust bedding and pillows for comfort.

16. Leave signal cord within easy reach.

17. Put on gloves.

18. Remove receptacle from commode and cover. Close lid of commode.

19. Take receptacle to bathroom. Note contents and measure if required.

20. Empty and clean per facility policy. Replace in commode. Remove and dispose of gloves properly.

20. Put commode in proper place.

21. Carry out each procedure completion action.

REVIEW

A. True/False.

Mark the following true or false by circling T or F.

1. T F Plastic dentures should be stored in an antiseptic solution.

2. T F Backrubs are routinely given as part of the bath procedure.

3. T F A padded footboard is used to prevent foot drop.

4. T F Routine oral hygiene should be carried out once daily.

5. T F Proper oral hygiene helps prevent tooth decay.

6. T F When not in the patient's mouth, dentures should be left on the bedside stand.

7. T F Patients should never be awakened abruptly.

8. T F When giving PM care, the bottom sheet should be tightened and the top linen straightened.

9. T F Disposable gloves should be used by a nursing assistant giving oral care.

10. T F The unconscious patient needs no oral care because he is not eating.

B. Matching.

Choose the correct word from Column II to match the phrases in Column I.

Column I	Column II
11. _____ bad breath	a. oral hygiene
12. _____ mouth care	b. caries
13. _____ tooth cavities	c. dentures
14. _____ means of relieving pressure	d. bridging
15. _____ artificial teeth	e. halitosis
	f. foot drop

C. Completion.

Complete the statements in questions 16–20 by writing in the correct word from the following list.

arm	name
breakfast	PM care
down	removed
early AM care	surgery
hand	

16. After PM care, the bed should be left with the back rest _____.

17. _____ should be completed before sleep medication is given.

18. The best way to awaken a patient is to place your _____ on the patient's arm and say his _____.

19. Patients are not wakened early if they are going to have _____.

20. Early morning care awakens the patient before _____.

D. Multiple Choice.

Select the one best answer for each question.

21. Which of the following patients should be given special mouth care?
  a. One who can brush her own teeth
  b. One who is drinking water ad lib
  c. One who has a broken leg
  d. One who has a high fever

22. To warm lotion before giving a backrub,
  a. hold it under running water.
  b. soak it in a basin of warm water.
  c. let the patient hold the bottle for a few minutes.
  d. none of these.

23. The best way to support a patient in a side-lying position is to
  a. use a footboard to keep the feet aligned.
  b. place a pillow doubled under the head.
  c. place two pillows lengthwise between the legs.
  d. double a pillow lengthwise behind the back.

24. When brushing a patient's teeth, the best technique includes
  a. inserting the toothbrush with the bristles in a downward position.
  b. brushing in a circular motion.
  c. inserting the toothbrush with bristles facing the teeth.
  d. brushing the teeth in a downward motion only.

25. Backrubs are given
  a. routinely as part of the bed bath.
  b. following use of the bedpan.
  c. when changing the position of the helpless patient.
  d. all of these.

E. Nursing Assistant Challenge.

Your patient, Mrs. Ubanan, has a history of heavy smoking and breathes through her mouth. She has plastic dentures and her care plan indicates that she needs assistance with denture care. Complete the following statements regarding this patient.

26. State two reasons why special oral hygiene has been ordered for Mrs. Ubanan.
  a. _____
  b. _____

27. Where are the dentures stored when not in use? _____

28. Should the dentures be kept dry or wet? _____

29. Should you wear gloves when removing dentures? _____

30. Will you clean the dentures in cool or hot water? _____

Principles of Nutrition and Fluid Balance

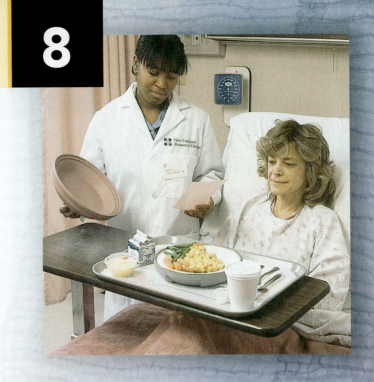

UNIT 25
Nutritional Needs and Diet Modifications

Nutritional Needs and Diet Modifications

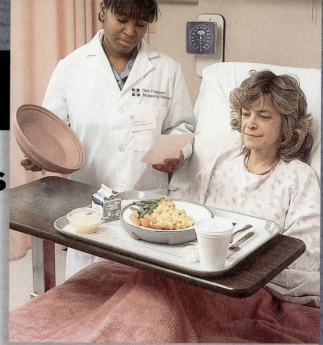

As a result of this unit, you will be able to:

- Spell and define terms.
- Define normal nutrition.
- List types of alternative nutrition.
- List the essential nutrients.
- Name the six food groups and list the foods included in each group.
- State the liquids/foods allowed on the five basic facility diets.
- Describe the purposes of the following diets:
  - clear liquid
  - full liquid
  - soft
- State the purposes of therapeutic diets.
- Describe the nursing assistant actions when patients are unable to drink fluids independently.
- Demonstrate the following procedures:
  - Procedure 75 Assisting the Patient Who Can Feed Self
  - Procedure 76 Feeding the Dependent Patient

VOCABULARY

Learn the meaning and the correct spelling of the following words and phrases:

amino acids	edema	gastrostomy feeding	nutrients
aspiration	emesis	graduate	nutrition
carbohydrates	enteral feeding	hyperalimentation	protein
cellulose	essential nutrients	intake and output	push fluids
clear liquid diet	exchange list	(I&O)	soft diet
defecation	excrete	intravenous infusion	supplement
dehydration	fats	(IV)	therapeutic diets
diaphoresis	fluid balance	minerals	total parenteral
digestion	force fluids	nasogastric feeding (NG	nutrition (TPN)
diuresis	full liquid diet	feeding)	vitamins

INTRODUCTION

Nutrition is the entire process by which the body takes in food for growth and repair and uses it to maintain health. The signs of good nutrition include:

- Shiny hair
- Clear skin and eyes
- A well-developed body
- An alert expression
- A pleasant disposition
- Healthy sleep patterns
- Appropriate appetite
- Regular bowel habits
- Body weight appropriate to height

NORMAL NUTRITION

Food is normally taken into the body through the mouth. The mouth is the beginning of the digestive tract. Digestion is the process of breaking down foods into simple substances that can be used by the body cells for nourishment. These substances are called essential nutrients.

ESSENTIAL NUTRIENTS

To be well nourished, we must eat foods that:

- supply heat and energy.
- build and repair body tissue.
- regulate body functions.

These foods are called nutrients. The six nutrients essential to maintain health are:

- Proteins
- Carbohydrates
- Fats
- Minerals
- Vitamins
- Water

Protein

Protein is an essential nutrient. It is the basic material of every body cell. It is the only nutrient that can make new cells and rebuild tissue. The foods that contain the greatest amount of protein come from animals. They include:

- Meat
- Poultry
- Eggs
- Milk
- Cheese

Proteins are made of small building blocks called amino acids. The body can manufacture some of the amino acids, but not all of them.

- *Complete proteins* are proteins that contain all the amino acids the body cannot manufacture. Examples of complete proteins are meat, fish, eggs, and poultry.
- *Incomplete proteins,* although still important, do not contain all the essential amino acids. Essential amino acids are those that must be obtained through foods. Examples of incomplete proteins are corn, soybeans, peas, and nuts.

Carbohydrates and Fats

Carbohydrates and fats are called energy foods because the body uses them to produce heat and energy. When a person eats more energy foods than the body needs, the remainder is stored as fat. Foods that contain the greatest amount of carbohydrates come from plants. They include:

- Fruits
- Vegetables
- Foods that are made from grains, such as breads, cereals, and pasta products

Carbohydrate foods also supply the body with fiber or roughage (cellulose). Cellulose is important in maintaining bowel regularity.

Fats come from both plants and animals. Examples of foods that are rich in fat include:

- Pork
- Butter
- Nuts
- Egg yolk
- Cheese

Vitamins and Minerals

Vitamins and minerals are present in a wide variety of foods. The best way to be sure that you are getting enough vitamins and minerals is to include a variety of foods in your daily diet.

Vitamins are substances that regulate body processes. They help to:

- build strong teeth and bones.
- promote growth.
- aid normal body functioning.
- strengthen resistance to disease.

You probably know the vitamins by their letter names:

- Vitamin A
- B-complex vitamins
- Vitamin C
- Vitamin D
- Vitamin E
- Vitamin K

Fat-soluble vitamins do not dissolve easily in water. They can be stored in the body. Vitamins A, D, E, and K are fat-soluble vitamins.

Vitamins B and C are water soluble. Water-soluble vitamins dissolve in water, so they can be lost in the cooking process.

In general, these vitamins are not stored in large amounts in the body. Deficiencies in water-soluble vitamins are more common.

Minerals help to build body tissues, especially the bones and teeth. They also regulate the chemistry of body fluids such as the blood and digestive juices. Minerals needed in the daily diet include:

- Calcium
- Phosphorus
- Iodine
- Iron
- Copper
- Potassium

THE SIX FOOD GROUPS

The U.S. Department of Agriculture revised the recommendations for a balanced food intake. The guidelines now include:

- Eat a variety of foods.
- Maintain a healthy body weight.
- Select foods low in fat, saturated fat, and cholesterol.
- Select plenty of vegetables, fruits, and grain products.
- Use sugar in moderation.
- Use salt and sodium in moderation.
- Drink alcoholic beverages in moderation, if at all.

Food Guide Pyramid

Figure 25-1 shows the six food groups. The guide to daily food choices recommends:

- 6–11 servings daily from the bread, cereal, rice, and pasta group
- 2–4 servings from the fruit group
- 3–5 servings from the vegetable group
- 2–3 servings from the milk, yogurt, and cheese group
- 2–3 servings from the meat, poultry, fish, dry beans, eggs, and nuts group
- Use fats, oils, and sweets sparingly

The food pyramid is used to represent the need for the foods at the bottom (grain foods) and gives equal importance to fruit and vegetables. Persons eating the lowest number of servings from each group would take in about 1600 calories daily if low-fat foods are chosen. This may be adequate for most older women and some older men. Younger and more active people would need more calories and can obtain them by choosing the larger number of servings.

Average servings of foods include:

- One medium-size fruit or its equivalent
- 1/2 cup cooked fruit or vegetable
- 3–4 ounces of meat
- 2–3 ounces of pasta/bread

Table 25-1 shows average servings for selected foods.

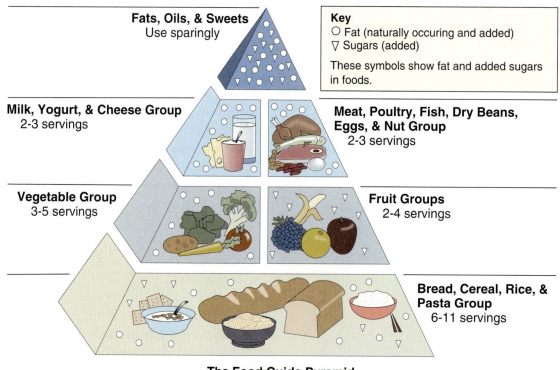

Fats, Oils, & Sweets
Use sparingly

Key
○ Fat (naturally occuring and added)
▽ Sugars (added)

These symbols show fat and added sugars in foods.

Milk, Yogurt, & Cheese Group
2-3 servings

Meat, Poultry, Fish, Dry Beans, Eggs, & Nut Group
2-3 servings

Vegetable Group
3-5 servings

Fruit Groups
2-4 servings

Bread, Cereal, Rice, & Pasta Group
6-11 servings

The Food Guide Pyramid
A guide to daily food choices

FIGURE 25-1 The food guide pyramid. *Courtesy of USDA*

TABLE 25-1 AVERAGE SERVINGS FOR SELECTED FOODS

Food	Serving Size
Fruit	
Apple	1 medium
Banana	1 medium
Peach	1 medium
Apricots	2–3
Figs	2–3
Canned—	
Grapefruit	1/2 can
Pineapple	2 slices
Peaches	1/2 cup
Juice	6 ounces
Vegetables	
Fresh	3–4 ounces
Cooked	1/2 cup
Milk	8 ounces
Eggs	1–2 medium
Meat, Fish, Poultry	3–4 ounces, cooked
Cereal (dried)	1 ounce (2/3 cup)
Bread	2 slices
Pasta	2 ounces (uncooked)

Vegetable Group

- Select three to five servings. Include:
  — Dark green or yellow vegetables
  — Tomatoes
  — Leafy, green, and yellow vegetables
- Use vegetables raw, cooked, frozen, or canned.
- This group provides vitamin A, vitamin C, B-complex vitamins, calcium, and iron.
- Leafy green vegetables furnish riboflavin and niacin, which are both B vitamins.

Three to Five Servings Daily

asparagus	celery
beans	corn
broccoli	cucumber
brussels sprouts	eggplant
cabbage	escarole
carrots	kale
cauliflower	leeks
lettuce	potatoes
other greens	pumpkin
mushrooms	radishes
mustard greens	rutabaga
okra	spinach
onions	squash
parsley	sweet potatoes
parsnips	tomatoes
peas (green)	turnips
peppers	

Fruit Group

- Select two to four servings daily.
- Use foods in this group raw, cooked, frozen, canned, or dried.
- When eaten in fairly large amounts, foods in this group provide thiamine, vitamins A and C, calcium, and phosphorus.

Two to Four Servings Daily

apples	kumquats
apricots	lemons
artichokes	limes
avocados	oranges
bananas	peaches
berries	pears
cantaloupe	persimmons
cherries	pineapple
cranberries	plums
currants	prunes
dates	raisins
figs	rhubarb
fruit juice	strawberries
grapefruit	tangerines
grapes	

Milk, Yogurt, Cheese Group

- This group provides calcium, phosphorus, riboflavin, protein, vitamin A, and fat.
- People need varying amounts of the nutrients in dairy foods at different periods of their lives.
  — Children should have three or four glasses of milk daily.
  — Teenagers need four or more glasses.
  — Adults should drink two or more glasses.
  — Pregnant women should drink at least one quart of milk, or the nutritional equivalent, daily.
  — Nursing mothers should increase the amount of milk in their diet to 1-1/2 quarts daily.
- Daily calcium requirement for postmenopausal women is 1,500 mg.

- Cheese, ice cream, and other milk-made foods can be substituted for part of the milk requirement. (This increases fat and sodium content.)

The following dairy foods contain calcium equal to that in one cup of milk and may be substituted for milk:

Milk Substitutes

1 ounce cheddar-type cheese

4 ounces cream cheese

12 ounces cottage cheese

1-3/4 cups ice cream

1 cup yogurt

Milk is available in the following forms:

whole milk

skim milk

evaporated milk

condensed milk

buttermilk

dried milk

Grain Group

- Select six to eleven servings daily.
- This group provides carbohydrates, thiamine, niacin, iron, and roughage (fiber).

Six to Eleven Servings Daily

breads: whole wheat, dark rye, enriched cornmeal, whole grain enriched, or oatmeal

rolls or biscuits made with whole wheat or enriched flour

flour: enriched, whole wheat, other whole grain

grits, enriched cereals: whole wheat, rolled oats, brown rice, converted rice, other cereals, if whole grain or restored

noodles, spaghetti, macaroni

Meat Group

- Select two to three servings daily.
- Alternate dried beans, peas, or nuts. These are incomplete protein foods.
- This group provides protein, some fat, iron, phosphorus, and B-complex vitamins.
- Choose low-fat items.
- Remove skin from poultry and trim fat from meat.

Two to Three Servings Daily

beef	goose, turkey
eggs	fish, shellfish
lamb	lunch meats, such as
game	bologna
veal	dried beans
pork (except bacon and fatback)	dried peas
	lentils
poultry: chicken, duck,	nuts

peanuts	soybeans
peanut butter	soya flour and grits

BASIC FACILITY DIETS

The food you will serve to patients in the health care facility will be prepared by the dietary department (Figure 25-2). It will include the essential nutrients. The way in which it is prepared and its consistency will depend on the individual patient's condition and needs. Sometimes very strict dietary control is needed.

The trays will usually be delivered to the patient floors in large food containers. Each tray will be labeled with the patient's name and type of diet. You will:

- Prepare the patient for the meal.
- Check the tray card for the patient's name.
- Check the tray card against the patient's armband.
- Serve the tray to the patient.
- Assist with feeding as necessary.

Health care facilities usually have many types of diets. Four common diets are:

- Regular or house, sometimes called a general diet (Figure 25-3)
- Full liquid
- Clear liquid
- Soft

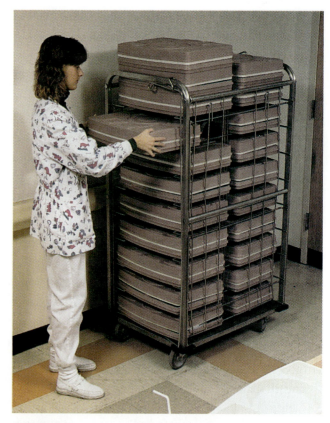

FIGURE 25-2 Patient diets are prepared in the dietary department.

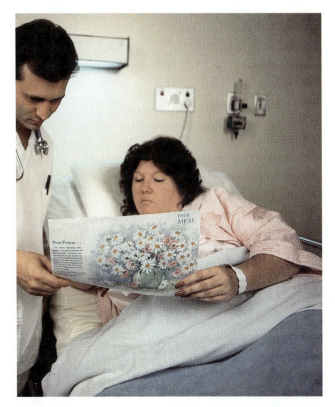

FIGURE 25-3 Patients on a house diet can select foods from a menu.

The progression of diets a patient is allowed following surgery is as follows:

1. Ice chips/sip of water
2. Clear liquids
3. Full liquids
4. Soft diet
5. Regular diet

In addition, the dietary department prepares special or **therapeutic** (treatment) **diets**. Therapeutic diets are discussed later in this unit.

Regular Diet

The regular-select or house diet is a normal or full diet based on the six food groups. The regular diet:

- Includes a great variety of foods.
- Excludes only very rich foods: pastries, heavy cakes, fried foods, and highly seasoned foods, which might be difficult for inactive people to digest.
- Has a lower caloric count, because an inactive person does not require as many calories as an active person.

In many health care facilities, patient may select foods from a menu.

Liquid Diets

Clear Liquid Diet. A **clear liquid diet** is a temporary diet because it is an inadequate diet. It is made up primarily of water and carbohydrates for energy. Feedings are given

every two, three, or four hours as prescribed by the physician. It replaces fluids that may have been lost by vomiting or diarrhea. When a clear liquid diet is held up to the light, you can see through it. The clear liquid diet consists of liquids that do not irritate, cause gas formation, or encourage bowel movements (**defecation**).

Foods allowed on the clear liquid diet include:

- Tea, coffee with sugar but without cream
- Strained fruit or vegetable juice with gelatin (occasionally)
- Fat-free meat broths
- Ginger ale (usually), 7Up®, Coke®, strained grape or apple juice
- Gelatin (occasionally)

Full Liquid Diet. The **full liquid diet** does supply nourishment and may be used for longer periods of time than the clear liquid diet. Six to eight ounces are usually given every two to three hours.

The full liquid diet is given to:

- Those with acute infections
- Patients who have difficulty chewing
- Those who have conditions that involve the digestive tract

The diet includes all of the foods allowed on the clear liquid diet, in addition to the following:

- Strained cereal (gruel)
- Strained soups
- Sherbet
- Gelatin
- Eggnog
- Malted milk
- Milk and cream
- Plain ice cream
- Strained vegetables and fruit juices
- Junket
- Solids that liquefy at room temperature
- Yogurt

Soft Diet

The **soft diet** usually follows the full liquid diet. Although this diet nourishes the body, between-meal feedings are sometimes given to increase calorie count. Foods allowed on the soft diet are:

- Low-residue, which are almost completely used by the body
- Mildly flavored, slightly seasoned, or unseasoned
- Prepared in a form that requires little digestion

The diet includes liquids and semisolid foods that have a soft texture and are easily digested (Figure 25-4). It is given to patients who:

- Have infections and fevers
- Have difficulty chewing

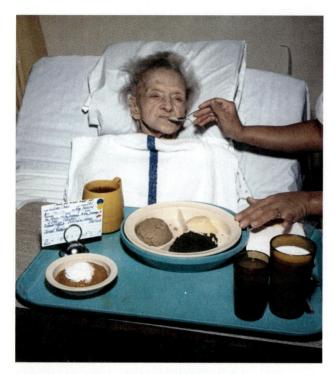

FIGURE 25-4 Soft diets include foods that require little chewing and are easy to digest.

- Have conditions that involve the digestive tract
- Are on a progressive postoperative dietary regime

The following foods are usually allowed on the soft diet:

- Soups
- Cream cheese and cottage cheese
- Crackers, toast
- Fish
- White meat of chicken or turkey (boiled or stewed)
- Fruit juices
- Cooked fruit (sieved)
- Tea, coffee
- Milk, cream, butter
- Cooked cereals
- Eggs (not fried)
- Beef and lamb (scraped or finely ground)
- Cooked vegetables (mashed or sieved)
- Angel or sponge cake
- Small amounts of sugar
- Gelatin, custard
- Pudding
- Plain ice cream

Foods to be avoided include:

- Coarse cereals
- Spices
- Gas-forming foods (onions, cabbage, beans)
- Rich pastries and desserts
- Foods high in roughage/fiber

- Fried foods
- Raw fruits and vegetables
- Corn
- Pork (except bacon)

SPECIAL DIETS

Special diets are planned to meet specific patient needs. Patients may need special diets because of religious preferences or health needs.

Religious Restrictions

Religious practice requires changes in diet for some patients. For example, persons of the conservative Jewish faith follow strict food laws.

- There are strict prohibitions against shellfish and nonkosher meats such as pork.
- Certain fishes, such as tuna and salmon, are permitted.
- Foods may not be prepared in utensils that have been used for nonkosher food preparation.
- There are strict rules regarding the sequence in which milk products and meat may be consumed.

Some other faith restrictions are summarized in Table 25-2.

Therapeutic Diets

Standard diets can be changed to conform to special dietary requirements. For example, an order might be written for a low-sodium soft diet when a patient has poor dentures and heart disease. These therapeutic diets are prepared for patients with individual health problems.

Commonly prescribed therapeutic diets include the diabetic diet, sodium-restricted diet, and low-fat diet.

The Diabetic Diet

Diet is an integral part of the therapy of the patient with diabetes mellitus. The diet is nutritionally adequate. It provides enough energy in the form of calories for a 24-hour period. Sometimes a proper diet is all that is needed to control the disease. Usually, however, the food intake is balanced by the administration of insulin or hypoglycemic drugs.

It is important for you to accurately evaluate and report the patient's intake. Foods and liquids have a major impact on diabetes management. Illness increases the need for insulin because the liver releases more glucose in response to the stress. Dehydration is a particularly serious problem for the diabetic. This can occur when not enough foods and fluids are taken in. Insulin administration may depend on your observations. Not all physicians prescribe dietary intake in the same way.

- Some physicians prescribe a very carefully balanced diet and insulin to maintain the level of blood sugar (glucose) within normal limits. All foods must be measured and repeated injections of insulin are required.
- Other physicians are much more liberal in their approach. They permit an unmeasured diet, limiting

TABLE 25-2 RELIGIOUS DIETARY PRACTICES

Faith	Coffee	Tea	Alcohol	Pork/Pork Products	Caffeine-Containing Foods	Dairy Products	All Meats
					Restricted Food		
Christian Science	•	•	•				
Roman Catholic							1 hour before communion, Ash Wednesday, Good Friday
Latter Day Saints (Mormons)	•	•	•		•		
Seventh Day Adventist	•	•	•	•	•		
Some Baptist	•	•	•				
Greek Orthodox (on fast days)						•	Fasting from meat and dairy products on Wed./Fri. during Lent and other holy days
Jewish Orthodox				• Also shellfish		Certain holy days	Forbids the serving of milk and milk products with meat; regulates food preparation; forbids cooking on the Sabbath
Moslem, Islamic		•	•	•			Fasting during Ramadan during day, feasting at night
Hindu							Some are vegetarians
Buddhist							Meat must be blessed and killed in special ways; some sects are vegetarians

only sugar and high-sugar foods. This diet is known as a no-concentrated-sweets diet. It may be balanced by insulin or hypoglycemic drugs.

- Many physicians treat diabetes with an approach that is midway between the preceding two methods. They prescribe the American Dietetic Association diets with specific calorie levels, such as the 1,200-calorie diet or the 1,500-calorie diet. The dietician teaches the patient about the diet and acts as a major resource for health care providers. The diet is balanced by insulin or hypoglycemic drugs.

The Exchange List. The exchange list method of balancing the diabetic diet:

- is based on standard household measurements to make it easier to measure.
- excludes sugar or high-sugar-content foods to prevent rapid swings in blood sugar.
- divides foods into six groups.

- allows equivalent exchanges to be made within a group but not from group to group.

The six groups are:

- Milk exchanges
- Vegetable exchange: Group A, Group B
- Fruit exchange
- Bread exchange
- Meat exchange
- Fat exchange

Sodium-Restricted Diet

Sodium-restricted diets may be ordered for patients with chronic renal failure and cardiovascular disease. Diets that are moderately, mildly, or severely restricted in sodium content may be prescribed. This latter diet is one of the most difficult for patients to follow. Processing may add significant levels of sodium to foods. This factor is considered in planning and selecting foods for the sodium-restricted diet. It is important to carefully read the labels for the contents of all commercially prepared foods.

Some foods naturally contain relatively large amounts of sodium. These foods may be restricted for this diet. They include:

- Meat
- Fish
- Poultry
- Milk and milk products
- Eggs

Avoid:

- Pork
- Potato chips
- Pop (soda)
- Pickles
- Processed meats
- Canned foods, such as vegetables and soups

Some foods are naturally low in sodium. They can be used more liberally. They are:

- Some cereals, such as shredded wheat
- Vegetables
- Fruits

Calorie-Restricted Diet

As long as activity remains constant, a person must take in approximately 500 calories a day less than usual (3,500 calories deficit per week) to lose one pound.

Calorie-restricted diets are prescribed for patients who are overweight. These diets are planned to meet general nutritional needs. They take into consideration the patient's energy output, general nutritional state, and weight goal.

In planning the calorie-restricted diet, the dietitian tries to create a realistic balance between fats, proteins, and carbohydrates. This type of diet encourages the patient to develop better, more consistent eating habits. Exact amounts of the three nutrients are not uniformly prescribed, but they may be balanced as follows:

- Proteins, 20%
- Fats, 25–35%
- Carbohydrates, 45–65%

Some physicians use a factor of 10 calories multiplied by the desired weight in calculating the daily calorie requirements. For example:

- Desired weight 120 lb. × 10 = 1,200 calories per day
- Desired weight 160 lb. × 10 = 1,600 calories per day

Low-Fat/Low-Cholesterol Diet

Low-fat/low-cholesterol diets are prescribed for patients who suffer from vascular, heart, liver, or gallbladder disease, and for those who have difficulty with fat metabolism. Fats are limited and calories are balanced by increasing proteins and carbohydrates. Foods are baked, roasted, or broiled, and the skin is removed from chicken. Low-fat foods include:

- Low-fat cottage cheese (no other allowed)
- Skim milk, buttermilk, yogurt
- Lean meats, fish, chicken
- Vegetables and fruits
- Jams, jellies, ices
- Cereals, pasta, bread, potatoes, rice
- Carbonated beverages, tea, coffee

SUPPLEMENTS AND NOURISHMENTS

Many patients receive a nutritional **supplement** or between-meal nourishments. Supplements are ordered by the physician and have a definite therapeutic value. Patients who have wounds may receive supplements high in protein to facilitate healing. These supplements may be liquid or in any form that is easy to eat and digest. It is essential that the patient consume the entire serving. Between-meal nourishments are snacks served to patients to provide the required nutrient daily intake or to prevent between-meal hunger.

Serving between-meal snacks and supplements is an important function of the nursing assistant (Figure 25-5). Between-meal nourishments are usually served:

- Midmorning—between 9:30 and 10:00 AM
- Midafternoon—between 2:30 and 3:00 PM
- At bedtime—between 8:00 and 10:00 PM

Snacks served include:

- Milk
- Juices

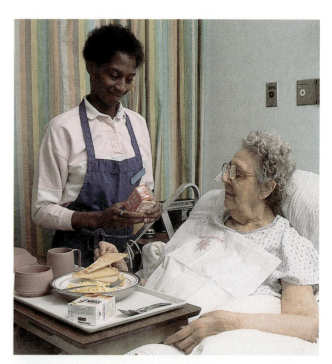

FIGURE 25-5 Nourishments are served between meals.

- Gelatin
- Custard
- Ice cream
- Sherbet
- High-protein drinks
- Fruits

The physician may order a commercial thickener for patients who have trouble swallowing. A thickener is a white powder that is mixed into liquids. The resulting consistency depends on the amount of powder that is added. It is important to add the amount that has been ordered.

To serve nourishments:

- Wash your hands.
- Check the nourishment list of each patient for any limitations or special dietary instructions.
- Allow patients to choose from the available nourishments whenever possible.
- Assist those who are unable to take their nourishment alone.
- Remember to pick up used glasses and dishes after the patient has finished and return them to the proper area.
- Notice what the patient was or was not able to take.
- Record on intake and output (I&O) sheet if required.

FLUID BALANCE

Fluid balance is the balance between liquid intake and liquid output. Because two-thirds of the body's weight is water, there must be a balance between the amount of fluid taken into the body and the amount lost under normal conditions. Generally, we do not need to concern ourselves about this balance. It usually takes care of itself.

The metric system is used for fluid measurements: milliliters (mL) or cubic centimeters (cc). A mL and a cc are the same amount. Table 25-3 provides a comparison of U.S. customary and metric measurements.

TABLE 25-3 COMPARISON OF U.S. CUSTOMARY AND METRIC MEASUREMENTS

U.S. Customary Units	Metric Units
1 minim	0.06 milliliter (mL)
16 minims	1 mL
1 ounce	30 mL
1 pint	500 mL
1 quart	1000 mL (1 liter)
2.2 pounds	1 kilogram (kg)
1 inch	2.5 centimeters (cm)
1 foot	30 cm

Intake

We take in approximately 2-1/2 quarts (2500 mL) of fluid daily:

- In liquids such as water, tea, and soft drinks
- In foods such as fruits and vegetables
- Artificially, such as by intravenous infusions or gavage.

Most adult patients will need to consume an average 600 to 800 mL of fluid during each eight-hour shift. Because patients may sleep during most of the night shift, additional fluids must be provided during waking hours to keep the body in balance. Excessive fluid retention is called edema. Inadequate fluid intake results in dehydration, or the lack of sufficient fluid in body tissues. Some disease conditions may change the amounts of fluid the patient is allowed to have.

Output

Typical output equals about 2-1/2 quarts daily in the form of:

- Urine, 1-1/2 quarts (1,500 mL)
- Perspiration
- Moisture from the lungs
- Moisture from the bowel

Excessive fluid loss results in dehydration. This can occur through:

- Diarrhea
- Vomiting
- Excessive urine output (diuresis)
- Excessive perspiration (diaphoresis)

Recording Intake and Output

An accurate recording of intake and output (I&O), or fluid taken in and given off by the body, is basic to the care of many patients. Intake and output records are kept when specifically ordered by the physician and when patients:

- are dehydrated.
- receive intravenous infusion.
- have recently had surgery.
- have a urinary catheter.
- are perspiring profusely or vomiting.
- have specific diagnoses such as congestive heart failure or renal disease that require accurate monitoring of I&O.

Fluid intake may need to be encouraged in some patients. This is called push fluids or force fluids. In some situations (as in kidney disease), fluid intake may have to be restricted.

Fluid intake and output is calculated by measuring and recording the fluids the patient takes in and the fluids the patient excretes (eliminates from the body) (Table 25-4). Because the fluids taken in by the patient cannot actually be measured, an estimate is made and recorded. This is done by:

- Knowing what the liquid container holds when full.

Note: Sizes of containers vary. Learn the fluid content of the containers used at your facility. Remember that there are 30 mL per ounce (240 mL ÷ 30 mL = 8 oz).

TABLE 25-4 COMPUTING INTAKE AND OUTPUT	
Intake	
IV	3,000 mL
By mouth	2,000 mL
Total	5,000 mL
Output	
Urine	2,000 mL
Vomitus	500 mL
Drainage	600 mL
Total	3,100 mL

- Coffee/tea cup, 8 oz = 240 mL
- Water carafe, 16 oz = 480 mL
- Foam cup, 8 oz = 240 mL
- Water glass, 8 oz = 240 mL
- Soup bowl, 6 oz = 180 mL
- Jello, 1 serving = 130 mL
- Ice chips, full 4 oz glass = 120 mL
- Estimating how much is gone from the container (what the patient drank), such as one-third of a glass of juice or half of a cup of coffee

- Converting this to mL

Example: A water glass holds 240 mL when filled. The patient drinks 3/4 of the glass of water. 3/4 × 240 = 180 mL. Intake for the glass of water is recorded as 180 mL. Fluids that are calculated and recorded include all liquids such as water, juices, soda, coffee, tea, milk, and soup. Also included are foods that melt at room temperature: ice cream, sherbet, and gelatin.

Note: Containers may vary from one facility to the next. Each facility should have a chart available that tells you what each size of glass, cup, and bowl holds when full.

Fluids taken by mouth, through intravenous infusion, or through gastric feeding are all recorded separately (Figure 25-6). At the end of each eight-hour shift and the end of 24 hours, the figures are totaled.

Fluid output is obtained by measuring all fluids excreted from the body. This includes urine, **emesis** (vomitus), and drainage from body cavities, such as gastric drainage. A container called a **graduate** is marked in mL or cc. The substance is poured into the graduate to determine the amount of output. Urine and any other excretion are recorded separately.

Note: Standard precautions must be followed when measuring any body excretion. Gloves are required for measuring all forms of output (Figure 25-7).

Date	Time	Method of Adm.	Solution	Intake Amounts Rec'd	Time	Output Urine Amount	Others Kind	Amount
7/16	0700	PO	water	120 mL		500 mL		
	0830	PO	coffee	240 mL				
			or. ju.	120 mL				
	1030	PO	cran.ju.	120 mL				
	1100					300 mL		
	1230	PO	tea	240 mL				
	1400	PO	water	150 mL				
Shift Totals	1500			990 mL		800 mL		
	1530	PO	gelatin	120 mL				
	1700	PO	tea	120 mL				
			soup	180 mL				
	2000					512 mL		
	2045						vomitus	500 mL
	2205						vomitus	90 mL
Shift Totals	2300			420 mL		512 mL		590 mL
	2345						vomitus	80 mL
	0130	IV	D/W	500 mL				
	0315					400 mL		
Shift Totals	0700			500 mL		400 mL		80 mL
24 Hour Totals				1910 mL		1712 mL		670 mL vomitus

FIGURE 25-6 Sample intake and output sheet

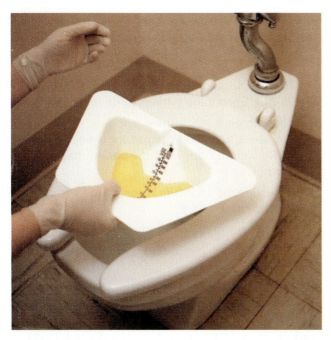

FIGURE 25-7 Gloves are required for measuring patient output.

CHANGING WATER

It is important to provide fresh water for patients, because water is essential to life. In all cases, you should know whether a patient is allowed ice or tap water and if water is to be especially encouraged. Even without an order to force fluids, you must encourage patients to take 6 to 8 glasses of fluids daily, unless the patient is NPO (nothing by mouth) or on restricted fluids. Give special attention to confused patients, patients who may not be able to reach a source of water, and the elderly. The need for adequate water intake cannot be overstressed. Because patients often do not drink enough water, sometimes the physician will leave orders that fluids are to be forced to a specific number of mL per day. Providing fresh water is one way to encourage the patient to increase intake of fluids. The procedure for providing fresh water varies greatly.

- In some hospitals, the water pitcher and glass are replaced with a new sterilized set each time water is provided.
- In others, the pitcher and glass are washed, refilled, and returned to the patient's bedside table.

In all cases, be sure you know whether a patient is allowed ice or tap water.

FEEDING THE PATIENT

Eating should be an enjoyable experience. (See Procedures 75 and 76.) Prepare the patient for his tray before it arrives by:

- Offering the bedpan or helping the patient to the bathroom.
- Assisting the patient to wash hands and face.
- Assisting with oral hygiene, if needed.
- Raising head of bed, if permitted, or assisting patient out of bed and into a chair, if permitted.
- Adjusting the in-bed patient's position with pillows.
- Clearing away anything that is unpleasant, such as emesis basin and bedpan.
- Clearing the overbed table.
- Encouraging the patient to do as much as possible.

When you have served the tray and after you have washed your hands, assist the patient as needed by:

- Being unhurried and pleasant.
- Opening pre-packaged items.
- Cutting meat.
- Pouring liquids.
- Buttering bread.
- Explaining the arrangement of the tray as if items were on the face of a clock, if patient cannot see.

There are times when you will be responsible for the entire feeding procedure.

 Note: Carry some extra straws with you during meal times. It can save you steps.

PROCEDURE **75**   OBRA

ASSISTING THE PATIENT WHO CAN FEED SELF

1. Carry out each beginning procedure action.
2. Assemble equipment:
   - bedpan/urinal
   - disposable gloves
   - wash water
   - oral hygiene items
   - tray of food
3. Offer bedpan/urinal. (If used, follow Procedure 72 in Unit 24—"Giving and Receiving the Bedpan.") Use standard

continues

PROCEDURE **75** *continued*

precautions if you anticipate contact with blood, body fluids, mucous membranes, or nonintact skin when assisting the patient with elimination or feeding.

4. If permitted, elevate head of bed or assist patient out of bed.

5. Provide washcloth to wash patient's hands and face.

6. Assist with oral hygiene or assist with dentures.

7. Remove and discard personal protective equipment, if used, according to facility policy.

8. Clear overbed table and position in front of patient (Figure 25-8A). Remove unpleasant equipment from sight.

9. Wash your hands. Obtain meal tray from dietary tray conveyor.

10. Check the diet with the dietary card and with the resident's identification band (Figure 25-8B).

11. Place tray on overbed table and arrange food in a convenient manner.

12. Assist in food preparation as needed (Figure 25-8C). Encourage patient to do as much as possible.

13. Remove tray as soon as patient is finished. Make sure to note what the patient has and has not eaten.

14. Record fluids on intake record, if necessary. Record food intake.

15. Push overbed table out of the way.

16. Carry out each procedure completion action.

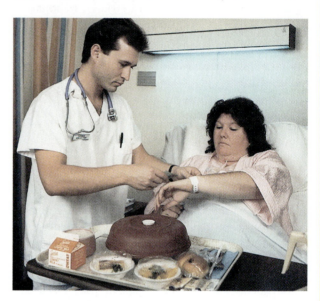

FIGURE 25-8B Check patient's arm band against tray card.

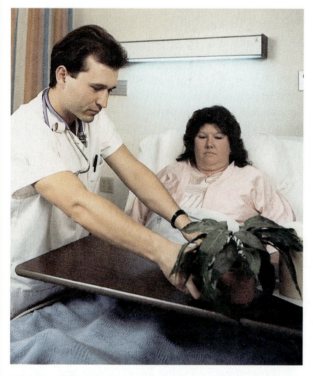

FIGURE 25-8A Patients eat better when properly prepared for their meal. Prepare overbed table for the meal tray.

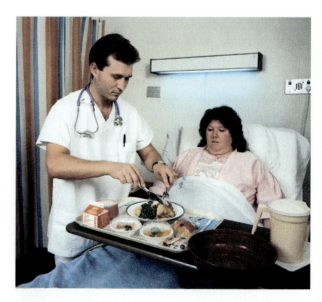

FIGURE 25-8C Assist patient in food preparation as needed.

PROCEDURE **76** OBRA

FEEDING THE DEPENDENT PATIENT

1. Carry out each beginning procedure action.

2. Assemble equipment:
   - bedpan/urinal
   - wash water
   - oral hygiene items
   - tray of food

3. Offer bedpan or urinal. (If used, follow Procedure 72 in Unit 24—"Giving and Receiving the Bedpan.") Follow standard precautions.

4. Provide oral hygiene, if desired.

5. Remove unnecessary articles from the overbed table.

6. Elevate head of bed with patient's head slightly bent forward.

7. Place towel or protector under patient's chin (Figure 25-9A).

8. Obtain meal tray and check diet against patient's identification band and dietary card.

9. Place tray on overbed table (Figure 25-9B).

10. Butter bread and cut meat. Do not pour hot beverage until patient is ready for it.

11. Use different drinking straws to give each fluid, or use a cup. Thick fluids are more easily controlled by using a straw. Use adaptive devices as indicated on care plan.

12. Sit down while you are feeding the patient, so you are at eye level.

13. Holding spoon at a right angle:
    - Give solid foods from point of spoon (Figure 25-9C).
    - Alternate solids and liquids.
    - Ask the patient in what order she would like the food.
    - Describe or show patient what kind of food you are giving.
    - If patient has had a stroke, direct food to unaffected side and check for food stored in affected side. Watch patient's throat to check for swallowing.
    - Test hot foods by dropping a small amount on the inside of your wrist before feeding them to patient.
    - Never blow on patient's food to cool it.
    - Never taste patient's food.
    - Do not hurry the meal.

14. Allow patient to assist to the extent that patient is able.

15. Use napkin to wipe patient's mouth as often as necessary.

16. Remove tray as soon as patient is finished. Record percentage of food eaten. Record fluid intake.

17. Carry out each procedure completion action.

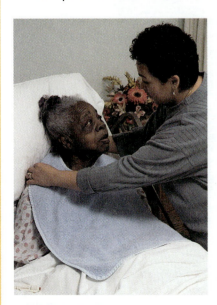

FIGURE 25-9A Place a towel or protector over patient.

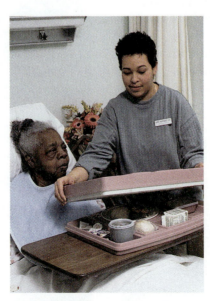

FIGURE 25-9B Uncover food and arrange on overbed table.

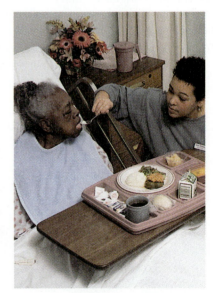

FIGURE 25-9C Give solid foods from the tip of the spoon.

ALTERNATIVE NUTRITION

There may be situations in which the patient is unable to take in food in the usual way. This may occur if the patient:

- is unconscious.
- has a disease of the digestive tract.
- has persistent vomiting and cannot hold down food.
- is unable to swallow without **aspiration** (choking).

To maintain life, the body must meet its requirements for daily essential nutrients. This may be done by:

- administration of **total parenteral nutrition** (**TPN**) (also called **hyperalimentation**), which is a form of **intravenous infusion** (**IV**), or by
- **enteral feedings** (tubes inserted into digestive tract).

Total Parenteral Nutrition

TPN is a technique in which high-density (concentrated) nutrients are introduced into a large vein such as the subclavian or the superior vena cava. This method of feeding is used for patients with diseases of the digestive tract. Caring for patients with TPN is discussed in Unit 34 (Subacute Care).

Enteral Feedings

Enteral feedings may be administered by a tube that is

- Inserted through the nose and into the stomach (**nasogastric** or **NG feeding**) (Figure 25-10).
- Inserted directly through the abdominal skin and into the stomach (**gastrostomy feeding**) (Figure 25-11).

Many different types of tubes may be used for these feedings. The nurse or physician inserts the feeding tube. Specially prepared solutions contain all the nutrients required by the body. The feeding may be administered intermittently or it may run continuously. In either case, the container of solution is hung from an IV (intravenous) pole and is usually attached to a device that automatically controls the administration (Figure 25-12).

When caring for the patient with tube feedings, you need to:

- Keep the head of the bed elevated 45° to 60° during feeding and for half an hour after feeding.

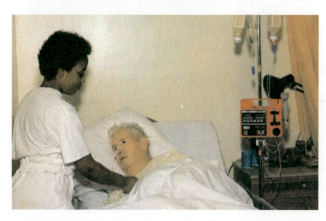

FIGURE 25-10 An NG tube is inserted through the nose and into the stomach.

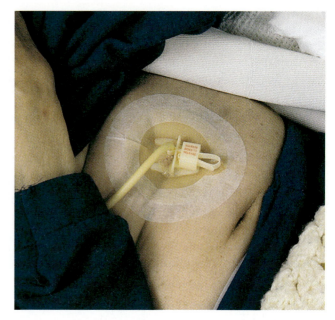

FIGURE 25-11 Gastrostomy tubes are inserted through the skin and directly into the stomach.

- Check the taping of tubes. If tape is loose, or pulls, or is causing skin irritation, inform the nurse.
- Report any retching, nausea, or vomiting immediately.
- Check tubing for kinks. Be sure patient is not lying on tubing.
- Provide frequent mouth hygiene.
- Notify nurse if controlling device alarm sounds.

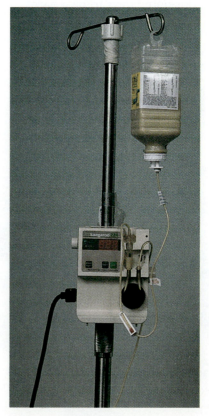

FIGURE 25-12 Enteral feedings are usually controlled by a device that sets off a warning signal if problems arise.

REVIEW

A. True/False.

Mark the following true or false by circling T or F.

1. T F Vitamins are nutrients that help regulate body activities.

2. T F The exchange lists are used by patients on low-salt diets.

3. T F Fats are one of the six essential nutrients.

4. T F Ice cream would be served to a patient on a clear liquid diet.

5. T F Labels of canned foods must be checked when planning their use in low-sodium diets.

6. T F A gastrostomy tube introduces nutrients directly into the stomach.

7. T F Carbohydrate foods are used to make new body cells and build tissues.

8. T F Green leafy vegetables are a good source of calcium, iron, and B vitamins.

9. T F Complete protein foods like poultry contain all of the essential amino acids.

B. Matching.

Match the correct term from Column II with the words and phrases in Column I.

Column I

10. _____ calcium

11. _____ roughage

12. _____ encourage liquid intake

13. _____ all the processes involved in taking in food and building and repairing the body

14. _____ treatment

Column II

a. therapeutic

b. mineral

c. nutrition

d. forcing fluids

e. cellulose

f. vitamin

C. Multiple Choice.

Select the one best answer for each question.

15. Feeding the patient through a nasogastric tube is known as a/an
    a. intravenous infusion.
    b. gastrostomy feeding.
    c. gavage.
    d. lavage.

16. Which of the following is a water-soluble vitamin?
    a. Vitamin C
    b. Vitamin E
    c. Vitamin A
    d. Vitamin D

17. An example of a fat-soluble vitamin is
    a. vitamin C.
    b. vitamin B-complex.
    c. vitamin D.
    d. vitamin N.

18. An average serving of meat is
    a. 1 ounce.
    b. 3 to 4 ounces.
    c. 8 ounces.
    d. 16 ounces.

19. Which of the following is part of the meat group?
    a. Peas
    b. Nuts
    c. Poultry
    d. All of these

20. Foods naturally high in sodium include
    a. milk.
    b. cereals.
    c. vegetables.
    d. fruits.

21. Supplemental nourishments might include
    a. hot fudge sundaes.
    b. mashed potatoes.
    c. scrambled eggs.
    d. high-protein drinks.

22. A serving of cooked vegetables would be approximately
    a. 1/2 cup.
    b. 3/4 cup.
    c. 1 cup.
    d. 1-1/2 cups.

23. It is especially important to report to the nurse that the patient only ate two-thirds of her meal when the patient is on a
    a. low-salt diet.
    b. calorie-restricted diet.
    c. diabetic diet.
    d. house diet.

D. Nursing Assistant Challenge.

Mrs. Gole is one of your assigned patients. She is 72 years old, is on a 1,500-calorie diabetic diet, and is a member of the Seventh Day Adventist Church. She also has Parkinson's disease with tremors of her hands, and occasionally has trouble swallowing. Mrs. Gole sometimes eats food brought in by family and friends that is not on the 1,500-calorie diet. Consider Mrs. Gole's care:

24. Discuss safety issues that you need to think about when Mrs. Gole is eating.

25. Are there conflicts between the ordered diet and the dietary restrictions of her church? If so, what are the conflicts and how might they be resolved?

26. Do you anticipate that Mrs. Gole will have any problems feeding herself? If so, what are those problems, and what can you do to help her eat independently?

27. Discuss the issues of Residents' or Patients' Rights and the conflict between her desire to eat more food and what the physician has prescribed.

SECTION 9

Special Care Procedures

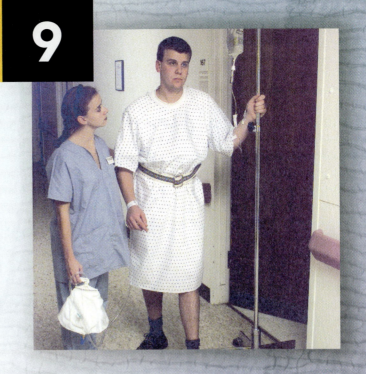

UNIT 26
Warm and Cold Applications

UNIT 27
Assisting with the Physical Examination

UNIT 28
The Surgical Patient

UNIT 29
Caring for the Emotionally Stressed Patient

UNIT 30
Death and Dying

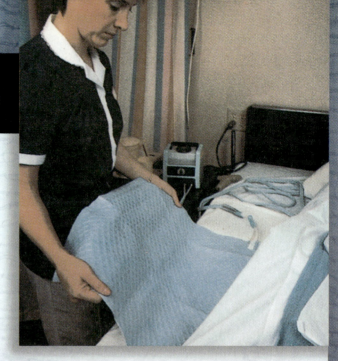

UNIT 26

Warm and Cold Applications

OBJECTIVES

As a result of this unit, you will be able to:

- Spell and define terms.
- List the physical conditions requiring the use of heat and cold.
- Name types of heat and cold applications.
- Describe the effects of local cold applications.
- Describe the effects of local heat applications.
- List safety concerns related to application of heat and cold.

- Demonstrate the following procedures:
  - Procedure 77 Applying an Ice Bag
  - Procedure 78 Applying a Disposable Cold Pack
  - Procedure 79 Applying an Aquamatic K-Pad®
  - Procedure 80 Performing a Warm Soak
  - Procedure 81 Applying a Warm Moist Compress
  - Procedure 82 Assisting with Application of a Hypothermia Blanket

VOCABULARY

Learn the meaning and the correct spelling of the following words and phrases:

Aquamatic K-Pad®	hypothermia	ice bag	vasodilation
diathermy	hypothermia-	thermal blanket	warm soak
hemorrhage	hyperthermia blanket	vasoconstriction	wet compress

INTRODUCTION

Heat and cold applications are used only on written orders from the physician or nurse for a specific length of time. Some facilities allow only professional personnel to apply heat and cold. **Some states have laws against nursing assistants applying heat or cold in a home health setting**. In other facilities, nursing assistants who have been specially trained are permitted to carry out these procedures under the supervision of the nurse. Be sure you know and follow the policy of your facility and are adequately prepared and *supervised*.

THERAPY WITH HEAT AND COLD

The physician orders the use of heat or cold applications to:
- relieve pain.
- combat local infection, swelling, or inflammation.
- control bleeding (**hemorrhage**).
- reduce body temperature.

Local applications of heat and cold are made with:
- Ice bags.
- Electronically operated Aquamatic K-Pads®. K-Pads® come in many shapes and sizes. They can be used to apply dry heat. By using an attachment, they can also be used for cooling.
- Pre-packaged, single-use units for the application of hot and cold. A single hit on the surface activates the contents, providing a controlled temperature.
- Gel packs that can be cooled or heated as needed.

General treatments of heat and cold consist of thermal mattresses known as **hypothermia-hyperthermia blankets**. These are widely used to:
- lower body temperature when there is fever.
- elevate body temperature in cases of hypothermia.

Applications of warm and cold may be either dry or moist. Moisture makes both heat and cold more penetrating. Therefore, moist heat or moist cold is more likely to cause injury. Extra care must be taken to protect the patient when moist treatments are used. Be sure you know:
- Exact method to be used
- Correct temperature and placement
- Proper length of time the warm or cold application is to be performed
- How often the area being treated is to be checked

Table 26-1 summarizes types of warm and cold applications.

Commercial Preparations

Easy-to-use commercial warm and cold packs are available for dry applications. For one type of pack, a single hit or blow to the pack before application activates it. The pack is discarded after one use. Reusable packs are also available, but infection control issues make them less desirable.

TABLE 26-1 WARM AND COLD APPLICATIONS

Dry Warm Applications	Dry Cold Applications
Aquamatic K-Pad®	Ice cap
Disposable warm pack	Ice bag
Electric heating pads	Disposable cold pack
	Aquamatic K-Pad®
	Hypothermia blanket
Moist Warm Applications	**Moist Cold Applications**
Warm soaks	Compresses
Compresses	Soaks
Tub baths	Packs
Sitz baths	

GUIDELINES *for*

Warm and Cold Treatments

You must be very watchful when applying cold or warm treatments. When assigned to this task, keep in mind the following:
- The age and condition of the patient. Give extra care to:
  - Young children
  - The aged
  - Patients with cognitive impairment
  - Patients who are uncooperative
  - Patients who are unconscious
  - Patients who are paralyzed
  - Patients with tissue damage
  - Patients with poor circulation
- An electric heating pad must not be used with moist dressings unless a rubber cover is placed over the pad. If the wires become damp, a short circuit may result. The patient must not lie on the pad, because severe burns can result. Sensitivity to heat varies, so patients receiving heat treatments must be checked frequently. Although heating pads are not used in health care facilities, they are used by individuals in homes.
- Heat is not applied to the head because it could make blood vessels in the area dilate, causing headaches.
- Heat should not be applied to the abdomen

continues

GUIDELINES
continued

if there is any chance that the patient has appendicitis, because it would increase the chance of the appendix rupturing.

- Areas where cold treatments are used should be carefully and frequently checked for discoloration and numbness. If the area is discolored or numb, discontinue the treatment and report to the nurse.
- Rubber or plastic should never touch the patient's skin. Be sure all appliances are covered with cloth.

USE OF COLD APPLICATIONS

Applications of cold are given only with a physician's order. The application of cold:

- Constricts or decreases the size of blood vessels (vaso-constriction) and reduces swelling
- Decreases sensitivity to pain
- Reduces temperature
- Slows inflammation
- Reduces itching

Cautions

Remember, moisture intensifies the effect of cold just as it does heat. Caution must be used in the application of moist cold.

- Excessive cold can damage body tissues.
- Report color changes such as *blanching* (turning white) or *cyanosis* (becoming bluish).
- Report feelings of numbness or discomfort experienced by patient.
- Stop the cold treatment if the patient starts to shiver. Cover the patient with a blanket and report immediately to the nurse.

(See Procedures 77 and 78.)

Dry Cold Applications

There are several methods for applying therapeutic cold. Careful attention to the application is needed to prevent injury.

- **Disposable cold pack**—This single-use commercial pack can be stored until needed. Reusable commercial packs are also available (for both warm and cold applications). The pack remains effective for approximately 15 to 30 minutes. If the cold pack must be activated, follow the manufacturer's instructions exactly. When activating the pack, do not hold it in front of your face. If the pack leaks or bursts, the chemicals inside the pack may splash. Check the area being treated every 10 minutes.
- **Ice bag**—This reusable, waterproof, canvas container can be filled with ice to provide temporary local cold. An ice bag is never placed directly on the affected area because the weight of the bag will cause the patient discomfort.
- **Thermal blanket**—This is a large, fluid-filled blanket that is placed over or around the patient. The temperature of the fluid in the blanket may be raised or lowered. The blanket is used to lower or raise the patient's body temperature. However, it is most often used in care facilities to lower the body temperature. This process is called inducing **hypothermia**. A licensed professional usually monitors the use of this type of blanket.

Moist Cold Applications

- **Wet compresses** are moistened with a solution and placed on the affected area.
- A syringe may be used to add water to the compresses to keep them moist.
- The compresses can be kept cold by placing a covered ice bag against the affected area.
- Each time the pad is removed and replaced, be careful to reposition the protective covering.

Follow facility policy for:

- method of applying the treatment.
- length of time treatment is to be applied.
- how often patient is to be checked for condition of skin in the treatment area and general response to the treatment.
- signs that treatment should be discontinued.

PROCEDURE | **77**

APPLYING AN ICE BAG

1. Assemble equipment:
   - ice bag
   - cover (usually cotton, such as a towel, or cover specified by your facility)
   - paper towels
   - spoon or similar utensil
   - ice cubes or crushed ice
2. Prepare ice bag as follows:

continues

a. Fill ice bag with cold water and check for leaks.

b. Empty the bag.

c. If ice cubes are used, rinse them in water to remove sharp edges. The use of crushed ice makes the bag more flexible and is more comfortable for the patient.

d. Fill ice bag half full, using ice scooper, paper cup, or large spoon (Figure 26-1). Avoid making ice bags too heavy. Do not allow scoop to touch ice bag.

e. To remove air from ice bag:

- Rest ice bag flat on a paper towel on a flat surface.
- Put top in place, but do not screw on.
- Press bag until air is removed (Figure 26-2).

f. Fasten top securely.

g. Test for leakage.

h. Wipe dry with paper towels. Place in cloth cover.

Note: As an alternative, a gel pack stored in the freezer can be used for cold applications. These packs can be refrozen and reused if this is facility policy.

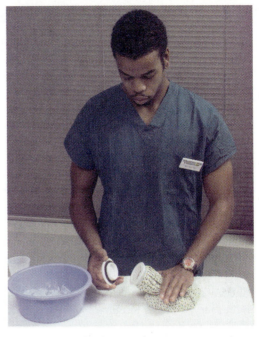

FIGURE 26-2 With the ice bag on a towel on the overbed table, press the bag gently with your flat hand to remove the air.

3. Take equipment to bedside on tray. Carry out each beginning procedure action.

4. Apply ice bag to the affected part.

5. Refill ice bag before all ice is melted.

6. Check skin area under ice bag every 10 minutes. Report to supervising nurse immediately if skin is discolored or white or if patient reports that skin is numb.

7. Continue the cold application for the amount of time specified by your supervisor. If patient feels cold, cover with a blanket, but do not cover the area being treated.

8. Carry out each procedure completion action.

9. When the treatment is complete, wash the bag with soap and water, rinse, dry completely, and then screw top on. Wipe with a disinfectant if this is your facility policy. Leave air in ice bag to prevent sides from sticking together.

10. If a reusable cold pack is used, wash it thoroughly with soap and water or wipe with a disinfectant, according to facility policy. Return pack to the refrigerator. Discard a disposable pack.

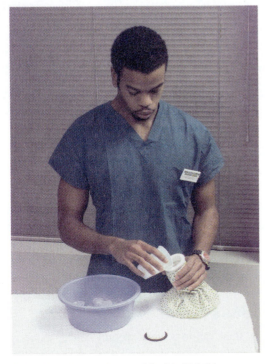

FIGURE 26-1 The ice bag is filled half full.

APPLYING A DISPOSABLE COLD PACK

1. Carry out each beginning procedure action.

2. Assemble equipment:
   - disposable commercial cold pack
   - cloth covering (towel, warm water bag cover, or other cover specified by the facility)
   - tape or rolls of gauze

3. Expose area to be treated. Note condition of area.

4. Place cold pack in cloth covering (Figure 26-3).

5. Strike or squeeze cold pack to activate chemicals. (Follow manufacturer's instructions.)

6. Place covered cold pack on proper area and cover with a towel (Figure 26-4). Note time of application.

7. Secure cover with tape or gauze, if necessary, to hold in place.

8. Leave patient in comfortable position with signal cord within easy reach.

9. Return to bedside every 10 minutes. Check area being treated for discoloration or numbness. If these signs and symptoms occur, discontinue treatment and report them to your supervisor.

10. If no adverse symptoms occur, remove pack in 30 minutes, or after the amount of time given in your instructions. Note condition of area. Continuous treatment requires application of a fresh pack.

11. Remove pack from cover and discard according to facility policy. Return unused gauze and tape.

12. Put cover in laundry hamper.

13. Carry out each procedure completion action.

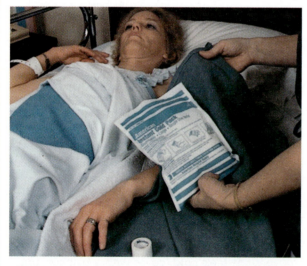

FIGURE 26-3 Cover the disposable cold pack with a towel before applying it to the patient.

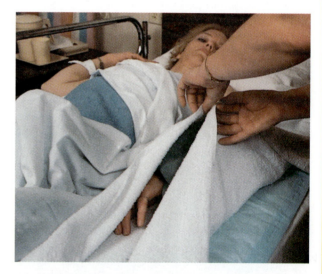

FIGURE 26-4 Once the cold pack is in place, cover the entire application with a towel.

USE OF WARM APPLICATIONS

Warm applications are ordered to:
- relieve muscle spasms.
- reduce pain.
- promote healing.
- combat local infection.
- improve mobility before exercise periods.
- soothe the patient.

The value of heat treatments (**diathermy**) is that heat dilates or increases the size of blood vessels (**vasodilation**). This brings more blood to the area to promote healing. Warmth is very soothing when there is pain.

There must be a specific order for a warm application. Some groups of people require extra care when they receive warm applications. (See Procedures 79 to 81.)

Cautions

Follow these cautions when working with patients:
- Constant warmth must be carefully monitored.
- Moisture intensifies the effect of warmth. Use extra caution.

- Never allow a patient to lie on a constant heat unit, because heat may be trapped and build up to dangerous levels.
- Temperature of a constant heat unit should be between 95° and 100°F.
- Always use a bath thermometer to check solution temperatures.
- Always remove the body part being soaked before adding warm solution.
- Always stay with the patient during the treatment.
- Protect areas not being treated from excessive exposure.
- Warmth is not applied to the head because it could cause blood vessels in the area to dilate, resulting in headaches.
- Rubber or plastic should never touch the patient's skin. Be sure all appliances are covered with cloth.

Dry Warm Applications

The **Aquamatic K-Pad®** is commonly used to provide dry warmth. It consists of a plastic pad with fluid-filled coils and a control unit that maintains a constant temperature of the fluid. The fluid in the pad is distilled water that is supplied from a reservoir in the control unit. The control unit is placed on the bedside stand and is plugged into an electrical outlet. In most facilities, the temperature is preset by the central supply department. The temperature is usually set at 95° to 100°F.

Moist Warm Applications

 Remember: Moisture intensifies heat and you must use extra care. For each of the warm treatments, follow the facility policy for:

- method of applying the treatment.
- length of time treatment is to be applied.
- how often patient is to be checked for condition of skin in the treatment area and general response to the treatment.
- signs that treatment should be discontinued.

Moist warm treatments include:

- **Warm soaks**—The patient, or the part of the patient's body that is being treated, is immersed in a tub filled with water at a specific temperature, usually 105°.
- **Wet compresses**—The same cautions apply to warm compresses as to cold compresses. They may be kept wet with a syringe and warm by covering them with an Aquamatic K-Pad®.

APPLYING AN AQUAMATIC K-PAD®

1. Carry out each beginning procedure action.
2. Assemble equipment:
   - K-Pad® and control unit
   - distilled water
   - covering for pad
3. Check the cord for frayed or damaged insulation. Also check that the tubing between the control unit and the pad is intact.
4. Place the control unit on the bedside stand (Figure 26-5).
5. Remove the cover of the control unit and check the level of the distilled water. If it is low, fill the unit two-thirds full or to the fill line using distilled water. Tilt the unit back and forth gently to clear the tubing of air.
6. Screw the cover in place and loosen it one-quarter turn.
7. If the temperature was not preset, check with the nurse for the proper setting before turning on the unit. Remove the key after setting the temperature.
8. Plug in the unit.

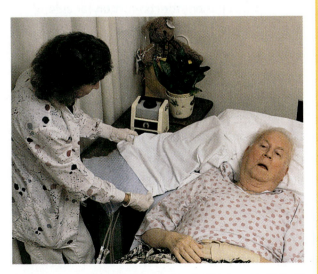

FIGURE 26-5 The control unit for the Aquamatic K-Pad® maintains a steady temperature.

continues

PROCEDURE   79   *continued*

9. Cover pad with an appropriate cover, according to facility policy or as specified by the manufacturer of the unit. Do not use pins to hold the cover in place.

10. Expose the area on patient to be treated. Place the covered pad on patient and note the time.

   ● Be sure the tubing between the control unit and the pad does not hang over the side of the bed. It should be coiled on the bed to promote the flow of liquid.

11. Following facility policy, periodically check the skin under the pad.

12. Check the level of the water in the control unit. Refill if necessary to the fill line.

13. Remove the pad after the prescribed amount of time.

14. Carry out each procedure completion action.

PROCEDURE   80

PERFORMING A WARM SOAK

1. Carry out each beginning procedure action.

2. Assemble equipment:
   ● bath thermometer
   ● soak basin
   ● pitcher
   ● large plastic sheet
   ● bath towel
   ● bath blanket

3. Bring equipment to bedside.

4. Cover patient with bath blanket.

5. Fanfold bedding to foot of bed.

6. Expose limb to be soaked.

7. Position patient for comfort on far side of bed (opposite the part to be soaked). Be sure side rail is up and secure.

8. Cover bed with plastic sheet and towel.

9. Fill soak basin half full with water at prescribed temperature (usually 105°F). Check temperature with bath thermometer.

10. Take soak basin from overbed table and position on bed protector.

11. Assist patient to gradually place limb in basin (Figure 26-6).

12. Check temperature every 5 minutes. Use pitcher to get additional water and add to soak basin to maintain temperature. Remember to remove patient's limb before adding water.

13. Discontinue procedure at end of prescribed time.

   a. Lift patient's limb out of basin.

   b. Slip basin forward and allow limb to rest on bath towel.

   c. Place basin on overbed table. Gently pat limb dry with towel.

14. Remove plastic sheet and towel.

15. Adjust bedding and remove bath blanket. If treatment is to be repeated, fold bath blanket and place in bedside stand. Leave unit tidy and call bell within reach.

16. Lower head of bed and make patient comfortable.

17. Take equipment to utility room. Clean and store according to facility policy.

18. Carry out each procedure completion action.

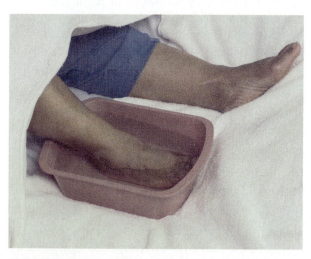

FIGURE 26-6 The patient is receiving warm soak therapy.

PROCEDURE   **81**

APPLYING A WARM MOIST COMPRESS

1. Carry out each beginning procedure action.

2. Assemble equipment:
   - disposable gloves
   - syringe
   - bed protector
   - compresses
   - bath thermometer
   - binder or towel
   - pins or bandage
   - basin with prescribed solution at temperature ordered

3. Bring equipment to bedside.

4. Expose only the area to be treated.

5. Protect bed and patient's clothing with bed protector (Figure 26-7A).

6. Put on disposable gloves.

7. Moisten the compresses; remove excess liquid (Figure 26-7B). Apply to treatment area (Figure 26-7C).

8. Secure the dressings with bandage or binder. Dressing must be in contact with skin.

9. Help patient to maintain a comfortable position throughout the treatment.

10. Unscreen unit. Leave unit neat and tidy with signal cord within easy reach.

11. Maintain proper temperature and moisture.
    - If dressings are to be kept warm, a K-Pad® may be applied.
    - If dressings are to be kept cool, an ice bag may be applied.
    - A syringe may be used to apply more solution to keep dressings wet.

12. Remove dressings when ordered. Change as ordered or once in 24 hours. Check skin several times each day.

13. Discard compresses.

14. Remove and dispose of gloves according to facility policy.

15. Carry out each procedure completion action.

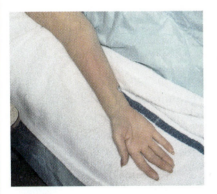

FIGURE 26-7A Protect bed with a towel or other protector.

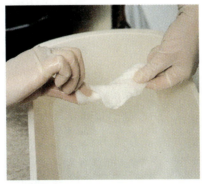

FIGURE 26-7B Dip compress into basin of water (105°F). Grasping edges, squeeze out excess liquid.

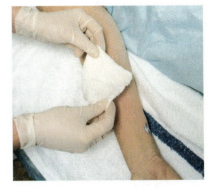

FIGURE 26-7C Apply open compress to inflamed area.

TEMPERATURE CONTROL MEASURES

Excessively high or low body temperatures are treated in acute care facilities by placing hypothermia-hyperthermia blankets (Figure 26-8) over and under the patient. These blankets are units filled with water. The temperature of the water can be adjusted higher or lower depending on whether the patient's body temperature is to be raised or lowered. This is a professional nursing responsibility. (See Procedure 82.)

Hypothermia

Hypothermia is a drop in core body temperature below 95°F (35°C) rectally. This can occur:

- when people are exposed to cold without adequate protection.

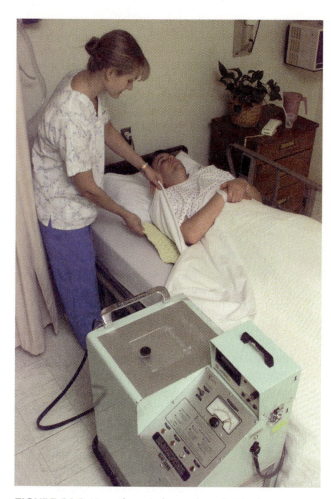

FIGURE 26-8 Hypothermia-hyperthermia blanket

- in the elderly, when a person is exposed to external temperatures as warm as 60°F.
- as deliberately induced before surgery to slow body metabolism.

Indications of hypothermia to report include:

- Drop in body temperature
- Poor coordination and confusion
- Slurred speech
- Decreased respiratory and heart rates

Nursing Assistant Actions

- Report observations to the supervisor.
- Check the environmental temperature and adjust it.
- Provide external warmth with a sweater or blanket.
- Reduce drafts with screens or curtains.
- If permitted, give something warm to drink.
- Check vital signs.

Hyperthermia

Hyperthermia is an elevation of core body temperature to 104°F (40°C) rectally or higher. This can occur:

- when a person is exposed to high external temperature.
- with serious injuries such as burns.
- when there is damage to the temperature control center in the brain.
- with infections.

Indications of hyperthermia to report include:

- Elevated body temperature
- Hot, flushed skin
- Faintness
- Headache
- Nausea
- Convulsions

Fever or *pyrexia* is when core body temperature rises to at least 101°F (rectally). Fever is often associated with infections, injury, surgery, and serious trauma. Indications of fever are the same as those for general hyperthermia.

Note: In children, temperatures tend to rise higher than in adults. This puts children at greater risk for seizures.

Nursing Assistant Actions

- Report observations to the supervisor.
- Check environment temperature and adjust it.
- Reduce external warmth. Cover the patient only with a gown or sheet.
- If permitted, give cooling drink.
- Carry out cooling procedures as ordered. For example, give cooling baths or enemas.
- Check vital signs frequently.

PROCEDURE 82

ASSISTING WITH APPLICATION OF A HYPOTHERMIA BLANKET

Applying a hypothermia blanket and monitoring a patient receiving a hypothermia treatment is a professional nursing responsibility. The nurse will supervise the procedure and monitor the patient throughout the treatment. The nurse will check the specific gravity of the patient's urine, vital signs, and nervous system response. The nursing assistant may be asked to assist in setting up equipment, positioning the patient and the thermal blanket, observing the patient during the treatment, and keeping the patient comfortable. In addition, the nursing assistant may be asked to transport equipment to and from the central supply service.

1. Wash hands, collect equipment, and take equipment to bedside.

2. Assemble equipment:
   - disposable gloves
   - hypothermia-hyperthermia control unit
   - fluid for control unit
   - thermometer probes (rectal or skin)
   - adhesive tape
   - sphygmomanometer
   - stethoscope
   - hypothermia-hyperthermia blanket (disposable or reusable), one or two as ordered
   - bath blanket or sheet, one or two as ordered
   - lanolin-based skin cream

3. Follow manufacturer's directions for setting up the equipment. Check equipment for safety. Be sure the control unit is grounded.

4. Connect blanket(s) to control unit and set control.

5. Turn on control unit and add liquid.

6. Allow blanket(s) to precool as you prepare patient.

7. Carry out each beginning procedure action.

8. Place patient in hospital-type gown with ties.

9. Measure vital signs and record.

10. Place hypothermia-hyperthermia blanket on bed and cover with sheet. Position patient on the sheet-covered thermal blanket in the recumbent position, with head on pillow that does not touch blanket.

11. Wash hands. Put on gloves.

12. Insert rectal thermometer probe into rectum (unless contraindicated) and tape in place. (Alternatively, place skin probe into axilla and tape in place.)

13. Plug end of probe into proper jack on control panel.

14. Place second sheet over patient and place second thermal blanket over sheet, if ordered.

15. Apply lanolin-based cream to patient's skin where it contacts the blanket.

16. Remove gloves. Discard according to facility policy. Wash hands.

17. Monitor vital signs, neurologic response, and intake and output every 5 minutes until desired body temperature is reached, and then every 15 minutes as ordered.

18. Report color changes in skin or excessive shivering.

19. Patient should be repositioned every 30 minutes to 1 hour. Reapply skin cream as necessary. Covering sheets should be changed if they become moist. Put on gloves each time you care for patient. At the end of care, remove gloves, discard according to facility policy, and wash hands.

20. At completion of treatment, follow manufacturer's instructions for turning off unit, disconnecting blanket(s), and returning them to storage.

21. Put on gloves. Continue to monitor patient as you remove the equipment.

22. Replace any damp bedding or garments and cover patient. Continue to monitor patient every 30 minutes until stable for 2 hours.

23. Clean thermometer probe and store according to facility policy.

24. Remove gloves and discard according to facility policy.

25. Carry out each procedure completion action.

REVIEW

A. True/False.

Mark the following true or false by circling T or F.

1. T F Heat and cold treatments should be supervised by the nurse.

2. T F If a patient has a possible diagnosis of appendicitis, heat should not be applied to the abdomen.

3. T F The temperature of a warm soak solution should be approximately 100°F.

4. T F Special blankets used to alter the patient's temperature are called infrared blankets.

5. T F A patient who is unconscious must receive special attention during a heat treatment.

6. T F Hyperthermia is an elevation of core body temperature to below 95°F.

7. T F Heat is frequently applied to the head.

8. T F When charting an application of cold, always include the length of time of the application.

9. T F Aquamatic K-Pads® are usually set at 115°F.

B. Multiple Choice.

Select the one best answer for each question.

10. Heat affects the body by
    a. causing vasodilation.
    b. increasing blood supply to the area.
    c. promoting healing.
    d. All of these.

11. Special care with heat and cold treatments must be taken when the patient is
    a. aged.
    b. very young.
    c. uncooperative.
    d. All of these.

12. Dry cold is provided by
    a. compresses.
    b. hyperthermia blanket.
    c. ice caps.
    d. soaks.

13. Cold affects the body by
    a. reducing pain sensations.
    b. stimulating life processes.
    c. promoting inflammation.
    d. promoting healing.

14. Moist cold is applied with
    a. ice bags.
    b. ice caps.
    c. ice collars.
    d. soaks.

C. Matching.

Choose the correct word from Column II to match each statement in Column I.

Column I	Column II
15. _____ excessive blood loss	a. diathermy
16. _____ increase in size of blood vessel	b. vasoconstriction
17. _____ heat treatment	c. vasodilation
18. _____ heat treatment given only by persons specially trained in the procedure	d. hypothermia blanket
19. _____ used to lower body temperature	e. hemorrhage
	f. infrared

D. Nursing Assistant Challenge.

Peggy, 17 years of age, was admitted to your unit from the emergency room. She fractured an ankle and will require internal repair with screws and wire. You will care for her prior to surgery. The physician has ordered an ice bag for her ankle and her leg is to be elevated. Answer the following questions.

20. What are two reasons for applying the ice bag?
21. How full should the ice bag be filled?
22. Why should ice cubes be rinsed?
23. How should the metal cap be positioned when the ice bag is placed on the patient?
24. When should the ice bag be refilled?
25. How is the ice bag held in place?
26. What important observation should be reported immediately to the nurse?

Assisting with the Physical Examination

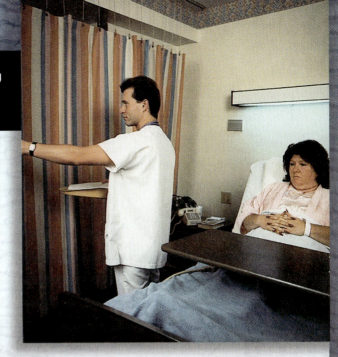

OBJECTIVES

As a result of this unit, you will be able to:

- Spell and define terms.
- Describe the responsibilities of the nursing assistant during the physical examination.
- Name the positions for the various physical examinations.

- Drape patient for the various positions.
- Name the basic instruments necessary for physical examinations.
- Demonstrate the following procedure:
  - Procedure 83 Assisting with a Physical Examination

VOCABULARY

Learn the meaning and the correct spelling of the following words:

dorsal lithotomy position	dorsal recumbent position	ophthalmoscope	speculum
	knee-chest position	otoscope	Trendelenburg position
		percussion hammer	

INTRODUCTION

Physical examinations are done in the physician's office, in clinics, after the patient's admission to the facility, and in the patient's home. Remember to carry out each beginning procedure action and procedure completion action as you assist.

The physical examination helps the physician:

- evaluate the patient's current status.
- establish a diagnosis.
- determine the patient's progress and response to therapy.

Nursing physical assessments will be performed by the nurse in the facility after the patient is admitted. This information is used by the nurse to establish a nursing diagnosis.

Both of these procedures are carried out in a similar manner. The responsibilities of the nursing assistant include:

- providing for the comfort and privacy of the patient.
- trying to anticipate the examiner's needs.
- draping and positioning patients.
- using proper body mechanics and exposing only the part of the patient being examined.
- preparing equipment that might be needed.
- reassuring the patient.
- caring for and labeling specimens.
- handing equipment as needed.
- cleaning equipment after use.
- adjusting lighting.
- remaining available during the examination.
- assisting the patient after the examination.

POSITIONING THE PATIENT

When the physical examination takes place on an examination table, extra attention must be given to safety. The examination table may be raised or lowered in sections and stirrups and shoulder braces applied to assist in positioning. Be sure you know how to properly operate the examination table before positioning a patient on it. In Figures 27-2 to 27-9, an examination table is shown.

Modifications

Some of the positions discussed here may be modified and used for other purposes. For example, they might be used to change the position of a patient who is confined to bed, or to perform specific procedures. Pillows must be used to support a patient who is to be kept in position for a period of time. Remember, the patient who "feels" covered and comfortable will be able to cooperate more fully. Providing privacy for the patient is one of your tasks (Figure 27-1).

Dorsal Recumbent Position

The **dorsal recumbent position** is the basic examination position.

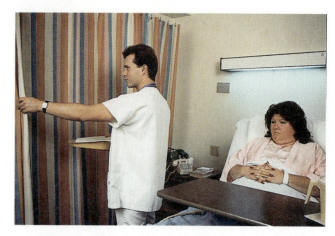

FIGURE 27-1 Before the examination begins, close the curtains to provide privacy.

- Assist the patient to be flat on the back, with knees flexed and slightly separated. The feet should be flat on the bed or table (Figure 27-2).
- Place a small pillow under the patient's head.
- Loosen the gown at the neck.
- Cover the patient with a sheet.

Supine or Horizontal Recumbent Position

- Assist the patient to lie flat on the back. The legs are extended and slightly separated (Figure 27-3).

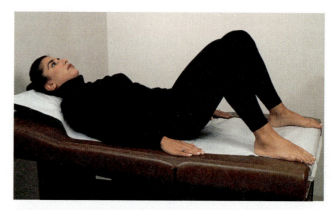

FIGURE 27-2 Dorsal recumbent position. (Draping has been omitted for clarity.)

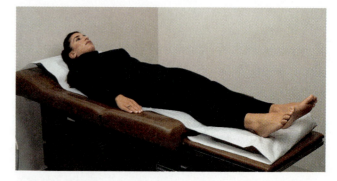

FIGURE 27-3 Supine or horizontal recumbent position

- Place a pillow under the patient's head.
- Cover the patient with a sheet.
- Loosen the gown at the neck.

Knee-Chest Position

The **knee-chest position** may be used to examine the rectal or vaginal areas and to relieve pain following childbirth. This is a difficult position to maintain, so never leave the patient alone. Position the patient in a prone position until the examiner is ready.

- Draping may be done with one or two sheets.
- Place a small pillow under the patient's head.
- Assist the patient to turn and lie on the abdomen with head turned to one side.
- Have the patient flex the arms and bring them up on either side of the head.
- Assist the patient to flex the knees and draw them up as far as possible toward the chest (Figure 27-4).

Prone Position

This position is used to examine the patient's back.

- Assist patient to lie on the abdomen with head turned to one side.
- Place a small pillow under the patient's head.
- Arms may be extended at the patient's side or flexed and brought up on either side of the head (Figure 27-5).
- One sheet is used for draping.

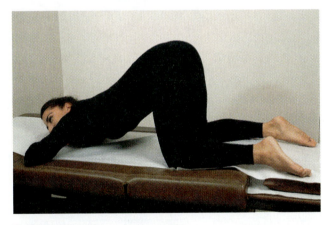

FIGURE 27-4 Knee-chest position

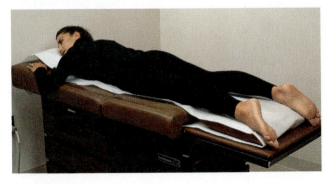

FIGURE 27-5 Prone position

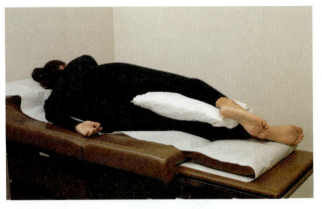

FIGURE 27-6 Sims' position

Sims' Position

This position is used for vaginal and rectal procedures, including enema administration.

- Assist patient to turn on the left side with head turned to the same side on a small pillow.
- Position the left arm extended behind the body.
- Flex the right arm and position it in front of the patient.
- The left leg is slightly bent, while the right leg is sharply flexed (Figure 27-6).
- One drape is usually adequate.

Semi-Fowler's Position

This is a common position for head and neck examinations of the in-bed patient.

- Assist patient to a semi-sitting position with back rest elevated at a 45-degree angle to the bed.
- The knees are supported in a slightly flexed position (Figure 27-7).
- The arms rest at the sides.
- One drape is usually enough.

Trendelenburg Position

The **Trendelenburg position** encourages circulation to the patient's heart and brain. It is used when the patient is in shock.

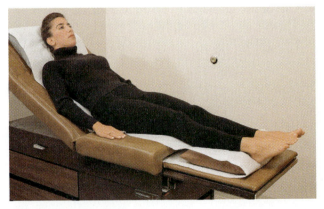

FIGURE 27-7 Semi-Fowler's position

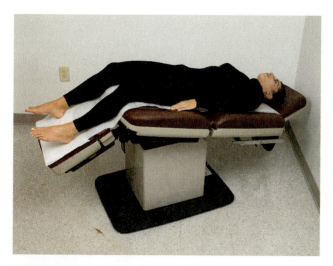

FIGURE 27-8 Trendelenburg position

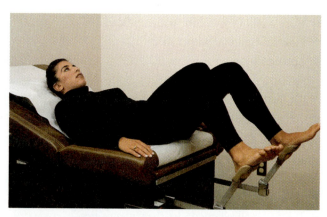

FIGURE 27-9 The patient's feet are placed in stirrups for the dorsal lithotomy position, so that the knees are well flexed and separated.

- Assist patient to lie flat on the back with the head lower than the rest of the body.
- If possible, the lower half of the bed or table is tilted so the legs are slightly flexed (Figure 27-8). In an emergency, the entire bed frame may be supported on blocks, tilting the bed to a 45-degree angle.
- Beds that are electrically powered may be adjusted to this position.
- Shoulder braces may be needed to prevent the patient from slipping.
- One drape is usually sufficient.

Dorsal Lithotomy Position

The **dorsal lithotomy position** is frequently used for the pelvic examination of female patients. This is a difficult examination for most women, so make sure your draping makes the patient feel covered.

- Make sure the patient voids her bladder before the examination.
- The patient is positioned on her back.
- The knees are well separated and flexed.
- Usually this position is achieved by placing the feet in stirrups (Figure 27-9).
- One or two drapes may be used to cover the patient. The draping may be similar to draping for the knee-chest position.

PHYSICAL EXAMINATION

Some health care facilities have examining instruments and equipment collected on trays. At other facilities, you will gather the necessary equipment and assemble it (Figure 27-10).

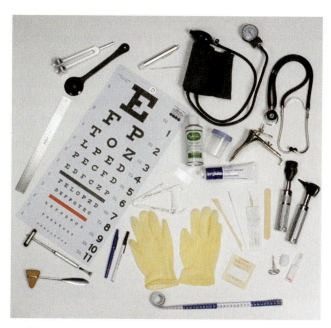

FIGURE 27-10 Basic equipment for the physical examination

PROCEDURE   83

ASSISTING WITH A PHYSICAL EXAMINATION

1. Carry out each beginning procedure action.
2. Assemble equipment:
   - gloves
   - flashlight or penlight
   - **percussion hammer** (tests nerve reflex)
   - tongue depressors
   - thermometer
   - cotton balls
   - emesis basin (lined with paper towel)
   - specimen cup
   - vaginal speculum
   - cervical brush
   - cotton-tip applicator
   - cervical spatula
   - slide and fixative
   - lubricant
   - tape measure
   - nasal speculum
   - sterile needle
   - **otoscope** (used to examine ears)
   - **ophthalmoscope** (used to examine eyes)
   - blood pressure cuff (sphygmomanometer)
   - stethoscope
   - visual acuity chart
   - tuning fork
   - pen and paper
   - marking pen
   - guaiac material
   - goniometer

   📝 *Note: A **speculum** is an instrument used to spread a body opening. If only a female pelvic examination is to be performed, the following equipment will be needed (Figure 27-11).*

   - gloves
   - linens for draping
   - microscope slides and cover slips
   - fixative spray
   - reagents
   - cotton-tipped applicators
   - vaginal speculum
   - spatulas
   - cytobrushes
   - lubricant

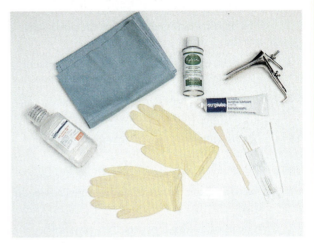

FIGURE 27-11 Equipment for pelvic examination

3. Ask patient to void if ambulatory. If patient is in bed, follow procedure for giving the bedpan or urinal.
4. Help patient onto examination table.

   📝 *Note: If examination is in bed, cover the patient with the bath blanket and fanfold the top bedding to the foot of the bed.*

5. Cover patient with a drape.
6. Assist as examination is performed.
   a. Provide privacy.
   b. Position patient and equipment as necessary.
   c. Hand equipment required to examiner.
   d. Adjust lighting as necessary.
7. After examination is complete, help patient to:
   a. Sit up slowly.
   b. Get off table and stand.
   c. Dress.
   d. Return to unit or office.
8. Wash hands and return to examination room.
9. Put on gloves.
10. Clean equipment according to facility policy.
11. Care for specimens according to facility policy.
12. Remove gloves and dispose of properly.
13. Wash hands.

REVIEW

A. True/False.

Mark the following true or false by circling T or F.

1. T F The physical examination helps the physician establish a nursing assessment.

2. T F A patient who feels covered is able to cooperate more fully.

3. T F Positions used for the physical examination can only be used for that purpose.

4. T F The nursing assistant performs the actual physical exam.

5. T F When a patient is placed in the Trendelenburg position, the feet must be at the same level as the knees.

6. T F When positioning a patient for a physical examination, you must maintain proper body mechanics.

7. T F Once you have the patient positioned for a physical examination, you should leave the room.

8. T F The nursing assistant assists in the physical assessment by draping and positioning the patient.

9. T F Lighting may have to be adjusted during the examination.

10. T F The semi-Fowler's position encourages blood flow to the head and heart.

B. Multiple Choice.

Select the one best answer for each question.

11. The basic examination position is
    a. Sims'.
    b. dorsal recumbent.
    c. dorsal lithotomy.
    d. Trendelenburg.

12. The patient is to have a pelvic examination. In what position should she be positioned?
    a. Sims'
    b. Lithotomy
    c. Trendelenburg
    d. Semi-Fowler's

13. Your female patient is to have a pelvic examination. Which instrument would you be sure to have ready?
    a. Otoscope
    b. Vaginal speculum
    c. Nasal speculum
    d. Ophthalmoscope

14. The patient has vaginal bleeding and the physician orders you to place her in a position that will increase blood flow to the head. Which position would you prepare for?
    a. Sims'
    b. Semi-Fowler's
    c. Trendelenburg
    d. Lithotomy

15. Stirrups are used in which position?
    a. Dorsal lithotomy
    b. Semi-Fowler's
    c. Sims'
    d. Trendelenburg

C. Matching.

Choose the correct word from Column II to match the word or phrases in Column I.

Column I	Column II
16. _____ instrument to examine the ear	a. apprehensive
17. _____ instrument to examine the eye	b. drape
18. _____ instrument to spread (dilate) a body opening	c. ophthalmoscope
19. _____ full of fear	d. otoscope
20. _____ covering	e. speculum
	f. percussion hammer

D. Nursing Assistant Challenge.

Robert Ubek is to have a physical examination in the doctor's office. He is 88 years of age and appears very nervous. He tells you he fears he has prostate cancer. You are to assist the doctor. Complete the following statements using words from the following list.

anticipate	off
dorsal recumbent	on
drape	reassure

21. One of your responsibilities will be to _____ the patient.

22. Because of Mr. Ubek's age, you will be especially careful in assisting him to get _____ and _____ the table.

23. You can help him feel more comfortable if you _____ him properly.

24. You can help the examination go more smoothly if you _____ the examiner's needs.

25. You will position Mr. Ubek in the _____ position to begin the examination.

The Surgical Patient

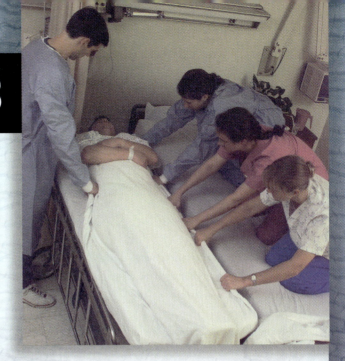

As a result of this unit, you will be able to:

- Spell and define terms.
- Describe the concerns of patients who are about to have surgery.
- List the various types of anesthesia.
- Shave the area to be operated on.
- Prepare the patient's unit for the patient's return from the operating room.
- Prepare a recovery bed.

- Demonstrate the following procedures:
  - Procedure 84 Shaving the Operative Area
  - Procedure 85 Assisting Patient to Deep Breathe and Cough
  - Procedure 86 Performing Postoperative Leg Exercises
  - Procedure 87 Applying Elasticized Stockings
  - Procedure 88 Applying Elastic Bandage
  - Procedure 89 Assisting Patient to Dangle

VOCABULARY

Learn the meaning and the correct spelling of the following words and phrases:

ambulation	drainage	perioperative	stable
anesthesia	embolus	postanesthesia care unit	surgical bed
anti-embolism hose	general anesthetic	(PACU)	TED hose
aspirate	hypoxia	postoperative	thrombophlebitis
atelectasis	local anesthetic	preoperative	thrombus
dangling	nosocomial	prosthesis	umbilicus
depilatory	NPO	recovery room	vertigo
disruption	operative	singultus	
distention	orifice	spinal anesthesia	

INTRODUCTION

Patients facing any surgical procedure tend to be fearful. Remember that these patients require great emotional as well as physical support (Figure 28-1). Such support should be given from the time the patient is admitted through the discharge.

Patients are concerned with:

● Disfigurement
● Pain
● Loss of control as they undergo anesthesia
● What serious conditions might be found
● Length and cost of recovery
● Possibility of death

Surgery is often associated with anxiety, pain, and discomfort. For this reason, medications are given before, during, and after surgery.

PAIN PERCEPTION

When a person feels pain sensations, the:

● pain receptors record the sensation.
● sensation is sent by the spinal nerves to the spinal cord and then to the brain.
● sensation is received and interpreted in the brain.

Before surgery, the patient is given medication to promote relaxation. During surgery, anesthetics are given to prevent pain (Figure 28-2). After surgery, medications are given to reduce discomfort.

ANESTHESIA

Anesthesia is given to prevent pain, to relax muscles, and to induce forgetfulness. The anesthetic agent (drug) and method of administration used are determined by the location and type of surgery to be performed, the length of time needed for surgery, and the patient's physical condition.

There are two main types of anesthetics:

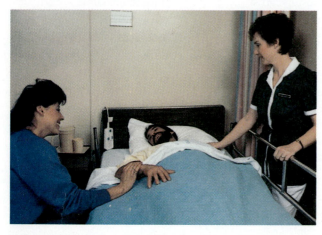

FIGURE 28-1 Patients and their families need support during the preoperative period.

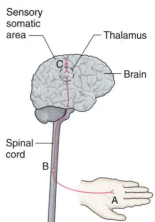

A Pain messages are picked up by free nerve endings in the skin. Local anesthetic blocks this.

B Message is carried into the spinal cord. Spinal anesthetic blocks this.

C Message is then carried to the cortex of the brain. General anesthetic blocks this.

FIGURE 28-2 Pain may be blocked through the action of anesthetics at points A, B, or C.

1. **General anesthetics**—These induce the patient to become unconscious.
2. **Local anesthetics**—These induce loss of feeling in a specific area.

General Anesthetics

General anesthetics block reception of pain in the brain. They are usually given in one of two ways:

1. Inhalation—Some gases that are used as anesthetics include nitrous oxide and cyclopropane.
   - Inhaled anesthetics are apt to make the patient secrete more mucus and to experience nausea.
   - Special attention must be given after surgery to keep the respiratory tract clear.
   - There is a real danger that the patient may **aspirate** (inhale) vomitus into the respiratory tact.
2. Intravenous—Drugs are introduced directly into the veins.
   - These drugs, such as sodium pentathol, act rapidly.
   - The patient quickly loses consciousness.
   - IV anesthetics are often used with other types of anesthesia for short operations.

Local Anesthetics

Local anesthetics act by:

1. Blocking pain receptors in the operative area.
   - Drugs such as procaine hydrochloride may be injected into the patient around the operative area.
   - These drugs stop the sensation of pain only in that area.
   - The patient remains awake but free from pain during the operation.
2. Blocking transmission of the pain sensation at the level of the spinal cord.
   - A drug injected into the spinal canal prevents feeling in any point below the level of the injection.

— The patient remains awake.

— This type of anesthesia is commonly used for abdominal surgery because it produces good relaxation of the muscles.

— This technique is called spinal anesthesia.

After getting this type of anesthetic, the patient is unable to feel or move the legs for a period of time. If not prepared ahead of time, the patient may be frightened by this experience.

SURGICAL CARE

The care of the surgical patient (perioperative) can be divided into three parts:

- Preoperative (before surgery)
- Operative (in the operating room)
- Postoperative (after surgery)

PREOPERATIVE CARE

Preoperative care begins when surgery is planned by the physician with the patient. Your responsibilities begin when the patient is admitted to the hospital. Remember that you may answer general questions that the patient asks, but you must refer specific questions about the surgery, its possible outcome, and anesthesia to your team leader.

Although it is the responsibility of the physician and nurse to answer questions and give explanations, it is helpful if you are aware of the information that has been given. Refer any questions the patient has to the nurse.

Teaching

Time spent with the patient in the preoperative period is very helpful. Patients who are prepared are able to cooperate more successfully in their recovery. Ideally, this time is spent shortly after the patient's admission. Sometimes much of the information is given in the doctor's office or clinic.

During the preoperative period, the nurse will determine the patient's specific needs. The nurse also does preoperative teaching. The other staff members support this effort.

- Tests, medications, and preoperative procedures are explained.
- Questions regarding the postoperative period are answered.
- The patient is taught and given an opportunity to practice postoperative exercises, such as leg exercises and respiratory exercises.
- The patient and staff discuss the events of the preoperative period, and what the patient may experience while being taken to the operating room and being given anesthesia.
- The recovery period is outlined and the purpose of special procedures or equipment, such as tubes or intra-

venous fluid lines, that may be used after surgery is explained.

- Play therapy may be used to explain to children.
- Every effort is made to teach ways of decreasing discomfort and to assure the patient that means for pain relief will be available.
- Planning for the discharge period begins now.

Psychological Preparation

The nursing staff spends as much time as possible helping patients deal with their emotional stress.

All members of the health team need to be sensitive and responsive to the psychological needs of the patient. Because you will be in frequent contact with the patient, you may be the first person to recognize signs of fear or concern. Listen to what the patient says and observe the patient's body language carefully. Report your observations to the nurse so that appropriate nursing intervention may be carried out.

Build patient confidence by:

- Performing your work in an efficient, calm manner.
- Being available to listen.
- Explaining what you plan to do before carrying out any procedure.
- Encouraging the patient to participate in his own care as much as possible. This helps the patient feel he still has a measure of control over his life.
- Immediately transmitting requests for clergy visits.

Physical Preparation

The Evening Before Surgery. If the patient is in the hospital the evening before surgery, part of the surgical preparation may be done then. It usually includes:

- Bath or shower with surgical soap
- Enema
- Surgical prep (shaving of the operative site)
- Special tests
- Medication to ensure a good night's rest, when indicated
- Insertion of special tubes for draining body cavities
- Being placed on NPO (nothing by mouth) orders after midnight
- Removal of the water pitcher from the bedside table and having the NPO notice posted over the bed, bedside stand, on the door, on the patient's chart, and on the Kardex.

Nosocomial infections are those acquired during the hospital stay. It is known that such infections:

- are more likely to occur the longer the patient is in the hospital.
- add days to the hospital stay.
- increase the cost of hospitalization.
- can be life-threatening.

To decrease costs and the potential for nosocomial infections, patients are often admitted on the morning of surgery and are sometimes discharged on the day of surgery or the day after. In this circumstance, much of the preoperative care must be done at home or immediately upon admission. This is called outpatient or "short-term" surgery.

The Surgical Prep Area. Skin preparation before surgery may or may not include hair removal. There is a trend away from removing the hair unless its thickness will interfere with the surgery. In fact, some studies have shown more infections among shaved patients compared with unshaved patients.

If shaving is ordered, it must be done according to the procedure provided. (See Procedure 84.) It must be performed skillfully in a well-lighted area. Also, the area to be washed and shaved will be larger than the surgical incision area (Figure 28-3). In some cases, a **depilatory** (hair-removing) cream will be ordered for use the night before surgery. If a depilatory is to be used, check the skin for sensitivity. Apply a small amount to the skin of the forearm and wait 10 minutes. If redness occurs, do not continue, but report to the nurse.

Skin preparation may be performed by:
- Special surgical prep team
- Operating room (OR) staff in the OR
- Nursing staff in the patient's unit just prior to surgery

To prepare the surgical area by shaving:
- Make sure you know exactly what area is to be shaved. Most hospitals have routine prep areas.
- Do not shave the neck or face of a female patient. If in doubt, check with the nurse.
- Be aware that the preparations for cranial surgery are usually performed after the patient has been medicated and taken to the operating suite. Doctors have special preferences in this regard.
- Remember that if a spinal anesthesia is to be given, the back may also be shaved.

Calm the patient's fears by explaining that the area prepared is much larger than the actual incision area. This is to prevent contamination of the surgical site, which may lead to possible complications after surgery.

Immediate Preoperative Care. Approximately one hour before surgery, the patient will be given additional medication by the nurse. Your responsibilities regarding the patient must be completed before this time. You may be asked to do the following:
- Take and record vital signs (Figure 28-4) (see Section 6).
- Take care of valuables according to hospital policy. Remove dentures and any other **prosthesis** (artificial

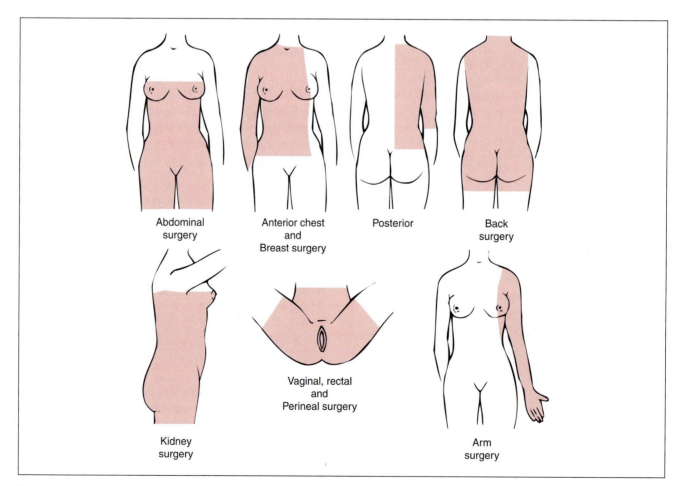

Abdominal surgery

Anterior chest and Breast surgery

Posterior

Back surgery

Kidney surgery

Vaginal, rectal and Perineal surgery

Arm surgery

FIGURE 28-3 Shaded areas are those usually shaved preoperatively.

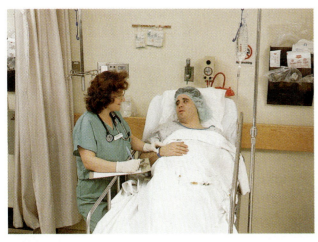

FIGURE 28-4 Taking vital signs is part of preoperative care.

part), such as a hearing aid or glasses. See that they are safely marked with the patient's name and cared for.

- Remove nail polish, makeup, hairpins, and jewelry. Long hair should be neatly braided or capped. Plain wedding bands may be taped in place.
- Dress the patient in a gown and cover the hair with a surgical cap.
- See that the patient voids and measure the urine. Drain Foley bag, if present.
- Make sure that the room is quiet and comfortable, with television off.

As soon as the nurse gives the preoperative medication:

- Elevate the bed to stretcher level.
- Be sure the side rails are in place for safety.
- Remove all unnecessary equipment.

PROCEDURE 84

SHAVING THE OPERATIVE AREA

1. Carry out each beginning procedure action.
2. Assemble equipment:
   - disposable gloves
   - bath blanket
   - individual prep pack, *or*
   - tray with razor and new razor blades, *or*
   - electric clipper—make sure heads are disposable or, if reusable, that they have been sterilized
   - 2 small bowls
   - applicators
   - cleansing soap
   - lighting—for example, a spotlight or gooseneck lamp
   - 4 × 4 sponges
   - paper towels
   - towels or disposable Chux® (bed protector)
3. Determine exact area to be prepped.
4. In utility room:
   a. Fill small bowls with warm water.
   b. Add cleansing soap to one.
   c. Adjust razor and blade.
   d. Make sure razor and blade are tight.
5. Cover tray and take to bedside.

6. Drape patient with bath blanket. Place towel or bed protector under area to be shaved.
7. Put on disposable gloves.
8. If a safety razor and blade are used, soften hairs with soapy solution and wait 1 minute. This makes hair removal easier and helps avoid skin injury.
9. Holding skin taut with one hand, lather area to be shaved. If hair is very long, such as on the pubis and axilla, it may be clipped with scissors before shaving. Take care when clipping—do not nick the skin. If an electric clipper is used, attach heads and check for security.
10. Shave area with strokes in same direction as the hair grows. Be careful not to cut the skin or to remove any warts or moles. Work carefully around such areas.
11. Using the applicators, clean the **umbilicus** (navel) and shave it if it is in the operative area.
12. Check carefully for hairs after shaving is complete.
    - Unattached hairs are easily removed by gently pressing a piece of tape against the area.
    - Discard hair in paper towel.

continues

PROCEDURE 84 *continued*

13. Cleanse the skin with warm, soapy water. Rinse and dry thoroughly.

14. Dispose of equipment according to facility policy.

15. Remove the towel from under patient.
- Make sure side rails are up.

- Make sure linen is dry.
- Change, if necessary.

16. Remove and dispose of gloves according to facility policy.

17. Carry out each procedure completion action.

- Push the bedside table, overbed table, and chair out of the way to make room for the stretcher when it arrives from surgery.
- Complete the surgical checklist:
    1. Admission sheet
    2. Surgical consent
    3. Sterilization consent (if necessary)
    4. Consultation sheet (if necessary)
    5. History and physical
    6. Lab reports (pregnancy test also if necessary)
    7. Surgery prep done and charted, if required
    8. Latest TPR and blood pressure charted
    9. Preoperative medication has been given and charted (if required)
    10. Name tape on patient
    11. Fingernail polish and makeup removed
    12. Metallic objects removed (rings may be taped)
    13. Dentures removed
    14. Other prostheses removed (such as artificial limb or eye, wigs and hairpieces)
    15. Bath blanket and head cap in place
    16. Bed in high position and side rails up after preop medication is given
    17. Patient has voided
    — Check off those duties to which you were assigned.
    — Note the time your patient leaves for surgery.
- Follow facility policy regarding visitors. Sometimes they are allowed to wait quietly with the patient. Sometimes they need to be directed to the visitors' waiting room.

The nurse and surgical attendant will check the patient's identification and surgical checklist before the patient is moved. A staff member, and sometimes a family member, accompanies the patient to the doors of the operating room. You will probably be asked to assist in transferring the patient from the bed to the stretcher and, after surgery, from the stretcher to the bed. Review Procedures 24 and 25 in Unit 15.

DURING THE OPERATIVE PERIOD

While the patient is in the operating room, you will prepare the room for the patient's return.

- A special surgical bed will be prepared. This was described in Unit 22. The **surgical bed** is also called a postop bed or recovery bed.
- Everything should be removed from the top of the bedside stand except an emesis basin, tissue wipes, tongue depressors, and equipment to check vital signs.
- A pencil and small pad to record the signs should also be available.
- Check with your team leader for any special equipment, such as oxygen, IV poles, suction, or drainage bags, that might be necessary for your patient.
- Be watchful while carrying out your other assignments for the return of your patient from surgery.
- Follow facility policy regarding the location of visitors and family during surgery. They are sometimes permitted to wait in the patient's room. In most cases they are directed to a special waiting area.

POSTOPERATIVE CARE

During the immediate postoperative period, the patient recovers from anesthesia. For this period, the patient is placed in a special area called the **recovery room** (Figure 28-5). The recovery room is located next to the operating room and is sometimes called the **postanesthesia care unit** (**PACU**).

When the patient's condition is stabilized, the patient is returned to the unit. Upon the patient's return from the recovery room, you should:

- Identify the patient.
- Assist in the transfer from stretcher to bed (see Unit 15).
- Never leave the unconscious patient alone at any time.
- Learn from your team leader any special instructions to be followed.

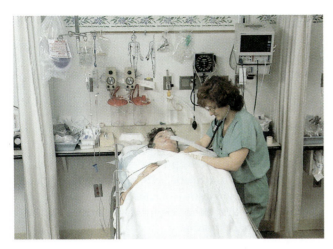

FIGURE 28-5 Following surgery, the patient remains in the recovery room until vital signs are stable.

- Realize that the patient may be drowsy for several hours after return.
- Have an extra blanket available—many patients complain of feeling cold upon return (Figure 28-6).

The following are routine instructions to be followed unless otherwise ordered.

- Always wear gloves and follow standard precautions when contact with blood, body fluids, mucous membranes, or nonintact skin is likely.
- Take vital signs of the patient upon arrival on the unit (Figure 28-7) and every 15 minutes for four readings

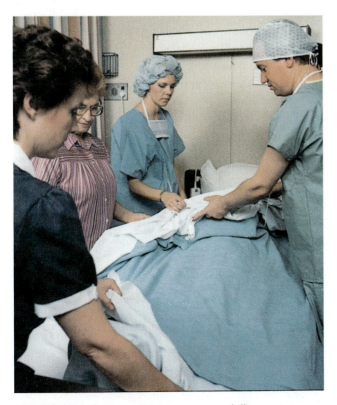

FIGURE 28-6 Cover patient to prevent chilling.

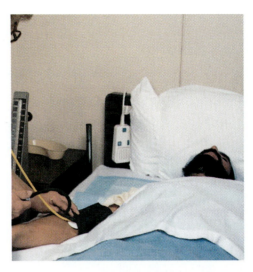

FIGURE 28-7 Check vital signs carefully until they are stable.

(see Section 6). The patient's temperature may not always be taken at this time. If signs are **stable** (approximately the same) at the end of this time, repeat in one hour. Note the patient's state of consciousness (unresponsive, drowsy, alert).

- Check dressings for amount and type of any drainage. The nurse may reinforce them as necessary.
- Check IV solution for flow rate. Restrain infusion site whenever ordered by the physician and report to the charge nurse. Remember that the flow rate is ordered by the physician.
- Encourage the patient to breathe deeply, cough, and move in bed. Position should be changed every 2 hours.
- Turn the patient's head to one side and support if vomiting. Have emesis basin ready, as well as tissues and wet cloth. If patient is conscious, allow patient to rinse mouth with water after vomiting. Note type and amount of vomitus.
- Check pulses distal to operative site. Inform the nurse if the pulse is weak or cannot be felt.
- If the patient was given a spinal anesthetic:
  - Give extra care in turning frequently and maintaining proper alignment.
  - Remember the patient will be unable to move independently until sensation and motor functions return. Make sure to calm the patient's fear about this.
  - Some physicians require that the patient remain flat on the back and without a pillow for 8 to 12 hours following spinal anesthesia to avoid headaches.
  - Any complaints of a headache following spinal anesthesia should be reported promptly.
  - Provide extra blankets if patient is cold.
- Be sure all drainage tubes have been connected (the nurse will usually attend to this). If you notice a tube clamped shut, check with your team leader.

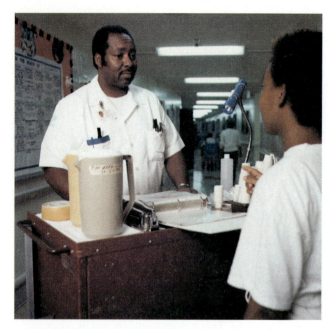

FIGURE 28-8 Report complaints of discomfort and pain to the nurse.

- Measure and record the first postoperative voiding. Inform nurse.
- Report any patient complaints of discomfort and pain to the nurse (Figure 28-8).

Tubes

Patients often return from surgery with a variety of tubes and drains in place.

- Some tubes may deliver materials into the patient. Examples of these are oxygen tubes or intravenous tubes.
- Other tubes may have been placed in the patient to provide **drainage** from wounds or body cavities. Examples of these are drains in the incision or urinary catheters.

The following are some special precautions to be taken:

- Always wear gloves if contact with drainage from the tube is likely.
- Learn the type, purpose, and location of each tube.
- Check drainage for character and amount.
- Check for obstructions to the tube system.
- Check flow rate of infusions from intravenous lines.
- Keep **orifices** (body openings) clear of secretions and discharge.
- Never disconnect tubes or raise drainage bottles above the level of the drainage site.
- Never lower infusion bottles below the level of the infusion site.
- Never put stress on the tubes when moving the patient or giving care.
- Restrain infusion sites as necessary to prevent dislocation.

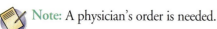 Note: A physician's order is needed.

- Monitor levels of infusions and report to the nurse before they run out.
- Report any signs of leakage or disconnected tubes immediately.
- Report pain, discoloration, or swelling at sites or drainage and infusion.

Drainage

When a body cavity is the operative site, it may be necessary to drain fluid such as blood, pus, serous drainage caused by tissue trauma, or gastric contents from it before or after surgery. Always wear gloves if contact with drainage is likely. The drainage outlet may be a:

- Catheter
- T-tube
- Jackson-Pratt (J–P)® drain
- Penrose drain
- Cigarette drain

When such a drain is in place, the drainage accumulates on the dressing (Figure 28-9). You should:

- note the amount and character of the drainage.
- inform the nurse when the dressing needs to be changed or reinforced.

At times, the withdrawal of fluids is controlled by attaching the drainage tube to a connecting tube and then a suction apparatus. The drainage accumulates in a container. The container is emptied and the contents measured at the end of each shift. The Jackson-Pratt® or Hemovac drains are closed drainage systems. The drains are placed directly in the wound, and drainage goes directly into an expandable container. A record of the amount and character of the drainage is entered in both the output chart and the nurses' notes.

It is your responsibility to:

- Report either heavy or light drainage.

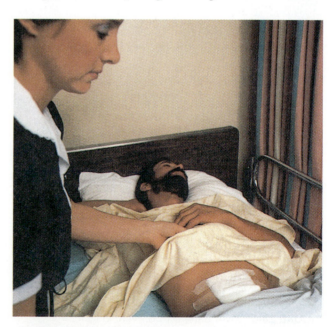

FIGURE 28-9 Check dressings for drainage or bleeding.

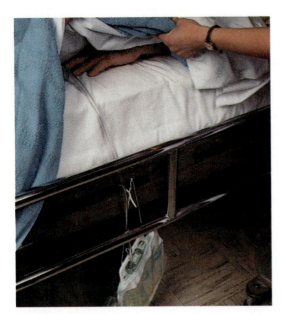

FIGURE 28-10 Check to be sure all drainage tubes are free of obstructions.

- Report a change in the character or amount of the drainage.
- Make sure that the flow of drainage is not blocked by kinking of the tube (Figure 28-10).

Never assume responsibility for chest drainage or attempt to empty chest bottles. Chest bottles and irrigations require the nurse's or physician's attention.

Careful preoperative preparation and postoperative care can help limit the extent of postoperative discomfort and complication.

The patient must be carefully observed, especially during the first 24 hours, for possible complications. Possible postoperative discomfort and complications and appropriate nursing assistant actions are summarized in Table 28-1.

When the patient has responded sufficiently and vital signs are stable, the patient may be refreshed by:

- washing the hands and face.
- changing the linen.
- being given a light backrub.

The patient is now ready to participate more actively in recovery. Exercises taught in the preoperative period are practiced, including:

- Deep breathing and coughing
- Leg exercises.

Deep Breathing and Coughing

Deep breathing and coughing clear the air passages. This helps to prevent postoperative respiratory complications such as pneumonia and atelectasis, which is the collapse of the alveolar air sacs. This may be an uncomfortable task when the patient has a new incision and feels fatigued. (See Procedure 85.) You can best assist the patient by:

- Explaining the value of the exercise and carrying out the following procedure.

TABLE 28-1 POSTOPERATIVE COMPLICATIONS AND NURSING ASSISTANT ACTIONS

Possible Discomfort	Report	What You Can Do*
Thirst	Patient complaints of dryness of lips, mouth, and skin	Carefully check I&O. Increase fluid intake by mouth with permission. Monitor IV if ordered. Give mouth care. Check BP and pulse. Watch for signs of shock and hemorrhage.
Singultus (hiccups)—intermittent spasms of the diaphragm	Incidence of hiccups	Allow patient to rest; hiccups can be tiring. Support incisional area. Assist patient to breathe into paper bag.
Pain	Location, intensity, type	Change position. Apply warmth if instructed. Monitor carefully for and report effects of medication given by nurse.
Distention (accumulation of gas in bowel)	Distention of abdomen, complaints of pain	Increase mobility. Insert a rectal tube if instructed and permitted.
Nausea, vomiting	Nausea, character of vomitus	Keep emesis basin at bedside. Monitor IV fluids, which are substituted for oral fluids. Give mouth care. Limit fluids by mouth. Encourage patient to breathe deeply.
Urinary retention	Amount and time of first voiding. Distention, restlessness, imbalance between I&O	Monitor I&O carefully. Check for distention.

continues

TABLE 28-1 *continued*

Complication	Report	What You Can Do*
Hemorrhage (excessive blood loss)	Fall in blood pressure; cold, moist skin; weak, rapid pulse; restlessness; pallor/cyanosis; condition of dressing; thirst	Report immediately to nurse. Keep patient quiet. Check vital signs.
Shock	Fall in blood pressure; weak, rapid pulse; cold, moist skin; pallor	Report immediately to nurse. Keep patient quiet. Monitor ordered oxygen. Be prepared to follow additional instructions.
Hypoxia (lack of oxygen)	Restlessness, dyspnea, crowing sounds to respirations, pounding pulse, perspiring	Report immediately to nurse. Monitor oxygen, if ordered.
Atelectasis (failure of lungs to expand)	Dyspnea; cyanosis/pallor	Report immediately to nurse.
Wound infection	Increased pain in incisional area; fever; chills, anorexia, increased drainage on dressing	Be observant. Report findings promptly to nurse. Check dressing.
Wound disruption (separation of wound edges)	Pinkish drainage. Complaints by the patient that he "feels open," "broken," "given away"	Report immediately to nurse. Keep patient quiet. Support incisional area.
Pulmonary emboli	Anxiety, difficulty breathing; feelings of "heaviness in chest," cyanosis, chest pain	Keep patient quiet. Report immediately to nurse. Elevate head of bed.

*In all cases, be prepared to follow the nurse's additional instructions.

PROCEDURE   85

ASSISTING PATIENT TO DEEP BREATHE AND COUGH

1. Carry out each beginning procedure action.
2. Assemble equipment:
   - disposable gloves
   - a pillowcase-covered pillow or binder, if ordered
   - tissues
   - emesis basin
3. Elevate head of bed and assist patient to assume a comfortable semi-Fowler's position.
4. Have patient place hands on either side of his rib cage or over operative site (Figure 28-11). A pillow over the operative site can be used to support an incision during respiratory exercises.

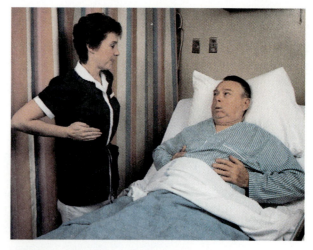

FIGURE 28-11 Encourage patient to perform deep breathing exercises taught before surgery.

continues

PROCEDURE **85** *continued*

5. Ask patient to take as deep a breath as possible and hold it for 3 to 5 seconds; then exhale slowly through pursed lips.

6. Repeat this exercise about five times unless the patient seems too tired. If so, stop procedure and report to nurse.

7. Place the pillow across the incision line as a brace. Have patient hold pillow on either side or have patient interlace fingers across incision to act as a brace.

8. Pass tissues to patient and instruct patient to take a deep breath and cough forcefully twice with mouth open, collecting any secretions that are brought up in tissues (Figure 28-12).

9. Put on disposable gloves to handle tissues.

10. Dispose of tissues in emesis basin.

11. Assist patient to assume a new, comfortable position.

12. Clean emesis basin.

13. Remove and dispose of gloves according to facility policy.

14. Carry out each procedure completion action.

15. Report to nurse number of times patient performed each exercise, how patient tolerated the exercise, and the type and amount of any sputum coughed up.

   - Be sure the patient does not become overly fatigued.

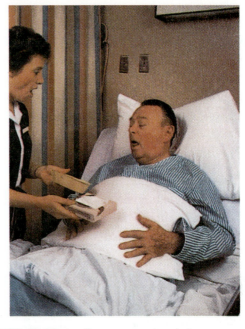

FIGURE 28-12 A pillow across the abdomen supports the incision during deep coughing.

- Encourage the patient to cough and clear the respiratory passages.
- Report to your team leader if the patient seems overly fatigued during the procedure.
- Carefully observe and report any unusual responses such as pain, dizziness, or throat and airway irritation.

- Checking with the nurse to see if medication for pain is to be administered before the exercise. If so, wait for 45 minutes after the medication has been given before carrying out the exercise.
- Learning from the nurse how many deep breaths and coughs should be attempted. The usual number is 5 to 10 breaths and 2 to 3 coughs.
- Using a pillow or binder to support the incision during the procedure.

Leg Exercises

Leg exercises following surgery encourage steady circulation. This helps to prevent another serious complication of the postoperative period—the development of blood clots. (See Procedure 86.)

A blood clot or **thrombus** could develop in the venous system and block the essential blood flow. A small piece of thrombus broken off (**embolus**) could travel throughout the vascular system and block a vessel in the lungs.

A specific order must be written for leg exercises when there has been surgery on the legs themselves. Otherwise, leg exercises are routinely performed by the patient. If the patient is very weak, you may need to assist.

- Encourage leg exercises and be sure they have been performed.
- Each exercise should be performed 3 to 5 times at least every 1 or 2 hours and at other times as well.
- Carry out leg exercises as you assist position changes.
- Apply or reapply support hose (TED) after exercises if ordered.

PROCEDURE   86

PERFORMING POSTOPERATIVE LEG EXERCISES

1. Carry out each beginning procedure action.

2. Explain how the exercise is to be performed. Have patient:
   a. Brace the incisional area with laced hands.
   b. Rotate each ankle by drawing imaginary circles with toes.
   c. Dorsiflex (bring toes toward knee) and plantar flex (point toes and foot down) each ankle (Figure 28-13).
   d. Flex and extend each knee.
   e. Flex and extend each hip.
   f. Repeat each exercise 3 to 5 times. Assist as needed.

3. Lower side rail.

4. Cover with bath blanket and draw top bedding to the foot of the bed.

5. Supervise exercises or assist. Apply or reapply support hose (TED hose) as ordered after exercises.

6. Draw bedding up and remove bath blanket.

7. Fold bath blanket and place in bedside stand for reuse.

8. Carry out each procedure completion action. Report to nurse number of exercises done and how they were tolerated by patient.

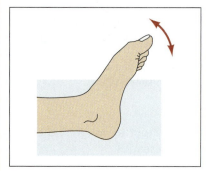

A. Curl the toes down and up. Repeat 5 times.

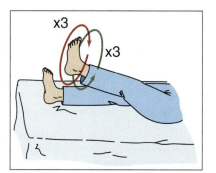

B. Make circles with the feet clockwise 3 times and counterclockwise 3 times. Repeat 5 times.

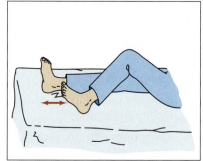

C. Slide one leg up and down in bed. Do the same with the other leg. Repeat 5 times.

FIGURE 28-13 Help the patient perform leg exercises to encourage circulation.

Elasticized Stockings

Elasticized stockings, called **TED hose** or **anti-embolism hose**, or Ace bandages that extend from the ankle or foot to calf or mid-thigh, are often applied during the preoperative and postoperative periods to support the veins of the legs.

This reduces the incidence of **thrombophlebitis**, which is inflammation of the veins that can lead to blood clots. The stockings must be applied smoothly and evenly before the patient gets out of bed. They should be removed and reapplied at least every eight hours—more often if necessary or as ordered. (Refer to Procedure 87.)

PROCEDURE   87

APPLYING ELASTICIZED STOCKINGS

1. Carry out each beginning procedure action.
2. Assemble equipment:

   • elasticized stockings of proper length and size

continues

PROCEDURE **87** *continued*

3. Always apply stockings with patient lying down. Expose one leg at a time.

4. Grasp stocking with both hands at the top and roll toward toe end (Figure 28-14A).

5. Adjust over patient's toes, positioning opening at base of toes (unless toes are to be covered) (Figure 28-14B). Remember that the raised seams should be on the outside.

6. Apply stocking to leg by rolling upward toward body (Figure 28-14C).

7. Check to be sure stocking is applied evenly and smoothly and there are no wrinkles (Figure 28-14D and E).

8. Repeat procedure on opposite leg.

9. Carry out each procedure completion action.

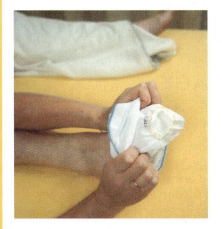

FIGURE 28-14A Grasp stocking with both hands at stocking top, gather, and slip stocking over patient's toes.

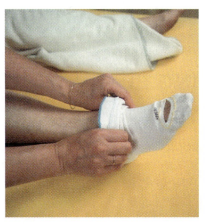

FIGURE 28-14B Position opening on top of foot at base of toes.

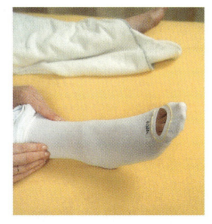

FIGURE 28-14C Draw stocking smoothly toward knee.

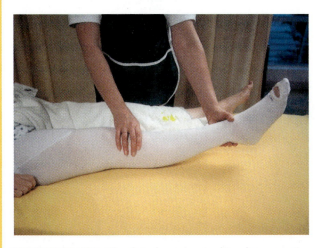

FIGURE 28-14D Check to be sure stocking has no wrinkles.

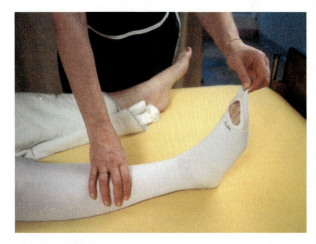

FIGURE 28-14E Check material on toes to be sure it is not too tight.

Elastic Bandage

An elasticized bandage (Ace bandage) may be used to keep dressings in place, especially on an extremity or on the head. You may need to remove and reapply the bandage once or twice on your shift. Elastic bandages are also used on non-surgical patients to promote venous blood flow in the legs and for injuries of the musculoskeletal system to reduce swelling. Elastic bandages come in 2-inch to 6-inch widths and in 4-foot and 6-foot lengths (Figure 28-15). Check with the nurse for the appropriate size bandage. (Refer to Procedure 88.)

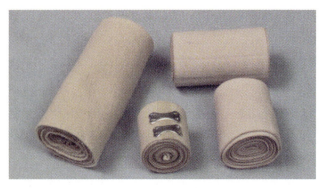

FIGURE 28-15 Elastic bandages come in a variety of widths.

Initial Ambulation

Some time after surgery, a patient is permitted to sit up with the legs over the edge of the bed. This position is called **dangling**.

● Watch carefully for signs of fatigue or dizziness (**vertigo**).

● Assist the patient to assume the position slowly.

The first **ambulation** (walk) is usually short. The patient usually dangles for a short time before ambulating. Dangling is an important part of postoperative care because it stimulates circulation and helps prevent the formation of blood clots (thrombi). (Refer to Procedure 89.)

PROCEDURE   88

APPLYING ELASTIC BANDAGE

1. Carry out each beginning procedure action.

2. Assemble equipment:
   ● appropriate size bandage (check for cleanliness)
   ● tape, pins, or self-closures that come with bandage

3. Check area to be bandaged.

   a. If there are lesions or signs of skin breakdown, report to nurse before bandaging.

   b. If there are dressings underneath the bandage, the nurse may want to check them before you reapply the bandage.

   c. If an arm or leg is to be bandaged, elevate it for 15 to 30 minutes before application to promote venous blood flow.

   d. Apply bandage so two skin surfaces do not rub together (toes, fingers, under breasts and arms). Place gauze or cotton to prevent friction (Figure 28-16A).

4. Hold the bandage with the roll facing upward in one hand and the free end of the bandage in your other hand (Figure 28-16B).

   a. Hold the roll close to the part being bandaged so pressure is even.

   b. When bandaging an extremity, always wrap from the distal (far) area to the proximal (near) area (Figure 28-16C).

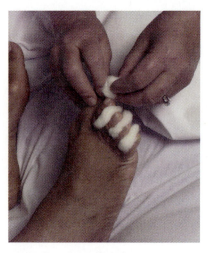

FIGURE 28-16A Place cotton or gauze to prevent two skin surfaces from rubbing together.

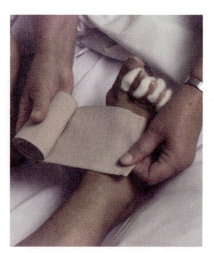

FIGURE 28-16B Hold the bandage with the roll facing upward in one hand and the free end of the bandage in your other hand.

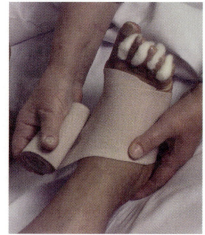

FIGURE 28-16C Always wrap from the distal area to the proximal area.

continues

PROCEDURE 88 *continued*

c. Unroll the bandage as you wrap the body part. Never unroll the entire bandage at once.

5. Use appropriate bandaging technique (Figure 28-16D). Overlap each layer of bandage by one-half the width of the strip (Figure 28-16E).

6. When finished rolling, secure bandage with pins, tape, or self-closures. Avoid using the clips that may come with the bandage. They tend to come loose and could injure the patient's skin. The bandage should be smooth and wrinkle-free (Figure 28-16F).

7. Check distal circulation after bandage is applied and once or twice every 8 hours (check skin under bandage for color and temperature; note complaints of patient of burning, tingling, or other discomfort).

8. Remove and reapply the bandage every shift, or more often if needed. The patient should have two bandages so that they can be laundered daily. Ask the nurse whether the bandage is to be worn continuously or only at specified times.

9. Carry out each procedure completion action.

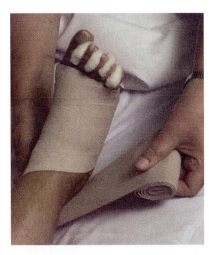

FIGURE 28-16D Use the appropriate bandaging technique.

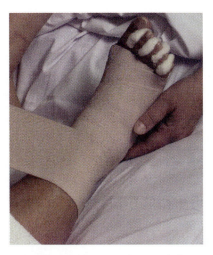

FIGURE 28-16E Overlap each layer of bandage by one-half the width of the strip.

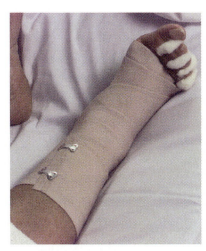

FIGURE 28-16F The bandage should be smooth and wrinkle-free.

PROCEDURE 89

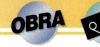

ASSISTING PATIENT TO DANGLE

1. Carry out each beginning procedure action.

2. Assemble equipment:
   - bath blanket
   - pillow

3. Check the pulse (see Unit 15).

4. Lower side rail nearest to you. Lock bed at the lowest position.

5. Drape patient with bath blanket and fanfold top bedcovers to foot of bed.

6. Gradually elevate head of bed.

7. Help patient to put on bathrobe.

8. Place one arm around patient's shoulders and the other arm under the knees.

continues

9. Gently and slowly turn patient toward you. Allow patient's legs to hang over the side of the bed.

10. Roll pillow and tuck firmly against patient's back for support.

11. After putting slippers on patient, ask patient to swing the legs.

12. Have the patient dangle as long as ordered.
    - If patient becomes dizzy or faint, help him lie down.
    - Report to the supervising nurse immediately.

13. Check patient's pulse.

14. Rearrange pillow at head of bed. Remove patient's bathrobe and slippers.

15. Place one arm around patient's shoulders and the other arm under the knees. Gently and slowly swing patient's legs onto the bed.

16. Check patient's pulse. Lower head of bed and raise side rails.

17. Carry out each procedure completion action. Remember to wash your hands, report completion of task, and document time dangled (duration), pulse, and patient reaction.

The patient may need assistance the first few times he stands up to ambulate. The anesthesia and medications administered before, during, and after surgery may affect the patient's balance, endurance, and strength. There may be drainage tubes or an intravenous feeding that must be moved with the patient (Figure 28-17).

GUIDELINES
for

Assisting the Patient in Initial Ambulation

- Check with the nurse to see if a transfer belt can be used.
- Assist the patient to sit on the edge of the bed with bed in low position.
- Take the patient's pulse before and after standing. If there is more than 10 points difference, return the patient to bed and inform the nurse.
- If the patient becomes dizzy or faint, return the patient to bed and inform the nurse.
- Walk with the patient as instructed in Unit 16.

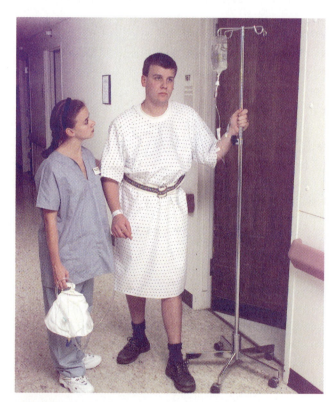

FIGURE 28-17 Drainage tubes or intravenous feedings may be in place and must be moved with the surgical patient.

REVIEW

A. True/False.

Mark the following true or false by circling T or F.

1. T F Patients receiving local anesthetics lose consciousness during the surgery.

2. T F When spinal anesthetics are used, patients may lose feeling and movement in their legs.

3. T F Preoperative teaching has little effect on the patient's postoperative recovery.

4. T F You help build patient confidence when you explain what you plan to do when carrying out procedures.

5. T F Skin preparation involves shaving an area larger than the size of the incision.

6. T F The nursing assistant has no responsibilities related to the patient while the patient is in surgery.

7. T F Patients should be dangled without incident before initial ambulation.

8. T F Patients who are unconscious following surgery should not be left alone.

9. T F Nosocomial infections do not affect the cost or length of hospital stay.

10. T F Patients who are faced with surgery are often filled with apprehension and fears.

B. Matching.

Choose the correct word or phrase from Column II to match each question in Column I.

Column I	Column II
11. ____ inflammation of a vein with clot formation	a. ambulation
	b. orifice
12. ____ period before surgery	c. nosocomial
13. ____ medicine given to prevent pain	d. recovery room
	e. umbilicus
14. ____ hospital-acquired	f. vertigo
15. ____ opening	g. anesthesia
16. ____ walking	h. preoperative
17. ____ dizziness	i. aspiration
18. ____ lung collapse	j. embolism
19. ____ blood clot	k. atelectasis
20. ____ area where immediate postoperative care is given	l. thrombophlebitis

C. Nursing Assistant Challenge.

Mr. Dovetski is a 47-year-old patient on the surgical unit. He has had abdominal surgery. When he is returned to his room from surgery, you note that he has a Foley catheter, an intravenous feeding running, dressings on the abdominal incision, and elastic stockings. Think about what procedures you will include in your care of Mr. Dovetski.

21. How often will you take his vital signs? Which procedures are included in vital signs? What are the "normal" ranges for each vital sign for a person of this age? If there are changes in the vital signs, these changes may be indications of what complications?

22. What observations will you make regarding the Foley catheter? Why do you think he has the catheter in place?

23. What observations will you make regarding the intravenous feeding? Why do you think the physician ordered an IV?

24. You know you will need to have Mr. Dovetski perform deep breathing exercises and deep coughing. Why is this important? How can you help him do the exercises with the least discomfort?

25. Why do you think he has elastic stockings on? How often should you take the stockings off and reapply them? What do you need to remember when putting the stockings back on?

26. How will you report any complaints of pain?

27. How will you check for bleeding from the incision?

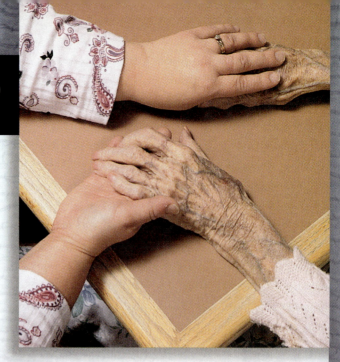

UNIT 29

Caring for the Emotionally Stressed Patient

INTRODUCTION

There are varying degrees and differing aspects of health. A person who is in poor physical health may be mentally healthy. Because of good mental health, the person may be self-reliant and able to make decisions and to live an effective, productive life (Figure 29-1).

In contrast, a person with good physical health may not be able to cope with and adapt to changes. This inability limits the person's chances to participate successfully in society.

MENTAL HEALTH

Mental health means exhibiting behaviors that reflect a person's **adaptation** or adjustment to the multiple stresses of life, such as:

- Illness
- Hospitalization
- Loss of a loved one
- Loss of a job
- Loss of status

Stresses or **stressors** are situations, feelings, or conditions that cause a person to be anxious about his or her physical or emotional well-being. Good mental health leads to positive adaptations. Poor mental health is demonstrated by maladaptive behaviors (behaviors that harm the person or her adjustment).

Physical and mental health are interrelated. Physical illness is often preceded by stressful life situations. Ill health causes emotional stress. It is easy to understand that each of these factors contributes to the total health pattern of each person.

Ways of **coping** with (handling) stressful situations (Figure 29-2) are learned early in life. As people grow, they find these behaviors that work best for them. They learn to use those behaviors to reduce stress and protect self-esteem. These coping patterns become part of the individual's habitual responses, becoming more and more obvious as the person ages.

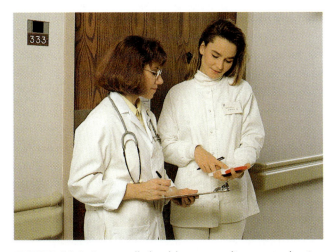

FIGURE 29-1 A mentally healthy person lives a productive life.

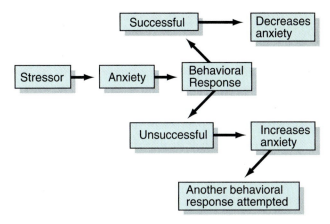

FIGURE 29-2 Individuals learn to cope with stress in different ways.

DEFENSE MECHANISMS

When any person feels unable to cope with stress and the situation threatens self-esteem, the person tends to act in protective ways. These ways are called **defense mechanisms**. A diagnosis of cancer, for instance, may be so overwhelming that a person must temporarily defend himself against acknowledging the truth. Everyone uses these defense-oriented behaviors from time to time to protect themselves. You use them. Patients use them. Your coworkers use them.

You must recognize and understand the need to use defense mechanisms. Do not be critical of their occasional use. Most people do not use one mechanism all the time. They usually rely on a combination of defenses. They may not even be aware that they are behaving in a defensive way.

Defensive behavior becomes harmful only when it is the major means of coping with stress. In such cases, the person continuously avoids recognizing and responding to reality with problem-solving methods. The person's stress is temporarily reduced, but the stressor (feeling or situation) is not resolved. Such a person needs counseling from a trained mental health provider.

Some of the commonly used defense mechanisms include:

- **Repression**—The involuntary exclusion from awareness of a painful or conflict-creating thought, memory, feeling, or impulse. For example, a woman has a lump in her breast, but refuses to go to a physician for examination and diagnosis. She has recently lost her husband, her house, and her job. She feels that she cannot "acknowledge" any other illness or crisis, so she unconsciously represses the knowledge of the lump in her breast. She is not going to take the chance that the lump may be cancer. She cannot face the possibility of a "terminal disease."

- **Suppression**—This mechanism differs from repression because the person is aware of the unacceptable feelings and thoughts but deliberately refuses to acknowledge them. For example, a man becomes immobilized with the fear of rejection by his wife if he tells her he has a diagnosis of AIDS. Therefore, he consciously suppresses the knowledge of the AIDS diagnosis because he cannot handle the anxiety associated with telling his wife.

- **Projection**—A person's own unacceptable feelings and thoughts are attributed to others. The person blames others for his own shortcomings. For example, a person blames his wife or family for his alcoholism and loss of jobs. He projects his failings onto his wife and children.

- **Denial**—Blocking out painful or anxiety-producing events or feelings. This is one of the most common defenses against the stress of diagnosis and illness. For example, a patient with very high blood pressure refuses to stop smoking. She continues to eat a diet high in fats. She cannot deal with her fear of disability and unemployment, so she refuses to accept the seriousness of her condition.

- **Reaction formation**—A person using this defense mechanism represses the reality of a situation and then behaves in a manner that is the exact opposite of the real feelings. For example, a woman dislikes one nursing assistant but is fearful that if she expresses that feeling, the assistant will be less caring. This patient may be overly friendly and cooperative with that assistant.

Other adaptive behaviors are as follows:

- Displacement—Substituting an object or person for another and behaving as if it were the original object or person.

  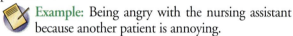 Example: Being angry with the nursing assistant because another patient is annoying.

- Identification—Behaving like another person whom one holds as an ideal.

  Example: Speaking to coworkers with the same tone the supervisor uses with you.

- Compensation—Excelling in one area to make up for feelings of failure in another.

  Example: The nursing assistant who overachieves in the skill area because her ability to read written directions is poor.

- Conversion—Offering a socially acceptable reason to avoid an unpleasant situation.

  Example: The nursing assistant who calls saying she cannot report for duty because she has the flu, when she is just tired from staying up too late.

- Fantasy—The use of imagination to solve problems.

  Example: The supervisor criticizes the nursing assistant, who then daydreams of a time when she is the head of nursing and can fire the supervisor.

- Undoing—A method of reversing something wrong that was done.

  Example: The person who used his hands to hurt another may wash his hands repeatedly to try to undo the deed.

ASSISTING PATIENTS TO COPE

Here are some ways to help patients become better able to cope and adapt:

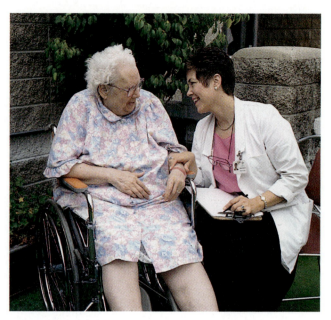

FIGURE 29-3 Staff can help patients find acceptable ways of coping.

- Be a good listener.
- Try to determine the source of stress so it can be removed and the stress reduced.
- Be sensitive to nonverbal messages (body language) that may give clues to the source of stress.
- Treat the person with respect, recognizing him as a unique individual.
- Understand the behavior in the same way the patient is viewing it, without labeling the behavior and passing judgment.
- Let the patient know you are reliable and you respect her privacy and feelings.
- Never argue, enter into a power struggle, or debate with a patient, even when you know the patient is wrong.
- Be supportive of the person's own attempts to overcome the stress (Figure 29-3).

Remember that illness, age, and separation from family and home are major stress factors.

THE DEMANDING PATIENT

In every nursing care situation, you will meet patients who are very demanding. This can be a difficult experience for everyone if it is not handled correctly.

Being demanding is another way that patients show their frustration. It is a coping behavior. Patients who are very demanding are usually frustrated by their loss of control. To be successful in caring for these patients, the nursing assistant must:

- Try to learn and understand the factors that are causing the demanding behavior.
- Show that you care about the patient's situation, but keep control of your emotions.

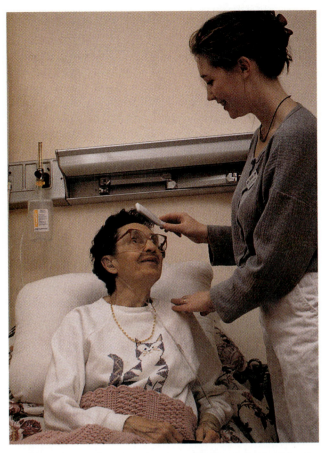

FIGURE 29-4 Being attentive and consistent builds the patient's security.

- Maintain open communications by listening to the patient's words and by being sensitive to the patient's body language.
- Provide opportunities that allow the patient to regain some control by making choices.
- Be consistent in the manner of care. This builds the patient's sense of security (Figure 29-4).
- Do not take the patient's demands personally.
- Report observations to the supervisor with suggestions for changes in the care plan.

ALCOHOLISM

Some people use alcohol as a means of coping with stress. The National Institute for Alcohol Abuse reports that two-thirds of the senior population uses alcohol. Fifteen percent of them become alcoholics. **Alcoholism** is regarded as a disease. Factors that contribute to the excessive use of alcohol include:

- Retirement
- Lowered income
- Grief
- Loss of spouse and/or friends
- Loneliness
- Stress in the family
- Decline in health

- Pain

Alcohol toxicity may be associated with an acute onset of:

- Altered levels of awareness
- Mild confusion
- Progressive stupor
- Acute delirium
- Disorientation similar to that seen in irreversible brain syndrome

Alcohol slows down brain activity. It impairs mental alertness, judgment, physical coordination, and reaction time—increasing the risk of falls and accidents.

Alcohol can affect the body in unusual ways. It can make it difficult to diagnose diseases and conditions of the cardiovascular system. It can mask pain that might otherwise serve as a warning sign of heart attack. Alcohol can also produce:

- Symptoms similar to dementia
- Forgetfulness
- Reduced attention
- Restlessness
- Impatience
- Agitation
- Confusion

Alcohol is a drug. It mixes unfavorably with many other drugs (Table 29-1). The use of alcohol can cause some drugs

TABLE 29-1 COMMON ALCOHOL-DRUG INTERACTIONS	
Drug Taken by Patient	**Effects to Report**
Narcotics	Increased central nervous system (CNS) depression with acute intoxication
Salicylates	Gastrointestinal bleeding
Sedatives and psychotropic drugs	Increased CNS depression with acute intoxication
Barbiturates	Decreased sedative effect after chronic alcohol abuse
Chloral hydrate	Prolonged hypnotic effects
Chlordiazepoxide (Librium, Librax)	Increased CNS depression
Chlorpromazine (Thorazine)	Increased CNS depression
Diazepam (Valium)	Increased CNS depression
Oxazepam (Serax)	Increased CNS depression
Antihistamines	Increased CNS depression
Antabuse	Flushing, vomiting, excessive sweating, hyperventilation, confusion, and drowsiness

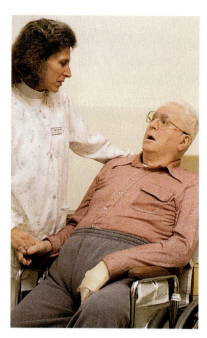

FIGURE 29-5 Listen with empathy.

to metabolize more rapidly, producing exaggerated responses. Such drugs include:

- Anticonvulsants
- Anticoagulants
- Antidiabetic drugs
- Diuretics

The alcoholic in withdrawal feels depressed and defensive. He needs to identify the stressors that bring on his need for alcohol and to find new ways of coping. This process takes professional skill, but you can:

- not allow the alcoholic to manipulate you.
- listen with empathy (Figure 29-5).
- reflect the person's ideas and thoughts.
- be sure alcohol is not available.
- be consistent in the limits that have been set.

Care of the intoxicated patient includes:

- caution during feeding to prevent choking or strangling.
- supervision of activities to prevent injury and falls.
- safety checks during bathing to prevent burns.
- close supervision if there is confusion or delirium.

Problem drinkers and alcoholics have a good chance for recovery. Getting help should start with the family physician, a member of the clergy, the local mental health association, or the local chapter of Alcoholics Anonymous.

MALADAPTIVE BEHAVIORS

Mental illness or **maladaptive behavior** occurs when behaviors and responses disrupt the person's ability to function smoothly within the family, environment, or community.

You must be careful about labeling anyone as mentally ill. Even when an official diagnosis of mental illness has been made, take care not to stereotype the patient.

Remember that stereotypes are often associated with *myths* (false beliefs). It is far better to view the person as an individual who is demonstrating poor behavioral responses.

As a nursing assistant, you need to be aware that sometimes signs and symptoms such as fatigue, loss of appetite, insomnia, and pain may reflect either physical or emotional stress. Note and report any unusual behavior or symptoms. Be careful, however, to be objective. Do not make judgments about your findings.

Remember also that confusion, disorientation, and aggressive behavior may only be temporary responses to a fever, drug interaction, or a full bladder. Continuation of such behavior may be the result of organic brain changes. Blaming and judging a patient is inappropriate and unhelpful.

Assessing the Patient's Behavior

An initial assessment of the patient's mental and emotional state will be made by the licensed care provider. Because you make frequent contact with the patient, you can make a valuable contribution to the nursing assessment process by making careful and sensitive objective observations.

Report observations regarding:

- Physical responses related to eating, personal hygiene, sleeping, participation in activities, or any strange or unusual behaviors
- Emotional responses related to interactions between the patient and yourself or between the patient and other patients, emotional outbursts, or inappropriate responses
- Patient's behavior as it relates to judgment and affects memory, comprehension, and orientation

When working in long-term care, you will find many people whose coping ability has failed and so are demonstrating maladaptive behaviors. The many losses these people have suffered add to their inability to cope. Physical problems make dealing with reality more difficult.

Common maladaptive responses result in:

- Depression
- Disorientation or delirium
- Agitation
- Paranoia

Depression

Depression is the most common functional disorder in older people (Figure 29-6), but younger people also may experience depression. Depression may be shown in a variety of ways:

- Preoccupation with constipation
- Flatulence
- Bad taste in the mouth
- Burning tongue
- Vague oral discomforts associated with dentures
- Burning on urination
- Pain in lower abdomen
- Crying spells

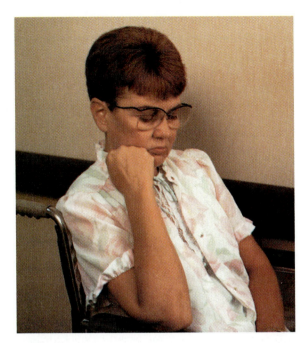

FIGURE 29-6 Withdrawal is common in a person who is depressed.

- Trouble sleeping (insomnia)
- Excessive sleep
- Loss of appetite or increased appetite
- Significant weight loss or weight gain
- Fatigue
- Headaches
- Backaches
- Stiff joints
- Apathy
- Impaired concentration
- Lethargy
- Agitation
- Poor personal hygiene
- Feeling of dejection
- Less interest in sex
- Depressed mood most of the day, nearly every day (irritability in children)
- Markedly diminished interest or pleasure in almost all activities, most of the day and nearly every day
- Psychomotor agitation or retardation
- Feelings of worthlessness or guilt
- Recurrent thoughts of death or suicide

Depression is often masked by symptoms that make it seem as though the patient is physically ill. Your observations are doubly important because a patient who is depressed may actually have minor or major illnesses. These infirmities may in turn cause depression. Remember, physical and mental health are interrelated.

Some drugs that are used to treat actual physical illness in the elderly may cause depression. They are:

- Digitalis
- Reserpine
- Inderal
- Diuretics
- Most of the antihypertensive drugs

If your patient is receiving any of these drugs, be alert for signs of depression. If the depression is drug-induced, it will be relieved when the drug is withdrawn.

Severely depressed patients may be treated with:

- Antidepressants
- Electroshock therapy (in severe cases)
- Talk therapy

A mental health clinical nurse specialist, psychologist, or psychiatrist will direct and support the staff efforts.

When depression is severe, suicidal thoughts and attempts are a real possibility. You must be sensitive to the possibility of such a situation and report and document your observations. The suicidal patient must be carefully protected. Watch for and report:

- Change in response such as deepening depression or sudden elevation of mood
- Evidence of withdrawal or secretiveness
- Sudden loss of a support system (such as the death of a family member)
- Repeated, prolonged, or sporadic refusal of food (oral or through nasal tubes), care, medications, or fluids
- Hoarding of medication (stockpiling of pills)
- Sudden decision to donate body parts to a medical school
- Changes in behavior, especially episodes of depression, screaming, hitting, throwing things, or a sudden failure to get along with family, friends, or peers
- Sudden interest or disinterest in religion
- Purchase of a gun
- Purchase of razor blades and hiding them
- Statements such as: "I just want out," "I want to end it all," "I'll never get well," "I'm going to kill myself," or "You would be better off without me."
- Increased use of alcohol and alcoholic drinks
- Behavioral manifestations of anger, hostility, belligerence, loss of interest, or inability to concentrate
- Inability to do simple tasks, confusion, slurred speech, or retarded motor skills
- Deep preoccupation with something that cannot be explained

Nursing Care of a Patient with the Potential for Suicide. Never assume that a suicide attempt is a means of getting the attention of the staff or family. At least 15% of people who try to commit suicide do it again. Keep in mind the at-risk individuals. These include:

- White males over the age of 65 who live alone
- The very old (75 years and above)
- Persons with a recent diagnosis of a terminal illness

GUIDELINES
for

Assisting the Patient Who Is Depressed

- Reinforce the person's self-concept by emphasizing her continued value to society and helping the patient to use the support systems that are available (Figure 29-7).
- Do not act in a pitying way. This only validates the person's depressed feelings.
- Make sure physical supports, such as eyeglasses and hearing aids, are in place. These help the person to focus on reality.
- Report all complaints so actual physical problems may be identified and corrected rather than being attributed to the depression.

- Provide the person with activities within her limitations to help her think beyond herself. For example, engage the person in some meaningful activity such as reading, making puzzles, or conversing with others (Figure 29-8).
- Avoid tiring activities.
- Use simple language and speak slowly when giving instructions.
- Monitor elimination carefully; constipation is common.
- Provide fluids frequently, because the depressed patient may be too preoccupied to drink.
- Be alert to the potential for suicide (the taking of one's own life).

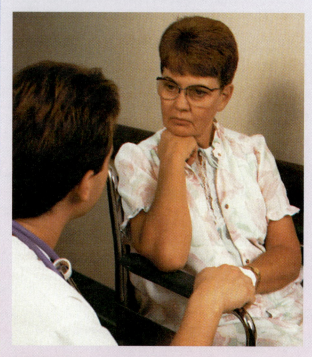

FIGURE 29-7 Try to reinforce the depressed person's sense of self-worth.

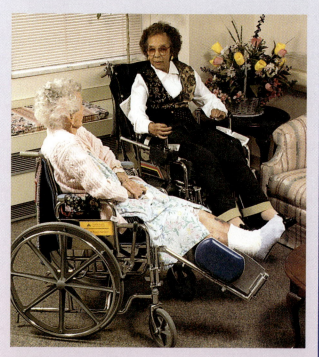

FIGURE 29-8 Socializing with others may help the person who is depressed.

- Those suffering the sudden loss of a spouse
- The elderly with recent multiple losses

Be aware that the suicide rate is higher in acute medical units than it is on psychiatric units. Most of the suicides occur while the patient is under the supervision of a health provider, who frequently either misses or ignores the clues of suicide. Suicide attempts may occur either when the patient is successfully recovering or is getting worse. It is the responsibility of all staff members to observe their patients carefully and immediately report any signs of depression and/or suicide. You should:

- Be observant for clues to suicide attempts, and report them to the appropriate person.
- Be consistent in approaches and care.
- Encourage the patient to review his life, emphasizing the positive aspects.
- Give the patient hope while being realistic (Figure 29-9).
- Work to restore the person's self-esteem, self-worth, and self-respect, to preserve positive self-concept.
- Help the patient find a support network within the family, religious groups, and self-help groups.

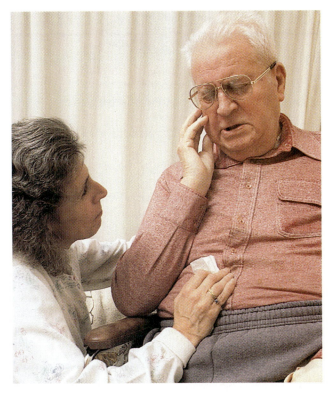

FIGURE 29-9 Be hopeful but realistic with the person who is depressed and may have a potential for suicide.

- Make the person feel accepted as a unique, valued person.
- Never ignore the person's statements or threats about suicide.

Disorientation (Disordered Consciousness)

Disorientation is a condition in which a person shows a lack of reality awareness with regard to time, person, or place (Figure 29-10). In some cases, the disorientation is mild, sometimes severe; sometimes temporary but at times pro-

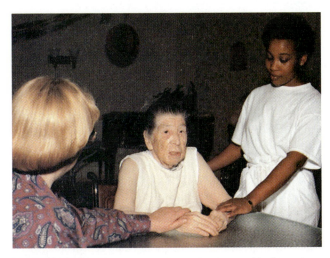

FIGURE 29-10 The person who is disoriented lacks awareness of reality.

longed. It is important to report patient behavior, actions, and responses. The disoriented person has impaired:

- Judgment
- Memory
- Comprehension
- Orientation

Physical ailments and stresses that can bring about a disoriented state include:

- Recovery from surgery
- Pneumonia
- Myocardial infarction
- Renal infection
- Head trauma
- Organic brain disease
- Fevers
- Dehydration
- Malnutrition
- Drug interaction

The signs and symptoms that identify the disoriented person are:

- Inability to think clearly
- Bewilderment
- Faulty memory
- Inability to follow directions
- Misinterpretation of stimuli
- Confusion about time
- Confusion about place
- Confusion about who he or she is

Nursing Assistant Responsibilities. The nursing assistant must realize that disoriented people cannot be responsible for their actions or for protecting themselves adequately. The patient's sensory misinterpretations (delusions or hallucinations) may put others at risk. The disorientation does not allow the patient to take action for self-protection. *Protection of the patient is the most important nursing responsibility.* In addition, you should:

- Be calm and gentle when approaching the patient. Disoriented patients are startled by even minor stimuli.
- Give instructions slowly, clearly, and in simple words.
- Give only one instruction at a time.
- Provide activities of short length that do not require much concentration.
- Build the patient's self-esteem with the reward of positive comments.
- Assist patients to participate in reality orientation activities (Figure 29-11). **Reality orientation** is making the disoriented patient aware of person, place, and time by visual reminders, activities, and verbal cues. See the guidelines for reality orientation activities.
- Maintain a constant, limited routine.
- Use restraints only when absolutely necessary and with a physician's order, making sure all safety practices are fol-

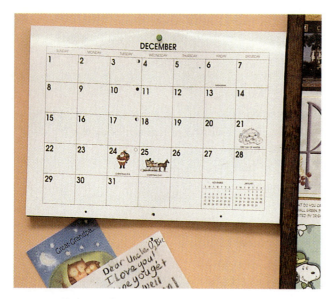

FIGURE 29-11 Calendars and clocks may help prevent disorientation.

lowed. Medications that chemically restrain patient responses and the presence of a friend or family member may make physical restraints unnecessary.

- Reduce disorientation by keeping rooms well lighted, cool, and quiet. Also, provide reality orientation according to the nursing care plan.

To maintain a safe environment for disoriented patients:

- Keep all sharps, such as knives, out of reach.
- Remove and store valuable or breakable items. If patient is at home, make sure the family knows where you put these items.
- Use sturdy chairs and couches.
- Put rails on windows that are close to the floor.
- Provide adequate lighting.
- Protect stairways with gates.
- Do not permit poisonous plants.
- Control matches and smoking materials.
- Supervise use of stoves and appliances.
- Keep all medications out of reach.

Agitation

Agitation is defined as inappropriate verbal, vocal, or motor activity due to causes other than disorientation or real need. It includes behavior such as:

- Aimless wandering
- Pacing
- Cursing
- Screaming
- Repeatedly asking the same question
- Spitting
- Biting
- Fighting constantly
- Demanding attention

Agitation is a significant problem for the elderly, their families, and the nursing staff. It is probably one of the foremost management problems in acute care hospitals, in home care, and in long-term care facilities.

The major factors contributing to agitation are:

- Noise
- Frustration at loss of control
- Feelings that the patient's space has been invaded
- Loneliness and need for attention
- Unresolved personal difficulties in the patient's past
- Drug interactions
- Organic brain disease
- Boredom
- Behavior of others around the patient
- Depression
- Constipation
- Restraints
- Too much sensory stimulation

Study this list carefully, because your awareness can lead to early intervention. Early intervention can often prevent serious problems.

Hypochondriasis

The patient suffering from **hypochondriasis** imagines or magnifies each physical ailment. Some authorities feel that hypochondriasis is an expression of depression and is one way these individuals reduce stress. These patients need reassurance and understanding but should not be encouraged to focus or believe in their supposed illnesses. However, the staff must be careful not to overlook real illness when it occurs, just

GUIDELINES *for*

Managing the Patient Who Is Agitated

- Do not argue with or confront the person.
- Make the environment safe (secure the windows and lock the doors).
- Make sure each patient wears an identification bracelet or patch, and that it is fastened securely.
- Keep a recent photo of the patient in case the patient wanders off.
- Notify the physician, the administrator, the family, or the police department if the patient wanders away from his unit, facility, or home.
- Assign the patient brief tasks.
- Engage the patient in games, walks, swimming, and other activities if not contraindicated. These should be activities that enhance the patient's self-esteem.
- Use bean-bag seats and rocking chairs in the parlors of the nursing home or the patient's home.
- Care for the patient—watch for injuries.
- Engage the patient in conversations and in reality therapy or remotivation groups.
- Engage the patient in short-term activities. Realize that the patient's attention span is short. Thus, the patient needs rewards for short-term activities.
- Prevent the patient from becoming exhausted.
- Carefully monitor the patient's activities, because the agitated patient is at risk for falls and injuries.

because they have become used to hearing the patient complain. Nursing assistants should report all complaints and never make a judgment that a patient is a hypochondriac.

Paranoia

Paranoia is another extreme maladaptive response to stress. It is characterized by a heightened, false sense of self-importance and delusions of being persecuted. Delusions are false beliefs about oneself, other people, and events. People with paranoia believe that everyone is against them. When treating the paranoid patient, you should:

- Find ways to reduce the patient's feelings of insecurity and misunderstanding.
- Keep the person as involved as possible in reality activities.
- Report and document observed responses to medication and psychotherapy.
- Monitor nutrition and fluid balance—these patients often refuse to eat or drink for fear of poisoning.
- Observe sleep patterns—the person may be fearful of being harmed while sleeping.
- Be direct and honest in all interactions.
- Not support any misconceptions or delusions that the person exhibits.
- Never argue with anyone who has delusions. It can trigger a serious confrontation.

REVIEW

A. True/False.

Mark the following true or false by circling T or F.

1. T F Mental health refers to the adaptations a person makes to the multiple stressors of life.

2. T F Stressors are the physical and emotional problems that a person encounters throughout life.

3. T F Defense mechanisms are used only by mentally unhealthy persons.

4. T F If you know that the patient is wrong about something she is saying, it is proper to debate the issue with the patient.

5. T F The best way to handle the demanding patient is by trying to determine the underlying factors causing the patient's distress.

6. T F Very few senior adults use alcohol and even fewer become alcoholics.

7. T F The use of alcohol impairs mental alertness, judgment, reaction time, and physical coordination.

8. T F It is dangerous for a person to drink alcohol when taking other medications.

9. T F Alcohol is a drug.

10. T F When intoxicated, a person could choke on food.

11. T F Alcoholics have a poor chance for recovery.

12. T F Maladaptive behaviors reflect the failure of usual defense mechanisms.

13. T F Depression is the least common of the functional disorders in older people.

14. T F The depressed patient needs to be encouraged not to be overactive.

15. T F Dehydration can lead the patient into a state of disorientation.

16. T F The disoriented patient needs a stimulating environment.

17. T F It is best to give a disoriented patient one instruction at a time.

18. T F If a patient threatens suicide, you need not be concerned.

19. T F The white male who is over age 65 and living alone is at high risk for suicide.

20. T F It is the responsibility of only the licensed staff to guard against suicide attempts.

21. T F Suicides are attempted only by patients in psychiatric institutions.

22. T F The patient who is agitated may ask the same question repeatedly.

23. T F Agitation is a significant problem for the elderly, their families, and facility staff.

24. T F Paranoia is a maladaptive response that usually requires medication and psychotherapy.

25. T F Paranoid individuals believe that others are out to get them.

B. Matching.

Choose the correct word from Column II to match each phrase or statement in Column I.

Column I	Column II
26. _____ conscious refusal to recognize the reality of the situation	**a.** repression
27. _____ excelling in one area to make up for feelings of failure in another	**b.** suppression
	c. projection
28. _____ blocking out painful or anxiety-producing events or feelings	**d.** denial
	e. identification
29. _____ involuntary exclusion of the awareness of reality	**f.** compensation
	g. conversion
30. _____ offering socially acceptable reasons to avoid an unpleasant situation	**h.** displacement
31. _____ substituting an object for another and behaving as if it were the original object	
32. _____ attributing one's own failing to another	
33. _____ behaving like another who is held in high regard	

C. Multiple Choice.

Select the one best answer for each question.

34. The patient tells you that her doctor says she has AIDS, but she knows that isn't possible. She most likely is using the defense mechanism of
    a. repression.
    b. displacement.
    c. projection.
    d. denial.

35. The best way to enhance the patient's capability to cope with an unpleasant situation that has developed with another patient is to
    a. tell him to ignore it.
    b. let him know he can talk to you safely.
    c. tell him everyone has problems, his aren't so important.
    d. suggest he discuss it with his clergyperson.

36. The patient who refuses to eat or drink because she is convinced that she is being poisoned is suffering from
    a. paranoia.
    b. depression.
    c. agitation.
    d. disorientation.

37. The patient is depressed. You can best help him by
    a. pitying him.
    b. keeping him from interacting with others.
    c. agreeing that he probably deserves the way he feels.
    d. stressing his continued value to society.

38. The best way to help the patient remain oriented to reality is to
    a. keep glasses in the bedside stand so they won't be broken.
    b. isolate the patient.
    c. place a clock and calendar nearby.
    d. explain things in detail.

39. The person holding a doll and acting as if it were a baby probably is experiencing
    a. repression.
    b. denial.
    c. projection.
    d. displacement.

40. Agitation may be demonstrated by
    a. repetitive questions.
    b. pacing.
    c. biting.
    d. all of these.

D. Nursing Assistant Challenge.

You are assigned to care for Mr. Simonson, who has recently been diagnosed with diabetes. He is a top executive in a large corporation and has a wife and three adult children. He is learning how to administer his insulin, how to plan his diet, and how to test his blood sugar. He has been very quiet and keeps his eyes closed most of the time, although he is not sleeping. One day as you enter the room, he screams at you to get out and then picks up his water pitcher and throws it. Think about what you learned in this unit about human behavior as you consider these questions.

41. What examples of nonverbal communication is Mr. Simonson displaying?

42. Do you think he is using defense mechanisms to cope with his diagnosis? If so, which ones?

43. If Mr. Simonson displays this kind of behavior again, what would be an appropriate response from the nursing staff?

44. How would you document this episode?

45. How can the nursing staff show respect and concern for this patient?

Death and Dying

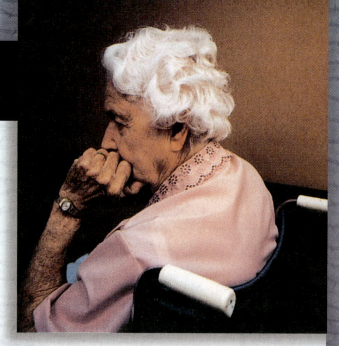

OBJECTIVES

As a result of this unit, you will be able to:
- Spell and define terms.
- Describe how different people handle the process of death and dying.
- List the signs of approaching death.
- Describe the nursing assistant's responsibilities for providing supportive care.
- Describe the spiritual preparations for death practiced by various religious denominations.
- Describe the hospice philosophy and method of care.
- Demonstrate the following procedure:
  - Procedure 90 Giving Postmortem Care

VOCABULARY

Learn the meaning and the correct spelling of the following words and phrases:

acceptance
advance directive
anger
autopsy
bargaining
cardiac arrest
cardiopulmonary
  resuscitation (CPR)

critical list
denial
depression
DNR
durable power of
  attorney for health
  care

harvested
hospice care
life-sustaining treatment
living will
moribund
no-code order
postmortem

postmortem care
rigor mortis
Sacrament of the Sick
supportive care
terminal

INTRODUCTION

Death is the final stage of life. It may come suddenly, without warning, or it may follow a long period of illness. It sometimes strikes the young but it always awaits the old. As a nursing assistant, you will be providing care throughout the period of dying and into the after-death (**postmortem**) period. Accepting the idea that death is the natural result of the life process may help you respond to your patient's needs more generously.

The concept of death and dying is handled differently by different people (Figure 30-1). There are many reactions to the diagnosis of a **terminal** (life-ending) illness:

- Some patients may have had time to prepare psychologically for their deaths. They may accept or be resigned to the inevitable.
- Some may actually look forward to relief from the pain and emotional burden of a long illness and await death calmly.
- Some may be fearful or angry and demonstrate moods that swing from outright denial to depression.
- Others may reach out, trying to verbalize feelings and thoughts of an uncertain future.
- In others, despair and anxiety may give way to moments of active hostility or periods of searching, groping questions.

None of the reaction states are predictable and no patient falls into one rigid pattern or another. You must accept the patient's behavior with understanding, interpret the patient's very real need for family support, and support the

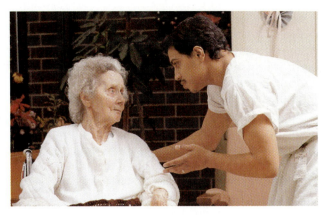

FIGURE 30-1 Each person handles death differently.

family in meeting their own needs during this adjustment period.

FIVE STAGES OF GRIEF

Dr. Elisabeth Kubler-Ross identified five stages of grief that can occur in the dying patient. They are denial, anger, bargaining, depression, and acceptance (Table 30-1). If there is adequate time and support, some patients may be able to move psychologically through each stage to a point of acceptance of their illness and death.

- **Denial** begins when the person is made aware that he is going to die. He may not accept this information as truth, and may instead deny it. Making long-range plans that are not likely to be fulfilled may indicate that the patient is in the denial stage. Most people with a termi-

TABLE 30-1 EMOTIONAL RESPONSES TO DYING	
Stages of Grief	**Response of the Nursing Assistant**
Denial	Reflect patient's statements, but try not to confirm or deny the fact that the patient is dying.
	Example: *"The lab tests can't be right—I don't have cancer."* *"It must have been difficult for you to learn the results of your tests."*
Anger	Understand the source of the patient's anger. Provide understanding and support. Listen. Try to meet reasonable needs and demands quickly.
	Example: *"This food is terrible—not fit to eat."* *"Let me see if I can find something that would appeal to you more."*
Bargaining	If it is possible to meet the patient's requests, do so. Listen attentively.
	Example: *"If only God will spare me this, I'll go to church every week."* *"Would you like a visit from your clergyperson?"*
Depression	Avoid clichés that dismiss the patient's depression ("It could be worse—you could be in more pain"). Be caring and supporting. Let the patient know that it is all right to be depressed.
	Example: *"There just isn't any sense in going on."* *"I understand you are feeling very depressed."*
Acceptance	Do not assume that, because the patient has accepted death, she or he is unafraid, or that she or he does not need emotional support. Listen attentively and be supportive and caring.
	Example: *"I feel so alone."* *"I am here with you. Would you like to talk?"*

nal illness must go through denial before they are able to eventually reach acceptance. This is a necessary and therapeutic stage. Other people should not try to convince the patient of his diagnosis or argue with the person. If denial begins to interfere with the person's adjustment, then professional counseling may be required.

- **Anger** comes when the patient is no longer able to deny the fact that she is going to die. The patient may blame those around her, including those who are giving care, for her illness. Added stresses, however small, are likely to upset the patient who is in the anger stage (Figure 30-2). Statements such as, "It's all your fault. I should never have come to this hospital," are typical of a patient in the anger stage. Remember, if the patient expresses anger, that she is angry about her diagnosis, not with you personally. Remain calm and avoid saying anything that may make her angrier. If you think the patient is angry about something other than the diagnosis, report this to the nurse so the situation can be remedied.

- **Bargaining** is the stage in the grief process in which the patient attempts to bargain for more time to live. He may ask to be allowed to go home to finish a task before he dies, or he may make private "deals" with God: "If you will let me live another two months, I promise I will try to be a better person." Bargaining frequently involves an important event that the patient has been looking forward to, such as a child's wedding or the birth of a grandchild. The patient in this stage is basically saying, "I know I'm going to die and I'm ready to die, but not just yet." This may be done in private and not stated verbally.

- **Depression** is the fourth stage identified in the grief process. During this stage, the patient comes to a full realization that she will die soon (Figure 30-3). She is

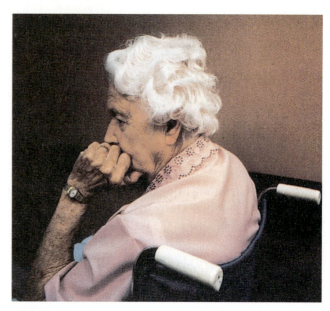

FIGURE 30-3 Depression is associated with the grieving process.

saddened by the thought that she will no longer be with family and friends, and by the fact that she may not have accomplished some goals that she had set for herself. She may also express regrets about not having gone somewhere or done something: "I always promised my husband that we would go to Europe and now we'll never go."

- **Acceptance** is the stage during which a patient understands and accepts the fact that she is going to die (Figure 30-4). During this stage, she may try to complete

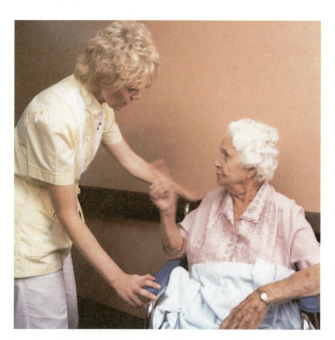

FIGURE 30-2 Patients may demonstrate feelings of frustration and anger.

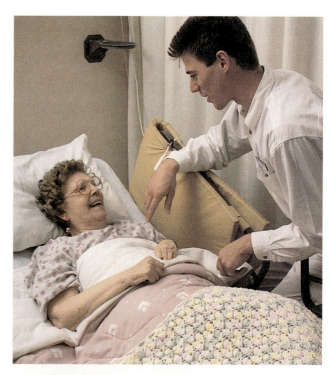

FIGURE 30-4 During the stage of acceptance, the patient may strive to complete unfinished business.

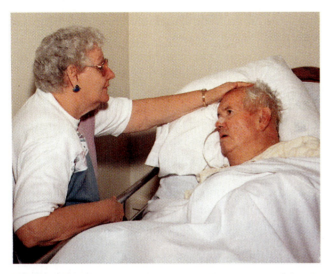

FIGURE 30-5 Dying patients need the support of family and friends.

unfinished business. Having accepted her eventual death, she may also try to help those around her to deal with it, especially family members.

Not all patients progress through these stages in sequential order. Nor does movement from one level to the next mean that the previous level will be completely left behind. The staff must be aware of the possible psychological positions and be able to identify the patient's current reactions. For example, a patient who displays anger one day may be full of optimism and denial the next.

Denial frequently comes first, followed by anger and despair. Frustrated by feelings of helplessness, the person lashes out at those who are nearby. If each of these stages is expressed with some degree of success, the person is then able to move on to a level of grieving, for himself and for loved ones. When all five stages have been passed, it is believed that the patient is better able to accept the termination of life. If there is adequate time and support (Figure 30-5), many patients can be helped to reach a more accepting frame of mind.

The family and staff move through these same stages, but not necessarily at the same time. It is particularly difficult when the patient is in one stage and the family is at another stage.

PREPARATION FOR DEATH

The knowledge of impending death comes to the patient directly from the physician or indirectly from the staff. A diagnosis of terminal illness is very difficult to conceal from the patient. The staff may, without realizing it, reveal the information by:

- Exhibiting false cheerfulness
- Being evasive
- Making fewer visits to the patient's room
- Spending less time with the patient

You must realize that most terminally ill patients do eventually come to accept that death is part of their near future. Keep the following in mind:

- Each patient reacts to this understanding in a unique way.
- How many feelings the patient wishes to share and with whom are very personal decisions.
- You should be available to listen, but do not force the issue.

Upon being told of the terminal diagnosis, the patient may proceed through several stages of emotional adjustment. Initially, the

- patient may react to the situation by denying the truth.
- patient may refuse all opportunities to discuss his illness with the staff or with family.
- patient's interpersonal relationships with family and staff may become greatly strained.
- patient may become defeated and full of despair, actively expressing a loss of hope.

THE PATIENT SELF-DETERMINATION ACT

The Patient Self-Determination Act of 1990 requires health care providers to supply written information about state laws regarding **advance directives**. An advance directive is a document that is put into effect if the patient later becomes unable to make decisions. All health care providers, including hospitals, long-term care facilities, and home health care agencies, must have policies and procedures covering these issues. The information must be provided before or at the time of admission.

Decisions often must be made when a patient is terminally or critically ill. These decisions involve provision of supportive care or life-sustaining treatment. The Patient Self-Determination Act was passed to assure patients and their families that their wishes will be followed. **Supportive care** means that the patient's life will not be artificially prolonged but that the patient will be kept comfortable physically, mentally, and emotionally. Supportive care includes:

- Oxygen to ease breathing if the patient needs it
- Food and fluids that the patient can consume by mouth
- Medications for pain, nausea, anxiety, or other physical or emotional discomforts
- The continuation of physical care such as grooming and hygiene, cleanliness, positioning, and range-of-motion exercises
- Caring and emotional support of staff

All patients deserve supportive care, but for terminally or critically ill patients, supportive care means the absence of life-sustaining treatment. **Life-sustaining treatment** means giving medications and treatments for the purpose of maintaining life. Life-sustaining treatments include all of the items listed under supportive care and may also include:

- Being placed on a ventilator to maintain breathing
- Receiving **cardiopulmonary resuscitation** (**CPR**) if **cardiac arrest** occurs (the heart and lungs stop functioning)

- Artificial nutrition through a feeding tube or hyperalimentation device
- Blood transfusions
- Surgery
- Radiation therapy
- Chemotherapy
- Other treatments that will maintain life

 Note: Radiation therapy and chemotherapy may also be given to relieve pain, not to extend life.

There are basically two types of advance directives: the living will and the durable power of attorney for health care. The **living will** is a request that death not be artificially postponed if the patient has an incurable, irreversible injury, disease, or illness that the physician judges to be a terminal condition. A living will must be witnessed by two other individuals who do not stand to benefit because of the person's death.

The **durable power of attorney for health care** is a directive that assigns someone else the responsibility for handling the patient's affairs and making medical decisions for the patient if the patient becomes unable to do so for himself. It must be signed by the *agent* (the person given the durable power of attorney) and by the *principal* (the person appointing the agent). It also must be signed by an adult witness. The durable power of attorney may indicate whether the person:

- Does not want his life to be prolonged and does not want life-sustaining treatment
- Wants his life prolonged and wants life-sustaining treatment to be provided unless the physician believes he is in an irreversible coma
- Wants his life to be prolonged to the greatest extent possible without regard to his condition

The durable power of attorney is one way to ensure that the wishes and rights of an individual will be followed and protected when the person is no longer able to make personal decisions. As a nursing assistant, you must be aware of the patient's status for supportive care or life-sustaining treatment. The person on supportive care will have a **no-code order** or **DNR** (do not resuscitate) order. This means that no extraordinary means, such as CPR to resuscitate the person, will be used to prevent death. This allows a person to die peacefully with maximum dignity. A no-code decision is reached after discussion by the patient with her family and physician. Once made, the no-code decision is entered in the patient's chart. All staff members are made aware of the decision, but it is kept confidential. If the patient changes her mind, the order in the chart is changed.

THE ROLE OF THE NURSING ASSISTANT

As a nursing assistant, you spend much time with the patient. You have a unique opportunity to be a source of strength and comfort. You must behave in a way that instills confidence in both the patient and the patient's family. Developing the proper attitude and approach for this type of situation is not easy. It will come with experience. There are some things to keep in mind:

- Your response should be consistent. It should be guided by the patient's attitude and the care plan.
- You must be open and receptive, because the terminal patient's attitude may change from day to day.
- Make sure you inform the nurse of incidents related to the patient that reflect moods and needs.
- Remember, each person's idea of death and the hereafter differs. You must be open to patients' ideas and not force your own upon them.
- Your own feelings about death and dying influence your ability to care for the dying patient. Honestly explore your feelings by talking about them with others until you can resolve any conflicts you may have. Your acceptance of death as a natural occurrence will enable you to meet patient needs in a realistic manner.
- Give your best and most careful nursing care, with special attention to comfort measures such as mouth care and fluid intake.
- You should be quietly empathetic and carry out your duties in a calm, efficient way.

When a patient's condition is critical, the physician will place his name officially on the **critical list**. Then the family and the chaplain will be notified.

Providing for Spiritual Needs

Many people find spiritual faith to be a source of great comfort during difficult times.

- Some religions have specific rituals that are carried out when a person is very ill or dying (Table 30-2). Your role is to cooperate with the patient, family, and clergyperson so that these rituals may be performed in a dignified, caring manner.
- Other religions do not have specific practices, but patients of those religions may spend time in prayer. Allow the patient and family privacy, but let them know you are close by if you are needed.
- Some patients may have no formal religious affiliation. This does not mean they do not have spiritual needs. They may request the services of a clergyperson and may not know who to call on. Relay this request to the nurse, because most health care facilities have chaplains to provide the services.
- Some patients do not believe in any higher spiritual being. This is their right and no one should try to change their feelings.
- Always respect the beliefs or nonbeliefs of any patient. Treat all religious items, such as Bibles, medals, and rosaries, with respect.
- When a Catholic patient is ill, a priest may be called for the **Sacrament of the Sick** (Figure 30-6). It is preferable that the family be present and leave the room only while the confession is heard. The practicing Catholic and her family consider it a privilege to have the opportunity for

TABLE 30-2 BELIEFS AND PRACTICES RELATED TO DYING AND DEATH FOR MAJOR RELIGIONS

Religion	Autopsy	Organ Donation	Beliefs and Practices
Judaism (Orthodox)	Only in special circumstances	With consultation of rabbi	Visits to the dying are a religious duty.
			Witness must be present if death occurs, to protect family and commit soul to God.
			Torah and Psalms may be read and prayers recited.
			Conversation is kept to a minimum.
			Someone should be with the body after death until burial, usually within 24 hours.
			Body must not be touched 8 to 30 minutes after death.
			Medical personnel should not touch or wash body unless death occurs on Jewish Sabbath; then care may be given by nurse wearing gloves.
			Water is removed from the room.
			Mirrors may be covered at family's request.
Hinduism	Permitted	Permitted	Priest ties thread around neck or wrist of deceased and pours water in the mouth.
			Only family and friends touch body.
Buddhism	Personal preference	Permitted	Buddhist priest is present at death.
			Last rites are chanted at the bedside.
Islam (Muslim)	Only for medical or legal reasons	Not permitted	Before death, read Koran and pray.
			Resident confesses sins and asks forgiveness of family.
			Only family touches or washes body.
			After death, body is turned toward Mecca.
Roman Catholic	Permitted	Permitted	Sacrament of the Sick administered to ill residents, to residents in imminent danger, or shortly after death.
Christian Scientist	Unlikely	Not permitted	No ritual is performed before or after death.
Church of Christ	Permitted	Permitted	No ritual is performed before or after death.
Jehovah's Witness	Only if required by law	Not permitted	No ritual is performed before or after death.
Baptist	Permitted	Permitted	Clergy ministers through counseling and prayers.
Episcopalian	Permitted	Permitted	Last rites are optional.
Lutheran	Permitted	Permitted	Last rites are optional.
Eastern Orthodox Christian	Not encouraged	Not encouraged	Last rites are mandatory and are given by ordained priest.

confession. Many patients recover completely, but this hope should not prevent the reception of this sacrament if this is the patient's wish.

- A Bible or spiritual reading of the patient's faith, if requested, may be of some spiritual help through this crisis. Be courteous and provide privacy when the patient's clergyperson visits.

Be aware that dying is a lonely business, a journey each person must finish alone. Until the final moment comes, privacy, but not total solitude, should be the guiding rule (Figure 30-7).

It is important to remember the family and other loved ones when a patient is dying. Check the policies of your health care facility and assist in the following actions:

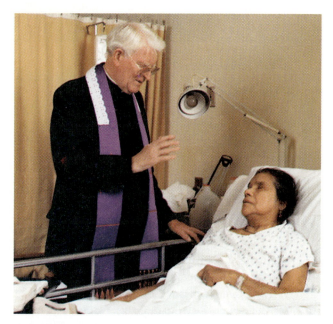

FIGURE 30-6 The Sacrament of the Sick is administered to gravely ill Roman Catholic patients.

- Allow the family to be with the patient as they desire.
- Allow the family to assist with some of the care, if they wish to do so; for example, moistening the patient's lips or giving a backrub.
- Inform the family where they can get a cup of coffee or a meal.
- Show the family where they can use a telephone in private.
- If a family member stays during the night, offer a pillow and blanket. Some facilities provide recliners or cots for family members.
- Avoid being judgmental of family members. Remember that each person grieves in his or her own way. The emotions that others see are not necessarily an accurate indication of what the individual is feeling.

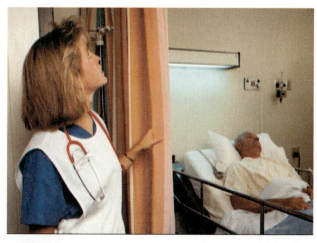

FIGURE 30-7 The dying patient needs privacy but not total solitude.

HOSPICE CARE

Hospice care has evolved around the philosophy that death is a natural process that should neither be hastened nor delayed and that the dying person should be kept comfortable. **Hospice care** is:

- Provided to terminally ill people with a life expectancy of six months or less
- Involved with direct physical care when needed
- Supportive to both the family and the patient
- Provided in special hospice facilities, in other care facilities, and at home
- Largely carried out by a home health assistant or a nursing assistant under the direction of professional health care providers
- Follow-up bereavement counseling to help survivors accept the death of a loved one
- A program in which volunteers play an important role, making regular personal visits to the patient and family

Hospice care is provided by teams who work in conjunction with the terminally ill person and his family. The team usually consists of a physician, professional nurse, nursing assistant, and other professionals (such as social workers and clergy) as needed and desired.

The goals of hospice care include:

- Control of pain so the individual can remain an active participant in life until death
- Coordinating psychological, spiritual, and social support services for the patient and the family
- Making legal and financial counseling available to the patient and family

Because hospice care is a philosophy, it becomes part of the guide for your actions when caring for the terminally ill. Hospice care is provided as you give your usual care. Some things to keep in mind, however, are:

- Report pain immediately and give close attention to comfort measures.
- Encourage the person to carry out as much self-care as possible.
- Be readily available to listen. Spend as much time with the patient as possible and desired by the patient.
- Get to know the family and be supportive to them.
- Give the same care you would if a terminal diagnosis had not been made.
- Carry out all activities with dignity and respect.

PHYSICAL CHANGES AS DEATH APPROACHES

As death approaches, there are notable physical changes. As these changes occur, report them immediately to the charge nurse.

- The patient becomes less responsive (Figure 30-8).
- Body functions slow down.

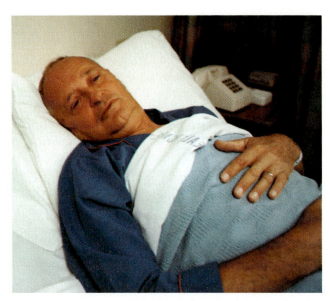

FIGURE 30-8 As death approaches, the patient becomes less responsive and bodily functions slow down.

- The patient loses general voluntary and involuntary muscle control.
- The patient may involuntarily void and defecate.
- The jaw tends to drop.
- Breathing becomes irregular and shallow.
- Circulation slows and the extremities become cold. The pulse becomes rapid and progressively weaker.
- Skin pales.
- The eyes stare and do not respond to light.
- Hearing seems to be the last sense to be lost. Do not assume that because death is approaching, the patient can no longer hear. You must be careful what you say.

In the period before death, the patient with a terminal diagnosis needs and receives the same care as the patient who is expected to recover. Attention is paid to physical as well as emotional needs.

As it becomes clear that death will occur very soon, you should call the nurse, who will supervise the care during the final moments of life.

Signs of Death

After death, changes continue to take place in the body. These changes are called **moribund** (dying) changes.

- Pupils become permanently dilated.
- There is no pulse or respiration.
- Heat is gradually lost from the body.
- The patient may urinate, defecate, or release flatus.
- Blood pools in the lowest areas of the body, giving a purplish discoloration to those areas.
- Within 2 to 4 hours, body rigidity, called **rigor mortis**, develops.
- Unless embalmed within 24 hours, there is indication of progressive protein breakdown.

POSTMORTEM CARE

The patient's body should be treated with respect at all times. Before death occurs, the limbs should be straightened and the head elevated on a pillow. The body should be cleaned by gently washing it with warm water. Discharges must be washed off and wiped away.

Care of the body after death is called **postmortem care** (Figure 30-9). This may be your responsibility. You may find it easier if you ask a coworker to assist.

- Use gloves when giving postmortem care. The body may continue to be infectious following death.
- Treat the body with the same dignity you would a living person.
- Some facilities prefer to have the patient left alone until the mortuary staff arrive. Your responsibility will be only to prepare the body for viewing by the family.
- Check the hospital procedure manual before proceeding with postmortem care.

The contents of morgue kits vary (Figure 30-10), but they usually include:

- A shroud of some kind (paper or cloth)
- A clean gown
- Two or three tags used to identify the body
- Gauze squares for padding
- Safety pins

One procedure for postmortem care is described here (refer to Procedure 90).

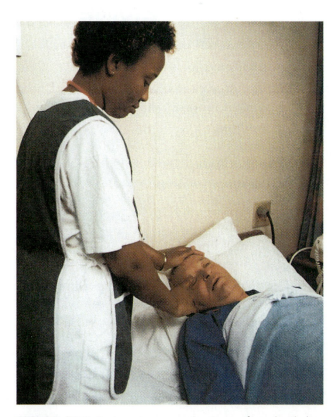

FIGURE 30-9 Postmortem care is given after death has occurred.

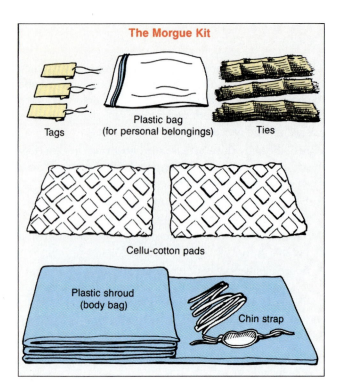

The Morgue Kit

Tags

Plastic bag
(for personal belongings)

Ties

Cellu-cotton pads

Plastic shroud
(body bag)

Chin strap

FIGURE 30-10 Supplies needed for postmortem care

ORGAN DONATIONS

Some people desire to share their organs with others after death. They use an organ donor card that is part of the driver's license. The card specifies if particular organs or the whole body is being donated. At times, because of a special need, the patient's family is asked for permission so that certain body organs may be removed and saved or removed and **harvested** (reused). Such a request is made by the physician or the nurse, never by the nursing assistant.

If the patient or family make their wishes known to you without your asking, it is important to report this to the nurse.

POSTMORTEM EXAMINATION (AUTOPSY)

In certain situations, the law requires a medical postmortem examination or **autopsy** of the body. At other times, the family and physician may desire such an examination to understand the reasons for the patient's death. It is possible that information learned from the examination can be used to protect other family members. As in the case of organ

---

P R O C E D U R E **90**

GIVING POSTMORTEM CARE

1. Carry out each beginning procedure action.

2. Assemble equipment:
   - shroud or clean sheet
   - basin with warm water
   - washcloth
   - towels
   - disposable gloves
   - identification cards (3)
   - cotton
   - bandages
   - pads as needed

3. Put on disposable gloves.

4. Remove all appliances, tubing, and used articles, if instructed to do so.

5. Work quickly and quietly; maintain an attitude of respect.

6. With bed flat, place the body on the back, with head and shoulders elevated on a pillow.

  a. Close the eyes by grasping the eyelashes, gently pulling the eyelids down, and holding shut for a few seconds.

  b. Replace dentures in patient's mouth, if used. Replace artificial eye, if used.

  c. The jaw may have to be secured with light bandaging.

  d. Pad beneath the bandage. Handle the body gently, as tight bandaging or undue pressure from the hands may leave marks.

  e. Straighten arms and legs and place arms by sides.

7. Bathe as necessary. Remove any soiled dressings and replace with clean ones. Groom hair.

8. Place a disposable pad underneath the buttocks. If the family is to view the body:

  a. Put a clean hospital gown on the patient.

  b. Cover the body to the shoulders with a sheet.

continues

PROCEDURE 90 continued

c. Remove disposable gloves and wash hands.

d. Make sure the room is neat.

e. Adjust the lights to a subdued level.

f. Provide chairs for the family.

g. Allow the family to visit in private.

9. Return to patient's room after the family leaves. Wash your hands and put on disposable gloves.

10. Collect all belongings and make a list. Wrap properly and label. Valuables remain in the hospital safe until they are signed for by a relative.

11. Put the shroud on patient.

12. Fill out the identification cards and fasten:

- One on the person's right ankle or right big toe.
- One on the patient's clothing and valuables (securely wrapped).
- One on the compartment in the morgue.

13. Transport the body to the morgue.

a. Call elevator to the floor and keep it empty.

b. Close patient corridor doors.

c. Empty the corridor.

d. With assistant, place the body on a gurney.

e. Keep patient supine, with a rubber head elevator under the neck.

f. Cover with a sheet.

g. Remove disposable gloves and discard according to facility policy. Wash your hands.

h. Take body to the morgue.

---

donations, however, requesting family permission for an autopsy is not part of the nursing assistant's responsibilities.

The nursing assistant is responsible for being supportive of the family and the decision that has been made.

REVIEW

A. True/False.

Mark the following true or false by circling T or F.

1. T F All people respond to a terminal diagnosis in the same way.

2. T F Hearing is the first sense to be lost in the dying patient.

3. T F Death is the final stage of life.

4. T F The nursing assistant should call the physician when the patient dies.

5. T F Sometimes the staff, without realizing it, allow the patient to learn of a terminal diagnosis through their behavior.

6. T F The dying patient receives the same complete care that would be given to someone expected to recover.

7. T F The hospice philosophy has pain relief as one of its goals.

8. T F Permanent dilation of the pupils is a moribund sign.

9. T F Hospice-type care is only possible in the acute care facility.

10. T F The dying person needs a great deal of understanding and realistic support.

B. Matching.

Choose the correct word from Column II to match each phrase or statement in Column I.

Column I	Column II
11. _____ refusal to accept reality	a. moribund
12. _____ after death	b. rigor mortis
13. _____ covering for the body after death	c. denial
14. _____ stiffening of the body after death	d. hospice
15. _____ dying	e. postmortem
	f. shroud
	g. anger

C. Multiple Choice.

Select the one best answer for each question.

16. Organs from a dead person may
   a. be harvested without permission.
   b. be obtained on an as-needed basis.
   c. be donated with permission of the family at the time of death.
   d. never be donated.

17. Postmortem examinations
   a. are never performed.
   b. may provide valuable information.
   c. are arranged by the nursing assistant.
   d. are forbidden by law.

18. As death approaches, changes include
   a. slower body responses.
   b. loss of voluntary and involuntary muscle control.
   c. slowing of circulation.
   d. all of these.

19. Moribund changes include
   a. permanent pupil constriction.
   b. increased body heat.
   c. both a and b.
   d. neither a nor b.

20. A "no code" order on a patient's chart means
   a. to start CPR immediately.
   b. do not resuscitate.
   c. begin postmortem care at once.
   d. to call the family if the patient seems in danger of dying.

D. Nursing Assistant Challenge.

Mrs. Goldstein is a patient in the hospital where you work. She was diagnosed with cancer of the ovaries two years ago. She has been at home but is admitted periodically for chemotherapy. You have taken care of her each time she has been in the hospital. The first time was right after Mrs. Goldstein was diagnosed. She seemed happy and made frequent comments like, "I'm glad I don't have cancer." The last time she was a patient, she refused to follow the suggestions of the nursing staff, but did allow her chemotherapy to be administered. When her family visited, she was irritated and hostile toward them. This time, she is agreeable with the staff on all matters and seems genuinely happy to see her family. She has told you that if she can live to see her granddaughter get married in two months, she will become a volunteer at the hospital so she can help other patients. She is not receiving chemotherapy anymore because the cancer is in an advanced stage. She is hospitalized for pain management now but plans to go home for hospice care. Consider these questions about Mrs. Goldstein:

21. Do you think she is preparing for her death?

22. How would you describe the stages of dying she has been experiencing?

23. What response is appropriate to her comments about the wedding?

24. Do you think hospice care will benefit Mrs. Goldstein? Give reasons for your answer.

25. Mrs. Goldstein is Jewish. What considerations must you give to her postmortem care?

Other Health Care Settings

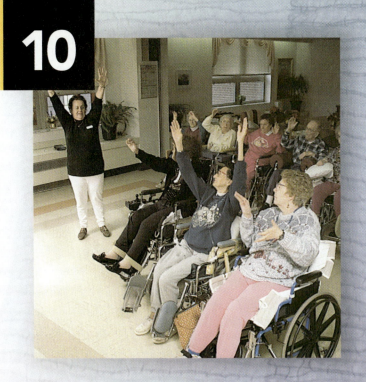

UNIT 31
Care of the Elderly and Chronically Ill

UNIT 32
The Organization of Home Care: Trends in Health Care

UNIT 33
The Nursing Assistant in Home Care

UNIT 34
Subacute Care

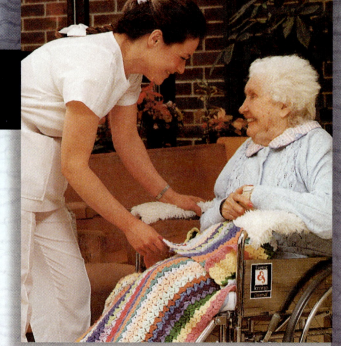

Care of the Elderly and Chronically Ill

See Appendix (page 667) for additional infection control information

OBJECTIVES

As a result of this unit, you will be able to:
- Spell and define terms.
- List the federal requirements for nursing assistants working in long-term care facilities.
- Identify the expected changes of aging.
- List the actions a nursing assistant can take to prevent infections in the long-term care facility.
- Recognize unsafe conditions in the long-term care facility.
- Describe actions to use when working with residents who have dementia.

VOCABULARY

Learn the meaning and the correct spelling of the following words and phrases:

Alzheimer's disease	diverticulitis	Medicaid	skilled care
assisted living	diverticulosis	Medicare	subacute care
catastrophic reaction	flatulence	pigmentation	sundowning
chronologic	hand-over-hand	reality orientation	superimpose
debilitating	technique	reminiscing	validation therapy
dementia	intermediate care	residents	vitality
diverticula	long-term care		

INTRODUCTION

Many individuals require continuing health care (Figure 31-1). These individuals are frequently elderly. This is because as people age, the risk increases of acquiring a chronic disease. A young person may also require continuing care for a chronic illness or severe injury. Persons of any age who are chronically ill or severely injured may require long-term care. This care is provided either in the patient's home or in a long-term care facility. This unit provides information about caring for the elderly and working in a long-term care facility. Units 32 and 33 will teach you about home care.

Nursing assistants are valuable members of the health care team in these facilities (Figure 31-2). The skills you use in acute care facilities, such as hospitals, are also used in long-term care facilities. There are some changes in the application of these skills because of the differences between long-term and acute care.

TYPES OF LONG-TERM CARE FACILITIES

Many types of facilities provide health care for persons with ongoing medical problems. Assisted living is designed for

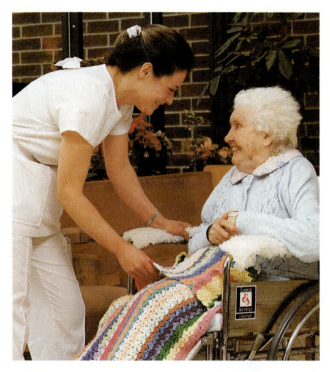

FIGURE 31-2 Nursing assistants are valuable caregivers in long-term care facilities.

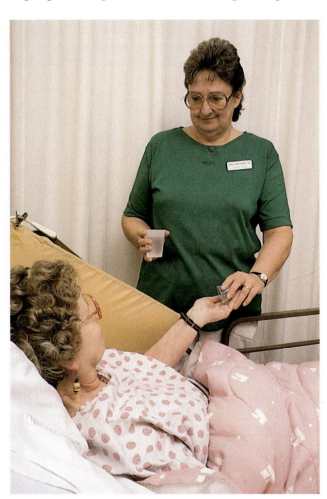

FIGURE 31-1 People of all ages require continuing health care.

persons who have conditions that require monitoring and who may require help taking medications. These people are ambulatory and can generally complete their activities of daily living independently. Intermediate care is available for people who have health problems that are stable and who need assistance with activities of daily living. Skilled care facilities are licensed to provide care to persons with unstable chronic health problems or who require specialized nursing care. Some skilled care facilities have units called subacute care. The subacute care unit may provide services to persons who need rehabilitation, special cancer treatments, or wound care. Subacute care is discussed in Unit 34. Subacute care units may also be located in some hospitals. Long-term care facilities used to be called nursing homes. The long-term care facilities of today bear little resemblance to those of the past. Employees must participate in staff development to maintain and update the knowledge and skills that are required to meet the needs of the consumers.

Some long-term care facilities specialize in the care of people with a specific diagnosis or unusual care needs. Some are licensed to care only for children. The majority care for adults with various diagnoses and problems.

One important issue facing our country today is the financing of long-term health care. Few hospital insurance policies cover expenses of a resident in a long-term care facility. Insurance specifically for long-term care is now available. People who pay for care from private funds may find that their money is soon used up.

Medicaid is a government reimbursement system through which the federal government issues money to the states. The states determine how to distribute the money to health care facilities. These funds are used for the care of people who have no money of their own.

Medicare is another government program that partially pays for health care for persons over the age of 65 or who are permanently disabled. However, Medicare covers only limited long-term care expenses.

These funds are available only to facilities that participate in the Medicaid and Medicare programs.

LONG-TERM CARE POPULATION

People living in long-term care facilities are usually called residents. This is because, for some residents, the facility is considered their home as well as a place to receive health care. Many admissions are permanent, but some residents are able to go home or to a less restrictive environment.

Residents are admitted to skilled-care facilities because they have problems that require ongoing monitoring and health care. They are not admitted just because they are old. The problems of residents are a result of a disease process and are not a natural part of aging. Most facilities also have younger residents who are mentally or physically disabled due to chronic disease or injuries (Figure 31-3). The number of people requiring long-term care is growing rapidly for several reasons:

- There are more people alive today.
- More people are living longer (Figure 31-4).
- Modern science has enabled people to recover from illnesses or injuries that would have been fatal in the past.
- The longer a person lives, the greater the risk for acquiring a chronic, degenerative disease.
- Families are unable to provide care because of geographic distances or because everyone in the family is employed.

Here are some examples of residents in a long-term care facility:

- Rose Johnson is 78 years old and had surgery in the hospital to repair a fractured hip. She is receiving reha-

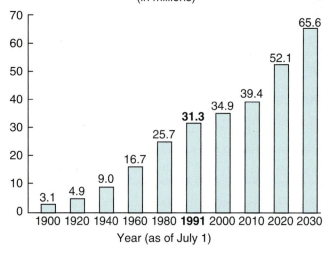

NUMBER OF PERSONS 65+: 1900 to 2030
(in millions)

FIGURE 31-4 Number of persons 65 years of age and older. *From* A Profile of Older Americans—1993, *American Association of Retired Persons, 1909 K Street NW, Washington, DC 20049*

bilitation to learn how to walk correctly on her affected leg. She will go back to her own home after the rehabilitation is completed.

- Antony Donali is 86 years old and has Alzheimer's disease. His family can no longer provide the 24-hour attention that he needs. He will remain in the facility for the rest of his life.

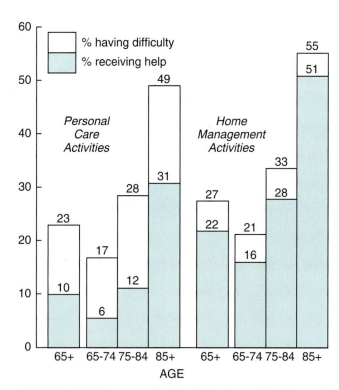

FIGURE 31-5 Percent of elderly having difficulty and receiving help with selected activities. *From* A Profile of Older Americans—1993, *American Association of Retired Persons, 1909 K Street NW, Washington, DC 20049*

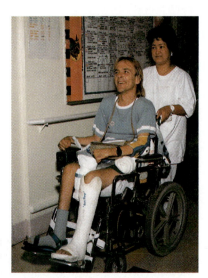

FIGURE 31-3 Most facilities also have young residents.

- Ted McMurry is 47 years old and has cancer of the lung. He is receiving chemotherapy. He may be able to go home after finishing the therapy unless his condition worsens.
- Jill Green is 18 years old and suffered severe, permanent head injuries in a motorcycle accident. She will never be able to care for herself and will need 24-hour-a-day care for the rest of her life. She will probably remain in the facility for this care.
- Tom Hernandez is 35 years old and has had multiple sclerosis for 10 years. The disease has progressed to the point where Tom can no longer care for himself. He will probably remain in the facility.
- Sara Pembkoski is 64 years old and has had a stroke. She is receiving intensive rehabilitation and hopes to return home. If she is not able to do so, she will be transferred to an assisted living facility.

The percentage of persons living in long-term care facilities is only 1 percent for those 65 to 74 years of age. However, this increases to 22 percent for people 85 years and older. As people grow older, the consequences of chronic disease increase. Varying degrees of functional deficits (disabilities) result. Therefore, the person requires assistance in performing the activities of daily living (Figure 31-5).

LEGISLATION AFFECTING LONG-TERM CARE

Federal legislation has brought about changes to improve the quality of long-term care. This legislation is called the Nursing Home Reform Act. It is the result of the Omnibus Budget Reconciliation Act of 1987 (OBRA). Each state is responsible for implementing this legislation.

Much of the OBRA content affects nursing assistants directly or indirectly:

- OBRA requires all nursing assistants working in long-term care to complete a course of at least 75 clock hours. The course must be approved by the state agency appointed to oversee OBRA regulations. Most states require more than the minimum of 75 hours.
- After completing the course, written and manual (skills) competency tests must be passed. The tests may be taken three times.
- Nursing assistants must complete specific hours of in-service education (12 hours) per year (Figure 31-6). (Some states may require more.)
- Nursing assistants who are not employed as such for 24 months must repeat the course and competency tests.

Federal regulations specify the content that must be included in a nursing assistant course:

- Residents' rights
- Communication and interpersonal skills
- Infection control
- Safety and emergency procedures
- Basic nursing skills

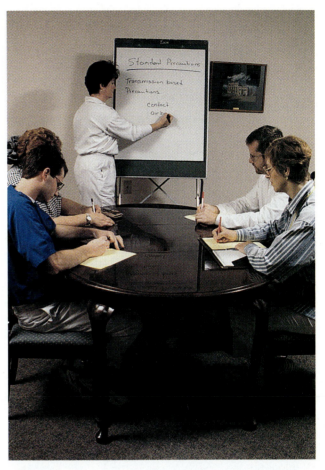

FIGURE 31-6 Nursing assistants in long-term care facilities must complete 12 hours of in-service education each year.

- Personal care skills
- Mental health and social service needs
- Care of residents with Alzheimer's disease or other dementias
- Basic restorative services

These topics are covered in other units of this textbook. This chapter provides specific information about long-term care and OBRA requirements.

ROLE OF THE NURSING ASSISTANT IN A SKILLED CARE FACILITY

As in the acute care facility, the nursing assistant carries out the procedures as taught, assisting in the health care of residents under the direct supervision of a nurse. Basic physical care, as well as special procedures, will be done to help these residents reach their maximum degree of well-being.

To be successful in this setting, you must:

- be patient and caring.
- understand the character of the older age group.
- be able to care for persons who may be your own age and have chronic illnesses.
- be comfortable with the thought of your own aging.

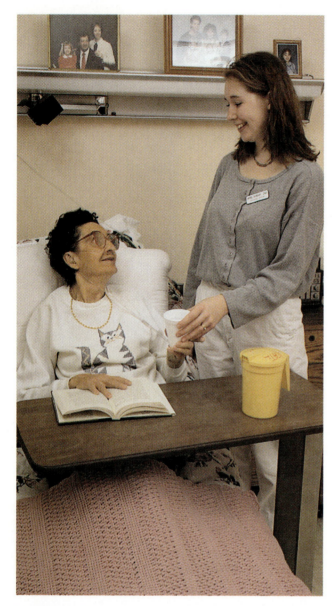

FIGURE 31-7 Persons working in long-term care facilities must have excellent communication skills.

- have the stamina to provide the assistance needed by the residents.
- be able to derive satisfaction from being part of a slow progress and small, if any, gains.
- have a sense of humor.
- be able to communicate effectively (Figure 31-7).

These attributes are important in any health setting, but in the long-term care facility they become very necessary.

Many of the residents will remain under your care for long periods of time, even for years. You will develop relationships that become important to both caregiver and care receiver. In those circumstances, communications take on greater importance. Greater significance may be attached to the attention to care or even the way thoughts are expressed in words. Thus, the long-term caregiver is a *very special person* who works in an important area of health care.

EFFECTS OF AGING

Many residents in the long-term facility are advanced in age and have one or more chronic, somewhat **debilitating** (weakening) conditions. Some are mentally alert. Others are confused and disoriented.

There are, however, some features of aging that are characteristic for most elderly residents. Do not expect every resident to exhibit the same characteristics at the same **chronologic** (year) age. Remember that aging is a natural, progressive process that begins at birth and extends to death. Remember also that every resident is unique and must be treated with dignity and respect.

Physical Changes in Aging

Some investigators believe we are born with a biological time clock. This clock is programmed for a specific life span, barring accidents and disease. As we move toward old age, changes that have been taking place gradually become more evident. For example, the elderly person:

- May lose vitality.
- May sleep less at night.
- May benefit from rest periods during the day.
- Stores less fluid in body tissue and is apt to become dehydrated. This results in a loss of elasticity and resiliency in tissues.
- Has fibrous tissue changes. These decrease the tone, mass, and strength of skeletal and smooth muscle.
- Has secretory and endocrine cells that become less functional and reduced nerve sensitivity.

Certain changes occur in every body system. They do not necessarily occur at the same rate in each system. These are listed in Table 31-1.

Emotional Adjustments to Aging

Emotional adjustments to aging are basically extensions of the adjustments the individual has made throughout life to the many changes in circumstances. Personality characteristics and ways of reacting to stress are developed fairly early in life and tend to become a constant in an individual's personality. In fact, as a person ages, personality traits become even more pronounced. The stress produced by the circumstances and illnesses that accompany old age do not drastically alter the individual's personality, but they do tend to magnify, and in some cases distort, the basic traits.

Old people have the same emotional needs and require the same supports for good mental health as young people (Figure 31-8). They need:

- to be loved.
- to have a sense of self-worth.
- to feel a sense of achievement and recognition.
- to have a degree of economic security.

Although these needs are common to all human beings, regardless of age, the means for achieving satisfaction and

TABLE 31-1 PHYSICAL CHANGES OF AGING

Body System	Physical Changes
Integumentary	• Hair loses color and becomes thinner • Skin dries, becomes less elastic; wrinkles develop • Skin is fragile and tears easily • Bruises easily (senile purpura common) • Fingernails and toenails thicken • Sweat glands do not excrete perspiration as readily • Oil glands do not secrete as much oil • There is increased sensitivity to cold • Skin discolorations (age spots) become more common
Nervous	• Problems with balance • Temperature regulation is less effective • Sensation of pain decreases • Deep sleep is shortened, more awakenings during the night • Brain cells are lost but intelligence remains intact unless disease is present • Decreased sensitivity of nerve receptors in skin (heat, cold, pain, pressure)
Sensory	• More difficult to see close objects • Night vision may decrease • Cataracts (clouding of the lens of the eye) are more common • Side vision and depth perception diminish • Hearing diminishes in most elderly persons • Smell receptors and taste buds are less sensitive, so foods have less taste
Musculoskeletal	• Less muscle strength • Less flexibility • Slower movements • Arthritis and osteoporosis common • Body becomes more stooped
Respiratory	• Breathing capacity lessens
Urinary	• Kidneys decrease in size • Urine production is less efficient • Emptying bladder completely may become more difficult • Stress incontinence may develop
Digestive	• Primary taste sensations of salt, sweet, and sour decrease • Constipation increases • Flatulence increases • Movement of food through the digestive system slows
Cardiovascular	• Blood vessels less elastic, more narrowed • Heart may not pump as efficiently, leading to decreased cardiac output and circulation
Endocrine	• Decrease in levels of estrogen, progesterone • Hot flashes, nervous feelings • Higher levels of parathormone and thyroid-stimulating hormone • Weight gain • Insulin production less efficient • Diabetes mellitus more likely
Reproductive	*Females:* • Ovulation and menstrual cycle cease • Vaginal walls are thinner and drier *Males:* • Scrotum less firm • Prostate gland may enlarge

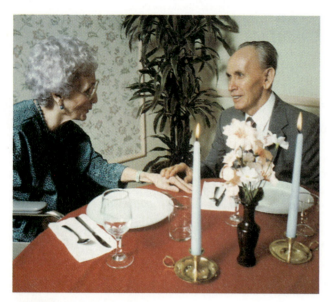

FIGURE 31-8 Older people have the same emotional needs as young people.

gratification of these needs are greatly reduced for older people. The opportunities for social exchange and sexual expression, the two major means of gratification, are lessened as the years advance. The need for them does not change, however.

The attitude of the Western world toward old people tends to relegate (place) them to positions of lesser and lesser significance. The older people become, the more their self-image is depreciated (devalued), both in their own eyes and in the eyes of others.

Physical ailments, far more common in the elderly because of slowed body processes, are **superimposed** (layered on top of) upon the changes brought about by the natural aging process. Change of body image and loss of the vigor and **vitality** (lively character) of former years are major losses the older person must accept—losses that further alter their self-image and self-esteem. The caregiver can make an important contribution by promoting the self-esteem of those being cared for.

In old age, some accommodations must be made in the attitudes or psychological outlooks of all persons. The most healthy emotional responses are based:

- on philosophies that accept aging as a natural progressive stage.
- in life attitudes that recognize the strengths as well as the limitations of the body.
- on a form of behavior that demonstrates interest in living here and now.

Healthy psychological adjustments mean both a realistic appraisal of the present circumstance and building on the positive values while coming to terms with the negative aspects.

Some of your long-term care residents will have already made these adjustments. Some will be in the process. Your supportive caring will be important and helpful to each.

Specific Emotional Responses. The elderly or infirm resident is apt to experience some common emotional responses. Frustration is an emotion frequently experienced by the elderly—frustration at physical limitations and at having less control over their own lives. That is why it is important to allow the elderly the opportunity to make as many decisions as possible. Signs of frustration are often demonstrated by:

- Aggressive behavior
- Anger
- Hostility
- Demanding behavior
- Complaining
- Crying

Some residents even resort to manipulating families, staff, or other residents in an attempt to relieve their feelings of helplessness (Figure 31-9).

Anxiety and fear may be expressed in periods of depression and withdrawal. The depression experienced by the elderly is easily understood. In many instances, they:

- are cut off from their social support systems.
- have had to make major adjustments in their lifestyles.
- may have lost loved ones and friends.
- may have very limited finances.
- may truly feel that they no longer have any control over their destinies or even of their day-to-day activities.

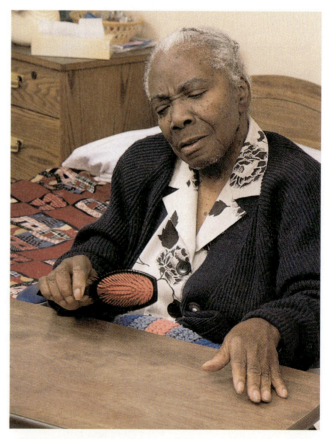

FIGURE 31-9 Residents may exhibit feelings of frustration and anger.

- may have stretched their coping ability to the breaking point because of physical weakness and disease processes.

Withdrawal, a common frustration response, is shown by:

- Lack of communication
- Temporary confusion
- General disorientation as to time and place

You can play a major role in helping residents move successfully through these periods by:

- reassuring them that they will not be abandoned now that they are no longer able to care for themselves.
- treating each person with respect to reinforce self-esteem.
- calmly helping your residents keep in touch with reality while conveying your own feelings of compassion and caring.
- reporting changes in behavior, mood swings, and emotional responses to your supervisor so that the entire staff can form a supporting network.
- responding to the residents' negative attitudes by being willing to listen and interact with them and emphasizing the positive.

NUTRITIONAL NEEDS

Malnutrition is a problem for the aged because the older person may develop an apathy toward food that becomes progressive. Factors that contribute to lack of appetite are:

- Decreased activity
- Inadequate teeth
- Bad dentures
- Decreased saliva
- Diminished smell and taste
- Poor oral hygiene
- Eating alone

The diet for the elderly person should:

- Be easy to chew and digest.
- Contain decreased amounts of refined sugars, fats, and cholesterol.
- Have adequate proteins and vitamins to provide for best bodily function and repair.
- Have many complex carbohydrates, found in fruits, vegetables, and grains (Figure 31-10). These foods also are good sources of vitamins and minerals, which tend to be deficient in the elderly diet.
- Be monitored for weight control. Obesity is a major nutritional problem among the elderly and those who are inactive. The excess weight increases the stress of existing conditions. Calories are generally limited to about 2,000 calories for the average woman and 2,400 to 2,500 calories for the average man.

Because of loss of muscle tone, three intestinal problems are seen. They are:

- Constipation—difficulty in eliminating solid waste
- Flatulence—gas production

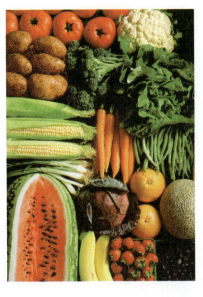

FIGURE 31-10
Elderly people require complex carbohydrates for a healthy diet. *From How to Eat for Good Health, Courtesy of National Dairy Council*

- Diverticulosis—small pockets (diverticula) of weakened intestinal wall

Dietary adjustments can help reduce these problems.

- Soft bulk foods, such as whole-grain cereals and fruits and vegetables, are helpful in overcoming the constipation.
- Skins and seeds should be avoided to prevent diverticulitis, which is an inflammation of the diverticula.

The presentation and service of food are important in stimulating appetites. Keep in mind the following:

- Several smaller meals seem to be more easily tolerated than three large meals.
- Residents should be allowed to feed themselves as much as possible. You may assist by cutting up the food into bite-sized pieces. Even if you must do most of the feeding, allow the resident to participate as much as possible.
- Adequate liquid is absolutely essential. This need is frequently neglected, leading to dehydration. You must encourage fluid intake and be sure that the resident actually drinks the fluids (Figure 31-11).
- Fruit and vegetable juices, eggnogs, and soups can serve the dual purpose of providing both nourishment and fluids.
- Fluids must be offered at frequent intervals between meals to ensure adequate intake.

PREVENTING INFECTIONS IN RESIDENTS

There are no additional or special infection control techniques in long-term facilities. Section 4 provides instructions on all infection control procedures performed in nursing homes. Effective and frequent handwashing is the best method for preventing the spread of disease from resident to resident, staff person to resident, or resident to staff person. Standard precautions should be implemented in the care of

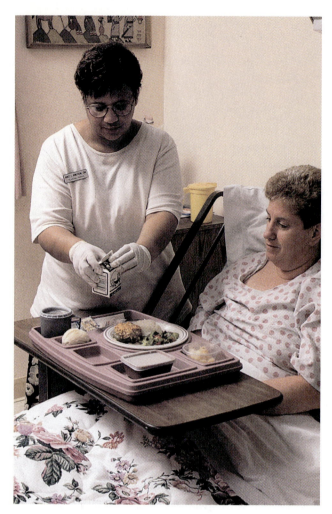

FIGURE 31-11 Encourage fluid intake.

all persons when contact with blood, body fluids, secretions, excretions, mucous membranes, or nonintact skin is anticipated. Isolation techniques are used for residents with known infectious diseases.

It is important to follow these procedures because it is easy for elderly people to get infections. There are a number of reasons for this:

- Body changes due to aging make older people more susceptible to infection. The skin offers less protection because of its fragility. Any break in the skin, such as a pressure sore or skin tear, can quickly become infected.

- Changes in the urinary system cause the bladder to empty less efficiently. Urine left in the bladder contributes to urinary tract infections.

- The ability to cough and raise secretions is reduced. As a result, there is decreased ability to get rid of bacteria from the lungs.

- Elderly people do not always eat well and may be undernourished.

- Elderly people have less resistance to disease because the immune system becomes less effective with age.

- Resistance to disease is reduced when residents have several chronic health problems.

The elderly do not readily show signs of infection. This means they may be sick for some time before you recognize the problem.

- The elderly do not always develop a fever with an infection. The average temperature for an older person may be one or two degrees less than that of a younger person. Therefore, average temperature may represent an increase or fever.

- Some elderly persons do not feel pain as acutely as younger people. They may feel no discomfort with a bladder infection, for example.

- The elderly do not readily develop signs of inflammatory response. A skin infection usually shows redness, swelling, heat, and pain. These signs may be missing or delayed in the elderly person.

- The elderly do not necessarily have an increase in the white blood cell count. This is usually a sign of infection but is often absent in the elderly.

- Elderly people do not cough as frequently when they have respiratory tract infections.

- Residents who are disoriented may not comprehend or be able to communicate feelings of pain or nausea.

The elderly are also more likely to develop serious complications from infections. A simple urinary tract infection can result in *bacteremia* (blood infection), causing the resident to become acutely ill. This can be fatal to a person who has little ability to cope with additional health problems.

Prevention of infection in residents is an ongoing concern. There are some steps that you can take to help in this process:

- Assist residents to maintain an adequate fluid intake. This helps prevent urinary tract and respiratory tract infections and keeps the skin healthier.

- Assist residents to maintain adequate nutritional intake. Report to the nurse when residents eat less or refuse food.

- Assist residents to perform exercise programs established by the nurse or physical therapist. Follow positioning schedules and orders for range-of-motion exercises and ambulation. This increases circulation, thus lowering the risk of pressure ulcers (a frequent source of infection). Exercise also improves breathing, thereby decreasing the risk of respiratory tract infections.

- Attend to residents' personal hygiene needs. Regular bathing and oral care help prevent infection. Inspect the body and mouth when performing these procedures.

- Toilet residents regularly who need assistance. This keeps the bladder empty and also assures residents that they will receive help when they need to urinate. Some residents hesitate to drink fluids for fear they will be incontinent. When caring for incontinent residents, be sure to wipe female residents using strokes from front to back. This avoids contaminating the urethra with stool or vaginal excretions.

- Perform catheter care as directed. Avoid opening the drainage system.

- Observe residents carefully and report any unusual signs or changes. Urinary tract infections may be discovered from changes in the urine or by incontinence. In some cases, the first sign of any infection is disorientation in people who are not usually disoriented. For persons with dementia, a change in behavior may indicate an infection. Incidents of falling often occur in residents with infections.

- You will be asked to collect urine specimens for culture and sensitivity. The specimen should be clean-catch (see Unit 42). You may need help when collecting the specimen. If it is contaminated because of inadequate cleaning or improper collection, the results will be altered.

Fighting infection in the long-term care facility is everyone's responsibility. As a nursing assistant, you can do your part by performing handwashing, universal precautions, isolation techniques, and all principles of medical asepsis on a routine basis. Help new employees to acquire these skills, and assist residents to maintain good personal hygiene practices.

See Appendix

KEEPING RESIDENTS SAFE

Each year an estimated 30 to 40% of all nursing home residents fall. There are several reasons for this:

- Changes in vision and hearing that most older people experience, which cause a loss of "warning systems."
- Problems with mobility resulting from arthritic changes, loss of flexibility, and endurance.
- Loss of balance related to inner ear changes.
- Frequency of urination, leading to fears of incontinence that result in unsafe toileting habits.
- Disorientation and faulty judgment in persons who are mentally incompetent.
- Dizziness that may occur when coming to a standing position too quickly.

External factors can also increase the risk of falls:

- Use of medications that affect mental status, balance, and coordination.
- Unsafe use of assistive mobility devices.
- Poorly planned environment.
- Staff delay in attending to the needs of residents.

In an effort to reduce the number of falls, the environment can be altered to meet the needs of elderly persons:

- Aging changes in the eye cause older people to be more sensitive to glare and to changes in lighting. They also have difficulty seeing colors at the blue-green end of the spectrum. To prevent falls due to faulty vision:
  - Use nonglare wax on floors.
  - Use blinds and curtains to prevent glare from windows.
  - Place mirrors to prevent glare.
  - Use nonglare glass in pictures.
  - Use bright nonglare lighting with constant, even illumination.
  - Use colors to mark the edges of steps and curbs that serve as caution reminders.
  - Use colors in the red and yellow range that increase residents' ability to see changes in walls and floors.
  - Encourage residents to wear sunglasses (if not contraindicated) and hats when they go outdoors.

- Noise increases disorientation and can create anxiety even in alert persons. This increases the risk of falls. Minimizing all noises reduces this risk.

- All tubs and showers should have chairs so residents can remain seated throughout the procedure. Lifts for tubs avoid the needs for the resident to stand in the tub. Avoid using oils that can make the tub bottom slippery.

- Check residents' clothing for fit. Loose shoes and laces, slippers, long robes, and slacks increase the risk of falling.

- Observe ambulatory residents when they get out of bed and chairs, off the toilet, and when they walk.
  - Give instructions to residents who have unsafe habits.
  - Residents who self-propel their wheelchairs need instructions on how to enter and leave elevators, how to use ramps, and reminders to use the brakes.
  - Dependent residents may benefit by learning self-transfer techniques. Check with the nurse to see if this is possible.
  - When you help dependent residents transfer, always use the method indicated in the care plan.

- Side rails are a frequent cause of falls. Many facilities leave side rails down on one side for residents who can safely transfer without help. In some situations, half rails are more effective.

Review Unit 14 for actions that can reduce the risk of falls and for guidelines regarding the use of restraints.

Other Safety Concerns

Elderly people are at risk for other injuries such as accidental poisoning, choking, thermal injuries, and skin injuries. These are discussed in Units 14 and 48.

Safety in long-term care facilities is a major concern. Unlike hospitals, residents are given the freedom to move about the facility as they desire. For this reason, the entire building must be free of hazards that contribute to accidents. All employees need to be constantly aware of the residents' safety.

EXERCISE AND RECREATIONAL NEEDS

Residents in long-term care facilities need the stimulation of planned recreation and exercise. The type of activity must be carefully tailored to the needs and abilities of the residents. Health workers in these facilities are often responsible for coordinating this aspect of care.

- Balding is an aging characteristic that first appears at widely varying ages. Again, genetics has a strong influence.

Hair care is important in maintaining the resident's overall personal appearance.

- Hair should be styled and neatly arranged.
- An order is required for a shampoo to be given once or twice a month.
- Dry shampoos are also available. They simplify shampoos for residents confined to bed.
- A mild conditioning shampoo is best.
  - A dryer will dry the hair quickly, decreasing the chance of chilling.
  - The resident must be kept out of drafts while the hair is being washed and dried.
  - Shampoos are more safely given in bed; if the person is seated, a shampoo board can be used. Bending is difficult for older persons and their decreased sense of balance is apt to result in a fall. Shampoos may also be given in the tub or shower.
- Hair care may be provided by a beautician or barber, if available, or by a family member or nursing assistant.

Facial Hair

Elderly women tend to have an increase in the growth and coarseness of the hair on their chins and upper lips. These can be removed:

- with tweezers.
- by electric needles used by a professional.
- by shaving, with a physician's order.

Facial hair may also be lightened by mildly bleaching it. Elderly men need to be shaved regularly, usually daily. You may need to:

- only provide the equipment.
- use a safety razor to shave the patient yourself.
- assist the person to obtain barbering services.

Mouth Care

The condition of the teeth affects the aged person's total health. Hygienic routines and observations are your responsibility when an individual is no longer able to do these things for himself. See Unit 24 for specific care procedures.

Natural Teeth. Poor oral hygiene can result in loss of appetite and weight, and may be the focus of any infection. Even if teeth are missing, the remaining teeth should be cleaned regularly. Dental checkups should be done as often as in younger years.

Dentures. False teeth, called *dentures,* must be cleaned daily (see Procedure 68 in Unit 24).

- Check the mouth and gums routinely for signs of irritation. Use a soft brush to clean mouth and gums.
- Teeth should be checked and polished during periodic dental examinations.

Mouth care is especially important for the bed resident who has lost teeth and is no longer able to keep dentures in the mouth. Check the mouth and gums for irritation. Dentures should be inspected for cracks, rough edges, and broken parts.

- A commercial mouthwash, a warm wash of saline solution, or baking soda should be used before and after meals.
- Glycerine and lemon, applied with applicators between meals, are very refreshing.
- Lips should be inspected for excessive dryness or fissures.
- Creams, petroleum jelly, or glycerine applied to the lips can prevent fissures from developing into deep sores and infections.

Eyes, Ears, and Nose

Eyes, ears, and nose should also be observed daily for any signs of irritation, redness, drainage, or excessive dryness of the skin that could lead to breaks and fissures. Observations of this nature by staff members should be part of routine care.

MENTAL CHANGES

Mental deterioration is not a normal part of aging. However, as people age, the risk of mental deterioration increases. Mental deterioration may stem from physical (organic) or emotional causes. A combination of both may occur in the residents in your care. Periods of mental confusion are often temporary. They may be due to unusual stress, such as an infection; sudden injury, such as a fracture; or transfer to an unfamiliar environment. In some situations, the changes may signify a progressive deterioration of mental abilities. The term dementia refers to any disorder of the brain that causes deficits in thinking, memory, and judgment.

CARING FOR RESIDENTS WITH DEMENTIA

You will care for many residents with dementia in the long-term care facility. Dementia is not a disease in itself, but is a group of symptoms seen in a number of different diseases. Alzheimer's disease is the most common form of dementia. Other types of dementias are related to cardiovascular disease, Parkinson's disease, and Huntington's disease and are listed in Table 31-2. The term *dementia* is used here when referring to symptoms, behavior, and nursing actions that are appropriate for people with any dementia. Alzheimer's is used when the information is specific to that dementia.

Alzheimer's Disease

Alzheimer's disease can begin during middle age, but is more common in older persons. The disease affects people of all races, levels of intelligence, education, and financial status. It is progressive and cannot be cured. It has been called a "slow death of the mind." In the past, the term *senility* was used to describe these symptoms. We know now that it is a disease of the brain cells and is not normal aging. The cause of

TABLE 31-2 DESCRIPTION OF MAJOR FORMS OF DEMENTIA

Disease	Features	Course
Alzheimer's disease	Lack of chemical in brain causing neurofibrillary tangles, neuritic plaques	Onset age: 60–80 Slowly progressive
Multi-infarct dementia	Interference with blood circulation in brain cells due to arteriosclerosis or atherosclerosis	Onset age: 55–70 Outcome depends on rate of damage to brain cells
Huntington's disease	Inherited from either parent who has gene for the disease	Onset age: 25–45 Average duration 15 years
Parkinson's disease	Deficiency of chemical in brain (dopamine)	Onset age: 55–60 Several years duration
Creutzfeldt-Jacob disease	Noninflammatory virus causes changes in brain	Onset age: 50–60 Rapidly progressive
Syphilis	Spirochete (bacteria) causes brain damage	Occurs 15–20 years after primary infection
AIDS dementia	HIV-1 infection	Symptoms sometimes precede diagnosis of AIDS

Alzheimer's is unknown. There is no diagnostic test. When symptoms appear, the person should have a medical workup to rule out other diseases. Nutritional problems, depression, medications, and metabolic diseases can all cause similar symptoms. However, these conditions can be reversed with treatment.

In Alzheimer's, changes occur in both the structure and function of the brain. The brain shrinks and becomes smaller. If an autopsy of the brain is performed after death, changes are noted in the brain cells. These changes are called *neuritic plaques* and *neurofibrillary tangles.*

Individuals with Alzheimer's often live as long as 20 years after the onset of the disease. Their bodies can be surprisingly healthy. Families and friends have difficulty believing that the person is ill. There is much that is unknown about this disease. Caregivers can increase the quality of life for those who have the illness.

The disease generally has three stages, with symptoms becoming progressively worse. The best learned skills tend to remain the longest. An English teacher, for example, may maintain verbal skills longer than usual. However, once a skill is lost, it is lost forever.

Stage I: Mild Dementia. During the first stage, most people remain at home if they have a supportive family to provide assistance. They are usually physically capable and can attend to the activities of daily living with supervision. Characteristics of Stage I include:

- Short-term memory loss
- Personality changes with loss of spontaneity and indifference (Figure 31-15)
- Decreased ability to concentrate and shortened attention span
- Disorientation to time and space

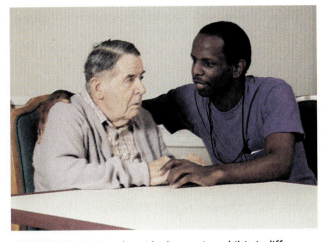

FIGURE 31-15 People with dementia exhibit indifference and loss of spontaneity.

- Poor judgment
- Carelessness in actions and appearance
- Anxiety, depression, and agitation
- Delusions of persecution—the person thinks that others are conspiring to do him harm

Stage II: Moderate Dementia. Symptoms of this stage are:

- Increased short-term memory loss and deterioration of memory for remote events.
- Complete disorientation.
- Wandering and pacing.
- Sundowning, which is confusion and restlessness that occur during the late afternoon, evening, or night (Figure 31-16).

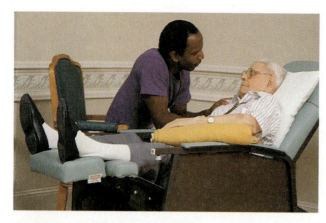

FIGURE 31-16 A recliner may be useful for a resident with sundowning.

- Sensory/perceptual changes. The person is unable to recognize and use common objects, such as eating utensils, combs, and pencils. Also, the person is unable to distinguish between right and left, up and down, hot and cold.
- Perseveration phenomena. This refers to repeating an action. Examples are repeating the same word or phrase, lip licking, chewing, or finger tapping.
- Problems with walking.
- Problems with speech, reading, writing.
- Good eating habits continue.
- Incontinent of bowel and bladder.
- Catastrophic reactions, hallucinations, delusions. A **catastrophic reaction** is the response of a person with dementia to overwhelming stimuli.

Most people with Alzheimer's are admitted to long-term care facilities during the second stage. Although they may still be healthy physically, they require constant care. Most families do not have the emotional resources and physical energy to cope. Admission is traumatic to families. Families are vital members of the interdisciplinary team. They can provide staff with valuable information about the resident and how to deal with the problems.

Stage III: Severe Dementia. The person in Stage III:

- is totally dependent.
- is verbally unresponsive.
- may have seizures.

Work with residents who have Alzheimer's disease or any dementia is challenging, rewarding, and gratifying. Caregivers must be compassionate, patient, calm, and have a sense of humor.

When you are caring for residents with dementia, remember to:

- protect residents from physical injury.
- allow residents to maintain independence as long as possible.
- provide physical and mental activities within residents' abilities.

- support residents' dignity and self-esteem.

To meet these goals, the care must be:

- consistent.
- provided with a structured but flexible routine.
- given in a peaceful, quiet environment that is simple, uncluttered, and unchanged.

It is helpful to:

- Make eye contact with residents.
- Use appropriate body language. Residents with dementia can "read" the staff. Therefore, residents' behavior will reflect the mood of the staff (Figure 31-17).
- Be able to "tune" into and accept residents without being judgmental or critical.
- Use touch appropriately. This can be soothing. But if a resident is surprised by the body contact, it can result in a catastrophic reaction.
- Avoid using logic, reasoning, or lengthy explanations.
- Remember that when the ability to use speech is lost, communication occurs through nonverbal means.
  - Biting, scratching, and kicking may be the only way the resident can express displeasure.
  - Watch for facial expressions and body language for clues to feelings and moods.
  - Learn what triggers agitation or anger. Work on preventing those situations.
- Use techniques of diversion and distraction. For example, calmly take the resident by the hand and walk

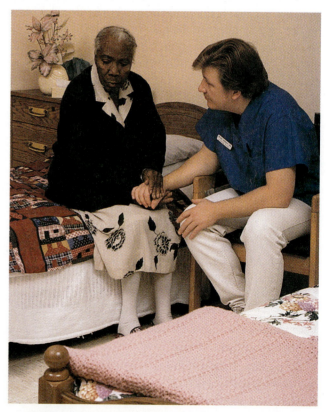

FIGURE 31-17 Residents can "read" the body language of caregivers.

GUIDELINES *for*

Activities of Daily Living for Residents with Dementia

- Allow the resident to do as much as possible.
  - Use the hand-over-hand technique for personal care and eating. The hand-over-hand technique means that the resident's hand is placed around an object, such as a glass. The caregiver then places a hand over the resident's hand and guides the object to the resident's mouth.
  - Give only one short, simple direction at a time.
- Observe the resident's physical condition. People with dementia are usually unaware of signs of illness.
- Assist residents to maintain a dignified, attractive appearance by helping them with grooming and dressing.
- Monitor food and fluid intake.
  - Too many foods at once are confusing.
  - Place one food at a time in front of the resident.
  - Do not use plastic utensils that can break in the resident's mouth.
  - Provide nutritious finger foods when the resident is unable to use utensils.
  - Avoid pureed foods as long as possible.
  - Check food temperatures.
  - Prepare foods for eating by buttering bread, cutting meat, and opening cartons.
  - Check the resident's mouth after eating for food. "Squirreling" food (hoarding food in the checks) can cause aspiration.
  - Weigh residents regularly to detect patterns of weight gain or loss.
  - The dining area should be quiet and calm.
- Persons with dementia eventually lose bowel and bladder continence. Taking residents to the bathroom every 2 hours keeps residents dry and prevents skin breakdown.
- Residents with dementia need activities geared to their abilities.
  - Avoid large groups or competitive activities.
  - In later stages, use sensory stimulation with quiet music, soft touching, and calm talk.

- Holding puppies or kittens (pet therapy) brings pleasure to severely impaired residents.
- Daily exercise should be planned according to residents' habits and abilities (Figure 31-18). The resident who wanders throughout the day may only need range-of-motion exercises.

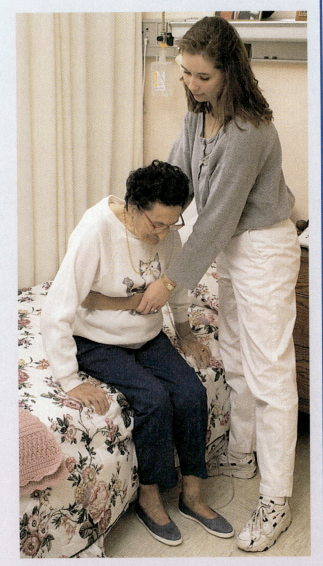

FIGURE 31-18 People with Alzheimer's or other dementias need daily exercise.

together or direct the resident's attention to another activity. These techniques work well because of the shortened attention span.

- Realize that people with dementia are not responsible for what they do or say.

- Their behavior is not intentional, and they cannot change.

- They are not aware of what they are doing.

- They lose the ability to control their impulses.

— Avoid confrontations and always allow them to "save face"—that is, keep their dignity.

— No one really knows what is happening in the minds of people with dementia.

Special Problems

Wandering and Pacing. Persons with Alzheimer's may wander or pace for hours at a time. No one knows why this occurs. Some reasons may be:

● They are looking for companionship, security, or loved ones.

● It is a way to handle stress.

● They realize they are in a strange environment and are looking for home.

When this behavior occurs:

● Allow them to wander. Using restraints only increases their anxiety and frustration, resulting in other problems.

● Adapt the environment to the residents, making it safe and secure. The problem may be getting lost rather than falling. When the resident walks off, walk with the resident, gradually returning to the direction of the facility.

● Watch wandering residents for signs of fatigue. They may have forgotten how to sit down and will need reminders and demonstrations of how to get into a chair or bed.

● Many companies now manufacture Alzheimer's chairs. These allow residents to rock without tipping over. A tray-table top keeps residents secure and can be used for hand activities.

● Nutritional needs increase with wandering, so additional food intake may be necessary.

Agitation, Anxiety, and Catastrophic Reactions. Agitation and anxiety are shown by an increase in physical activity, such as pacing, or the perseveration behaviors described for Stage II. If appropriate interventions are not implemented in time, a catastrophic reaction will likely occur (Figure 31-19). You may note any or all of the following.

● Increased physical activity

● Increased talking or mumbling

● Explosive behavior with physical violence

To avoid catastrophic reactions:

● Monitor behavior closely.

● Watch for signs of increasing agitation.

● Check to see if the resident:

— Is hungry

— Needs to go to the bathroom

— Is too hot or too cold

— Is overtired or in pain

— Has signs of physical illness

● Check the environment for:

— Too much noise

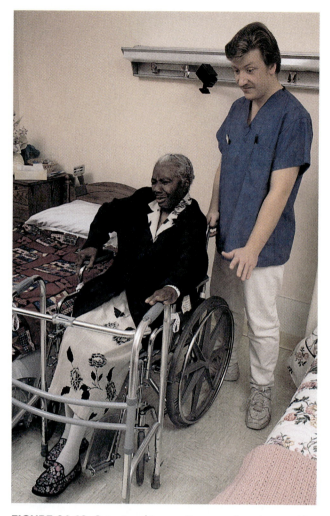

FIGURE 31-19 Catastrophic reactions can be triggered by environmental stimulation.

— Too many people

— Staff anxiety

— Television programs. People with dementia cannot distinguish fiction from reality.

● People with dementia cannot make decisions. For example, the question "What do you want to wear today?" may be more than they can handle.

When agitation or catastrophic reactions occur:

● Do not use physical restraints or force in any attempt to subdue the resident. This increases agitation and can result in injury to the resident or staff.

● Avoid having several staff persons approach the resident at the same time. This is frightening to the resident.

● Use a soft, calm voice. Do not try to reason with the resident. Using touch may or may not be appropriate. Some residents respond to smooth stroking of the arms or back. Others may react violently if they are already agitated.

Sundowning. As previously mentioned, *sundowning* means that the resident has increased confusion and restlessness during the late afternoon, evening, or night. It is sometimes prevented by avoiding too much activity before bedtime and by establishing a consistent bedtime routine.

- Overfatigue can cause sundowning. Encourage the resident to nap or rest in the early afternoon.
- Try to prevent the resident from sleeping too much during the day.
- The evening meal should be eaten at least 2 hours before bedtime. Eliminate caffeine from the resident's diet.
- Involve the resident in quiet evening activities, soft music, or interactions with a caregiver or family member.
- Provide a light bedtime snack that is easily chewed and digested.
- Take the resident to the bathroom. Allow sufficient time for bladder and bowel elimination.
- Give a slow back massage.
- Check with family members and continue the resident's established habits, such as wearing socks to bed, using two pillows, or having a night light.
- Check the lighting of the room. Shadows and reflections are disturbing.

- If the resident awakens during the night, repeat the bedtime routine. If this is ineffective and the resident does not remain in bed, try a recliner or Alzheimer's chair.

Pillaging and Hoarding. These events do not present a major problem unless residents collect items from other residents' rooms or they hide things that are difficult to find.

- Label all residents' belongings.
- If a missing item is located, note where it was found. The resident probably will choose the same hiding place the next time.
- Check the room daily for stale food.
- Keep the resident's hands busy. Activities like folding washcloths or "fiddling" with keys on a ring may help.
- Provide a "rummaging" drawer or box for the resident.

Reality Orientation

Reality orientation (R.O.) is used to help disoriented residents regain connections to the environment, to time, and to themselves. When it is used appropriately, it decreases anxiety in the resident. R.O. may be effective in the first stage and the early part of the second stage of

---

GUIDELINES for

Reality Orientation

- Always treat residents as adults, with respect and dignity, no matter how confused they are.
- Speak clearly and directly. Avoid the temptation to speak louder when they do not understand you.
- Give simple, brief instructions and responses.
- Establish and maintain a structured routine.
- Be polite and sincere.
- Give residents adequate time to respond.
- Allow residents to be independent as long as possible.
- Set residents' watches to the correct time.
- Make sure residents have clean eyeglasses and effective hearing aids if they need them.
- Place large numbered calendars in rooms and cross off the days as they pass.
- There should be clocks with large numbers around the facility.
- Signs with large letters and color codes on walls, floors, and equipment help residents find their way around the facility.
- Call residents by name. Disoriented residents usually respond to their first name more quickly.
- Tell residents your name—do not expect them to remember you.
- Use R.O. in conversation with the residents, for

example, "It's only March 5 today but it is warm outside."

When using R.O.:

- Do not put residents on the spot. For example, do not ask, "Do you remember who I am?" or "Do you know what day this is?" If you need to verify orientation, ask "What are your plans for today?"
- Answer questions honestly but avoid confronting the residents with information they are unable to handle. If a resident whose husband is deceased asks, "Is my husband coming today?" it is cruel to answer by saying, "Remember, your husband died two years ago." This response will likely trigger a catastrophic reaction. It is better to answer by asking another question, such as, "Tell me about your husband, Emma." She will receive pleasure from reminiscing and will probably work up to present time on her own.
- Never argue with a resident's reality. When a resident has a delusion, arguing increases the individual's anxiety and agitation. Many delusions are based on past experiences. Because the resident is disoriented, the experience seems to be happening now.
- Do not reinforce the resident's disorientation.
- Remember that a pleasant facial expression, relaxed body language, and a caring touch are the most important aspects of caring for confused residents.

Alzheimer's disease. In later stages it is meaningless and increases agitation.

Reminiscing

Reminiscing (remembering past experiences) is a natural activity for people of all ages. We tend to reminisce when we see old friends or get together with families.

- Past experiences are remembered and enjoyed as we think of pleasant times from the past.
- As people age, the tendency to reminisce increases, and the activity becomes more important.
- It is an appropriate activity for residents with dementia if long-term memory is still intact (Figure 31-20).
- Reminiscing may serve as a life review. Elderly people often review the past experiences of their lives. This can bring back unpleasant memories. If these experiences are resolved, peace of mind can be found.

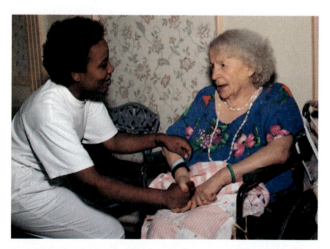

FIGURE 31-20 Reminiscing may be an appropriate activity for residents in the early stage of Alzheimer's disease.

- Reminiscing can help people adapt to old age. It helps to maintain self-esteem. It allows them to work through personal losses.
- When we listen to residents reminisce, we understand them better.
- Reminiscing therapy can be a group activity if done with a leader who is skillful and sensitive to the feelings of the members.

Validation Therapy

Validation therapy was developed by Naomi Feil. **Validation therapy** is a technique that tries to maintain the disoriented person's dignity by acknowledging the person's memories and feelings.

It is based on these ideas:

- Maintain the identity and dignity of the residents.
- Help disoriented people with dementia feel good about themselves.
- There is a reason for all behavior. What seems like confused behavior may be an acting-out of memories from long ago.
- Acknowledge feelings and memories.
- Disoriented people have the right to express feelings when they can no longer be oriented to reality.
- Living must be resolved in order to prepare for dying.
- Sometimes elderly persons have experienced so many losses during a lifetime that they have no coping abilities left.
- To live in reality is not the only way to live.
- Disoriented elderly have worth. We can give them joy by allowing them to express themselves.
- Within each confused person is a human being who was once a child and later an adult with hopes, joys, sadness, failures, and successes. They deserve to be cared for and loved in their final years.

REVIEW

A. True/False.

Mark the following true or false by circling T or F.

1. T F Older people have the same emotional needs for good mental health as young people.
2. T F Frustration is an emotion often experienced by the elderly.
3. T F As people age, they become less interested in sexuality.
4. T F Elderly people may not be aware of their need for fluids.
5. T F Infections are not a major cause of concern in the elderly.
6. T F The resident's mouth should be carefully inspected and cleaned each time the dentures are cleaned.
7. T F One of the best approaches when working with persons with dementia is to reason with them and use logic.
8. T F Calories should generally be increased in the diet of the elderly.
9. T F Elderly persons are generally fearful of death.
10. T F Daily tub baths or showers are not usually necessary or recommended for elderly residents.

B. Matching.

Choose the correct item from Column II to match each question in Column I.

Column I	Column II
11. _____ dementia	**a.** weakening
12. _____ validation therapy	**b.** remembering past experiences
13. _____ reminiscing	**c.** deficits in thinking, memory, judgment
14. _____ debilitating	**d.** tries to maintain disoriented person's dignity
15. _____ sundowning	**e.** wakefulness of person with Alzheimer's during evening and night

C. Multiple Choice.

Select the one best answer for each question.

16. Characteristics of the nursing assistant that are especially important while caring for older adults include
    a. patience.
    b. kindness.
    c. sense of humor.
    d. All of these.

17. Characteristics of the elderly include
    a. increased vitality.
    b. decreased night sleep.
    c. increased appetite.
    d. increased mobility and agility.

18. Which of the following nutrients should be increased in the diet of elderly persons?
    a. Fats
    b. Vegetables, fruits, and whole grains
    c. Calories
    d. Sugar

19. Which statement is true in regard to catastrophic reactions?
    a. They are unavoidable in persons with dementia.
    b. They may be precipitated by too much sensory stimulation.
    c. Providing activity will subdue the catastrophic reaction.
    d. They are always expressions of violence.

20. An appropriate approach to reality orientation is to
    a. ask the resident if he knows who you are.
    b. ask the resident what his plans are for the day.
    c. ask the resident if he knows the date.
    d. All of these.

D. Nursing Assistant Challenge.

Mr. Delgotti, 83 years old, is one of your assigned patients. Think about the changes that occur with aging and answer these questions.

21. What changes occur in the integumentary system?
22. Because of these changes, what complications could occur during his hospital stay?
23. What actions can you take to avoid these complications?
24. What possible complications can occur in the digestive system?
25. What observations are especially important for all the body systems because of Mr. Delgotti's age?

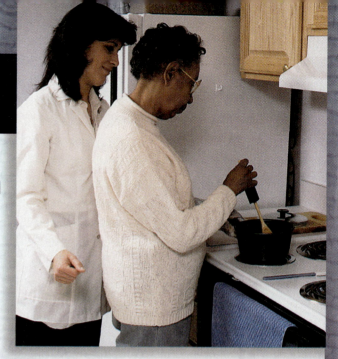

The Organization of Home Care: Trends in Health Care

As a result of this unit, you will be able to:

- Spell and define terms.
- Briefly describe the history of home care.
- Describe the benefits of working in home care.
- Identify members of the home health team.
- List guidelines for avoiding liability while working as a home health aide.
- Describe the types of information a home health aide must be able to document.
- Identify several time management techniques.
- List ways in which the home health aide can work successfully with families.

Learn the meaning and the correct spelling of the following words and phrases:

| client care records | intermittent care | time/travel records |

INTRODUCTION

The health care of persons (clients) in their own homes is an age-old tradition. It was not until the middle of the twentieth century that there was a massive trend to move patient care out of the home and into the community health care facility. The late nineteenth century saw the growth of medical schools and the licensing of physicians. Schools of nursing soon followed. Hospital staffing slots were filled with students enrolled in these programs. Although the permissive laws of the early 1900s gave requirements for nursing licensure, the laws did not restrict nursing practice. There were few legal restrictions for people who provided care in patients' homes. Almost anyone could hire out to provide such care. A few years later, laws were passed to control nurse education. These laws specifically stated the acts that a nurse could and could not perform. Anyone practicing nursing without a license could be held liable.

World War II brought with it:

- A gradual increase in the need for more technical care, as procedures and equipment became more complex
- Introduction of antibiotics and better techniques of infection control

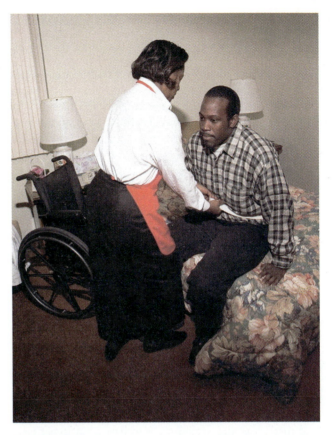

FIGURE 32-2 The high technology of hospital care has increased the cost, making home care a practical alternative.

- Growth of a new, supplementary force of workers (nursing assistants) to assist in providing nursing care
- Construction of many new health care facilities
- Hospital care of sick people

Today, the pendulum has swung back once more toward treating acutely ill people in hospitals and providing alternative care (such as home care, day care, or long-term care) for all others (Figure 32-1). Factors that foster this interest in home care include:

- Expensive high technology (Figure 32-2)
- Introduction of diagnosis-related groups (DRGs), resulting in earlier discharge from hospitals
- Growing population of chronically ill people
- The establishment of hospice care, enabling terminally ill people to choose to stay at home during their last months of life
- The preference of the health care consumer to remain at home if possible

PROVIDERS OF HOME HEALTH CARE

Because of the increasing demand for home care, there are many different types of home care providers:

- Government-sponsored agencies controlled by city or county governments

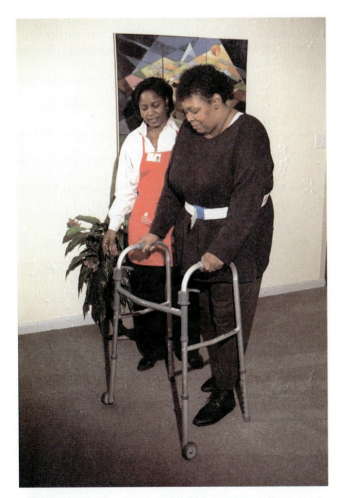

FIGURE 32-1 The trend toward home care is growing in response to increased numbers of people requiring continuing care.

- Private agencies; some are for-profit and others are non-profit
- Hospital-sponsored agencies

These providers employ several types of health care workers, including nurses, nursing assistants, therapists, and social workers. Each employer has personnel policies that regulate job descriptions, salaries, and benefits. The employer provides new employees with an orientation to the agency and to their responsibilities.

BENEFITS OF WORKING IN HOME HEALTH CARE

After you have completed your training, you may choose to join a group that provides home health care. There are advantages to working in such agencies:

- Satisfaction of giving complete care to one client at a time
- Satisfaction of caring for the same client over a period of time (Figure 32-3)
- Opportunity to work with greater independence
- Part-time employment, if desired

The person working in home care must have dependable transportation to the homes of the clients. In small towns and rural areas, the worker needs to have a car to get from one client to the next. In larger cities, the worker may be able to use public transportation.

SOURCE OF REFERRAL

Most persons using home care are patients being discharged from a hospital or skilled care facility. The health care team at the discharging facility completes a discharge plan and evaluates the person's need for continuing care at home. The physician must then write an order for home health care.

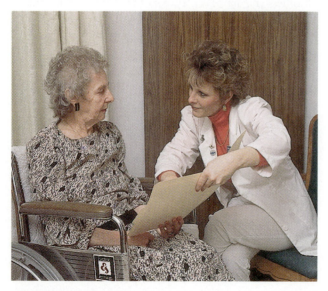

FIGURE 32-3 Caring for the same client over a period of time provides great satisfaction.

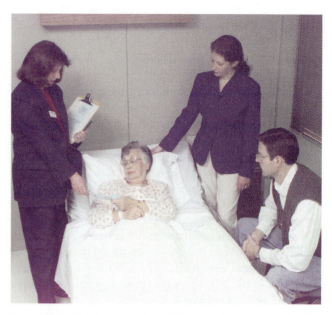

FIGURE 32-4 The patient and family select a home health care agency.

The discharge planner at the hospital or long-term care facility provides the patient and family with a list of agencies from which to choose the home care provider (Figure 32-4). (In some areas of the country, only one agency may be available.) The selected agency is given medical information about the patient and then begins to plan care.

PAYMENT FOR HOME HEALTH CARE

Home health care may be paid for by:

- Medicare, for persons over 65 years of age or for those who have been disabled for 2 or more years
- Medicaid (in some states)
- Private insurance companies
- Client's personal funds

Government programs and most insurance companies will only pay for home care that is considered "skilled" and is provided as **intermittent care**. This means that the nursing assistant or other caregiver goes to the home, performs certain procedures or treatments, and then leaves. If a family or client needs a caregiver for several hours a day, they will probably have to pay for the services with their own money. Because this is very costly, most home care is given on an intermittent basis.

THE HOME HEALTH CARE TEAM

The home health care team consists of the:

- Client (the person in need of care)
  - Clients are of various ages.
  - They need differing levels of nursing and physical care.

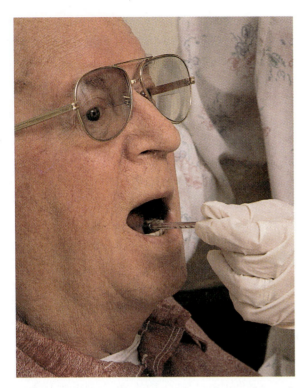

FIGURE 32-5 The home health aide provides direct client care.

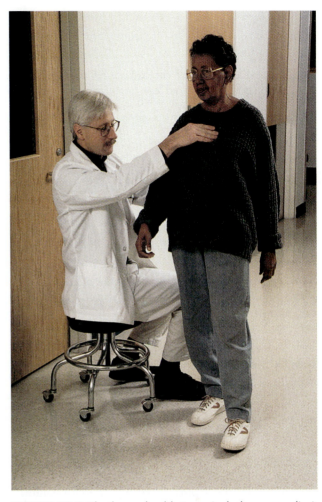

FIGURE 32-6 The home health team includes many disciplines, including physical therapy.

— They may have chronic, progressive ailments.
— They may be recovering from acute illness, surgery, or childbirth.
— They need assistance with activities of daily living.
— They usually require skilled services.
- Family
  — Family members may act as alternate caregivers.
  — They may live in the client's home.
  — They may or may not be supportive of the client.
- Nursing assistant
  — Provides direct client care (Figure 32-5).
  — Provides for client's safety and comfort.
  — Makes observations and reports them to the nurse.
  — Documents observations and care that was given.
- Supervising nurse
  — Completes periodic client assessments.
  — Plans the care.
  — Teaches and supervises nursing assistants.
  — Coordinates care and members of the home care team.
- Physician
  — Writes orders and acts as a consultant and guide.
- Other specialists, such as:
  — physical therapist (Figure 32-6)
  — occupational therapist
  — speech therapist
  — social worker

THE ASSESSMENT PROCESS

The nurse does an assessment of the client during the first visit. Other health care professionals assigned to the case also complete assessments. After the assessments are finished, the nurse and other team members:

- Identify the client's problems
- Determine approaches to resolve the problems
- Establish goals for the client
- Evaluate the home situation for safety concerns
- Determine the amount of time needed for each visit and the length of time the services may be required

The nurse discusses the plans with the client. The nurse includes the client's wishes as much as possible within the available payment plan. The nurse then develops the assignment for the nursing assistant. You may be assigned to care for several clients or a particular client for a:

- Specified number of hours daily
- Specified period two or three days per week
- Long-term period
- Brief period

LIABILITY AND THE NURSING ASSISTANT

You need to be aware of the responsibilities involved in home care and how to avoid legal problems associated with caregiving.

RECORDKEEPING

Be sure you know exactly what documentation you are expected to do, what types of records you should keep, and the forms you need to use. All documentation must be accurate, complete, and up-to-date. Medicare and insurance companies frequently audit these records to decide whether to pay for the services.

Two types of records are compiled by the nursing assistant giving home care. They are time/travel records and client care records.

Time/travel records (Figure 32-8) are a record of how you spend your time in the client's home. The information recorded includes:

- Time of arrival
- Time of departure
- Length of time required for specific activities
- Travel time if working in more than one home
- Mileage or transportation costs

Keeping a time/travel record requires accuracy and some calculations. Fill in the record as you complete each assignment. Do not wait until the end of the day or your assigned time and then try to rely on your memory.

To compute mileage (round off to the nearest full mile):

- Record the car odometer reading before starting to your assignment.
- Record the odometer reading when you arrive at the client's home.
- Subtract the starting odometer reading from the arrival reading.
- Record this difference as the mileage.

For example, if the reading on your car odometer before starting was 45,061 and upon arrival at the client's home it is 45,068, the mileage should be recorded as 7 miles (45,068 − 45,061).

Client care records (Figure 32-9) are a record of:

- Care given, such as bathing, positioning, range-of-motion exercises
- Client's responses to care
- Housekeeping tasks completed, if assigned to you by nurse
- Observations:
  - Condition of skin
  - Vital signs
  - Elimination; bowel and urine
  - Food and fluid intake

GUIDELINES *for*

Avoiding Liability

- Be sure you are given a job description upon employment that lists your specific duties and responsibilities. In some areas, home health aides are only allowed to do certain assigned tasks when working with an insurance company or Medicare. Auditors check the tasks assigned and confirm what is actually done in the client's home.
- Carry out procedures carefully and do them as you were taught.
- Always keep safety factors in mind and be on the lookout for possible hazards.
- Be familiar with client's rights.
- Ask for assistance if you are assigned to a procedure that you have never performed before.

Make sure the procedure is within the legal boundaries of nursing assistant practice.

- Do only those tasks that are assigned to you.
- Know how to contact the supervising nurse for questions and issues related to the care of your client. Do not overstep your authority.
- Know how and when to contact emergency services for the client (Figure 32-7).
- Document your care and observations carefully and completely.
- Participate in care conferences with the other team members.

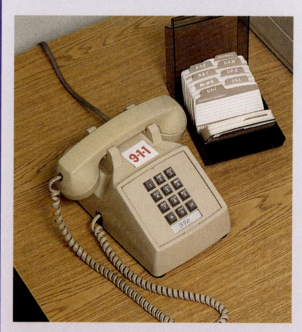

FIGURE 32-7 The home health aide needs to know when and how to contact emergency services.

RIVERVIEW HOME HEALTH SERVICE
8987 Walkman Ave
Parkhurst, Nebraska
Time and Travel Log

CARE GIVER NAME ___Siadto, Laura CNA___   TITLE ___Home Health Assistant___   EMPT. NO. _62718_   DATE _Aug. 29_

CLIENT NAME/ADDRESS (Last, first)	SERVICE PROVIDED	VISIT CODE	NON BILL CODE	TIME IN	TIME OUT	CLIENT CONTACT TIME	ODOMETER READING	MILES
Volheim, Eleonore	Bedbath, Shampoo	4		8^{15}	9^{05}	50 min	From: 45,061 To: 45,068	7 miles
Jaronello, Sharri		1		9^{30}	9^{45}	15 min	From: 45,068 To: 45,083	15 miles
Doyle, Kindra	Enema, bedbath, amb	4		10^{10}	11^{30}	1 hr. 20 min.	From: 45,083 To: 46,001	18 miles
Hammond, Rachel	Ass't c̄ colostomy cath care, bath, ROM	4		11^{50}	1^{20}	1 hr. 30 min.	From: 46,001 To: 46,017	16 miles
Minzey, Aimee		2		1^{30}	1^{35}	—	From: 46,017 To: 46,025	8 miles
Galloway, Rosa		5		1^{50}	2^{00}	10 min	From: 46,025 To: 46,028	3 miles
							From: To:	

Total Visits __6__   Total Mileage __67__   Parking Fees __—__

Visit Code
1 IE Initial Eval & Rx   4 HC Home Care
2 FV Follow Up Visit   5 Hospital/Hospice
3 DV Discharge Visit   6 MC Maternal/Child

Supervising Nurse: _Bruce Davenport R.N._

Nonbill Code
1. Refused Care
2. Patient Not Home
3. Non-Bill
4. Expired
5. Delivered Supplies

FIGURE 32-8 Example of a time/travel record

— Appetite

— Incidents such as client falls

— Any observation that indicates a change in the client's health status

— Mental status: orientation, alertness, mood, and behavior

You may be expected to keep reports that cover a longer period of time. For example, you may need to keep a weekly or monthly record of daily blood testing results for a client with diabetes. The physician may change the schedule of insulin based on your long-term report.

TIME MANAGEMENT

As a home health care aide, you are responsible for planning your assignment and completing the client's care within a certain amount of time. You may have several clients to see during your shift. They will be expecting you at a specific time of the day. There are several actions you can take to make the best use of your time:

● Be sure you have everything you will need for your assignments before you leave home. This might include a thermometer, watch with second hand, stethoscope, blood pressure cuff, forms for documenting, pen.

● Have a work plan in mind before you arrive at the client's home. For example, will you give the client a bath first or help him with his exercises first?

● Organize your supplies before you begin your assignment. Gather together the linens, client clothing, and other items you will need.

● Avoid being distracted by the family. There are many things you may need to discuss with the family, but you probably will not have time for lengthy conversations.

● Call your next client if you find you will be arriving later than expected.

● Avoid getting bogged down in tasks that you are not expected to perform.

RIVERVIEW HOME HEALTH SERVICE
8987 Walkman Ave
Parkhurst, Nebraska
Client Care Plan / Progress Notes

HOME HEALTH ASSISTANT _YOLANDA BROWN, CNA_

CLIENT NAME _NICHOLAS FRENCH_   SOC. SECURITY # _728-24-8884_

ADDRESS: _529 MAPLE AVE.   PARKHURST, NEBRASKA_

ACTIVITY

Time	Activity
0800	Arrived, Determined needs, planned activities Client seemed fatigued "Slept poorly". On nasal O_2 2.5L
0830	Circumoral pallor noted. Vital signs checked. Dyspneic on exertion.
0900	Put laundry into washing machine. Started breakfast. Client ate 1 sl. toast, 8 oz oatbran cereal / milk 6oz orange juice
0930	Prepared equipment for A.M. care – complete bath, shave and denture care.
1000	Asst to commode, soft brown formed stool.
1030	Made comfortable in easy chair. Reading newspaper. Nasal O_2 Cleaned kitchen including refrigerator
1100	Linen changed – dusted and dust mopped bedroom. Vacuumed living room.
1130	Prepared lunch.
1200	Client ate 1/2 chicken sandwich, 8 oz. tea, chocolate pudding, 8 oz. tomato soup.
1230	Client returned to bed for nap
1300	Cleaned lunch dishes and prepared salad, jello for evening meal
1330	Put washed laundry into dryer.
1400	Cleaned bathroom, washed kitchen floor Put bed linen into washer.
1430	Made out shopping list for A.M.
1500	Client awake. Assisted into living room. Watching T.V. Ordered O_2 tank replacement.
1530	Folded and put clean laundry away. Put washed linens in dryer.
1600	Client seems more rested. Color improved. Resp. easier. Notified supervisor of client's progress.
1630	Left client's home @ 3²⁵ P.M.

Y. Brown CNA

VITAL SIGNS	T	P	R	B/P
	97⁴	92	26	
INTAKE				
OUTPUT				

SUP. SIGNATURE _____

FIGURE 32-9 Examples of client care records

RIVERVIEW HOME HEALTH SERVICE
8987 Walkman Ave
Parkhurst, Nebraska
Client Care Plan / Progress Notes

WT. _146_ TEMP. _98_ BP _114/80_ P _70_ R _14_   MD CONTACT _C. Boylston_

HOMEBOUND DUE TO _Spinal Cord Injury – Paraplegia_   MEN. STATUS _Alert – Coherent_

PROBLEMS	INTERVENTIONS	TIME	PLAN	OUTCOME
① Potential altered	Maintain high-calorie, low-residue, high protein diet		Morning Care	Tol. Well
nutrition: less than	Reduce high calcium and gas-producing foods.	0700	Breakfast	ate entire meal
body requirements	Provide balanced meals and supplements morning and evening	0815	Commode	soft formed stool
		0900	Bath, Cath Care,	
		0945	ROM	
			up in wheelchair	Tolerated well
② Potential for disuse	Exercise to tolerance Avoid fatigue ROM	1030	6oz High Cal drink	
syndrome related to	Turn and reposition q 1 hr.	1045	Returned to Bed	
effects of immobility	Up in wheelchair B.I.D.	1130	Positioned on Rt. Side	
	Encourage self-care activities to tolerance		Positioned on Back	
③ Alteration in bowel	Stool Softener, Glycerine	1230	Lunch	½ tuna sand/tea
elimination: constipation	Suppositories, enemas, PRN.			
	Check for BM q 3 day		up in wheelchair	
		1330	Returned to Bed	
④ Potential for infection	Routine catheter care	1430	Positioned on left side	
related to indwelling	Change per routine schedule		Watching T.V.	
Foley catheter		1500		
⑤ Self-concept disturbance	Encourage verbalization of feelings and fears.			
related to effects of	Encourage independence. Be positive and reassuring.			
limitations				

DAILY SUMMARY

Diet and supplements taken fairly well. Activity tolerated. Muscles soft but some tone. Soft formed stool.

Expressed frustration during transfers from bed to wheelchair. Enjoys reading and wathing T.V.

Seems to be gaining some confidence in transfer activities.

Visit Date _____   Pt. Last Name,   Employee

Nursing Supervisor Report   First Initial ___Mitchell, D.___   Signature _Ruthy Chek, CNA_

Joint Visit in Home _____   Patient's personal care and comfort measures by home aide are:

Conference _____   superior _____ ; good _____ ; satisfactory _____ ; need improvement _____ ;

Services provided were appropriate _____ ; inappropriate _____ .

Comments

FIGURE 32-9 *continued*

WORKING WITH FAMILIES

Clients may have a spouse or other family members who reside in the home. For other clients, their families may live elsewhere but stop in periodically. In some situations family members may live so far away that they can seldom visit. Family members may call or visit while you are there, seeking information on the client's condition. It is best to let the client speak with them directly if possible. If the client cannot do this, then remember to be objective in your comments. If you do not know the answer to a question, be honest and say so rather than providing false information. Refer all medical questions to the physician or the nurse.

Remember that as a home health aide, you are a guest of the family and client. You may be assigned to clients who have vastly different values and cultural beliefs than yours. It is not your role to try to change this. Report to your supervisor if you feel that there are family practices that are detrimental to the client's well-being and health. Families can be an excellent resource for you. They may be able to give you additional information about the client that will help you to give better care. This can avoid frustration for both you and the client. The family may also be able to tell you how they have cared for the client in the past.

Tact and courtesy are important when communicating with the family. They may wish to be involved in the caregiving, but it is important that you complete the tasks to which you have been assigned. The family has a right to know the progress the patient is making, but there may be some information that the client does not wish you to tell the family. You may need to discuss this issue with your supervisor. Families may feel overwhelmed and discouraged at times, particularly if the client has had a long illness. They need your support, so you must be realistic yet hopeful (Figure 32-10).

If you are spending an entire shift with the client, remember that you are getting paid to spend this time giving care. If all procedures are completed, take your cue from the client or family as to what activities you should complete for the rest of your tour of duty. Some clients may wish to be left alone to read (Figure 32-11) or watch television. Others may seek your companionship for visiting or playing cards. If you are working through the night, ask the client or family if you may read or do quiet activities such as needlework while the client is sleeping. Family members may ask you to do something that is not part of your assignment. Whether you can meet their request depends on:

- The nature of the request
- The time involved in filling the request
- The policies of the home care agency
- Whether you are assigned to intermittent visits to the client or assigned to work a full shift

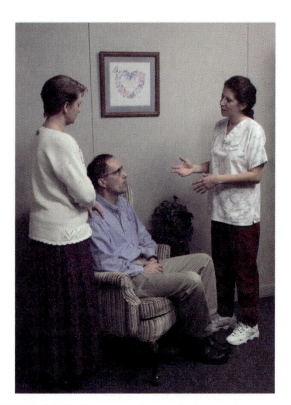

FIGURE 32-10 You must be realistic yet hopeful for families.

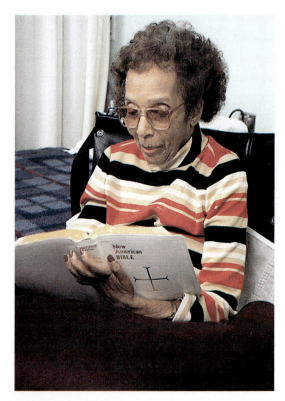

FIGURE 32-11 Some clients may wish to be left alone to pursue their own interests.

REVIEW

A. True/False.

Mark the following true or false by circling T or F.

1. T F World War I stimulated the enrollment of students in hospital-based nursing programs.

2. T F Many new hospitals were built after World War II.

3. T F Only nurses and nursing assistants are employed for home health care.

4. T F The physician acts as care coordinator for the client's home care.

5. T F Home health aides are expected to provide direct client care.

6. T F Documentation is an important responsibility of the home care aide.

7. T F The demand for home care has decreased within the last few years.

8. T F The client may receive the services of a physical therapist.

9. T F The home health care aide may have the opportunity for part-time employment.

10. T F The home health aide is responsible for completing periodic assessments of the client.

B. Multiple Choice.

Select the one best answer for each question.

11. World War II brought about
    a. an increase in the need for more technical care.
    b. the introduction of antibiotics.
    c. the growth of a supplementary work force.
    d. All of these.

12. Home care is increasing because
    a. hospitals are overcrowded.
    b. there are fewer physicians.
    c. people like being cared for in their own homes.
    d. families can do some of the nursing care.

13. The person receiving home health care is called the
    a. client.
    b. patient.
    c. resident.
    d. recipient.

14. Members of the home care team include
    a. the client.
    b. the family.
    c. health care givers.
    d. All of these.

15. Time management is important because
    a. you can get home earlier.
    b. you may have more than one client to care for during your shift.
    c. the client may have other business to tend to.
    d. the agency will make more money if you work faster.

16. Home care aides must be able to:
    a. treat the family with courtesy and tact.
    b. make accurate observations.
    c. document on a timely basis.
    d. All of these.

C. Nursing Assistant Challenge.

You are almost finished with your nursing assistant course and you are thinking about employment. You have been offered jobs in a home health agency and in a hospital and are having trouble making a decision. Your instructor advises you to think about both the advantages and disadvantages of working for each employer. Make a two-column list for each, labeling the columns "advantages" and "disadvantages."

The Nursing Assistant in Home Care

See Appendix (page 667) for additional infection control information

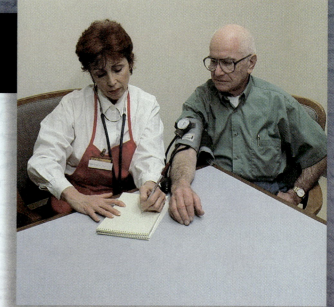

As a result of this unit, you will be able to:
- Spell and define terms.
- Describe the characteristics that are especially important to the nursing assistant providing home care.

- Describe the duties of the nursing assistant who works in the home setting.
- Describe the duties of the homemaker assistant.
- Carry out home care activities needed to maintain a safe and clean environment.

Learn the meaning and the correct spelling of the following words and phrases:

| home health assistant | home health aide | homemaker aide | homemaker assistant |

THE HOME HEALTH CAREGIVER

In the last unit you learned about the structure of home health care. In this unit you will learn more about the responsibilities of the nursing assistant (**home health aide**) working in the client's home.

The nursing assistant is an important part of the health team in the acute hospital and in the long-term care facility. The nursing assistant is part of an equally important team that provides home care.

The nursing assistant may be called:

* **Home health assistant** or home health aide, whose primary role is to provide assistance with nursing care.
* **Homemaker assistant** or **homemaker aide** when the primary role is to do housekeeping chores. The homemaker assistant carries out general household tasks, prepares meals, and runs errands such as food shopping.

The nursing assistant providing health care services may be asked to carry out homemaker assistant duties in some cases.

THE HOME HEALTH ASSISTANT AND THE NURSING PROCESS

You are part of the nursing process. During:

* *Assessment*, your observations and careful reporting can make a valuable contribution to the objective and subjective data from which the analysis of the client's needs is made. Make note of:
  - The client's response to your care
  - The interactions between family members and friends that could lead to stress on the client

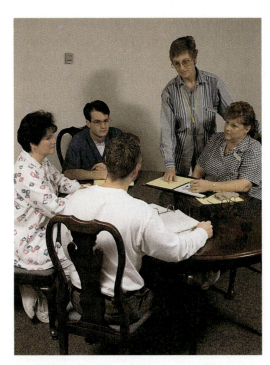

FIGURE 33-1 The home health aide participates in planning the client's care.

  - Support services that may be needed
* *Planning*, you contribute as you actively share in care conferences (Figure 33-1).
* *Implementation*, you spend the most time with the client. You are therefore responsible for seeing that the plan is carried out.
  - Report any difficulties in carrying out the plan.
  - Develop ways to organize your work to make the plan more efficient.
* *Evaluation*, you once more contribute to the nursing process when you share your observations about the success or lack of success of the care.
  - Be accurate and concise in your reporting.
  - Be honest in your appraisal of the client's progress and the point at which your services are no longer needed.

CHARACTERISTICS OF THE HOME CARE NURSING ASSISTANT AND HOMEMAKER ASSISTANT

The home care nursing assistant and homemaker assistant must have a full measure of the characteristics you have already come to associate with a successful hospital-based assistant. There are, however, some characteristics that need to be particularly strong in an assistant who works in clients' homes.

Remember that you will be working directly with the client and her personal possessions, without a supervising nurse constantly with you. This means you must demonstrate:

* Honesty, as you handle the client's possessions and shopping money. Treat the possessions with care and respect. Keep an accurate record of all money spent and receipts received.
* Self-starter ability. You must know and carry out your assigned tasks promptly and efficiently without needing someone to remind you.
* Self-discipline. Do not allow yourself to waste time on activities such as smoking, chatting with friends on the phone, and drinking coffee just because there is no supervisor to constantly check on your progress.
* Accuracy and attention to details, so that each task is performed exactly as you were taught.
* Organization, so that you plan your activities to make the best use of your in-home time. Plan your activities around the client's schedule, not your own.
* Maturity, so that judgment and assessments can be made properly.
* Insight that gives you the ability to see the whole client as an interactive member of a family unit and community.
* Observational skills. Be able to recognize and report abnormal signs and symptoms.

- Adaptability. Although you will need all the physical, emotional, and communication skills you learned and practiced in the clinical setting, you must be creative in adapting them to the home situation. For example, a cut-open plastic bag covered with a towel may be substituted for the bed protectors used in the hospital. Housekeeping chores may be performed as the client rests.
- Acceptance of clients and their home environments. Remember, your clients will be of all ethnic and religious groups and economic levels.
- Ability to perform independently, making decisions within the limits of your responsibilities and the scope of the assignment.

HOME HEALTH CARE DUTIES

The duties of the home health care assistant are planned around the family routine. These duties may include:

- Helping with the activities of daily living
- Giving special treatments, such as prescribed exercises
- Providing comfort measures, such as positioning and special mouth care
- Maintaining a safe environment
- Bathing the client
- Changing linen
- Interacting with family members

Homemaker duties may include:

- Light housekeeping
- Shopping for meals (Figure 33-2)
- Preparing meals

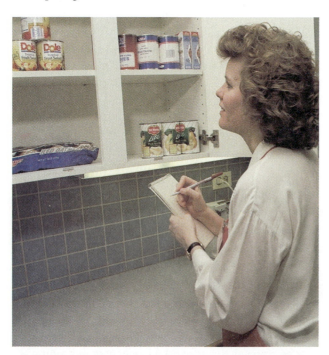

FIGURE 33-2 Homemaker duties may include shopping for groceries. Prepare a list of items needed before going to the market, to save time and ensure that you do not buy unneeded items.

You may also have to transport the client to clinic or therapy visits (Figure 33-3). You must have specific permission from your agency to perform activities outside of the home. The homemaker duties *do not* include:

- Doing heavy housework such as washing windows, waxing floors, or moving heavy furniture
- Making decisions about food purchases, unless the client is unable to do so
- Becoming involved in family disputes by offering opinions or taking sides

The skills you learned in the clinical setting can be adapted to the home environment (Figure 33-4). For example:

- Ice bags can be replaced by plastic bags sealed and wrapped in a towel.
- Reusable enema equipment can be substituted for disposable enema equipment.
- Extra pillows can be used to support position changes if the bed position cannot be changed.
- Some equipment may be rented from equipment rental companies (Figure 33-5) or borrowed from church groups or other organizations.
- The entire bed can be raised on blocks, to make caregiving easier if the patient is not ambulatory.
- A cotton blanket or lightweight spread can be used for a bath blanket.
- Plastic covered with a twin-size sheet can be used in place of a drawsheet.
- Apply the principles of standard precautions if contact with blood, body fluids, mucous membranes, or nonintact skin is likely.
- A cardboard box can be cut, taped, and padded for use as a back rest (Figure 33-6A).
- Two lightweight pieces of wood nailed at right angles can be padded and used as a footrest to hold bedding off the toes (Figure 33-6B).
- A bed tray can replace an overbed table for eating and activities.
- A paper bag can be taped to the bed springs to dispose of soiled tissues (Figure 33-6C). The entire bag can then be closed and properly handled for disposal.
- A shoe bag tucked under the mattress and hanging by the bedside (Figure 33-6D) can provide compartments for the patient's personal articles.
- A pillowcase hung on the back of a chair can serve as a laundry bag.

Most home health aides carry kits that contain:

- Plastic aprons
- Disposable gloves
- Observational equipment such as stethoscope, blood pressure cuff, and thermometers

The Home Environment

You are responsible for maintaining a safe and comfortable environment for the client. This means you must:

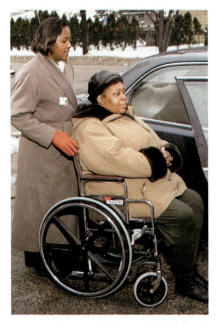

FIGURE 33-3 The home health aide may have to transport clients to clinics for additional care and therapy.

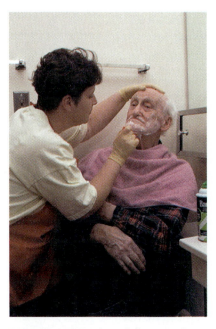

FIGURE 33-4 The skills you have learned may be adapted for care in the home.

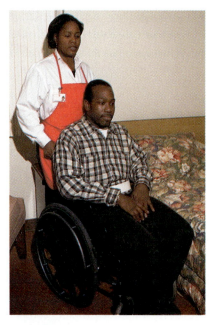

FIGURE 33-5 Equipment may be rented or borrowed from other organizations or agencies.

- be alert to unsafe situations.
- control the spread of infection.
- care for and maintain the client's furnishings, supplies, and appliances.

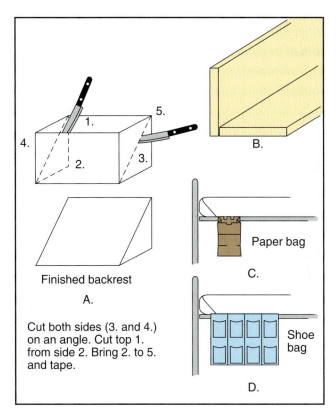

B.

Paper bag

C.

Finished backrest

A.

Cut both sides (3. and 4.) on an angle. Cut top 1. from side 2. Bring 2. to 5. and tape.

Shoe bag

D.

FIGURE 33-6 Making equipment using readily available materials.

SAFETY IN THE HOME

Your first visit to the home gives you an opportunity to check for safety factors. Tell a family member or supervising nurse about safety problems. For example, things to call to the attention of your supervisor include:

- Furniture or other items that obstruct the client's walkway
- Electrical cords that could cause the client to fall
- Stair railings and stair treads that need repair
- Unstable or lightweight chairs
- Highly polished floors that may be slippery
- The need to lock up specific items if the client is disoriented:
  - chemicals such as household cleaning supplies, paints, insecticides, and cleaning fluids
  - medications, both prescription and over-the-counter
  - aerosol cans
  - small appliances like toasters or irons that can be plugged in and used inappropriately
  - power tools
  - weapons or anything that could be used as a weapon
  - fragile, breakable, or valuable items
  - smoking materials that should only be used with supervision
  - electrical outlets that require covering
  - thermostats that may need guards over them
  - stove knobs
- Loose scatter rugs, which might cause a fall as the client ambulates

- Overloaded electrical outlets, which might cause a fire when you use equipment such as an electric lift
- Ambulatory aids that need repair or replacement, such as broken straps on braces or worn rubber tips on walkers, canes, and crutches
- Family or client smoking when oxygen is being used in the home

Your job is not to reorganize the client's home but to assure a safe environment. Discuss with the nurse any other conditions you feel are unsafe. For example, the client may need:

- Handrails installed by the toilet or the bathtub
- A commode to use if the bathroom is not easily accessible
- A raised toilet seat
- A trapeze to assist with bed mobility
- A mechanical lift for transferring out of bed

These items are readily available from durable equipment providers, and most insurance companies and Medicare will pay for equipment that is required for client care. However, the nurse must consult with the physician and an order must be written for the equipment.

Keep a list of emergency numbers close to the telephone. The list should include the:

- Agency
- Supervising nurse
- Physician
- Family member
- Emergency number 911 (in areas where this number is in use)

If the 911 number is not used in your area, you will need numbers for the:

- Ambulance
- Hospital
- Police department
- Fire department

Assisting with Medications

The physician may prescribe medications for clients receiving home health care. Nursing assistants are not legally responsible for giving medications. However, you may have to supervise the client as she self-administers the medications. The client may need assistance in opening the container. There are many types of containers available that will hold a week's doses in individual sections labeled for the days of the week. These containers simplify the process and it is easy to determine whether the medications have been taken.

ELDER ABUSE

As a home health aide, you may observe clients who might possibly have been abused. Unit 4 describes the various types of abuse that may be inflicted by staff members, family members, or other residents. These situations may also occur in the home:

GUIDELINES *for*

Supervising Self-Administration of Medications

- The medicine must be taken at the correct time. Note whether it should be taken before meals, with food, or after meals.
- Check the expiration date to be sure the medicine is not outdated.
- Note whether the client is also taking over-the-counter medications (nonprescription) and check with your supervisor to find out whether these medications will interact with the prescription drugs.
- Perform any monitoring activities required, such as checking the pulse, the blood pressure, or the blood sugar, *before* the drug is taken.
- Note how much medication is left in the container. Follow your instructions for getting the prescription refilled so that the patient does not run out.

- Some families provide loving, capable care for older, dependent relatives for many years without assistance. They may be emotionally stressed and may have also depleted their financial resources.
- In some cases there has been a long family history of one spouse abusing the other.
- Self-abuse may occur when a disabled person is unable to adequately carry out activities of daily living and is unwilling to accept help.

It is not the responsibility of the nursing assistant to determine if an individual has been abused or what type of abuse has been inflicted. It *is* the nursing assistant's responsibility to report to the nursing supervisor any signs or symptoms that might be the result of abuse. This includes:

- Statements of the client that reflect neglect or abuse
- Unexplained bruises or wounds
- Signs of neglect such as poor hygiene
- A change in personality

Remember, these indications do not necessarily mean that the person is being abused. However, they may signal a need for further investigation by your supervisor.

INFECTION CONTROL

Some of the methods used in daily cleaning help to control the spread of infection. Other requirements are:

- Washing your hands (Figure 33-7)
- Keeping the kitchen and bathroom clean
- Caring for food properly

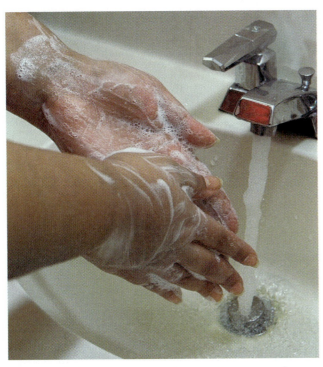

FIGURE 33-7 Handwashing is the most important infection control technique in the home (as it is in health care facilities).

- Disposing of tissues and other wastes properly
- Cleaning up dirty dishes
- Dusting daily
- Not allowing clutter to accumulate
- Wearing a plastic apron
- Wearing latex gloves for patient care if contact with blood, body fluids, mucous membranes, or nonintact skin is likely.
- Wearing utility gloves when cleaning environmental surfaces or doing laundry contaminated with blood, body fluids, secretions, or excretions.

See Appendix

HOUSEKEEPING TASKS

In some cases, the homemaker assistant (aide) will perform the housekeeping tasks. In other cases, the home health care nursing assistant may be assigned some or all of these duties.

Cleaning the Client's Room

Keeping the client's room clean is a way to prevent infection. It also helps raise the client's morale. Remember that you are not to rearrange the client's things without permission.

- Pick up things so clutter will not accumulate.
- Keep cleaning equipment in one place so you do not waste time gathering it for each job as you move from room to room (Figure 33-8).
- Clean and put equipment away as soon as you have finished with it.
- Dust the room daily.

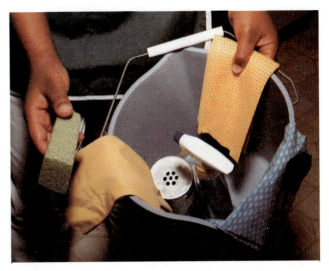

FIGURE 33-8 Keep cleaning equipment together for more efficient time management.

- Damp-dust noncarpeted floors weekly or vacuum carpeted floors.
- Remove used dishes and glasses when finished and rinse right away.
- Put clean clothes away after laundering. Hang up robes when not in use.
- Line wastepaper basket with a plastic bag and empty regularly.

Cleaning the Bathroom

The bathroom can be a source of infection, so you must be careful and thorough in your daily cleaning (Figure 33-9).

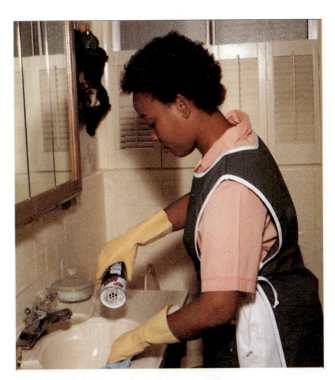

FIGURE 33-9 Clean the bathroom daily.

Use a disinfectant solution (family's choice) to clean the:
- Inside and outside of the toilet
- Shower or tub after each use
- Sink and faucets
- Countertops
- Floor; if carpeted, vacuum daily

Be sure dirty towels are put into the laundry. Replace them with clean towels and washcloths. Use a deodorant to keep the bathroom smelling fresh and clean.

Cleaning the Kitchen

The kitchen is another area that requires special attention. An unclean kitchen can be the source of infection.
- Clean up after each meal.
- Clean up dirty dishes immediately. Do not allow them to accumulate in the sink.
  - Rinse them and wash by hand in detergent and hot water.
  - Wash glasses first, then silverware, then dishes.
  - Rinse with hot water and allow to dry in drainer.
  - Put away when dry.
- You may wash them in the dishwasher by:
  - Rinsing well.
  - Adding recommended detergent to the dishwasher.
  - Loading washer; but do not run the dishwasher until it is full.
- Wash pots and pans by hand; most are not dishwasher-safe.
- Clean sink, countertops, and stove.
- Dispose of garbage properly. It may be put in an in-sink disposer if one is available. Do not include bones. Wrap those tightly in newspaper and put in trash or compactor if available.
- Sweep floor after each meal.
- Place leftover foods in small covered containers and refrigerate. Use or discard within a few days.

- Keep refrigerator clean and keep food covered. Clean spills in the refrigerator immediately (Figure 33-10).
- Keep the microwave oven clean (Figure 33-11). Use a damp cloth to wipe up spills immediately and to clean after each use. Make sure you heat food in microwave-safe dishes only. Do not use metal of any kind in a microwave oven. For example, dishes with metallic trim are *not* used.
- Wash the kitchen floor weekly, or more often if necessary.

Ask the client or a responsible family member for instructions on operating appliances before using.

Other Duties

Two other tasks are frequently your responsibility in the home situation. They are food management and laundry.

Food Management. Plan food purchases with the client or a family member. If consultation is not possible, keep these guidelines in mind:
- Plan menus a week in advance. Base them on good nutrition.
- Take into consideration the client's preferences, cultural background, and any religious prohibitions.
- Spend only what the client's budget allows.
- Buy only what you need and what can be used. Large quantities are not a bargain if much of it goes unused or is wasted.
- Look for quality bargains.
- Keep track of all money spent and a list of items purchased; keep receipts.
- Make an accounting of all money handled.

Using the weekly menu, prepare foods in such a way that the client's dietary needs are met. Also:
- Wash fresh fruits and vegetables that are to be used soon and store in the refrigerator; store unwashed if they are not to be used right away. Remember to wash before use.

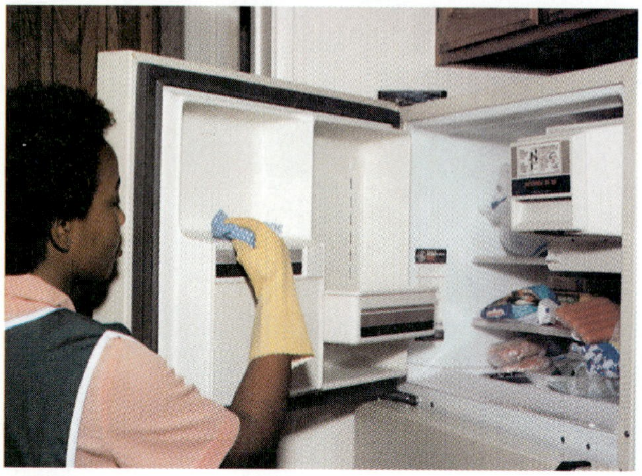

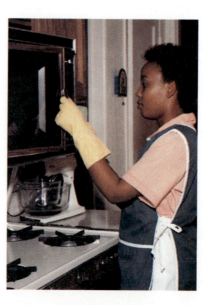

FIGURE 33-10 Clean spills immediately.

FIGURE 33-11 Clean the microwave oven after each use.

- Keep dairy products and meats refrigerated until use.
- Allow frozen meats to thaw in the refrigerator before use.
- Take into consideration the client's ordered diet, any digestive problems, and preferences.
- Keep dried and canned foods in cabinets.

Laundry. Carefully launder the client's clothes. They represent a sizable investment. This may have to be done daily. Always:

- Read labels before laundering. Some clothes must be dry cleaned or washed at special temperatures.
- Use the client's choice of detergent and read the label for instructions on amount to use.
- Wear gloves when sorting clothing and loading the washing machine if contact with blood, body fluids,

secretions, or excretions is likely.
- Separate light and dark fabrics and wash them separately.
- Wash drip-dry fabrics separately so they can be hung and dried or folded.
- Be sure clothes can be dried in a dryer, and use the proper setting.
- Hang clothes after wiping off clothesline, if dryer is not available.
- After laundering, fold, iron, or hang clothes.
- Check for needed repairs and do mending before storing clothes.
- Ask client or responsible family member for operating instructions before using washer or dryer.

REVIEW

A. True/False.

Mark the following true or false by circling T or F.

1. T F The home health care nursing assistant may be responsible for both nursing care and household tasks.
2. T F The home health care nursing assistant makes no contribution to the nursing process, because care is given at the client's home and not in the hospital.
3. T F Self-discipline is an important characteristic of the nursing assistant who works in a home.
4. T F When washing dishes, wash the plates first, then the pots and pans, and then the glassware.
5. T F As a home health aide, your primary role is to do the housework and cooking.
6. T F Your observations are important for monitoring the patient's progress.
7. T F Because the client is your responsibility, you need not be concerned with the client's family.
8. T F If the client smokes, it is permissible for the home health aide to smoke with the client.
9. T F Adaptability is an important characteristic for home health aides.
10. T F You should clean the bathroom daily.

B. Multiple Choice.

Select the one best answer for each question.

11. A special characteristic needed by a home health care nursing assistant working in a home is
    a. self-discipline.
    b. being a follower.
    c. being a fast worker.
    d. being able to take shortcuts.
12. Which household tasks would the home health care nursing assistant *not* be required to do?
    a. Shop for food.
    b. Move heavy furniture.
    c. Carry out nursing procedures.
    d. Prepare food for the client.
13. Home health aide responsibilities include all but which of these?
    a. Washing windows
    b. Cleaning the bathroom daily
    c. Documenting the care given
    d. Shopping for the client
14. The home health aide should carry a kit that contains
    a. disposable gloves.
    b. thermometers, stethoscope, blood pressure kit.
    c. plastic apron.
    d. all of these.
15. Daily tasks may include
    a. sweeping the floor after each meal.
    b. watering the lawn and shrubs.
    c. shampooing the carpets.
    d. all of these.

C. Nursing Assistant Challenge.

You are working for a home health agency and Mrs. Fernandez is one of your patients. She has had a stroke and needs assistance with all activities of daily living. Your assignment includes: a bath, personal care, dressing, making the bed, making her breakfast, making her lunch so she can have it after you are gone, cleaning the bathroom, and general "picking up" around her apartment. She asks if you will go to the drugstore before you leave to get her prescriptions refilled. Make a work plan that includes all of these tasks, as well as any other routine tasks you need to complete.

Subacute Care

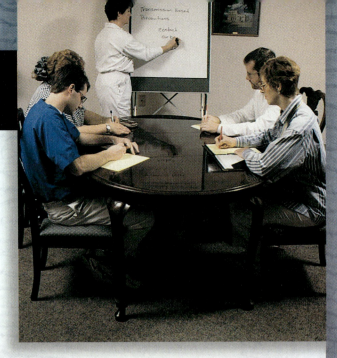

OBJECTIVES

As a result of this unit, you will be able to:

- Spell and define terms.
- Describe the purpose of subacute care.
- List the differences between acute care, subacute care, and long-term care.

- Describe the responsibilities of the nursing assistant when caring for patients receiving the special treatments in subacute care.
- Demonstrate the following procedure:
  - Procedure 91 Changing a Gown on a Patient with a Peripheral Intravenous Line in Place

---

VOCABULARY

Learn the meaning and the correct spelling of the following words and phrases:

alopecia
anorexia
central venous (CV)
  catheter
chemotherapy
dialysis
epidural catheter

fistula
graft
hemodialysis
narcotic
oncology
patient-controlled
  analgesia (PCA)

peripheral intravenous
  central catheter
  (PICC)
peritoneal dialysis
piggyback
pulse oximetry
radiation therapy

subacute care
tracheostomy
transcutaneous electrical
  nerve stimulation
  (TENS)
transitional care

DESCRIPTION OF SUBACUTE CARE

Subacute care is a type of "step-down" care given to persons who have been acutely ill. These individuals are out of the acute phase of illness but still need monitoring and ongoing treatment and services. Subacute care is sometimes called transitional care. The purpose of subacute care is to provide the care a person still needs but at a lower cost than in an acute care facility (hospital). Subacute care units are usually located in a section of a skilled nursing facility. Hospitals may also have separate subacute care units. Most patients are in these special units for three to four weeks. Patients being treated for cancer or AIDS may be there for a longer time. Patients may be discharged to:

- Their homes
- A skilled care or intermediate care facility
- An assisted living facility

On a subacute care unit, there are:

- More medications and treatments to administer than on a regular skilled unit
- More frequent physician's visits than in a skilled care unit
- More sophisticated types of equipment than in a skilled care unit

Types of Care Provided in a Subacute Care Unit

Most subacute care units provide specialized care in one or two areas. Some examples are:

- Rehabilitation—all therapies are provided and the patient participates in rehabilitation for 5 hours a day, 6 or 7 days a week.
- Peritoneal dialysis—a method of ridding the body of wastes for a person who has kidney failure.
- Ventilator weaning and tracheostomy care for persons who have been unable to breathe without the help of a ventilator
- Cardiac monitoring for persons who have a myocardial infarction or acute heart failure
- Pain management and control for persons who have acute or chronic pain
- Oncology—the care of persons with cancer who are receiving treatments such as radiation or chemotherapy
- Wound management for persons with stage 3 or stage 4 pressure ulcers, ulcers related to peripheral vascular disease, or burns
- Specialized care for persons who have suffered brain damage resulting from trauma
- AIDS care
- Hospice care
- Postoperative care for persons who have other complicating conditions such as chronic obstructive pulmonary disease or diabetes

If you work on a subacute care unit, you will participate in special staff development classes to prepare you to meet the needs of patients in your care. A nursing assistant on a subacute unit is expected to:

- work closely with registered nurses who are specialists in critical care or in a specific area of nursing, such as rehabilitation or wound care.
- have extensive knowledge of the types of patients in the unit.
- care for patients receiving complicated treatments.
- have excellent observational skills, because of the complex conditions of the patients.
- be a member of an interdisciplinary team that includes professionals in physical therapy, occupational therapy, speech therapy, respiratory therapy, and social services.

It is important that the staff on a subacute care unit be able to provide for the patients' emotional well-being. Many of these patients will be able to return to their own homes. For them, this is a time of rejoicing and for making plans for the future. These patients may still have concerns if they will have to rely on community services or family members to meet some of their needs. Some of the patients will have an uncertain future. For example:

- Will the patient receiving dialysis receive a kidney transplant in time?
- Will the cancer be cured in the patient receiving oncology treatments?
- Will the patient on a ventilator be able to be weaned off the ventilator, or will it be a lifelong need?
- Will the patient receiving rehabilitation recover enough independence to be able to go home?

SPECIAL PROCEDURES PROVIDED IN THE SUBACUTE CARE UNIT

You will be assigned to care for patients who are receiving special treatments because of their health problems. These treatments may require the use of equipment that is unfamiliar to you. As a nursing assistant, you will not be expected to be responsible for these procedures. However, you will be providing the same personal care and procedures that you would with any patients.

Rehabilitation

Patients may require intense rehabilitation because they have had:

- a stroke that affected their mobility, their ability to complete the activities of daily living, or their speech.
- orthopedic surgery or an amputation.
- an accident that resulted in neurological or orthopedic problems.

All caregivers working with these patients must have a knowledge of rehabilitation as well as a knowledge of the underlying condition (stroke, brain injury, etc.). You need to know what the goals are for the patients and what approaches you will be using to help the patients reach their goals. Consistency is the key to successful rehabilitation.

Pulse Oximetry

Patients receiving oxygen may be monitored with pulse oximetry. **Pulse oximetry** is used to monitor the level of oxygen in arterial blood. Red and infrared light is sent through an artery in the fingertip. A photodetector is placed over the finger. The photodetector measures the transmitted light as it passes through the blood (Figure 34-1). The nurse is responsible for this procedure.

Intravenous Therapy

Intravenous (IV) therapy refers to medication or solutions administered directly into a vein. Standard intravenous therapy is given into a peripheral vein (a large vein in the arm) (Figure 34-2). This is called an IV. The IV may consist of a single bag of solution connected to a simple tubing with a needle or small catheter on the end. Sometimes an additional small bag of fluid is attached to tubing that is connected to the main (primary) tubing. This is called a **piggyback**. The small bag contains medication such as an antibiotic that is intermittently dispersed into the vein (Figure 34-3).

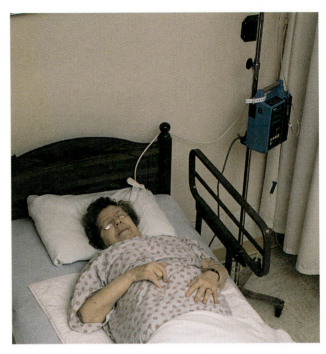

FIGURE 34-2 Standard intravenous therapy is given into a peripheral vein in the arm.

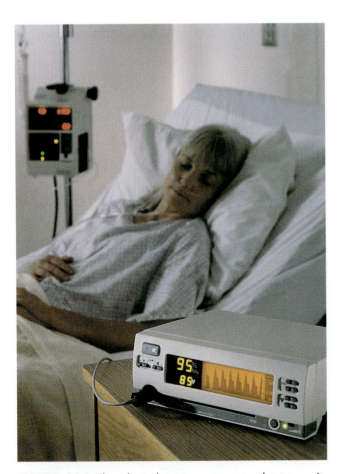

FIGURE 34-1 The photodetector measures the transmitted light as it passes through the blood. *Courtesy of Ohmeda, Louisville, CO*

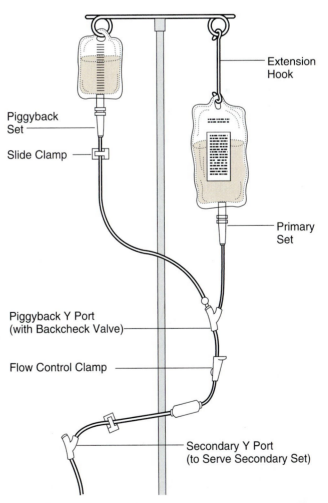

Extension Hook

Piggyback Set

Slide Clamp

Primary Set

Piggyback Y Port (with Backcheck Valve)

Flow Control Clamp

Secondary Y Port (to Serve Secondary Set)

FIGURE 34-3 The small bag (piggyback) contains medication that is given through the vein.

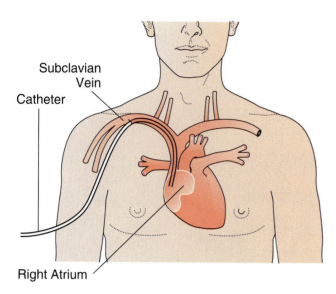

Subclavian
Vein

Catheter

Right Atrium

FIGURE 34-4 Central venous insertion

Central Venous Insertion

IV therapy can also be administered through a **central venous (CV) catheter**. A special catheter is inserted into a vein near the patient's collar bone (Figure 34-4). The catheter tip ends in or near the heart chamber. CV therapy is used to administer medications or to provide total parenteral nutrition.

Peripheral Intravenous Central Catheter Line

A **peripheral intravenous central catheter** or **PICC** line consists of a catheter that is inserted into a peripheral vein and threaded upward through the vein to the jugular or subclavian vein. It is used to administer medications or to provide total parenteral nutrition.

Total Parenteral Nutrition

Total parenteral nutrition (TPN) is also called hyperalimentation. TPN is given to a patient whose bowel needs complete rest. All required nutrients (carbohydrates, proteins, and fats) are given directly into the vein so the bowel does not have to work to digest food. Patients receiving TPN may need to be weighed daily or every other day. This should be done at the same time of day with the patient wearing the same type of clothing. The patient may be gradually switched over to enteral feedings. With an enteral feeding, liquid nourishment is administered through a tube inserted into the patient's stomach (Figure 34-5).

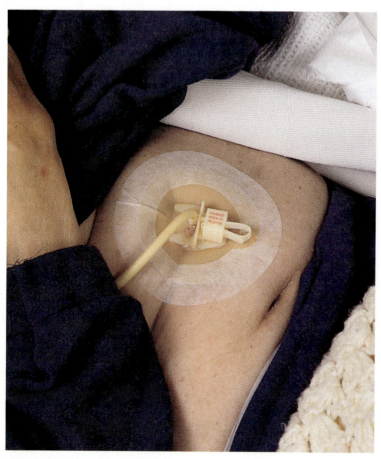

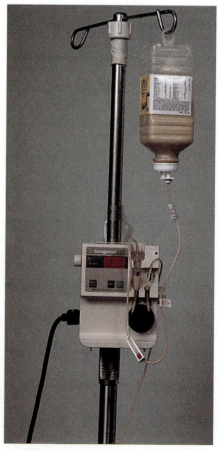

FIGURE 34-5 Nourishment may be given through a gastrostomy tube inserted into the patient's stomach.

GUIDELINES *for*

Caring for Patients with Intravenous Lines

- Know the drip rate in the drip chamber. Notify the nurse if the rate changes or the drip chamber is full.
- Avoid pulling or twisting tubing. Make sure the patient does not lie on the tubing.
- Observe area of needle insertion for signs of swelling, redness, or warmth.
- Note signs of moisture that may indicate the tubing is leaking.
- Make sure all junctions in the tubing are securely connected.
- Report immediately to the nurse:

— Signs of dyspnea, cyanosis, chest pain, or back pain
— Complaints of pain or burning at site of needle insertion

- Remember that all IV procedures are sterile. If you are assisting a nurse with any of these procedures, you must never contaminate the sterile field or supplies.
- When caring for patients with any type of IV therapy, NEVER:
— Change the drip rate
— Disconnect any tubing
— Manipulate the needle or tubing
— Remove, change, or manipulate any dressing over the site

PROCEDURE　91

CHANGING A GOWN ON A PATIENT WITH A PERIPHERAL INTRAVENOUS LINE IN PLACE

Note: *This procedure is used only when the IV is not run through an electric pump. When a pump is used, the patient may wear a gown that snaps at the shoulder. In this case, the gown can be removed without touching the IV bag or tubing. If the patient is wearing a nonsnap gown, call the nurse if the gown is to be changed. Never disconnect the tubing from the pump.*

1. Carry out each beginning procedure action.
2. Assemble equipment:
   - clean gown
3. Make sure windows and door are closed, to prevent chilling and to provide privacy.
4. Remove gown from the arm without the IV and bring gown across patient's chest to other arm.
5. Place clean gown over patient's chest to avoid exposure.
6. On the arm with the IV, gather material of gown in one hand so there is no pull or pressure on the line and slowly draw the gown over tip of fingers (Figure 34-6).

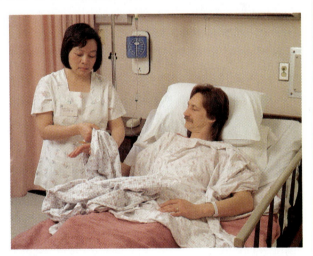

FIGURE 34-6 Gather material of gown in one hand so there is no pull or pressure on the IV line. Slowly draw gown over tips of fingers.

7. With free hand, lift IV free of standard and slip gown over bag of fluid (Figure 34-7), removing gown from patient's body. **Never allow the bag of fluid to be lower than the patient's arm.**

continues

PROCEDURE **91** *continued*

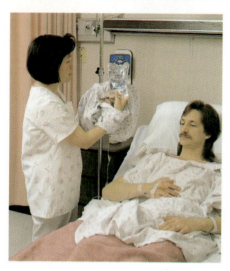

FIGURE 34-7 With free hand, lift IV free of standard and slip gown over bag of fluid.

8. Take sleeve of clean gown and slip it over the bag of fluid, the tubing, and up the patient's arm.

9. Replace bag of fluid on IV standard.

10. Remove soiled gown and place at end of bed. Finish putting clean gown on patient's other arm. Secure neck ties.

11. Place soiled gown in laundry hamper.

12. Make sure that IV is dripping and that tubing is not kinked or twisted.

13. Carry out each procedure completion action.

Note: If you are changing a gown for a patient with a centrally inserted line, you will not need to lower the fluid container. Change the gown in the usual manner, taking care not to manipulate the tubing.

PAIN MANAGEMENT PROCEDURES

Pain management may be the major reason why some patients are in a subacute unit. Other patients may be undergoing pain management related to conditions such as recent surgery or cancer. Both drug and nondrug treatments can be successful in helping to prevent and control pain. Various types of relaxation techniques are also used for pain management.

Patient-Controlled Analgesia

Patient-controlled analgesia (PCA) is used for acute, chronic, or postoperative pain. *Analgesia* means pain relief. A device is inserted into the patient's vein. It is connected to a solution that contains a narcotic. A narcotic is a drug such as morphine that is used for pain relief. The dosage is controlled by equipment that has been preset by the nurse. The patient or the nurse pushes the PCA button at times of discomfort. Report to the nurse if you note any change in the patient's:

● Level of consciousness
● Rate and pattern of respirations
● Pupil size
● Skin color

Pain Management with an Epidural Catheter

An epidural catheter is implanted beneath the patient's skin. It is inserted near the spinal cord at the first lumbar (L1)

space. A local anesthetic is administered either intermittently or continuously through the catheter. The patient may have leg numbness and weakness for the first 24 hours after the catheter is inserted. Report to the nurse at once if:

● the catheter becomes dislodged from the insertion site.
● you note changes in respiration rate and pattern.
● the patient complains of itching.
● the patient vomits or complains of nausea.

Transcutaneous Electrical Nerve Stimulation

Transcutaneous electrical nerve stimulation (TENS) is a nondrug method of pain relief. Mild, harmless electrical current stimulates nerve fibers to block the transmission of pain to the brain. Electrodes are taped to the patient's skin. The location of the electrodes depends on the areas related to the pain. The electrodes are attached to wires that are in turn attached to a control box (Figure 34-8). The intensity of the stimulation is set on the control box by the nurse.

CARING FOR PATIENTS WITH TRACHEOSTOMIES

A tracheostomy is a tube that is inserted into a surgical opening in the patient's trachea (windpipe). A tracheostomy is performed when the patient is unable to breathe in air through the nose. The tube allows the patient to breathe as air goes directly into the trachea and then into the lungs. A person who is on a ventilator for a long time will have a tracheostomy that is connected to the ventilator. The patient

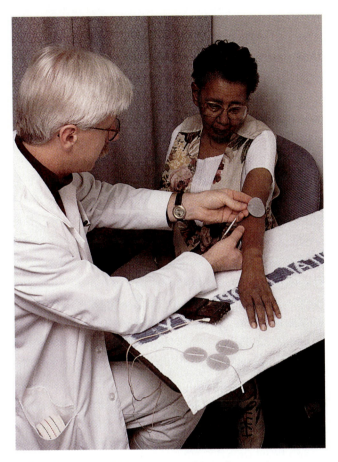

FIGURE 34-8 A TENS unit is used to relieve pain.

may have secretions coming from the chest and through the tube. The nurse will use suction to remove these secretions.

The tube may be made of plastic or metal. Tracheostomy tubes consist of an inner, removable tube called a *cannula* and an outer tube called a *neckplate* that is held in place with neck ties. The neckplate rests between the clavicles (breastbones). There is a slot on each side. Tracheostomy ties are inserted here to secure the tube in place (Figure 34-9). Patients with tracheostomies can usually take a bath or shower but must keep the water from entering the opening. Avoid using powders, sprays, or shaving cream around the

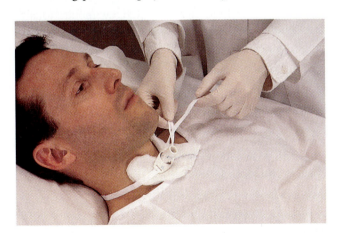

FIGURE 34-9 A tracheostomy tube is held in place with ties.

tube. When you care for a patient with a tracheostomy, observe for:

- changes in respiratory rate, depth, and quality.
- changes in mental status, such as confusion, restlessness, or irritability, that indicate the patient's brain is not getting adequate oxygen.

Report to the nurse immediately if the:

- Tube becomes dislodged from the opening
- Patient is having trouble breathing
- Patient needs suctioning

Be sure you know how the patient communicates. The opening in the trachea interferes with the patient's ability to talk.

CARING FOR THE PATIENT RECEIVING DIALYSIS TREATMENTS

Dialysis is a process by which the blood is artificially cleansed of liquid wastes when the kidneys are unable to remove the wastes. This procedure is needed when a person has kidney failure. Without dialysis, the person would die as the waste products accumulate in the blood stream. Dialysis is usually considered a temporary treatment that is used until a suitable organ is found for a kidney transplant. The two types of dialysis are hemodialysis and peritoneal dialysis.

Hemodialysis

During hemodialysis treatment, the patient's blood is circulated outside of the body into an artificial kidney machine. In the dialysis machine, the blood is cleansed with a liquid substance called dialysate. After the waste products have been removed, the blood is returned to the patient's body. Most persons needing hemodialysis are treated in a dialysis center. However, you may care for patients in the subacute unit who go as outpatients to the dialysis center for their treatments. Dialysis is usually done three to four times a week and each treatment takes several hours.

To do dialysis, a connection must be made between the patient's circulatory system and the artificial kidney machine. Minor surgery is done to create either a fistula or a graft. The fistula (Figure 34-10) is created by attaching a

A.V. Fistula

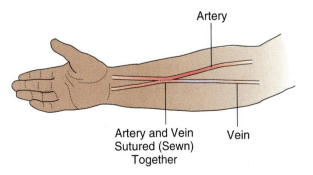

Artery

Vein

Artery and Vein
Sutured (Sewn)
Together

FIGURE 34-10 Fistula used for hemodialysis

Graft

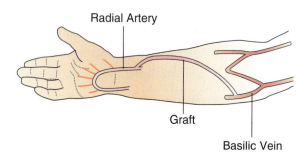

Radial Artery

Graft

Basilic Vein

FIGURE 34-11 Graft used for hemodialysis

vein to an artery, either in an arm or a leg. When a **graft** is used (Figure 34-11), synthetic material is inserted to form a connection between an artery and a vein. Two needles are inserted for treatment with either a fistula or a graft. The needles are connected to tubes that go to and from the artificial kidney machine.

As a nursing assistant, you are not expected to care for the fistula or the graft. You need to be aware that the patient on dialysis will:

- Have fluid restrictions
- Have dietary restrictions for calories, sodium, protein, potassium, calcium, and phosphorus
- Need all fluid intake and output measured accurately and recorded
- Need to be weighed regularly at the same time of day and with the same type of clothing
- Need to be monitored and have vital signs taken frequently after dialysis. Remember that blood pressure should not be taken in the arm used for dialysis.

Report to the nurse if the patient has:

- Swelling (edema) of the hands, feet, or face
- Changes in vital signs
- Changes in weight
- A change in intake or output measurements
- Shortness of breath
- Complaints of pain at the site of the fistula or graft

Peritoneal Dialysis

Peritoneal dialysis is also a process of cleansing the blood. In peritoneal dialysis, the process takes place within the patient's body in the peritoneal (abdominal) cavity, rather than outside the body in a machine. During dialysis, the dialysate is introduced into the abdominal cavity, allowed to stay in for some time, and then drained out. As blood flows through the vessels in the peritoneum, waste products are fil-

tered and excess fluids are removed. The nurse instills the dialysate through a catheter that is surgically implanted through the wall of the abdomen into the abdominal cavity. This is done using sterile technique.

Nursing assistants are not expected to administer peritoneal dialysis. You may be responsible for monitoring the patient's vital signs every 10 to 15 minutes for the first 1 to 2 hours after a treatment and then every 2 to 4 hours. Notify the nurse if there are any changes in vital signs.

ONCOLOGY TREATMENTS

Oncology is the care and treatment of persons with cancer. Cancer may be treated with surgery, radiation, chemotherapy, or a combination of any of these.

Radiation Therapy

Patients receiving radiation therapy in a subacute care unit may be transported to a special cancer treatment center or to a hospital to receive this therapy as outpatients. **Radiation therapy** is the use of high-energy radiation to kill cancer cells. It is considered a local therapy because it kills only the cancer cells in the area being treated. Patients receiving radiation may complain of fatigue and lack of appetite. When caring for patients receiving radiation therapy:

- report signs of redness, pain, or peeling of the skin in the area being treated.
- do not remove markings made on the skin for treatment purposes.
- do not use any heat or cold treatments on the area being treated.
- wash the area only with tepid water and a soft washcloth; do not apply any soaps, powders, deodorants, perfumes, makeup, lotions, or skin preparations to the area.
- instruct the patient to avoid wearing tight clothing over the area.

Chemotherapy

Chemotherapy is the use of drugs to kill cancer cells within the body. The drugs may be given by mouth (orally), through the vein (IV), or in the muscle (intramuscular [IM]). The nurse or physician administers the drugs. The person receiving chemotherapy may have side effects including nausea, vomiting, **anorexia** (loss of appetite), or **alopecia** (loss of hair). Modern treatment techniques have minimized the side effects of chemotherapy, but loss of hair is still common. However, the hair usually comes back after treatments are completed. Some persons prefer to wear wigs during this time. Respect the patient's wishes regarding personal appearance.

REVIEW

A. Multiple Choice.

Select the one best answer for each question.

1. Subacute care is given to persons who
   a. have been acutely ill.
   b. have had a long, progressive illness.
   c. require only custodial care.
   d. require intensive care.

2. The purpose of subacute care is to
   a. increase the population of long-term care facilities.
   b. discharge patients from the hospital as quickly as possible.
   c. provide the care a person needs at a lower cost.
   d. all of these.

3. Patients treated in subacute care include persons
   a. requiring dialysis.
   b. requiring high levels of rehabilitation.
   c. receiving wound care.
   d. all of these.

4. A nursing assistant working in subacute care would need to
   a. learn how to start intravenous feedings.
   b. have excellent observational skills.
   c. learn how to administer chemotherapy.
   d. instruct patients in pain management techniques.

5. If you accept a position in a subacute care unit, you may need to learn
   a. why hyperalimentation is given.
   b. your responsibilities for patients receiving dialysis.
   c. more about the rehabilitation process.
   d. all of these.

6. The procedure to measure the level of oxygen in arterial blood is called
   a. hemodialysis.
   b. pulse oximetry.
   c. total parenteral nutrition.
   d. intravenous therapy.

7. A central venous catheter is inserted into
   a. a vein in the patient's arm.
   b. an artery in the patient's arm.
   c. the jugular or subclavian vein.
   d. the epidural space.

8. Total parenteral nutrition (TPN) is used for patients
   a. who need to lose weight.
   b. who are unconscious.
   c. who refuse to eat.
   d. whose bowel needs complete rest.

9. The nursing assistant's responsibility for caring for patients with intravenous feedings is to
   a. insert the needle into the vein.
   b. add medication to the bag of fluid.
   c. observe for complications.
   d. change the drip rate if it is going too fast or too slow.

10. Patient-controlled analgesia is used
    a. for acute, chronic, or postoperative pain.
    b. for administering narcotics for pain.
    c. to allow the patient to receive medication when it is needed.
    d. all of these.

11. An epidural catheter is used for
    a. pain management.
    b. administering nutrition.
    c. emptying the bladder.
    d. intravenous feedings.

12. When caring for patients with tracheostomies, you should
    a. not allow the patient to bathe or shower.
    b. observe for changes in respiratory rate, depth, and quality.
    c. maintain the patient on a liquid diet.
    d. be responsible for changing the tracheostomy tube.

13. Dialysis is a procedure for
    a. cleansing the blood of liquid wastes.
    b. relieving postoperative pain.
    c. administering oxygen.
    d. giving total parenteral nutrition.

14. A patient on dialysis will have
    a. fluid restrictions.
    b. dietary restrictions.
    c. frequent weights taken.
    d. all of these.

15. When caring for patients on dialysis, you should observe for
    a. edema of the face, hands, and feet.
    b. changes in vital signs.
    c. shortness of breath.
    d. all of these.

16. Oncology is the care and treatment of patients with
   a. severe wounds.
   b. kidney failure.
   c. cancer.
   d. terminal illness.

17. When caring for patients receiving radiation therapy, you should
   a. remove the markings made on the skin for treatment purposes.
   b. apply cold treatments to the area.
   c. avoid applying soaps, powders, lotions, deodorants, or other substances to the treated area.
   d. wrap the treatment area with an elastic bandage.

B. Word Choice.

Choose the correct word or phrase from the following list to complete each statement in questions 18–25.

   dialysis
   enteral
   hyperalimentation
   piggyback
   pulse oximetry
   transcutaneous electrical nerve stimulation
   narcotic
   transitional care

18. Subacute care is also called _____.

19. A procedure for removing liquid wastes from the blood is called _____.

20. _____ is used for measuring the oxygen level in arterial blood.

21. A _____ refers to a small bag of fluid containing intravenous medication that is connected with a tube to the primary tubing.

22. Total parenteral nutrition (TPN) is also called _____.

23. A feeding administered through a tube into the patient's stomach is called an _____ feeding.

24. A _____ is a potent drug used for pain relief.

25. The use of electrical current to treat pain is done with a procedure called _____.

C. Nursing Assistant Challenge.

You have completed your nursing assistant course and have been working the night shift for three months in a skilled care facility. The director of nursing calls you into her office and asks you if you would like to work the day shift in the new subacute care unit of the facility. You tell her you would like to think about it for a day and then give your decision. Consider the types of care that are given in subacute care and then answer these questions.

26. What would your duties be in the new unit?

27. You feel confident of your nursing assistant skills. However, you know you will need to do some learning in order to care successfully for subacute care patients. What new information or skills will you need to acquire?

28. How do you plan to go about obtaining this learning?

Body Systems, Common Disorders, and Related Care Procedures

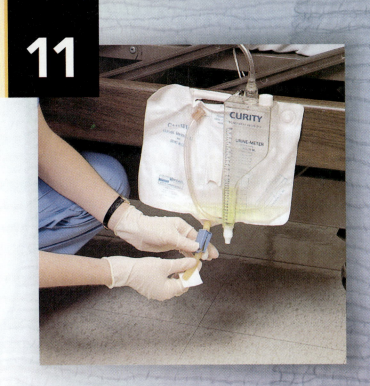

UNIT 35
Integumentary System

UNIT 36
Respiratory System

UNIT 37
Circulatory (Cardiovascular) System

UNIT 38
Musculoskeletal System

UNIT 39
Endocrine System

UNIT 40
Nervous System

UNIT 41
Gastrointestinal System

UNIT 42
Urinary System

UNIT 43
Reproductive System

Integumentary System

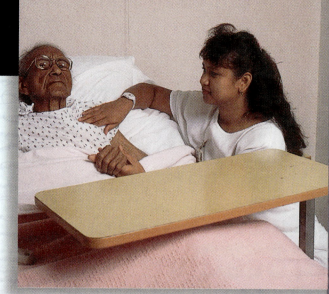

As a result of this unit, you will be able to:
- Spell and define terms.
- Review the location and function of the skin.
- Describe some common skin lesions.
- List three diagnostic tests associated with skin conditions.
- Describe nursing assistant actions relating to the care of patients with specific skin conditions.
- Identify persons at risk for the formation of pressure ulcers.
- Describe measures to prevent pressure ulcers.
- Describe the stages of pressure ulcer formation and identify appropriate nursing assistant actions.
- List nursing assistant actions in caring for patients with burns.

Learn the meaning and the correct spelling of the following words and phrases:

allergen	dermal ulcer	macule	rubra
allergies	dermis	necrosis	sebaceous gland
anaphylactic shock	epidermis	obese	shearing
contraindicated	eschar	pallor	subcutaneous tissue
crust	excoriation	papule	sudoriferous gland
cyanotic	integument	pressure ulcer	vesicle
debride	lesion	pustule	wheal

INTEGUMENTARY SYSTEM STRUCTURES

The integumentary system (Figure 35-1) includes:

- Skin
- Hair
- Nails
- Sweat glands
- Nerves
- Oil glands

The outermost layers of the skin make up the epidermis. The dermis lies under the epidermis. The subcutaneous tissue that attaches the skin to the muscles lies under the dermis.

The nails are horny cell structures found on the dorsal, distal surfaces of the fingers and toes. They protect the sensitive fingers and toes. The teeth are formed from the tissues of the integument (body shell).

Epidermis

The epidermis consists of dead outer cells that are constantly shed as new cells move upward from the dermis. There are no blood vessels in the epidermis, so injury to this layer does not cause bleeding. Nerve endings reach into this outer layer. The nerves are sense organs that keep us in contact with changes in the environment. Nerve endings called *receptors* receive information about:

- Heat
- Cold
- Pain
- Pressure

Dermis

The dermis contains blood vessels, nerve fibers, and two kinds of glands:

- Sweat glands (sudoriferous glands)
- Oil glands (sebaceous glands)

Sweat Glands

The sweat glands produce perspiration that reaches the skin surface through tubes or ducts that end in openings called *pores.* Heat from deep in the body is brought to the skin by blood vessels. This heat is transferred to the perspiration. At the skin surface, the perspiration and the heat are lost through the pores to the air. The heat of the body is controlled by changes in the size of the blood vessels in the skin.

- When the central opening of a blood vessel becomes enlarged (dilated), more heat is brought to the body surface.
- When the central opening of a blood vessel becomes smaller (constricted), less heat is brought to the body surface.

Oil Glands and Hair

Oil glands lubricate and keep flexible the hairs found in the skin. Hair covers almost all body surfaces except for the palms of the hands and the soles of the feet.

SKIN FUNCTIONS

The skin has many functions that are critical to the well-being of the body:

- Protection—forms a continuous membranous covering for the body and regulates body temperature
- Storage—stores fat and vitamins
- Elimination—loses water, salts, and heat through perspiration
- Sensory perception—contains nerve endings that keep us aware of environmental changes

The skin tells us much about the general health of the body.

- A fever may be indicated by hot, dry skin.
- Unusual redness—rubra, or flushing of the skin—often follows strenuous activity.
- Pallor, which is less color than normal, is a sign associated with many conditions.
- The oxygen content of the blood can be noted quickly by the color of the skin. When the oxygen content is very low, the blood is darker and the skin appears bluish or cyanotic.

AGING CHANGES

As a person ages, changes become evident in the skin and its elements. These changes include:

- Glands that are less active
- Decreased circulation
- Dryness, thinning, and scaling
- Thickening of fingernails and toenails
- Loss of fat and elasticity

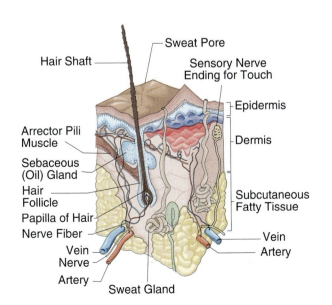

FIGURE 35-1 Cross section of the skin.

- Loss of hair color
- Development of skin irregularities such as skin tabs, moles, and warts

SKIN LESIONS

Injury or disease can cause changes in skin structures. These changes are called **lesions**. The lesions may be caused by disease, trauma, wear, or the aging process. When caring for patients with skin lesions, standard precautions are followed. Some of the most common skin lesions or eruptions are:

- **Macules**—flat, discolored spots, as in measles (Figure 35-2)
- **Papules**—small, solid, raised spots, as in chickenpox
- **Pustules**—raised spots filled with pus, as in acne
- **Vesicles**—raised spots filled with watery fluid, such as a blister (Figure 35-3)
- **Wheals**—large, raised, irregular areas frequently associated with itching, as in hives
- **Excoriations**—portions of the skin appear scraped or scratched away
- **Crusts**—areas of dried body secretions, such as scabs

Skin lesions may be a result of systemic responses:

- Communicable disease—diseases that are easily transmitted, directly or indirectly, from person to person. Measles and chickenpox are two such diseases. Each has characteristic skin lesions called *skin eruptions* or *rashes.*
- Immune system problems—Persons whose immune systems are depressed, such as those suffering from HIV infection, may develop a specific type of cancer called *Kaposi's sarcoma.* It appears as lesions in the skin and eventually in other organs. The skin lesions begin as macules, papules, or violet areas that gradually become bigger and darker. They are frequently seen on the trunk, neck, and head (especially on the tip of the nose). Progression of the disease may be slow or rapid.
- **Allergies**—also called *sensitivity reactions,* may have associated skin lesions. The vesicles of poison ivy are well known. The material causing the sensitivity is called an

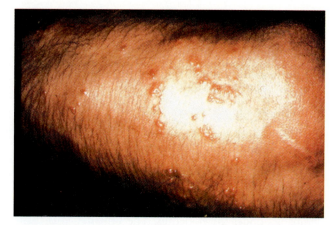

FIGURE 35-3 The fluid-filled vesicles of poison ivy. *Courtesy of the Centers for Disease Control and Prevention (CDC), Atlanta, GA*

allergen. Individuals respond to allergens in different ways.

- **Anaphylactic shock**—a severe, sometimes fatal, sensitivity reaction.

Observation of the skin and accurate descriptions of what you see must be carefully charted.

Diagnosing Skin Lesions

Your careful observations and accurate description of any skin lesions provide valuable information about the patient's condition. There are several diagnostic tests that may be ordered by the physician to help establish the cause of the lesion. These tests include:

- Studying scrapings from the skin lesion under the microscope.
- Culturing the skin lesion if an infection is suspected.
- Performing skin testing if sensitivities are suspected, by introducing small quantities of substances (allergens) known to bring about an allergic (hypersensitivity) reaction in humans. Allergens include pollens, foods, dust, animal dander, and medications.

Care of Skin Lesions

When skin lesions are present, certain general nursing care is indicated. Take the following precautions when caring for these patients.

- Closely observe the patient's skin on admission, but do not remove any dressings. Any changes noted should be reported immediately and described accurately.
- Soap and water and rubbing lotions are often **contraindicated** (not permitted). Check the nursing care plan before bathing the patient or giving a backrub.
- Wear gloves when contact with blood, body fluids, or nonintact skin is likely.
- Do not attempt to remove any crusts from skin lesions without special instruction from your supervisor.
- Handle the patient gently. Avoid rubbing the skin.

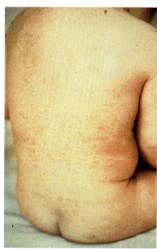

FIGURE 35-2 The macules of German measles. *Courtesy of the Centers for Disease Control and Prevention (CDC), Atlanta, GA*

Pressure Ulcers (Dermal Ulcers)

Pressure ulcers, commonly called bedsores or **dermal ulcers**, may occur in patients of any age. They are particularly common in patients who are:

- Elderly
- Very thin
- Overweight (**obese**)
- Unable to move
- Incontinent
- Debilitated
- Poorly nourished
- Confined to bed or wheelchairs
- Disoriented
- Dehydrated
- In prolonged contact with moisture
- Circulation-impaired
- Subjected to shearing

Shearing occurs when the skin moves in one direction while the structures under the skin, such as the bones, remain fixed or move in the opposite direction. This can happen when patients are dragged rather than lifted up in bed, when positions are changed, or when patients slide down in bed or in a wheelchair (Figure 35-4). Blood vessels become twisted and stretched, causing the tissues being served to lose essen-tial oxygen and nutrients, leading to breakdown. In addition, shearing may cause actual tears in fragile skin. These skin tears are painful, a portal of entry for infectious pathogens, and commonly lead to further breakdown.

Pressure ulcers are caused by prolonged pressure on an area of the body that interferes with circulation. The tissue first becomes reddened. As the cells die (undergo **necrosis**) from lack of nourishment, the skin breaks down and an ulcer forms. The resulting pressure ulcers may become large and deep.

Pressure ulcers occur most frequently over areas where bones come close to the surface. The most common sites (Figure 35-5) are the:

- Elbows
- Heels
- Shoulders
- Sacrum
- Hips
- Ankles
- Ears
- Knees (inner and outer parts)

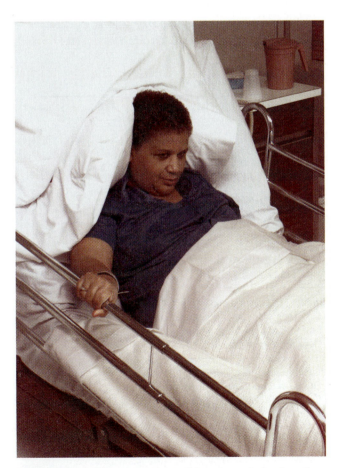

FIGURE 35-4 When a patient slides down in bed, or in a wheelchair, shearing occurs with potential skin damage.

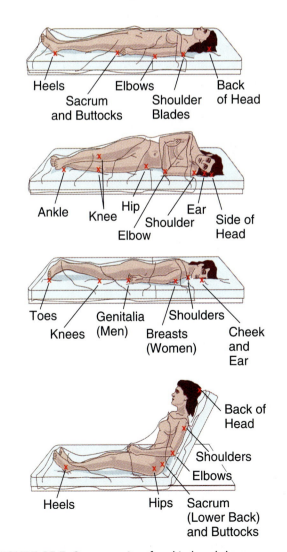

FIGURE 35-5 Common sites for skin breakdown.

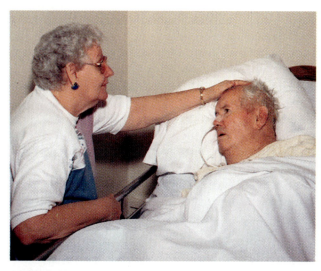

FIGURE 35-6 The rubbing of nasal catheters, nasogastric tubes, or urinary catheters can cause breakdown of skin.

Patients tend to develop pressure ulcers where body parts rub and cause friction. Common sites are:

- Between the folds of the buttocks
- Legs
- Under the breasts

- Abdominal folds
- Ankles
- Knees

The rubbing of tubing and other equipment used in the care of patients over a long period can also cause pressure sores (Figure 35-6).

Preventing Pressure Ulcers. Because pressure ulcers are far easier to prevent than to cure, everyone participating in the patient's care has a responsibility to prevent skin breakdown.

When a patient is admitted, the nurse will assess the patient's current status and potential for skin breakdown. This assessment gives a baseline against which all future assessments may be measured. The assessment may be described on the patient's chart in words, pictures, diagrams, or as a score (Figures 35-7A and 35-7B). If a nursing diagnosis of actual or "potential impairment of skin integrity" is made, every staff member must make extra efforts to prevent skin breakdown, limit any breakdown that has already occurred, and promote the healing process.

Development of Pressure Ulcers

Tissue breakdown occurs in four stages. Nursing intervention at each stage can limit the process and prevent further

---

PATIENTS AT RISK TO DEVELOP PRESSURE SORES: Identify any patient at risk to develop pressure sores by assessing the seven clinical condition parameters and assigning a score. Any patient with intact skin, but scoring **8 or greater** should have nursing diagnosis **"Potential Impairment of Skin Integrity"** identified.

Clinical Condition Parameters—Risk of Pressure Sores

Clinical Condition Parameters	Score	Clinical Condition Parameters	Score
General Physical Condition (health problem)		**Mobility (extremities)**	
Good (minor)	0	Full active range	0
Fair (major but stable)	1	Limited movement with assistance	2
Poor (chronic/serious not stable)	2	Moves only with assistance	4
		Immobile	6
Level of Consciousness (to commands)			
Alert (responds readily)	0	**Incontinence (bowel and/or bladder)**	
Lethargic (slow to respond)	1	None	0
Semi Comatose (responds only to verbal		Occasional (≤ 2 per 24 hours)	2
or painful stimuli)	2	Usually (> 2 per 24 hours)	4
Comatose (no response to stimuli)	3	No Control	6
Activity		**Nutrition (for age and size)**	
Ambulant without assistance	0	Good (eats/drinks adequately $3/4$ of meal)	0
Ambulant with assistance	2	Fair (eats/drinks inadequately—at least $1/2$ of meal)	1
Chairfast	4	Poor (unable/refuses to eat/drink—less than $1/2$) . .	2
Bedfast	6		
		Skin/Tissue Status	
		Good (well nourished/skin intact)	0
		Fair (poorly nourished/skin intact)	1
		Poor (skin not intact)	2
		Total	

FIGURE 35-7A Assessing risk of pressure ulcers. *Courtesy of Artistic Press, Los Angeles, CA*

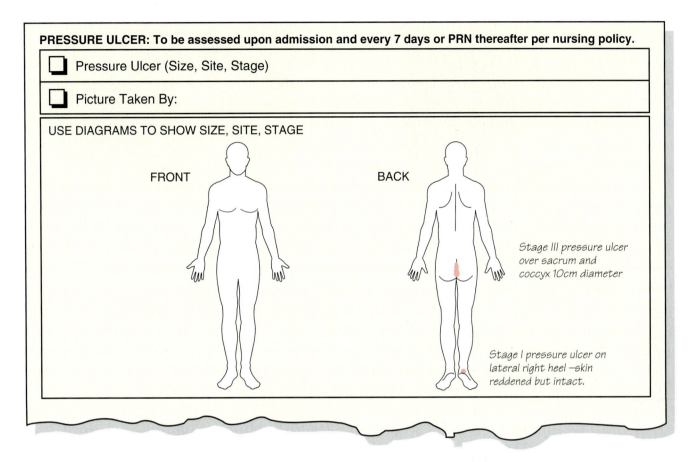

PRESSURE ULCER: To be assessed upon admission and every 7 days or PRN thereafter per nursing policy.

☐ Pressure Ulcer (Size, Site, Stage)

☐ Picture Taken By:

USE DIAGRAMS TO SHOW SIZE, SITE, STAGE

FRONT   BACK

Stage III pressure ulcer over sacrum and coccyx 10cm diameter

Stage I pressure ulcer on lateral right heel —skin reddened but intact.

FIGURE 35-7B Documentation of dermal ulcers is made on the patient's chart in words, pictures, and diagrams.

damage. Remember to continue all preventive measures throughout care.

Stage I. In Stage I, the skin develops a redness (Figure 35-8) or blue-gray discoloration over the pressure area. In dark-skinned people, the area may appear drier. If, after peripheral massage and relief of pressure, the blush has not subsided, it is probably the beginning of a pressure ulcer. Usually this stage of ulceration is reversible if the pressure is reduced or removed.

Stage II. In Stage II, the skin is reddened and there are abrasions, blisters, or a shallow crater at the site (Figure 35-9). The area around the breakdown site may also be reddened. The skin may or may not be broken. The epidermis alone or both the epidermis and the dermis may be involved. If this stage of involvement is neglected, further and deeper damage occurs.

Stage III. In Stage III, all the layers of the skin are destroyed and a deep crater forms (Figure 35-10). The

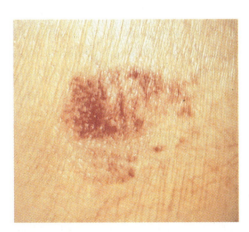

FIGURE 35-8 First indication of tissue damage (Stage I) is redness and heat over a pressure point. *Permission to reproduce this copyrighted material has been granted by the owner, Hollister Incorporated*

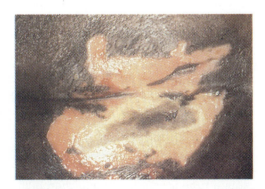

FIGURE 35-9 Stage II is marked by destruction of the epidermis and partial destruction of the dermis. *Permission to reproduce this copyrighted material has been granted by the owner, Hollister Incorporated*

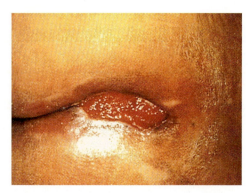

FIGURE 35-10 In Stage III, all layers of skin have been destroyed. A deep crater has formed. *Permission to reproduce this copyrighted material has been granted by the owner, Hollister Incorporated*

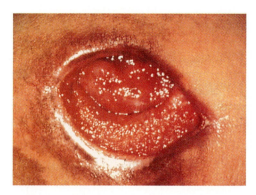

FIGURE 35-11 In Stage IV, tissue destruction can involve muscle, bone, and other vital structures. *Permission to reproduce this copyrighted material has been granted by the owner, Hollister Incorporated*

nurse documents the size of the lesion using a commercial scale.

Stage IV. In Stage IV, the ulcer extends through the skin and subcutaneous tissues, and may involve bone, muscle, and other structures (Figure 35-11). At this stage, the patient will experience fluid loss and pain and is at great risk for infection.

Actions to Take When Breakdown Occurs.

Nursing assistant actions when skin breakdown occurs include:

- Performing the actions listed in the guidelines to prevent further breakdown
- Following the care plan exactly

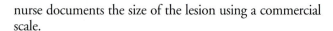

GUIDELINES *for*

Preventing Pressure Ulcers

Nursing assistant actions are vital in identifying potential causes of breakdown and eliminating or minimizing them. The following care should be given:

- Change the patient's position at least every two hours. Some patients will require positioning more often. A major shift in position is required. When positioning a patient, be careful to avoid friction, such as sliding the patient over bedclothes or against equipment. Use lifting devices to avoid dragging. The care plan for each patient must be followed carefully. The turning schedule will be posted in the care plan and in the room. Figure 35-12 shows an example of the sequence of turns.
- Encourage patients sitting in geri-chairs or wheelchairs to raise themselves every 10 minutes to relieve pressure, or assist patients to do so.
- Encourage proper nutrition and adequate intake of fluids. Breakdown occurs more readily and healing is delayed when the patient is poorly nourished. Proper nutrition may require tube feedings with enriched high-protein and high-vitamin supplements. Patients

who are able to eat should be encouraged to do so. Adequate fluids are a requirement.
- Immediately remove feces or urine from the skin, because they are very irritating. Wash and dry the area immediately.
- Whenever giving personal care to patients, carefully inspect areas where pressure ulcers (*decubiti*) commonly form. Report any reddened areas immediately.
- Inspect skin daily and report the condition.
- Keep the skin clean and dry at all times.

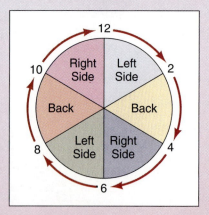

FIGURE 35-12 Example of a turning schedule with a position change every two hours

continues

GUIDELINES
continued

- Keep linen dry and free from wrinkles and hard objects such as crumbs and hairpins.
- Bathe patient frequently. Pay particular attention to potential pressure or friction areas. Avoid hot water and friction.
- Massage around reddened areas frequently with rubbing solution. Do not massage directly on the site and do not use alcohol. Apply moisturizers on dry skin by patting. Do not rub vigorously.
- Do not use lotion on broken skin.
- Separate body areas that are likely to rub together, especially over bony prominences, by using pillows or foam wedges according to the care plan.
- Use mechanical aids, such as foam padding, sheepskin, or an alternating-pressure mattress, to relieve pressure.
- Protect areas at risk, such as heels and elbows.
- Use a turning sheet to move dependent patients in bed.
- Elevate the head of the bed no higher than 30 degrees, to prevent a shearing effect on the tissues.

- Carry out range-of-motion exercises at least twice daily to encourage circulation.
- Check for improperly fitted or worn braces and restraints.
- Check nasogastric tubes and urinary catheters to be sure they are positioned so as not to be a source of irritation. Keep the nasal and urinary openings clean and free of drainage. These areas must be checked frequently and carefully.
- Use sheepskin and artificial sheepskin pads between patients and bottom linen, wheelchair backs, or wheelchair seats where excess pressure may be expected.
- For patients sitting in geri-chairs or wheelchairs, use foam, gel, or air cushions to reduce pressure on buttocks and sacrum. Routinely monitor such patients for skin problems.
- For patients in bed, relieve pressure on heels by supporting feet off the bed.
- Report signs of infection, such as fever, odor, drainage, inflammation, or bleeding, to the nurse.

- Reporting indications of infection, such as fever, odor, drainage, bleeding, and changes in size
- Keeping the area around the breakdown clean and dry
- Assisting with whirlpool baths, if ordered, to keep the area clean

The nurse or physician may perform other procedures to care for areas of skin breakdown. For example:

- The area may be covered with a dry, sterile dressing (DSD). Holding a DSD in place without causing additional injury is not easy. The skin of some patients may be sensitive to regular tape. In this case, silk tape, paper tape, cellophane tape, or other hypoallergenic tape may be used. To prevent injury when removing the tape for a dressing change, a saline solution is applied to loosen the tape.
- Patients may be placed on alternating-pressure mattresses or pressure-reducing mattresses or beds.
- In some facilities, open lesions are packed loosely with gauze soaked in a wound gel. The gel keeps the lesions moist, breaks down dead cells, and promotes healing.
- The area may be protected and kept moist by using special dressings. These dressings have a clear plastic covering that permits air to reach the tissues, but also keeps them moist to promote healing. The dressing must extend beyond the wound edge. It is held in place with a frame of either paper or silk tape. The dressing must

be changed every three to five days unless there is leakage or according to facility policy.

- The wounds may be cleaned by the nurse or physician with saline solution and **debrided** (dead tissue removed) using instruments and proteolytic enzymes (substances that react with skin proteins).
- Antiseptic sprays, antibiotic ointments, and dressings are used to control infection.
- Surgery may be needed to close the ulcerated area in severe cases.

Patients are encouraged to participate to whatever extent is possible in their own care. Attentive nursing care is essential in preventing skin breakdown. Remember that it is far easier to prevent pressure ulcers than to heal them!

Blood Circulation to Tissues. Ensuring adequate circulation to tissues is a major factor in preventing skin breakdown. This can be accomplished by:

- Positioning the patient properly
- Using mechanical aids
- Giving backrubs
- Performing active or passive range-of-motion exercises

Positioning. Five basic in-bed positions are used to relieve pressure as the patient's condition permits. Each position must be supported for comfort. The nursing assistant must remember that not all patients are able to assume the full range of positions, because of disabilities such as arthritis, contractures, and breathing limitations. Patients who sit in geri-chairs or wheelchairs for long periods of time must also change position to relieve pressure.

Patients with special problems require extra care when they are positioned in bed. For example:

- Be sure the patient can breathe properly.
- Remember that a fractured hip is never rotated over the unaffected leg.
- If the patient had a stroke, elevate the weak arm to reduce edema.
- Always maintain proper body alignment.
- The patient with a recent stroke is turned on the unaffected side.

The five basic positions patients assume in bed are:

- Supine position
- Semisupine position
- Lateral position
- Semiprone position
- Fowler's position

Mechanical Aids

Mechanical aids are used to reduce pressure. Examples are

- Sheepskin pads (or artificial sheepskin)
- Foam pads and pillows
- Protectors for areas such as heels (Figure 35-13A) and elbows (Figure 35-13B) that are subject to friction as the patient moves in bed
- Bed cradles
- Alternating-pressure mattresses
- Flotation mattresses
- Pillows
- Gel-filled mattresses

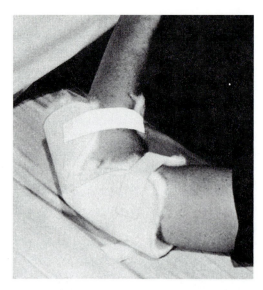

FIGURE 35-13B Elbow protector. *Courtesy of J. T. Posey Company, Arcadia, CA*

Sheepskin Pads (or Artificial Sheepskin). These absorb moisture and reduce friction when placed under the patient (Figure 35-13C).

Foam Pads and Pillows. These are used to bridge areas to reduce pressure. Watch patients for signs of disorientation that might be caused by the feeling of weightlessness. Adequate fluid intake to prevent urinary stasis must be provided and conscientious range-of-motion exercises must be carried out.

Bed (Foot) Cradles. Cradles can lift the weight of bedding but must be carefully positioned and may be padded, because injury can occur if the resident strikes them.

Alternating-Pressure Mattress (Air Mattress). This type of mattress (Figure 35-13D) is used in some facilities. Air pressure is reduced in a different area of the mattress on an alternating basis. The air-pressure alteration reduces pressure against the body so that no skin area is continuously subjected to pressure.

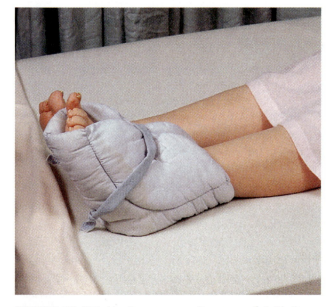

FIGURE 35-13A Heel protector. *Courtesy of J. T. Posey Company, Arcadia, CA*

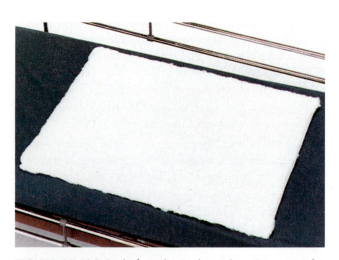

FIGURE 35-13C Pad of synthetic sheepskin. *Courtesy of J. T. Posey Company, Arcadia, CA*

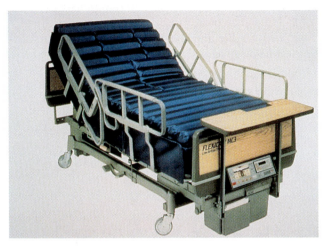

FIGURE 35-13D Alternating air pressure mattress overlay. Alternating air pressure in the mattress cells changes the pressure points against the patient's skin and gently massages the skin. *Courtesy of Hill-Rom, Charleston, SC*

Flotation Mattress. This is a water bed with controlled temperature (Figure 35-14). The weight of the resident's body displaces water so that pressure is consistently equalized against the skin. Sheets should not be tucked tightly over a flotation mattress because this will restrict its function.

Special Equipment. Specialized beds or overlays are available for residents who need continuous pressure relief. One type is the Clinitron® bed. It is filled with a sandlike material. Warm, dry air circulates through the material to maintain an even temperature and support the body evenly.

Gel-Filled Mattress. The gel in this type of mattress has a consistency similar to body fat. It allows a more equal distribution of body weight because it conforms to the body contours.

Pillows. Pillows are used in a technique called *bridging*. In bridging, body parts are supported by pillows so that spaces are left to relieve pressure on specific areas.

Burns

Whenever large sections of skin are destroyed, the body loses fluids and chemicals called electrolytes, and is vulnerable to infection. Burns are a common cause of loss of large amounts of skin.

Classification. The temperature and length of exposure determine the severity of a burn. Prognosis is based on the

extent of the burns. Burns are commonly classified as first-, second-, and third-degree. Burns may also be classified according to the depth of tissue involvement:

First-degree burns (partial thickness)

— Epidermis. When only the epidermis is involved, the skin is pink to red. There may be some temporary swelling and pain. There is usually no permanent damage or scarring.

Second-degree burns (partial thickness)

— Dermis. When both epidermis and dermis are involved in the burn, the color may vary from pink or red to white or tan. There is blistering and pain and some scarring.

Third-degree burns (full thickness)

— When the epidermis, dermis, and subcutaneous tissue are involved, the tissue is bright red to tan and brown. The area is covered with a tough, leathery coat (**eschar**). There is no pain initially because nerve endings have been destroyed. Later, pain and scarring will result from this injury.

— When the epidermis, dermis, subcutaneous tissues, muscles, and bones are involved, the tissue appears blackened. Scarring will be extensive.

Management of Burns. Once a burn patient is in the medical facility, the care will involve:

- Assessment of the burn damage
- Analgesia for pain
- Management of fluids and electrolytes
- Clean technique using cap, gown, mask, and gloves
- Complete reverse isolation technique in some cases
- Monitoring the patient for respiratory distress, shock, and anemia
- Cleaning of the burned areas and removal of all debris
- Application of topical antibiotics
- Emotional support

Some hospitals have established burn centers where specially trained personnel care for burn cases. One of two approaches is in common use:

- Open method—the burns are left uncovered. Sterile technique, also called reverse isolation technique, is used to care for the patient.
- Closed method—the burns are covered by special ointments, wrapped in layers of gauze. The part is checked for circulation distal to the dressing and maintained in proper alignment.

New techniques, such as keeping the patient submerged in a silicone solution, are also being used. Each method has its advantages and disadvantages. There are four goals of treatment, whatever method is selected:

1. Replacement of lost fluids and electrolytes to combat shock.
2. Relief of pain and anxiety.
3. Prevention of contractures, deformities, and infections.

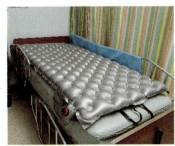

FIGURE 35-14 Mattress filled with water helps to minimize pressure points on the body.

A *contracture* is a shortening of a muscle, which limits motion and causes deformities. Plastic surgery may also be required.

4. Provision of emotional support and motivation.

Nursing Assistant Care. Special care emphasizes:

- Reporting pain so that appropriate analgesics may be prescribed and given.
- Maintaining proper alignment.
- Gentle positioning, as ordered, to prevent contractures.

Note: The burn patient may be on a CircOlectric® bed, Stryker frame, or Clinitron® bed to permit frequent rotation to relieve pressure.

- Encouraging a high-protein diet.
- Carefully measuring intake and output.
- Giving emotional support and encouragement.
- Carrying out procedures that prevent infection.
- Applying the principles of standard precautions and wearing gloves if contact with burned skin areas is likely.

REVIEW

A. True/False.

Mark the following true or false by circling T or F.

1. T F Obesity is a predisposing cause of pressure ulcer formation.

2. T F The sacrum is a common site for the development of pressure ulcers.

3. T F To avoid pressure ulcers, change the patient's position at least every two hours.

4. T F If an area is reddened, massage directly over the area.

5. T F The nails and hair are part of the integumentary system.

6. T F When only the epidermis is damaged by burning, the patient experiences no pain.

7. T F The skin stores carbohydrates and minerals.

8. T F When both the dermis and epidermis are damaged by burns, blisters are apt to form.

9. T F Reverse isolation technique is used when the closed method of burn treatment is prescribed.

10. T F The patient with burns needs great emotional support.

B. Matching.

Choose the correct item from Column II to match each question in Column I.

Column I	Column II
11. _____ redness	**a.** pressure ulcer
12. _____ skin	**b.** rubra
13. _____ thick leathery covering that forms in severe burns	**c.** tactile sense
	d. necrosis
	e. integument
14. _____ bedsore	**f.** obese
15. _____ feeling	**g.** eschar
16. _____ flat, discolored spots, as in measles	**h.** crusts
17. _____ raised spots filled with watery fluid	**i.** excoriations
	j. vesicles
18. _____ large, raised areas associated with itching, as in hives	**k.** papules
	l. macules
19. _____ areas of dried body secretions such as scabs	**m.** wheals
20. _____ areas where skin seems to be scraped or scratched away	

C. Multiple Choice.

Select the one best answer for each question.

21. Flat, discolored spots such as those seen in measles are called

 a. pustules.

 b. macules.

 c. papules.

 d. vesicles.

22. Raised spots filled with fluid, such as blisters, are called
  a. pustules.
  b. macules.
  c. papules.
  d. vesicles.

23. Anaphylactic shock is
  a. a severe sensitivity reaction.
  b. never fatal.
  c. a communicable disease.
  d. associated with partial-thickness burns.

24. When caring for patients with skin lesions,
  a. rub the skin vigorously.
  b. use soap and water when bathing.
  c. do not attempt to remove any crusts.
  d. use rubbing lotion.

25. To help ensure adequate circulation to prevent skin breakdown, you could
  a. change the patient's position frequently.
  b. use mechanical aids.
  c. provide back rubs.
  d. all of these.

D. Completion.

Complete the statements by filling in the correct word(s).

26. Three nursing assistant actions related to the care of patients with skin lesions are:
  a. _____   **c.** _____
  b. _____

27. Three diagnostic tests used to identify skin-related lesions are:
  a. _____   **c.** _____
  b. _____

28. Five types of patients at risk for the development of pressure ulcers are:
  a. _____   **d.** _____
  b. _____   **e.** _____
  c. _____

29. Name five common sites of pressure ulcer formation.
  a. _____   **d.** _____
  b. _____   **e.** _____
  c. _____

30. It is especially important to encourage proper nutrition and fluids in patients who have ulcers because _____.

E. Nursing Assistant Challenge.

Agnes Finlay has been transferred to your facility from a long-term care facility. She uses a wheelchair but fell and fractured her arm. You notice a reddened area around the base of her spine. Answer the following by selecting the correct word.

31. People sitting in wheelchairs should raise themselves every _____ minutes.
  (20) (10)

32. The head of the patient's bed should not be elevated more than _____ degrees.
  (30) (40)

33. While she is in bed, Ms. Finlay's position should be changed at least every _____ hours.
  (three) (two)

34. Range-of-motion exercises should be carried out at least _____ a day.
  (once) (twice)

UNIT 36

Respiratory System

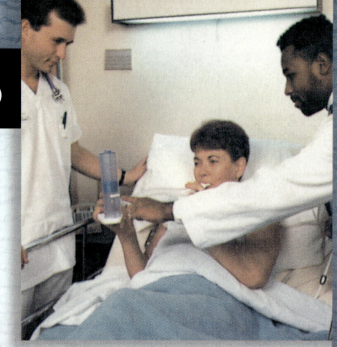

OBJECTIVES

As a result of this unit, you will be able to:

- Spell and define terms.
- Review the location and function of the respiratory organs.
- Describe some common diseases of the respiratory system.
- List five diagnostic tests used to identify respiratory conditions.
- Describe nursing assistant actions related to the care of patients with respiratory conditions.
- List five safety measures for the use of oxygen therapy.
- Demonstrate the following procedures:
  - Procedure 92 Refilling the Humidifier Bottle
  - Procedure 93 Collecting a Sputum Specimen

VOCABULARY

Learn the meaning and the correct spelling of the following words and phrases:

alveoli	dyspnea	orthopneic position	sputum
asthma	emphysema	oxygen	trachea
biopsy	expectorate	oxygen concentrator	tracheostomy
bronchi	high Fowler's position	oxygen mask	upper respiratory
bronchioles	incentive spirometer	pharynx	infection (URI)
bronchitis	larynx	pleura	ventilation
carbon dioxide	nasal cannula	pneumonia	vocal cords
chronic obstructive	nebulizer		
pulmonary disease			
(COPD)			

INTRODUCTION

Life cannot be maintained without oxygen, and carbon dioxide must be eliminated from the body. Diseases of the respiratory tract that interfere with this vital exchange of oxygen and carbon dioxide bring acute distress. Nursing care is directed toward making breathing easier and preventing transmission of infection.

STRUCTURE AND FUNCTION

The respiratory system (Figure 36-1) is sometimes called the lifeline of the body. It extends from the nose to the tiny air sacs (**alveoli**) that make up the bulk of the lungs.

The organs of the respiratory system include the:

- Nose
- Pharynx (throat)
- Larynx (voice box)
- Trachea (windpipe)
- Bronchi
- Lungs

The sinuses, diaphragm, and intercostal muscles between the ribs are called auxiliary structures.

Air is warmed, moistened, and filtered as it passes through the nasal cavities, which are separated by the nasal septum. The air passes through the **pharynx**, a passageway for both air and food, into the larynx and trachea. It then passes into the **bronchi** to join the upper respiratory tract to the lungs. Within the lungs, the bronchi branch into smaller and smaller divisions called **bronchioles**. The *alveoli* are tiny air sacs that extend from the bronchioles. It is at the level of the alveoli that the exchange of gases takes place (Figure 36-2).

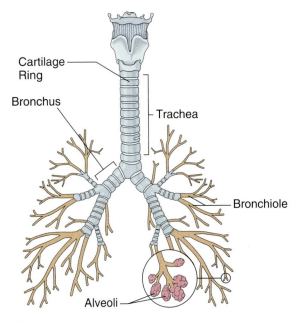

FIGURE 36-2 Ventral view of the structures of the lower respiratory tract

The alveoli, bronchioles, and the important pulmonary blood vessels form the lungs. The way in which oxygen and carbon dioxide are exchanged between the alveoli and the capillaries is shown in Figure 36-3.

The purpose of this system is to bring **oxygen** (O_2) into the body to meet cellular needs and to expel carbon dioxide (CO_2). **Carbon dioxide** is a gaseous, metabolic waste produced by the cells. It also functions in voice production (phonation).

Each cell in the body must have a constant supply of oxygen. The oxygen is used to produce the energy for cellular activity.

Nutrients + oxygen yields energy + water + CO_2

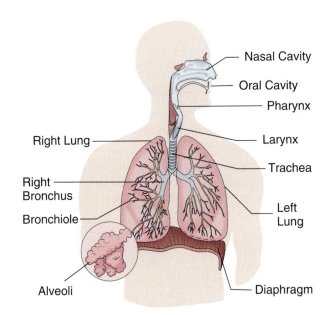

FIGURE 36-1 The respiratory system

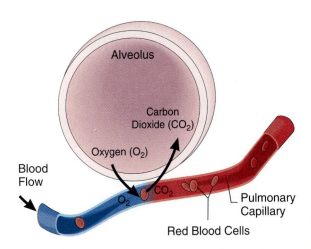

FIGURE 36-3 Oxygen and carbon dioxide are exchanged between the capillaries and each of the alveoli.

There is a close connection between the respiratory and circulatory systems. Cells depend on the bloodstream to carry gases to and from the lungs.

The Act of Respiration

Two lungs are located in the thorax. Each lung is surrounded by a double-walled membrane called the pleura. Between the layers of the pleura is a small amount of fluid that reduces friction as the lungs alternately expand and contract, filling with and then expelling air.

The size of the thorax depends on the contraction of the diaphragm and intercostal muscles. As the muscles contract, the thorax enlarges, expanding the lungs. Air carrying oxygen enters the lungs. When the muscles relax, the thorax resumes its normal size and the lungs recoil. Air carrying carbon dioxide leaves the lungs and is breathed out.

- *Inspiration* (or inhalation) is the act of drawing air into the lungs.
- *Expiration* (or exhalation) is the act of expelling air.
- Ventilation is the combination of these two actions.

Voice Production

The larynx, or voice box, is part of the respiratory tract. It is important in voice production. Two membranes called the vocal cords stretch across the inside of the larynx. As air moves upward through the larynx, it passes through an opening in the vocal cords. Changes in the shape of the vocal cords and the size of the opening permit controlled amounts of air to reach the mouth, nasal cavities, and sinuses, where specific speech sounds are made when formed by the teeth, lips, and tongue.

UPPER RESPIRATORY INFECTIONS

An upper respiratory infection (URI) follows invasion of the upper respiratory organs by microbes. The upper respiratory organs include the nose, sinuses, and throat. A common cold, which is caused by a virus, is an example of an upper respiratory infection. It is one of the most ordinary illnesses found in people. Symptoms include:

- Elevated temperature (fever)
- Runny nose
- Watery eyes

This usually self-limiting disease is best treated by:

- Use of a drug to reduce fever, such as acetaminophen
- Rest
- Increased fluid intake

Patients with respiratory infections should be taught to:

- cover the nose and mouth when coughing or sneezing.
- dispose of soiled tissues by placing them in a plastic or paper bag to be burned.
- turn face away from others when coughing or sneezing.
- wash hands after handling soiled tissues.

You must take special note of and report the following:

- Dyspnea (difficult breathing)
- Changes in rate and rhythm of respiration
- Presence and character of respiratory secretions, including color
- Cough
- Changes in skin color, such as pallor or cyanosis

URIs sometimes move down into the chest and develop into bronchitis or even pneumonia.

Pneumonia

Pneumonia is a serious inflammation of the lungs. It can be caused by a variety of infectious organisms. Three common causes of pneumonia are:

- Viruses
- *Streptococcus pneumoniae* (a bacterium)
- *Pneumocystis carinii* (a protozoan)

Pneumocystis carinii is most often seen in patients who have poorly functioning immune systems. Today, most pneumonias, though serious and potentially life-threatening, respond favorably to antibiotic therapy.

CHRONIC OBSTRUCTIVE PULMONARY DISEASE

Chronic obstructive pulmonary disease (COPD) is also called chronic obstructive lung disease (COLD). This term refers to conditions resulting from a prolonged impairment in the exchange of gases in the respiratory system. Several conditions can lead to COPD, including:

- Tuberculosis
- Frequent pneumonia
- Chronic asthma
- Chronic bronchitis
- Emphysema

Asthma

Asthma is a breathing disorder resulting from:

- Constriction of the muscles of the bronchioles
- Swelling of the respiratory membranes
- Production of large amounts of mucus that fill the narrowed passageways

A person having an asthma attack has labored breathing and frequent coughing. An attack may result when the person contacts an allergen or is under emotional stress. Common allergens are:

- Pollen
- Medications
- Dust
- Feathers
- Foods such as chicken, eggs, or chocolate

If a patient has known allergies (hypersensitivity to specific items), they should be marked in the patient's health record.

Long-term treatment consists of determining the allergen and eliminating it. To relieve the attack, the patient is given medication to decrease the swelling and dilate the bronchioles. Low levels of oxygen may also be given.

Chronic Bronchitis

Chronic **bronchitis** is prolonged inflammation in the bronchi due to infection or irritants. Signs and symptoms include:

- Swollen and red bronchial tissues, resulting in narrowed bronchial passageways
- Persistent cough, which may or may not produce sputum
- Respiratory distress

Treatment includes:

- Antibiotics to fight the infection
- Drugs to loosen the phlegm (secretions) deep in the respiratory tract
- Techniques to improve ventilation and drainage

Emphysema

Emphysema develops after chronic obstruction of the air flow to the alveoli. The air sacs:

- Become distended
- Lose their elasticity and recoil ability
- Finally become nonfunctional
- Lose ability to exchange gases

The patient can bring air into the lungs, but it becomes more difficult to expel air from the lungs (Figure 36-4). As a result, there is less and less room for air to reenter.

Several factors contribute to emphysema, including:

- Air pollutants, such as cigarette smoke, auto exhaust fumes, and insecticides
- Genetic predisposition to emphysema
- Recurrent infections, such as pneumonia and bronchitis
- Chronic asthma

People with emphysema are at greater risk for infections such as pneumonia. They experience:

- Chronic oxygen shortage and fatigue
- Increasing breathing difficulty (requires greater and greater effort)
- Productive coughing that may bring up large amounts of heavy mucous secretions (phlegm), or nonproductive coughing
- Dizziness and restlessness as carbon dioxide levels rise in the bloodstream
- Loss of appetite and weight loss
- Strain on the heart and blood vessels

General Care. The care of the emphysema patient includes all the care required of any patient with COPD:

- Assisting with the proper breathing techniques, such as pursed-lip breathing
- Encouraging breathing exercises

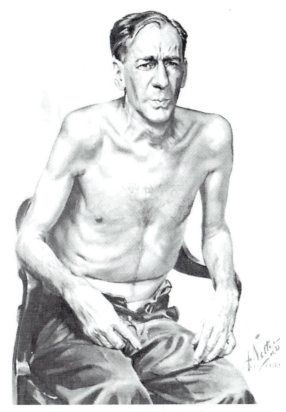

FIGURE 36-4 Characteristic posture of patient with emphysema. The patient leans forward on his arms and purses his lips. © Copyright 1968, CIBA-GEIGY Corporation. Reproduced with permission, from the Clinical Symposia, illustrated by Frank H. Netter, M.D. All rights reserved.

- Positioning to improve ventilation
- Assisting with use of an incentive spirometer
- Assisting with postural drainage
- Providing care during low-flow oxygen therapy
- Paying attention to nutrition and fluid intake
- Treating infections with antibiotics and drugs to loosen and thin respiratory secretions
- Encouraging patients to avoid crowds, especially during the flu season
- Encouraging patients not to go out of doors when the temperature is 35°F to 40°F or lower, because cold air can trigger spasms
- Encouraging patients not to smoke
- Maintaining humidity with a room humidifier if ordered

Wear gloves if your hands may contact the patient's respiratory secretions. Wear a gown, goggles or face shield, and a surgical mask if the patient is coughing and spraying respiratory secretions into the air.

MALIGNANCIES

Malignant tumors can develop in any part of the respiratory tract. Although the exact causes of malignancy are not fully

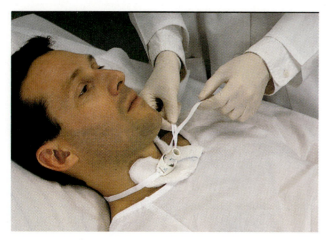

FIGURE 36-5 The tracheostomy stoma is a surgical opening in the trachea.

understood, cigarette smoking and exposure to cancer-producing agents in the environment are known to be contributing factors. Lung cancers are treated by surgery, radiation, or chemotherapy, or a combination of all three therapies.

Cancer of the Larynx

Cancer of the larynx may require removal of the larynx, resulting in the loss of the voice. The patient breathes through an artificial opening in the neck and trachea. The permanent opening (*stoma*) is called a **tracheostomy** (Figure 36-5).

Loss of voice is a major trauma for anyone. Just think for a moment of how frustrated you would feel if you could no longer use your voice to communicate your thoughts, feelings, wants, and needs to others.

Postsurgical care is given in the acute care hospital. At this time, writing is the major form of communication available to such patients. Later, the patient may be taught new ways to speak through esophageal speech or electronic speech.

Esophageal Speech. The patient learns to swallow air and then bring it back up through the esophagus into the mouth. Here the air is formed by the teeth and tongue into words, as it would be if it were being exhaled from the lungs. Esophageal speech is difficult to learn, but motivated patients can succeed.

Electronic Speech. Patients who cannot use esophageal speech may be able to use an electronic artificial larynx to create speech. Some patients may use a combination of both techniques.

Patients with laryngectomies (removal of larynx) need patience and understanding from all health care providers. Communication is possible, but the voice does not sound normal. More time is needed by the patient to formulate the sounds. A difficult psychological adjustment must be made by the patient. The loss of one's voice requires an adjustment similar to that experienced when grieving for the loss of a loved one. Expect periods of depression, anger, and hostility.

DIAGNOSTIC TECHNIQUES

Some techniques used to diagnose problems of the respiratory system include:

- Tissue **biopsy** (microscopic examination of specimen of tissue removed from patient)
- Cultures of secretions
- Volume studies that measure the amount of air entering or leaving the lungs during various respiratory movements
- Radiographic techniques such as x-rays, CAT scans, and MRIs
- Direct visualization procedures such as bronchoscopy

SPECIAL THERAPIES RELATED TO RESPIRATORY ILLNESS

Nursing assistants aid patient breathing by proper positioning and by helping provide moisture and oxygen. They also are assigned to collect sputum specimens for examinations.

Oxygen Therapy

Oxygen is often ordered by the physician. Remember that when oxygen is in use, special precautions are required to prevent fires and to administer the oxygen safely. Information about general fire control is presented in Unit 13.

Special safety measures must be emphasized in areas where oxygen is being used:

- Be certain that there are no open flames and that no one smokes or has matches.
- Post "no smoking" or "oxygen-in-use" signs.

Oxygen Source. Hospitals have oxygen piped from wall units directly into the patient's room (Figure 36-6). In some cases, the oxygen source is a tank that is brought to the

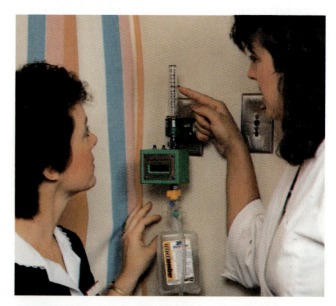

FIGURE 36-6 Oxygen is usually piped directly to each patient unit.

patient's room when therapy is ordered. The amount of oxygen (rate of flow measured in liters) is ordered by the physician. When caring for a patient receiving oxygen, you should:

- wear gloves and apply the principles of standard precautions if contact with the patient's oral or nasal secretions is likely.
- know the oxygen flow rate that was ordered and set for your patient.
- be able to read the flow meter for the rate of oxygen delivery if instructed to check the rate by the nurse.
- notify the nurse immediately if there is a change in the flow rate.
- check that the tubing is not obstructed in any way that would prevent oxygen from reaching the patient.
- check for proper position of the catheter, cannula, or mask and that the elastic band around the head is snug but not constricting.
- Check whether straps, catheter, cannula, or mask are causing skin irritation.

If a tank is used as the source of oxygen, be sure that:

- There is sufficient oxygen in the tank. Check the gauge each time you visit the patient (Figure 36-7).
- The oxygen is on.
- An additional tank is available to exchange for the tank in use when it is empty.
- Empty tanks are marked and stored according to facility policy.
- The tank is upright and secure on the carrier or in the stand.

Maintaining Moisture. Pure oxygen is very dry and thus is damaging to tissues. Therefore, oxygen should be moisturized by passing it through water before it reaches the patient. Be sure the level of water is maintained according to your facility policy. Figure 36-7 shows a humidifier into

which oxygen flows to pick up moisture before reaching the patient. Because many patients with respiratory difficulty breathe through their mouths, special attention to mouth care is essential.

Methods of Oxygen Delivery. Oxygen may be delivered to the patient by several different methods. The same basic care is required for each method, with modifications.

- *Nasal cannula:* Delivery of oxygen by **nasal cannula** is the most common method used today. The oxygen is delivered through a tube that has two small plastic prongs or nipples (Figure 36-8). The prongs are placed at the entrance to the patient's nose. A strap around the patient's head holds the prongs in place.
  - Make sure the strap is secure but not too tight.
  - Check for signs of irritation where the prongs touch the patient's nose.
  - Check that mucus has not blocked the prong openings. Clean if necessary.
  - Make sure the cannula is stored when not in use in such a way that it is not contaminated.
- *Mask:* The **oxygen mask** is a cuplike mask held in place by straps around the head (Figure 36-9).

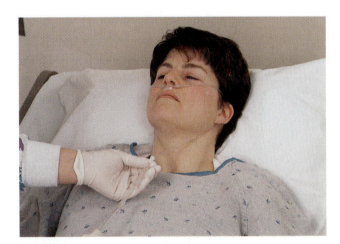

FIGURE 36-8 Oxygen administered by nasal cannula

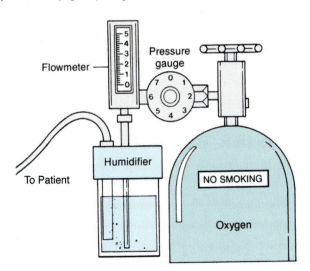

FIGURE 36-7 Note attachment of flowmeter gauge to oxygen tank. Check flowmeter and gauge whenever the patient is receiving oxygen. Note that the tank is green. Tanks of gas are color-coded for safety.

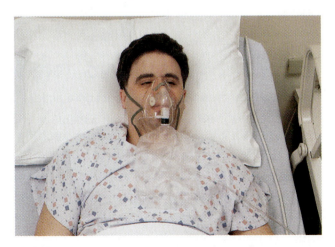

FIGURE 36-9 Oxygen administration by mask

— Place mask over nose and mouth.

— Be sure the straps are secure but not too tight.

— Periodically remove the mask. Wash the area under it and dry carefully.

- *Nasal catheter:* The catheter is a small plastic tube that is inserted into the nose (Figure 36-10).

  — Keep patient's face free of any nasal discharge.

  — Make sure that there are no kinks or undue pressure on the tubing. Tape is used to secure the catheter at the nose and temple. A linen tunnel around the tube allows patient mobility.

- *Tent:* An example of a tent is a Mistogen® unit (croupette). A *croupette* is a small, portable unit (see Unit 46).

- *Intermittent positive pressure breathing (IPPB):* Oxygen is administered intermittently under pressure by professional personnel such as respiratory therapists (Figure 36-11). This technique helps to expand the lungs.

Oxygen Concentrator

An oxygen concentrator takes in room air and removes impurities and gases other than oxygen, allowing the oxygen to become concentrated in the unit. The air delivered to the

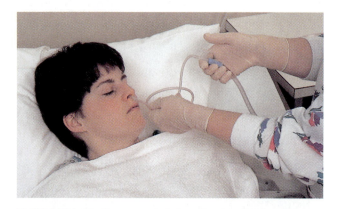

FIGURE 36-10 Oxygen administration by nasal catheter

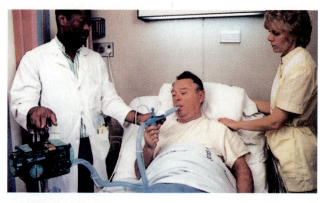

FIGURE 36-11 Oxygen administration by intermittent positive pressure breathing (IPPB).

patient from the concentrator is more than 90% oxygen. It is delivered by tubing attached to a nasal cannula or mask. The flow rate is usually 2 liters per minute (L/min). A humidifier bottle may be attached to the concentrator to offset the drying effect of the oxygen. (Refer to Procedure 92.)

General Oxygen Concentrator Precautions. Follow these precautions when a concentrator is used to supply oxygen to a patient:

- Place concentrator at least 5 feet away from any heat source and at least 4 inches away from the wall.
- Smoking is not permitted in the same room.
- Be sure the unit is plugged in and grounded.
- Do not use an extension cord with the concentrator.
- Never change the flowmeter setting.
- Notify the nurse if the alarm sounds.
- Be sure the fluid level in the humidifier (if used) is adequate.
- Wipe cannula or mask daily with a damp cloth (do not use alcohol- or oil-based products).
- Clean concentrator surfaces using a damp cloth only.
- Remove the filter weekly. Wash in warm soapy water, rinse, squeeze dry, and replace.

PROCEDURE   **92**

REFILLING THE HUMIDIFIER BOTTLE

1. Carry out each beginning procedure action.

2. Remove mask or cannula from patient, or connect it to a temporary oxygen source if constant oxygen is required.

3. Turn oxygen concentrator off.

4. Remove the lid from the humidifier bottle.

5. Remove the bottle and discard any remaining water.

6. Rinse bottle well with warm water. Shake dry.

7. Refill jar with distilled water to the fill line.

8. Replace bottle and reattach lid.

9. Turn on unit.

10. Position mask or cannula on patient.

11. Wash hands.

12. Carry out procedure completion actions.

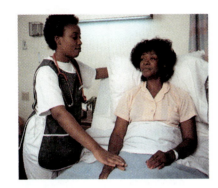

FIGURE 36-12
Patient is in a high
Fowler's position

Respiratory Positions

Positioning of the patient to permit expansion of the lungs and a straightened airway is helpful to patients with respiratory distress.

High Fowler's Position. In the high Fowler's position, the patient is sitting up with the back rest elevated (Figure 36-12).

- Position three pillows behind the patient's head and shoulders. Adjust knee rest.
- Keep feet in proper position.
- Check for signs of skin breakdown over coccyx due to shearing forces.

Orthopneic Position. The orthopneic position may be used as an alternative to the high Fowler's position (Figure 36-13).

- The position of the bed remains the same.
- The bedside table is brought across the bed and a pillow or two are placed on top.
- The patient leans forward across the table with arms on or beside the pillows.
- Another pillow is placed low behind the patient's back for support.

Incentive Spirometer

The physician may write orders for use of an incentive spirometer (Figure 36-14) to help the lungs expand fully. This prevents atelectasis (collapse of the alveoli) and also helps prevent pneumonia.

This procedure may be carried out with the patient in bed, with head and shoulders well supported, if permitted. The procedure usually is taught before surgery.

- The patient is instructed how to use the incentive spirometer by a respiratory therapist or nurse.
- For one type of spirometer, the patient exhales normally and then, with the lips placed tightly around the mouthpiece, inhales through the mouth strongly, enough to raise the balls in the chambers.
- The deep breath should be held as long as possible (or as ordered), thereby keeping the balls suspended.
- The patient then removes the mouthpiece and exhales normally.
- The exercise is repeated as many times as is ordered.

Although this procedure is started by the professional, you too have responsibilities:

- Observe the patient for correctness of procedure.
- Be sure the patient does not become overly fatigued.
- Encourage the patient to cough and clear the respiratory passages.
- Report to your team leader if the patient seems overly fatigued during the procedure.
- Carefully observe and report any unusual responses such as pain, dizziness, or throat and airway irritation.
- When patient has completed the pulmonary exercise, wash the mouthpiece in warm water, dry it, replace it in the plastic bag, and leave it at the bedside.

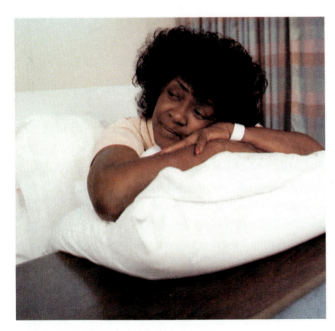

FIGURE 36-13 The orthopneic position

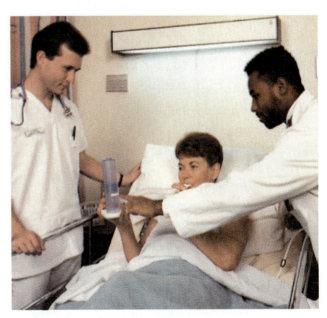

FIGURE 36-14 The nursing assistant may help the respiratory therapist or patient with equipment, but the incentive spirometer is a self-administered treatment.

- Patients should be praised for efforts. Many times this encourages greater effort the next time the incentive spirometer is used.

Other Techniques

Aerosol Therapy. **Nebulizers** deliver moisture or medication deep into the lungs. Drugs that thin the mucus (*mucolytics*) or dilate the bronchi are often prescribed. The stream of moisture or medication may be delivered by a hand-held nebulizer or driven by oxygen, compressed air, or compressor pump (Figure 36-15). The medication may be given in conjunction with an intermittent positive pressure breathing (IPPB) machine. If oxygen is used, the rate of administration and the depth of the patient's respirations must be carefully monitored. The treatment must be stopped if the respiratory rate and rhythm decrease by 25 percent.

Concentrations of 100 percent oxygen delivered continuously for 5 to 10 minutes can have a depressing effect on respirations. This is particularly hazardous to patients suffering from COPD.

After administering the mucolytics, nurses and therapists use various techniques to loosen the mucus and clear the air passageways.

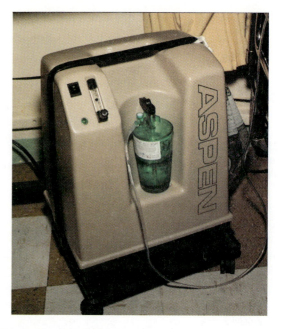

FIGURE 36-15 Nebulizers may be driven by compressed air instead of oxygen.

COLLECTING A SPUTUM SPECIMEN

You may need to collect a sputum specimen from the patient. **Sputum** is matter that is brought up (**expectorated**) from the lungs. A culture of the specimen identifies the cause of an infection.

You must be sure that the specimen comes from the lungs and is not saliva from the mouth.

If the patient cannot expectorate sputum, suctioning may be needed to obtain the specimen. (The nurse performs this procedure.) It is easier to collect the specimen when the patient wakes up in the morning and after taking two or three deep breaths. (Refer to Procedure 93.)

PROCEDURE 93

COLLECTING A SPUTUM SPECIMEN

1. Carry out each beginning procedure action.
2. Assemble equipment:
   - disposable gloves
   - container and cover for specimen
   - glass of water
   - label, including:
     - patient's full name
     - room number
     - patient number
     - date and time of collection
     - physician's name
     - examination to be done
     - other information as requested
   - tissues
   - emesis basin
   - biohazard specimen transport bag
   - laboratory requisition
3. Wash hands and put on disposable gloves.
4. Ask patient to rinse mouth with water and spit into emesis basin.
5. Ask patient to breathe deeply and then cough deeply to bring up sputum. The patient spits the sputum into the container.
   a. While coughing, have patient cover mouth with tissue to prevent spread of infection.
   b. Collect 1 to 2 tablespoons of sputum unless otherwise ordered.

continues

PROCEDURE 93 continued

c. Do not contaminate the outside of the container.

6. Remove gloves and discard according to facility policy.

7. Wash your hands.

8. Cover container tightly and attach completed label.

9. Place specimen container into biohazard transport bag and attach laboratory requisition.

10. Carry out each procedure completion action.

11. Follow facility policy for transport of specimen to laboratory.

REVIEW

A. True/False.

Mark the following true or false by circling T or F.

1. T F In asthma, there is increased production of mucus, which blocks the respiratory tract.

2. T F Drugs to reduce fever fight infection.

3. T F An allergen causes a sensitivity reaction.

4. T F URI stands for underrated respiratory injections.

5. T F The use of the incentive spirometer can help prevent pneumonia.

6. T F Always post a sign when oxygen is in use.

7. T F The oxygen flow rate is ordered by the physician.

8. T F Oxygen should always be moisturized before reaching the patient.

9. T F When oxygen is administered by mask, make sure the straps are very tight.

10. T F In the high Fowler's position, the patient leans forward across the overbed table.

B. Matching.

Choose the correct word from Column II to match each the phrase or statement in Column I.

Column I	Column II
11. _____ inflammation of the lungs	a. emphysema
12. _____ an example of COPD	b. sputum
13. _____ difficult breathing	c. pneumonia
14. _____ controlled	d. dyspnea
15. _____ material brought up from lungs	e. spirometer
	f. arrested

C. Multiple Choice.

Select the one best answer for each question.

16. Patients with respiratory disease should
    a. cover the nose and mouth when coughing.
    b. turn face toward others when sneezing.
    c. wash hands only after toileting.
    d. dispose of soiled tissues by dropping them in the nearest trash can.

17. When tank oxygen is in use
    a. mark empty tanks and store in patient's room.
    b. attach the tank to the patient's bed.
    c. make sure additional tanks are available.
    d. check the gauge indicating amount in tank once each shift.

18. You should know that
    a. patients receiving oxygen do not require special mouth care.
    b. oxygen need not be humidified when a mask is used.
    c. oxygen need not be moisturized when administered with a nasal catheter.
    d. oxygen is very drying to tissues.

19. When your patient is receiving oxygen, you should
    a. monitor intake and output.
    b. know the ordered rate.
    c. check the flow rate once each shift.
    d. check the flow rate every three hours.

20. When administering oxygen by mask, in addition to routine care and precautions, you should
    a. make sure straps are not too tight.
    b. periodically remove the mask to wash and dry under it.
    c. make sure mask covers nose and mouth.
    d. all of these.

D. Nursing Assistant Challenge.

Mrs. Harvey has had asthma all her life. She is sensitive to many allergens. She is admitted to your facility for emphysema. She is receiving respiratory assistance with an oxygen concentrator. Complete the following questions related to her care.

21. The flow rate of the concentrator is usually _____
(10 L/min) (2 L/min)

22. Smoking in the same room _____ permitted.
(is) (is not)

23. The flowmeter on a concentrator _____ be changed by the nursing assistant.
(may) (may not)

24. The concentrator should be placed at least _____ from a heat source.
(2 feet) (5 feet)

25. The concentrator filter should be cleaned _____.
(daily) (weekly)

Circulatory (Cardiovascular) System

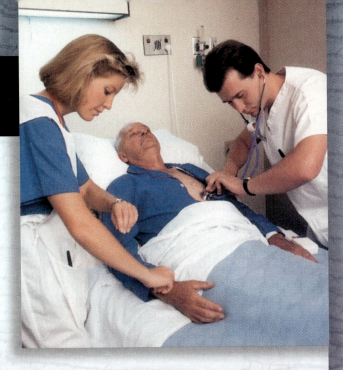

OBJECTIVES

As a result of this unit, you will be able to:

- Spell and define terms.
- Review the location and functions of the organs of the circulatory system.
- List five specific diagnostic tests for disorders of the circulatory system.
- Describe some common disorders of the circulatory system.
- Describe nursing assistant actions related to care of patients with disorders of the circulatory system.

VOCABULARY

Learn the meaning and the correct spelling of the following words and phrases:

anemia	coronary embolism	ischemic	phlebitis
angina pectoris	coronary occlusion	leukocytes	plasma
artery	coronary thrombosis	leukemia	sympathectomy
ascites	diuresis	lymph	TED hose
atheroma	dyscrasia	lymphatic vessel	thrombocytes
atherosclerosis	embolus	myocardial infarction	thrombus
atrium	endocardium	(MI)	transient ischemic
capillary	erythrocytes	myocardium	attack (TIA)
cardiac cycle	heart block	orthopnea	varicose vein
cardiac decompensation	hypertension	pacemaker	vein
compensate	hypertrophy	pericardium	ventricle
congestive heart failure	infarction	peripheral	
(CHF)			

INTRODUCTION

The circulatory system may be thought of as a transportation system. It takes nourishment and oxygen to the cells and carries away waste products. The closed system is kept in motion by the force of the heartbeat. Diseases that attack any part of this system interfere with the overall function. Long-standing diseases of the cardiovascular system eventually affect the pulmonary system as well.

STRUCTURE AND FUNCTION

The organs of the cardiovascular system include:

1. Heart—a central pumping station
2. Blood vessels
   a. **Arteries**—tubes that carry blood away from the heart. They
   - have muscular, elastic walls with smooth linings.
   - branch to form arterioles with thinner walls. Arterioles then become capillaries.
   - carry blood with a high concentration of nutrients and oxygen to the body cells.
   b. **Veins**—tubes that carry blood toward the heart. They
   - have thinner muscular walls.
   - carry blood back to the heart.
   - carry blood with a lower concentration of oxygen, more carbon dioxide, and more waste products.
   - have cuplike valves that help move the blood.
   c. **Capillaries**—tubes that connect arteries and veins. They
   - have walls only one cell thick.
   - are the site of exchange of nutrients and oxygen from the blood to the cells, and carbon dioxide and waste products from the cells to the blood.
3. **Lymphatic vessels**—tubes that carry lymph or tissue fluid to the bloodstream. Fluid from the bloodstream passes into the tissue spaces, where it is called *tissue fluid*. Some of the tissue fluid returns to the bloodstream by way of the capillaries. Some of it is first drawn off into the lymphatic vessels, where it is called **lymph**. Eventually the lymph is returned to general circulation and once more becomes part of the blood.
4. Lymph nodes—masses of lymphatic tissue along the pathway of the lymph. They filter the lymph.
5. Spleen—a lymphatic organ. The spleen produces some of the blood cells and helps destroy worn-out blood cells. It acts as a blood reservoir or blood bank.
6. Blood—a connective tissue made up of a liquid (plasma) and cellular elements.

The Blood

Blood is a red body fluid composed of plasma and cellular elements. The body contains 4 to 6 quarts (liters) of blood. Fifty-five percent of the blood is formed of the liquid plasma. **Plasma** is a watery solution containing:

- Antibodies (gamma globulin)—chemicals to fight infection
- Nutrients—such as glucose, amino acids, fats, salts
- Gases—such as oxygen and carbon dioxide
- Waste products—such as urea and creatinine

The blood cells are produced in the bone marrow and lymphatic tissues of the body. The bone marrow, liver, and spleen destroy worn-out blood cells. (See Unit 5.) The blood cells include red blood cells, white blood cells, and thrombocytes.

- Red blood cells (RBC)—**erythrocytes**—carry most of the oxygen and small amounts of carbon dioxide. There are 4.5 to 5 million RBC per cubic millimeter (mm^3).
- White blood cells (WBC)—**leukocytes**—fight infection. There are 7,000 to 8,000 WBC/mm^3.
- **Thrombocytes** (or platelets)—are not whole cells but only parts of cells. They seal small leaks in the walls of blood vessels and initiate blood clotting. There are 200,000 to 400,000 thrombocytes/mm^3.

The Heart

The heart is a hollow muscular organ about the size of a fist (Figure 37-1). It is divided into a right and left side by a muscular wall called the *septum* and into four chambers. There are three layers in the heart wall. The **endocardium** lines the heart chambers. The **myocardium** is the muscle layer. The **pericardium** is a membranous outer covering.

The four chambers are:

1. The right **atrium** (RA)—(right upper heart chamber) receives blood from all over the body. This blood has a low oxygen content and a relatively high carbon dioxide level. It is called *deoxygenated blood*.
2. The right **ventricle** (RV)—(right lower heart chamber) receives blood from the right atrium and sends it out to the lungs through the pulmonary artery to pick up oxygen and get rid of the carbon dioxide.
3. The left atrium (LA)—(left upper heart chamber) receives oxygenated blood from the lungs and sends it to the left ventricle.
4. The left ventricle (LV)—(left lower heart chamber) receives blood from the left atrium and sends it out through the aorta to the entire body.

Valves separate the chambers. They also guard the exit of the pulmonary artery and aorta to prevent backflow and maintain a constant forward motion. The pulmonary artery carries blood to the lungs. The aorta is the largest blood vessel in the body. The valves are located as follows:

- Tricuspid valve—between right atrium and right ventricle

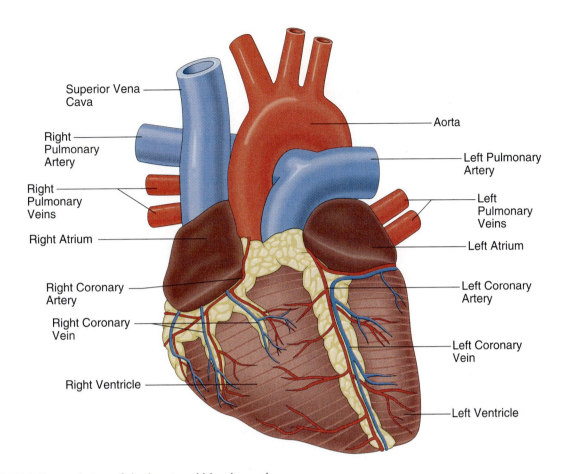

FIGURE 37-1 External view of the heart and blood vessels

- Bicuspid (mitral) valve—between left atrium and left ventricle
- Pulmonary semilunar valves—between right ventricle and pulmonary artery
- Aortic semilunar valve—between left ventricle and aorta

Nerve impulses make the heart contract regularly according to body needs. For example, when you run, your body cells need more oxygen. The cells signal the brain that they need more oxygen. The brain sends a signal to the heart through the nerves, telling it to supply more blood. These nerve impulses cause the heart to beat faster. Thus, more oxygenated blood is pumped to the body cells to supply the oxygen required. These impulses cause the heart to beat faster.

The Cardiac Cycle. The heart pumps blood through the body by a series of movements known as the **cardiac cycle**. First, the upper chambers of the heart, called *atria,* relax and fill with blood as the lower chambers contract, forcing blood out of the heart through the aorta and pulmonary arteries. Next, the lower chambers relax, allowing blood to flow into them from the contracting upper chambers. Then the cycle is repeated (Figure 37-2). Each cycle lasts about 0.8 second. This happens about 70 to 80 times per minute.

The pulse you feel at the radial artery corresponds to ventricular contraction. The sounds you hear when listening to the heart and when taking a blood pressure are the sounds made by the closing of the valves during the cardiac cycle.

The rate and rhythm of the cardiac cycle are regulated by the conduction system. The conduction system is made up of special neuromuscular tissue that sends out impulses. The impulses eventually reach the myocardial cells, which respond by contracting.

- The impulses begin at the S-A node in the right atrium and spread across the two atria.
- The atria contract.
- Impulses from the S-A node reach the A-V node in the right atrium.
- Messages from the A-V node then spread through the bundle of His in the septum. From there they go through the Purkinje fibers to the walls of the ventricles.
- The ventricles contract, forcing the blood forward.

An electrocardiogram, called an ECG or an EKG, is a test that traces the electrical impulses of the heart. Heart disease may be detected with this test.

Blood Vessels

Many large arteries and veins take their names from the bones they are near or from the part of the body they serve. For

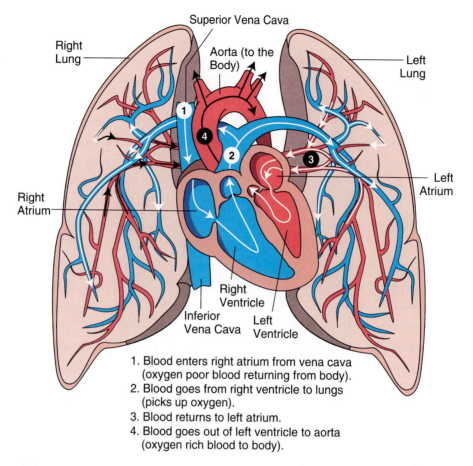

1. Blood enters right atrium from vena cava (oxygen poor blood returning from body).
2. Blood goes from right ventricle to lungs (picks up oxygen).
3. Blood returns to left atrium.
4. Blood goes out of left ventricle to aorta (oxygen rich blood to body).

FIGURE 37-2 Flow of blood from the heart to the lungs, to the body, and back to the heart to begin the cycle again

example, the femoral artery and vein run close to the femur (thigh bone). The subclavian arteries and veins are found under the clavicle. The axillary arteries and veins are found in the axillary (armpit) area. Figure 37-3 shows the arterial system that distributes blood from the heart. Figure 37-4 shows the venous system that returns blood to the heart.

COMMON CIRCULATORY SYSTEM DISORDERS

Common disorders of this system include:

- Diseases relating to the blood vessels
- Diseases of the heart
- Blood dyscrasias (abnormalities); these diseases can involve the bone, bone marrow, liver, or spleen.

Observations the nursing assistant is to report in patients with disorders of the circulatory system are:

- Color change, pallor or cyanosis, redness
- Cool to touch
- Hot to touch
- Changes in pulse rate or rhythm
- Changes in blood pressure

- Edema
- Disorientation

PERIPHERAL VASCULAR DISEASES

The blood vessels that serve the outer parts of the body, particularly those of the hands and feet, are referred to as peripheral (toward the outer part) blood vessels. Diseases of these vessels affect the parts of the body through which they pass. The health of these vessels also influences heart function.

Peripheral vascular diseases that affect the arteries diminish the flow of blood to the extremities. Tissues through which the narrowed arteries pass may not get the nourishment they need. Areas affected are the extremities: the arms, legs, and brain. The signs and symptoms associated with decreased peripheral circulation are:

- Burning pain during exercise
- Hair loss over feet and toes
- Thick and rigid toenails
- Dusky red skin or cyanotic, brownish skin
- Dry and scaly or shiny skin

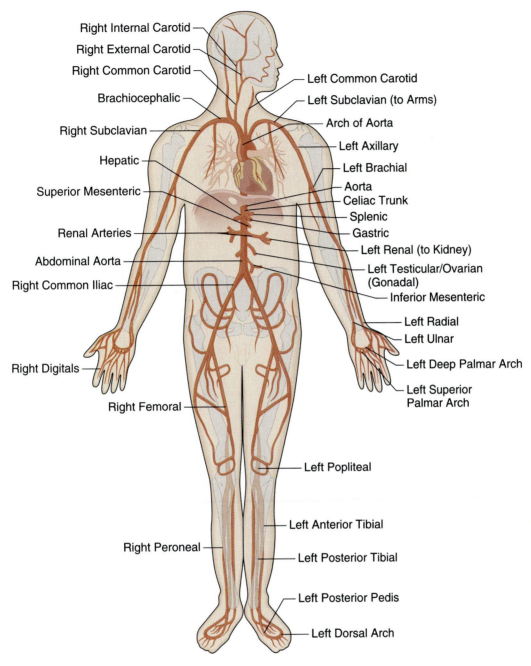

Right Internal Carotid

Right External Carotid

Right Common Carotid

Brachiocephalic

Right Subclavian

Hepatic

Superior Mesenteric

Renal Arteries

Abdominal Aorta

Right Common Iliac

Right Digitals

Right Femoral

Right Peroneal

Left Common Carotid

Left Subclavian (to Arms)

Arch of Aorta

Left Axillary

Left Brachial

Aorta

Celiac Trunk

Splenic

Gastric

Left Renal (to Kidney)

Left Testicular/Ovarian (Gonadal)

Inferior Mesenteric

Left Radial

Left Ulnar

Left Deep Palmar Arch

Left Superior Palmar Arch

Left Popliteal

Left Anterior Tibial

Left Posterior Tibial

Left Posterior Pedis

Left Dorsal Arch

FIGURE 37-3 Arteries of the body

- Chronic edema of the feet and legs
- Cool skin temperature of feet and legs
- Difficulty with ambulation

When the arteries are affected, the blood flow may be seriously interrupted. This condition requires immediate medical treatment. Vascular ulcers may occur. These are sores that start because of the poor circulation of the blood in the legs. These ulcers are difficult to treat and may take months to heal.

Treatment is aimed at:

- Increasing local circulation

- Positioning and specific prescribed exercises can promote arterial flow and venous return.
- Sometimes an oscillating (rocking) bed is employed to improve the circulatory flow. The oscillating bed rocks up and down in cycles, raising the patient's feet 6 inches above his head and then lowering them 12 to 15 inches. The steady rhythm provides both passive exercise for the patient and some circulatory stimulation.
- Nothing that would hamper the patient's circulation is permitted.
- Preventing injuries that heal poorly.

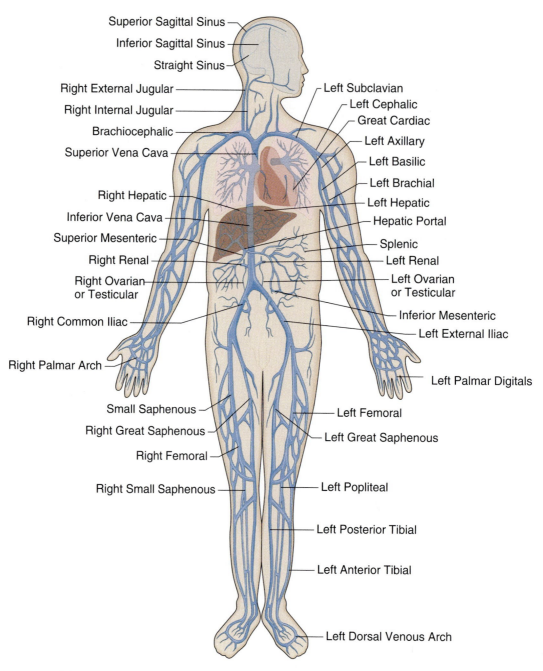

FIGURE 37-4 Veins of the body

Atherosclerosis

Atherosclerosis is a common form of vascular disease.

- Roughened areas known as **atheromas**, which are growths developed over deposits of fatty materials, form on the inner walls of the arteries and narrow the vessels.
- The vessels of the heart and brain, and those leading to the legs from the body, are often affected.
- The atheromas gradually grow larger until they eventually block blood flow to the parts and organs served by the affected vessels (Figure 37-5).

- Sometimes clots that have formed over the irregular areas in the vessel walls break off and travel as emboli to block distant vessels.
- The narrowing of vessels can lead to serious complications, such as:
  - Formation of blood clots
  - Angina pectoris
  - Myocardial infarction (MI)
  - Strokes (CVA) (also known as brain attacks)
  - Gangrene

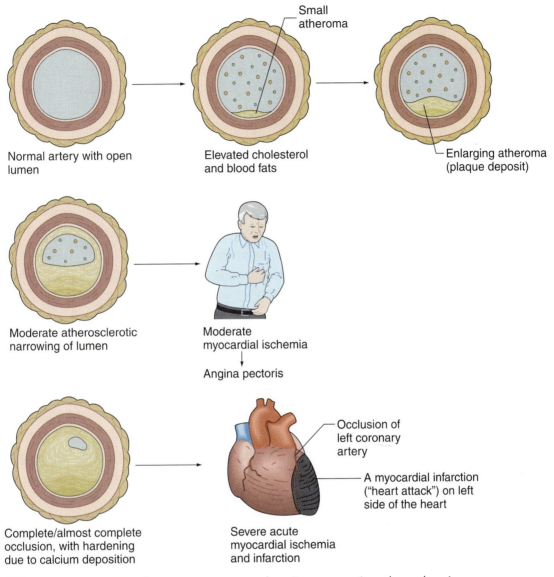

Normal artery with open lumen

Elevated cholesterol and blood fats

Small atheroma

Enlarging atheroma (plaque deposit)

Moderate atherosclerotic narrowing of lumen

Moderate myocardial ischemia

Angina pectoris

Complete/almost complete occlusion, with hardening due to calcium deposition

Severe acute myocardial ischemia and infarction

Occlusion of left coronary artery

A myocardial infarction ("heart attack") on left side of the heart

FIGURE 37-5 Cross-sections through a coronary artery undergoing progressive atherosclerosis

Refer to Figure 37-6.

The exact cause of this vascular disease is unknown, but several factors seem to increase the risk that a person will develop it. These factors include:

- Hypertension
- Diabetes mellitus
- Overweight
- Heredity
- Smoking
- Stress
- Lack of exercise
- Diets high in cholesterol and fats

Treatment includes:

- Exercise
- Proper diet
- Reduction of stress
- Control of smoking and obesity

Varicose Veins

The veins can also cause problems. **Varicose veins** form when the valves in the veins in the legs become weakened (Figure 37-7). This means:

- The blood does not flow through the veins as it should.
- The veins become distended and visible through the skin.
- The veins may become inflamed (**phlebitis**).
- A blood clot may form in the vein.

Report the following signs:

- Pain or aching in the legs
- Signs of inflammation (warmth and redness)

AFFECTED SITE   **COMPLICATION**

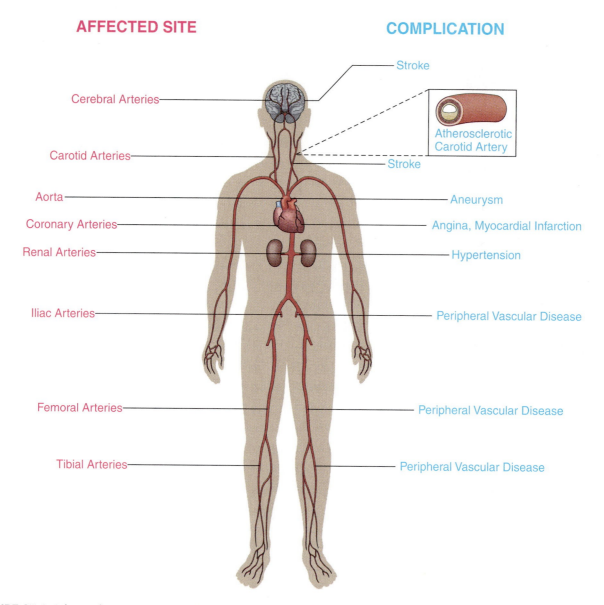

FIGURE 37-6 Atherosclerosis can cause disease in many parts of the body.

Remember that you *never* rub or massage the area of a varicose vein.

Transient Ischemic Attack

Transient ischemic attack (**TIA**) is a temporary interruption of the blood flow to part of the brain. The patient may experience:

- Weakness or paralysis of any extremity or the face
- Vision problems
- Difficulty with speech
- Difficulty with swallowing

These symptoms come on quickly and may last from just a few minutes to 24 hours. There are no permanent effects. However, a TIA is usually a warning that a brain attack will occur at some time. If a patient has any of the symptoms listed, report them to the nurse immediately.

Hypertension

Hypertension is another name for high blood pressure. It may have no known origin, or it may follow illnesses that affect such organs as the:

- Blood vessels
- Kidneys
- Liver

High blood pressure:

- Promotes the development of atherosclerosis, which further narrows the vessels. This increases the blood pressure even more.
- Increases the stress on the heart.
- Increases the damage to the blood vessel walls, so they are more apt to rupture.
- Further limits the blood flow to the organs of the body.

GUIDELINES *for*

Caring for Patients with Peripheral Vascular Disease

- Elevate the feet when the patient is sitting in a chair for a long time. When the feet are not elevated, make sure that the patient's feet are flat on the floor. If they are not, support the feet with a footstool. Discourage the patient from crossing the legs when sitting. Discourage the patient from using circular garters.

- Discourage smoking—it interferes with circulation.

- Avoid using the knee gatch of the bed.

- Avoid using heating pads or hot water bottles. The patient may not feel temperatures that are too hot.

- Maintain body warmth. Make sure the patient has warm clothes, including well-fitting socks. Provide blankets for the bed.

- Prevent injury to the feet:
  — Instruct the patient to wear shoes when out of bed.
  — Check to see that the shoes are in good repair and that they fit well.
  — Avoid pressure to the legs and feet from any source.

- Inspect the feet carefully when you bathe the patient or if the patient complains of any discomfort in the feet. Promptly report any signs of inflammation, injury, or circulatory problems:
  — Broken skin
  — Color change—redness, whiteness, or cyanosis
  — Heat or coldness
  — Cracking between toes
  — Corns or calluses
  — Swelling
  — Pain
  — Loss of function
  — Drainage

- Bathe the feet regularly.
  — Dry thoroughly and gently between the toes.
  — Use a moisturizing lotion on the feet and legs if the skin is dry.

- Do not cut the toenails of patients with peripheral vascular disease without instructions from the nurse.

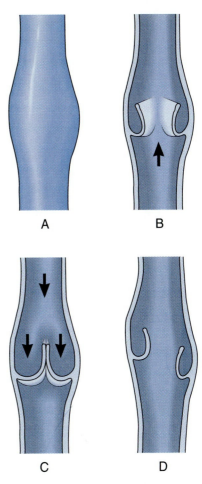

FIGURE 37-7 Veins contain valves to prevent the backward flow of blood. A. External view of the vein shows wider area of valve. B. Internal view with the valve open as blood flows through. C. Internal view with the valve closed. D. Vein with weakened valve causing a varicose vein.

Treatment may consist of:
- Drugs that lower the blood pressure
- Diet low in sodium
- Diet that promotes weight loss
- Regular exercise program
- Quitting smoking
- Surgical sympathectomy (a procedure in which the nerves that cause blood vessels to constrict are cut. When the nerves are cut, the blood vessels dilate.)
- Moderation in lifestyle
- Biofeedback techniques to lower the blood pressure

Report immediately any of the signs and symptoms of hypertension:
- Flushed face
- Dizziness
- Nosebleeds
- Headaches
- Changes in speech patterns
- Blurred vision

HEART CONDITIONS

Heart disease may sometimes be due to an infection, but most heart disease develops because of changes in the blood vessels. As the openings of the blood vessels become smaller, the heart must work harder and harder to do its job of pumping blood to the body.

Angina Pectoris

Angina pectoris is known as cardiac "pain of effort." You will recall that the blood vessels nourishing the heart are the coronary arteries. These vessels often are the site of atherosclerotic changes. In an angina attack, the vessels are unable to carry enough blood to meet the heart's demand for oxygen. This may develop:

- gradually over a period of time as atheromas develop.
- suddenly, as the vessels constrict.

Factors that precipitate (bring on) an attack include:

- Exertion
- Heavy eating
- Emotional stress

The signs and symptoms of angina pectoris that you should immediately report include:

- Pain when exercising or under stress. Stress causes a need for an immediate increase in coronary circulation. The pain is described as dull, with increasing intensity. It is usually centered under the breast bone (sternum), spreading to the left arm and up into the neck.
- Pale or flushed face.
- Patient who is freely perspiring.

Signs and symptoms may differ with individuals, but the symptoms are usually the same each time a person experiences an attack.

Treatment of angina pectoris consists of:

- Diagnosing hidden causes. A treadmill stress test is one method of doing this.
- Teaching the patient to avoid stress and sudden exertion.
- Drugs that relax the coronary arteries.
- Coronary artery bypass surgery.
- Angioplasty, a surgical procedure to open the vessels.

You may assist the patient who has angina pectoris by:

- helping the patient to avoid unnecessary emotional or physical stress.
- encouraging the patient not to smoke.
- reporting any signs or symptoms of an attack to the nurse at once.

Myocardial Infarction (Coronary Heart Attack)

The term myocardial infarction (MI), or heart attack, refers to a period in which the heart suddenly cannot function properly. There are different kinds of heart attacks.

They differ in their severity and prognosis (expected outcome). Remember that the heart is muscle tissue and may become tired just as any muscle may tire. The cells of the heart require nourishment and oxygen like all other cells.

An acute myocardial infarction occurs when the coronary arteries, which nourish the heart, are blocked. Part of the heart muscle supplied by these vessels becomes ischemic (loses its blood supply). Unless circulation is restored quickly, the cells die (infarction). If too much tissue dies, the person cannot survive. Coronary heart attack is also called:

- Coronary occlusion—blockage of coronary arteries
- Coronary thrombosis—when a thrombus (stationary blood clot) forms at the site, blocking the blood flow
- Coronary embolism—when a moving clot or insoluble particle (embolus), which originated elsewhere and has moved, becomes lodged in the artery

Signs and Symptoms.   The signs and symptoms of a heart attack include:

- Pain—may resemble severe indigestion. It is often described as "crushing" chest pain that radiates to the jaw and left arm (Figure 37-8).
- Nausea/vomiting.
- Irregular pulse and respiration.
- Perspiration (diaphoresis).
- Feelings of anxiety and weakness.
- Indications of shock, which include drop in blood pressure and pallor.
- Shortness of breath.
- Syncope (fainting).
- Restlessness.

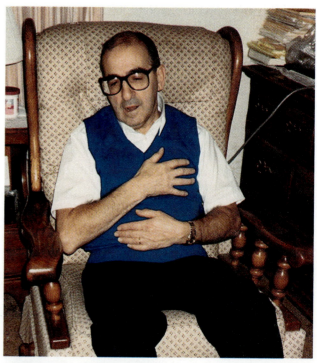

FIGURE 37-8 The patient having a heart attack often experiences crushing chest pain that radiates.

Immediate treatment has saved many people. The treatment is directed toward:

- Relieving the pain
- Reducing heart activity
- Altering the clotting ability of the blood
- Administering drugs to dissolve the clot

Nursing Care. During the acute stage, heart attack patients require professional care. Many hospitals provide intensive cardiac care units for these patients. Nursing care supports the therapy ordered. Special attention must be given to:

- Noting signs of a recurrence and reporting immediately to the nurse
- Watching for bleeding and reporting immediately
- Assisting with activities of daily living
- Monitoring vital signs

Congestive Heart Failure (CHF)

The heart, like any other muscle, will enlarge and tire if it has to work against increasing pressure. When blood vessels narrowed by atherosclerosis increase the resistance to blood flow, and when there is severe damage to major organs like the liver and spleen, it is more difficult to maintain the circulation. The heart muscle may also have been damaged and weakened by myocardial infarction. The heart must pump harder to maintain the internal flow of blood.

At first, the heart enlarges (**hypertrophy**) and makes up (**compensates**) for the additional workload. Eventually, however, it reaches a point when it can no longer compensate. Heart failure follows.

This form of heart disease is known as **congestive heart failure** (**CHF**) or **cardiac decompensation**.

Signs and Symptoms. The signs and symptoms are the result of the heart being unable to pump the blood with sufficient force.

- Hemoptysis (spitting up blood)
- Cough
- Dyspnea (difficulty breathing)
- **Orthopnea** (difficulty in breathing unless sitting upright)
- **Ascites** (fluid collecting in the abdomen)
- Neck vein swelling
- Fatiguing easily
- Hypoxia (inadequate oxygen levels)
- Confusion
- Edema (swelling), which develops in dependent tissues and slows blood flow, congesting the vessels and allowing more fluid to enter the body spaces and tissues
- Fluid accumulation in the lungs
- Cyanosis, which occurs because fluid in the lungs makes gas exchange less efficient
- Irregular and rapid pulse.

Treatment. Treatment involves:

- Drugs to help the heart beat more strongly and regularly and to increase the output of fluids (**diuresis**) by the kidneys.
- Low-sodium diet.
- Restriction of fluids, if ordered.
- Weighing patient daily to monitor level of fluid retention.
- Monitoring apical pulse and observing for pulse deficit (Figure 37-9).
- Positioning patient in orthopneic position or high Fowler's supported by pillows, or supported in a chair. The position must be changed frequently, but changes in position should be made slowly. Padded footboards help keep the weight of the bedding off the toes.
- Applying elasticized stockings or **TED hose**. TED hose are elastic anti-embolism stockings. TED hose and Ace bandages help channel blood to the deeper vessels. They must be checked often and reapplied every 6 to 8 hours. Check the extremities carefully for adequate circulation. The skin should be normal color and warm.
- Assisting with activities of daily living as needed.
- Attending to general hygiene. Complete bathing is tiring, but partial baths can stimulate circulation and provide comfort. Special attention must be given to the skin because the combination of position, edema, and poor circulation contributes to tissue breakdown.
- Assisting with oxygen therapy. Oxygen therapy may be provided either by face mask or nasal cannula. Because cardiac patients often breathe through the mouth, the mouth tends to be very dry. Special mouth care may be needed.
- Providing for elimination. A bedside commode is convenient. The use of a commode is less tiring for the patient than using a bedpan for elimination.

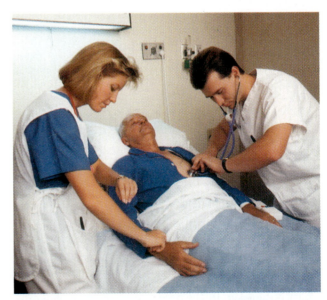

FIGURE 37-9 A pulse deficit may result from ineffective heart contractions.

- Encouraging adequate nutrition. Small, easily digested meals should be provided. You may need to assist in feeding the patient to prevent fatigue.
- Monitoring and recording fluid intake. Patients with acute heart failure may be given drugs that increase the output of urine and alter the heart rate. Measuring the intake and output and taking daily weights are ways of determining if fluid is being retained.
- Regularly checking vital signs. Sometimes the force of heart contraction, which propels the blood forward into the blood vessels, does not have enough strength to make the vessels expand.

Heart Block

Heart block is a condition that develops due to interference in the electrical current through the heart. (The flow of electrical current through the heart muscle makes the normal cardiac cycle possible.)

An electronic device called a pacemaker (Figure 37-10) is implanted under the chest muscles or in the abdomen. An electrode carries electrical current from the pacemaker directly into the heart muscle to replace the lost control. The

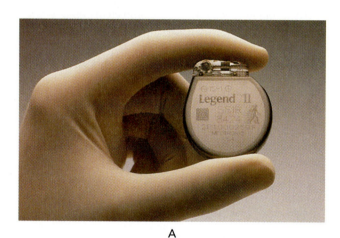

FIGURE 37-10 The electronic pacemaker sends electrical impulses to the heart muscle, causing it to contract. A. A typical pacemaker. B. The pacemaker is inserted under the skin with the electrode placed inside the heart, resting on the heart muscle. *Photo courtesy of Medtronic, Inc.*

electrical current signals the heart to contract. Some pacemakers send messages only if normal messages carried by the conduction system are delayed. This type of pacemaker is called a *demand pacemaker.* Other pacemakers send regular signals to keep the heart contracting at a preset rate.

When caring for a patient who has a pacemaker:

- count and record the pulse rate.
- report any irregularities or changes below the present rate.
- report any discoloration over the implant site.
- report hiccupping, because this may indicate problems.
- keep the patient away from microwave ovens and cellular phones, because they may disrupt the function of the pacemaker.

Patients usually function very well with pacemakers so long as they are adequately monitored.

BLOOD ABNORMALITIES

Blood abnormalities are often called *blood dyscrasias.*

Anemia

Anemia is a condition that results from a decrease in the quantity or quality of red blood cells. There are several causes, such as:

- Poor diet
- Low production of new red blood cells
- Blood loss, as in hemorrhage

Types of anemia include:

- Pernicious—inability to absorb vitamin B_{12} (most often seen in the elderly). Vitamin B_{12} is required by the body to produce red blood cells.
- Sickle cell—inability to form normal hemoglobin. Sickle cell anemia is transmitted genetically. It is seen most often in African Americans.
- Deficiency—inadequate intake of iron, inability to absorb iron, or excessive loss of iron.
- Dietary—inadequate intake of iron or vitamins in diet.

Signs and Symptoms. The person with anemia may:

- have little energy.
- be pale or jaundiced.
- have dyspnea.
- experience digestive problems.
- have a rapid pulse.
- complain of light-headedness.
- feel cold.
- experience dizziness.
- have an increased respiratory rate.

Treatment. Treatment is aimed at:

- Improving the quantity and quality of the blood by giving iron supplements
- Eliminating the basic cause of the disease
- Giving blood transfusions as needed

Leukemia

Leukemia is sometimes called cancer of the blood. The causes of the many forms of leukemia are not known. This disease may strike young or old. The number of white blood cells increases, but the white blood cells may be of poor quality. The number of erythrocytes and platelets decreases. Patients with leukemia are highly susceptible to infection. During the course of the disease, even minor trauma causes bleeding.

Treatment. Treatment is aimed at:

- Easing symptoms and keeping the patient comfortable.
- Maintaining normal blood levels. Transfusions may be needed to combat the anemia that accompanies the condition.
- Combating infection by using antibiotics.
- Slowing the production of abnormal white cells through chemotherapy and/or radiation therapy.

Special Care

Patients who have cancer or anemia require special care. You must:

- Check vital signs
- Encourage rest and a good diet
- Handle the patient very gently
- Give special mouth care, because the mouth and tongue become sensitive
- Be sure to report any signs of bleeding, such as bruises or discolorations, because further blood loss makes the condition worse
- Keep patient warm
- Protect patient from falls that may result from dizziness or weakness
- Change the patient's position often, at least every two hours
- Provide emotional support

DIAGNOSTIC TESTS

Some techniques used to diagnose problems of the cardiovascular system include:

- Blood chemistry tests, such as electrolyte panels
- Complete blood cell count (CBC)
- Electrocardiogram (ECG or EKG)
- Cardiac catheterization and angiogram—introduction of catheter and dyes into the vascular system under fluoroscopy
- Ultrasound—sound waves are bounced against tissues to reflect variations in tissue density

REVIEW

A. True/False.

Mark the following true or false by circling T or F.

1. T F The person with atherosclerosis is encouraged to smoke.
2. T F The treadmill test is done to detect hidden cardiac stress.
3. T F When warmth is needed by someone with peripheral vascular disease, a heating pad should not be used.
4. T F Another name for a heart attack is coronary infarction.
5. T F In leukemia, there is an increase in white cells.
6. T F The heart muscle shrinks as it undergoes hypertrophy.
7. T F An embolus is a moving blood clot.
8. T F Anemia is an example of a blood dyscrasia.
9. T F Hypertension is best treated with a high-sodium diet.
10. T F The person with CHF should be monitored for pulse deficit.

B. Matching.

Choose the correct word from Column II to match each phrase in Column I.

Column I	Column II
11. ____ largest artery in the body	a. hypertension
12. ____ death of the heart muscle	b. edema
13. ____ another term for stroke	c. myocardial infarction
14. ____ high blood pressure	d. plasma
15. ____ blocking of the blood supply to the heart	e. aorta
	f. CVA
	g. hypotension
	h. coronary occlusion

C. Multiple Choice.

Select the one best answer for each question.

16. Which of the following is not a predisposing cause of atherosclerosis?
    a. Emboli
    b. Diabetes mellitus
    c. Heredity
    d. Stress

17. You suspect the patient needs immediate attention for a possible heart attack because the person
 a. has chest pain.
 b. is perspiring profusely.
 c. feels anxious.
 d. all of these.

18. Nursing care of the patient with anemia might include
 a. blood letting.
 b. transfusions.
 c. frequent checking of vital signs.
 d. both b and c.

19. The patient with anemia has a
 a. high energy level.
 b. pink, rosy skin.
 c. low energy level.
 d. slower than normal respiratory rate.

20. An attack of angina pectoris could be brought about by
 a. heavy meals.
 b. physical exertion.
 c. emotional stress.
 d. all of these.

D. Completion.

Complete the statements in the spaces provided.

21. Five specific tests used to diagnose cardiac, vascular, or blood abnormalities are:
 a. ____   **d.** ____
 b. ____   **e.** ____
 c. ____

22. Six predisposing factors for atherosclerosis are:
 a. ____   **d.** ____
 b. ____   **e.** ____
 c. ____   **f.** ____

E. Nursing Assistant Challenge.

Mrs. O'Brien is only 38 years old, but has been diagnosed with hypertension. Recently she experienced dizziness and weakness and had difficulty speaking for a short period. The doctor suspects she had a TIA. Complete the statements in questions 23–30 by choosing the correct word from the following list.

> blurred vision
> brain
> discouraged
> encouraged
> exercise
> high
> hypertension
> low
> permanent
> potassium
> sodium
> stroke
> temporary

23. Hypertension means this patient has ____ blood pressure.

24. The TIA means there was a ____ interruption of the blood flow to the ____.

25. The diet for this patient should be low in ____.

26. Smoking should be ____.

27. The TIA indicates that a ____ will probably occur at some time.

28. Treatment for hypertension includes regular ____.

29. ____ is a sign that should be reported immediately.

30. Nosebleeds are a danger sign for people with ____.

Musculoskeletal System

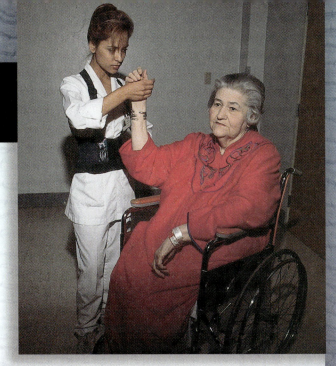

As a result of this unit, you will be able to:

- Spell and define terms.
- Describe the location and functions of the musculoskeletal system.
- Describe some common conditions of the musculoskeletal system.
- Describe the nursing assistant actions related to the care of patients with conditions and diseases of the musculoskeletal system.
- List seven specific diagnostic tests for musculoskeletal conditions.
- Demonstrate the following procedure:
  - Procedure 94 Performing Range-of-Motion Exercises (Passive)

VOCABULARY

Learn the meaning and the correct spelling of the following words and phrases:

abduction
adduction
amputation
arthritis
bursae
bursitis
cardiac muscle
cartilage
cervical traction
chymopapain
closed (oblique) fracture
comminuted fracture
compound (open)
  fracture
compression fracture

countertraction
degenerative joint
  disease (DJD)
dorsiflexion
eversion
extension
flexion
fracture
fusion
greenstick fracture
insertion
inversion
involuntary muscle
laminectomy
ligament

oblique (closed) fracture
open (compound)
  fracture
open reduction/internal
  fixation
origin
osteoarthritic joint
  disease (OJD)
pelvic belt traction
phantom pain
plantar flexion
pronation
radial deviation
range of motion
  (ROM)

rheumatoid arthritis
rotation
spica cast
stimulus
supination
tendon
total hip arthroplasty
  (THA)
trapeze
ulnar deviation
vertebrae
visceral muscle
voluntary muscle

THE MUSCULOSKELETAL SYSTEM

The bony frame of the body is called the skeleton. Tissue that is made up of contractile fibers (fibers that contract and relax) or cells that produce movement are called muscles. Together, the skeleton and muscles are termed the musculoskeletal system.

The musculoskeletal system includes:

- Skeletal muscles
- Bones
- Joints
- Tendons
- Ligaments

The system functions to:

- Give shape and form to the body
- Protect and support delicate body parts
- Permit movement
- Produce some blood cells
- Store calcium and phosphorus

When muscles, bones, or joints have been injured, a long period of rest and inactivity may be required for the part to heal. During this period, it is important that all other moving parts get sufficient exercise. Bones that are not stressed lose calcium and become less functional.

Structure and Function

Bones. It will be helpful for you to learn the names and general location of the bones of the body. To learn the names, study the skeleton in Figure 38-1A and the skull in Figure 38-1B. Note that the same number and kinds of bones are found on one side of the midline as on the other.

The bones:

- Number 206
- May share the same name. For example, there are:
  - 24 ribs helping to form the chest
  - 56 phalanges, the finger bones
  - 2 femurs, the thigh bones
  - 31 bones (**vertebrae**) in the spinal column. Small discs or pads of **cartilage** with soft, gel-like centers between the vertebrae help to cushion these bones. The anterior (front) of the vertebrae support the head and body. The posterior (rear) portions form a tunnel that surrounds the delicate spinal cord and nerves.
- Are of different shapes and sizes, such as
  - long, like the femur, humerus, ulna, and radius

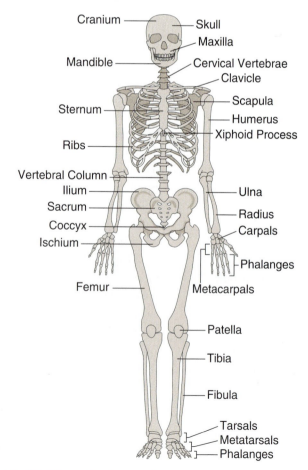

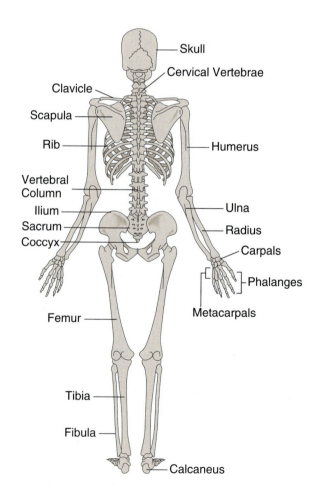

FIGURE 38-1A The human skeleton

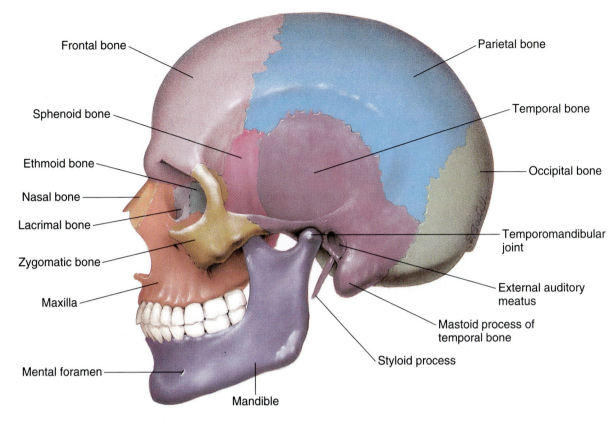

FIGURE 38-1B Bones of the skull

- short, like the phalanges, carpals, and tarsals
- flat, like the scapula and cranial bones
- irregular, like the vertebrae and mandible
● Meet one another to form joints

Joints. Joints are points where bones come together and there is the possibility of movement. Without movable joints, walking, bending, lifting, and sitting would not be possible. Joints are capable of different movements depending upon the type of joint (Figure 38-2). **Ligaments** are strong bands of fibrous tissues that hold the bones together and support the joints. **Bursae** are small sacs of synovial fluid that are located around joints and help reduce friction.

Special terms are used to describe the different movements in a diarthrotic joint.

● **Flexion:** Decreasing the angle between two bones (Figure 38-3A). For example, bending the elbow.

● **Extension:** Increasing the angle between two bones (Figure 38-3B). For example, straightening the elbow.

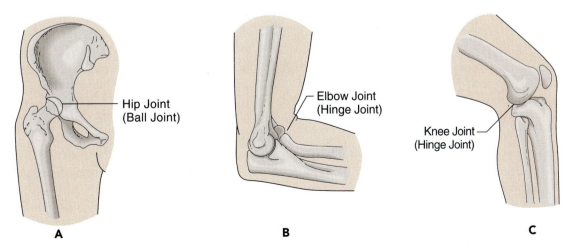

FIGURE 38-2 Types of joints: A. Ball joint. B. and C. Hinge joints

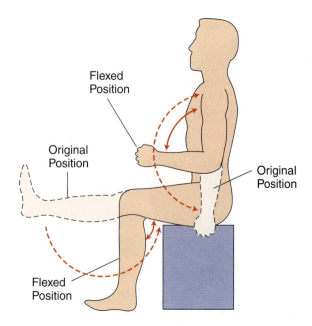

FIGURE 38-3A Flexion—bending a joint

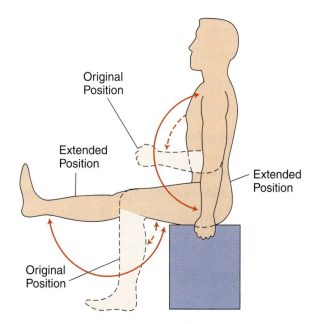

FIGURE 38-3B Extension—straightening a joint

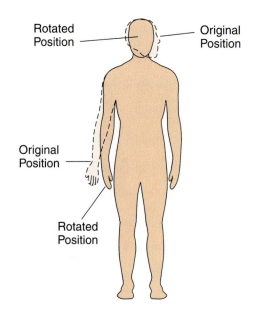

FIGURE 38-3C Rotation—circular motion in a joint

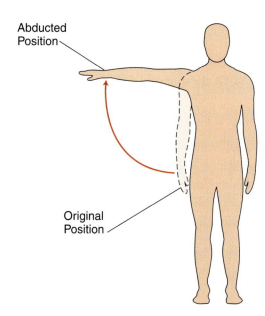

FIGURE 38-3D Abduction—moving an extremity away from the body

- **Rotation:** Circular motion in a ball-and-socket joint (Figure 38-3C). For example, the shoulder and hip joints, which can move in all directions.
- **Abduction:** Moving away from the midline (Figure 38-3D).
- **Adduction:** Moving toward the midline (Figure 38-3E).

Muscles. There are more than 500 muscles in the body (Figures 38-4A and B). The muscles work in groups. There are three kinds of muscles:

1. **Cardiac muscle** forms the wall of the heart.
2. **Voluntary muscles** are skeletal muscles that are attached to bones. When we wish to pick up some-

thing, for instance, we can make our muscles contract and perform the necessary movements.

3. **Involuntary** or **visceral muscles** form the walls of organs. These muscles operate without our conscious control.

Muscles receive their names in three ways:

1. Their location. For example, rectus femoris near the femur
2. Their shape. For example, trapezius—trapezoidal shape
3. Their action. For example, flexors—bring about flexion

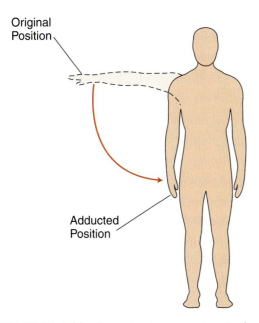

FIGURE 38-3E Adduction—moving an extremity back to the body

You can easily locate the major muscle groups responsible for an activity if you remember that:

- Muscles can only shorten (contract) and lengthen (relax). Contraction occurs when nerves bring the message (**stimulus**) to the muscle cells. Muscles relax when there is no stimulus.
- Muscles have two points of attachment to the bone. As they stretch from one point (**origin**) to the other (**insertion**), they cross over one or more joints.
- Muscles are not inserted directly into bones. Rather, they are connected to the bone by strong, fibrous bands of connective tissues called **tendons**. Ligaments support bones at joints.
- As muscles contract, they shorten, pulling their points of origin and insertion closer together. For example, bending the forearm at the elbow takes place when the biceps muscle contracts. The biceps muscle is on the anterior arm and extends from the shoulder to below the elbow. At the same time, the triceps muscle relaxes. This muscle is attached to the posterior shoulder and to the arm below the elbow. To straighten the arm at the elbow, the triceps contracts and the biceps relaxes.

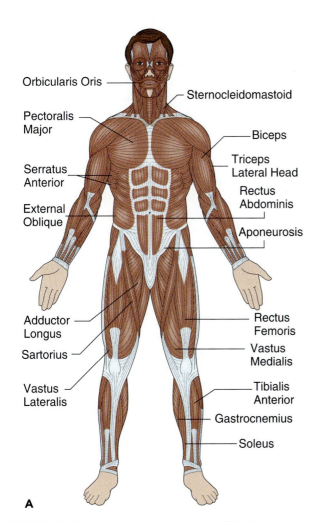

A

FIGURE 38-4A Major skeletal muscles of the body—anterior view

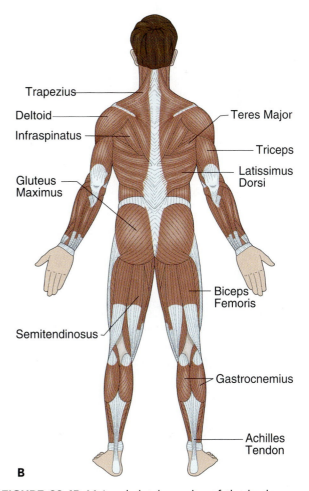

B

FIGURE 38-4B Major skeletal muscles of the body—posterior view

- The more muscles are used, the more powerful they become. The less muscles are used, the weaker they become.

COMMON CONDITIONS

There are many conditions that can affect the bones, muscles, tendons, ligaments, and joints. Often, when one of these structures is diseased or injured, the surrounding tissues are also involved.

Bursitis

Bursae are small sacs of fluid found around joints. They help to reduce friction when muscles move. At times, the bursae can become inflamed and the tissues around a joint may become painful. This condition is known as **bursitis**. Treatment of bursitis includes:

- Applications of heat to promote healing
- Immobilization so that the joint cannot move, to relieve pain around the joint
- Removal of excess fluid from the joint by aspiration with a needle
- Administration of steroids

Arthritis

The term **arthritis** (Figure 38-5) means inflammation of the joints. It may develop following an acute injury, or it may be chronic and progressive. There are two forms of chronic arthritis:

1. **Rheumatoid arthritis** affects the joint tissues and the joint lining, and can affect any other body system. It is a serious form of arthritis that can occur in persons of any age. The cause is not specifically known. It is believed to be an autoimmune response.

2. **Osteoarthritic joint disease** (**OJD**) or **degenerative joint disease** (**DJD**) affects the cartilage covering the ends of the bones which form a joint. Cartilage breaks

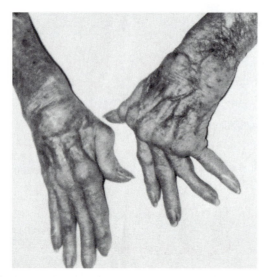

FIGURE 38-5 Joint deformities as a result of rheumatoid arthritis

down and the ends of the bones rub together, causing pain and deformity. The joints most often affected are the weight-bearing joints. Several factors seem to contribute to the disease process, including:

- Aging
- Trauma
- Obesity

Treatment of arthritis includes:

- Balance of rest and exercise
- Joint immobilization where there is pain
- Weight control to relieve pressure on the joints
- Medication to relieve pain and reduce the inflammation
- Physical therapy when inflammation subsides, to maintain joint mobility
- Replacement of badly damaged joints by surgery
- Use of adaptive equipment to enable the patient to get the most range of motion from injured joints
- Exercise of arthritic joints in warm water (with or without whirlpool action)

Fractures

A **fracture** is any break in the continuity of a bone. Falls are the most common cause of fractures. If the bone breaks through the skin, the injury is called an *open compound fracture.* If the bones do not break through the skin, the fracture is known as *closed.* There are several kinds of fractures (Figure 38-6).

- **Closed** or **oblique fractures**—those in which the bones remain in proper position (alignment).
- **Greenstick fractures**—in which the bone is not broken completely through. This is typical of fractures in young children. Children's bones are flexible because their growth is incomplete. Their bones tend to bend like young tree limbs, breaking on one side only. This gives rise to the name "greenstick."
- **Compression fractures**—seen in spongy bone such as the vertebral bodies. The bone is compressed or crushed.
- **Comminuted fractures**—result in a bone that is fragmented or splintered into more than two pieces.
- **Open** (**compound**) **fractures**—bone is broken and skin is open. The bone may poke through the open skin.

Treatment. Fractures of any kind are treated by keeping the part that is injured immobilized in proper position until healing takes place. Injured bones take from several weeks to several months to heal. Immobilization is achieved through the use of:

- Pins (Figure 38-7)
- Screws
- Bone plates
- Casting
- Traction

Special beds and attachments are used to make nursing care easier. The patient may be placed on a Stryker frame or the CircOlectric® bed.

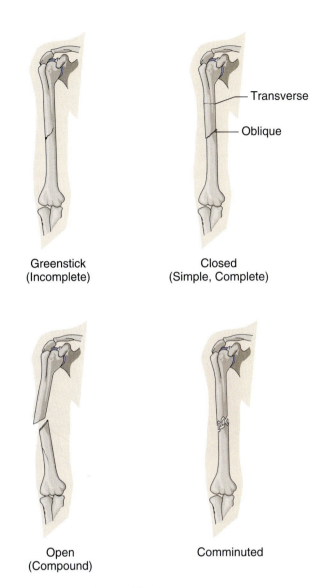

Greenstick
(Incomplete)

Closed
(Simple, Complete)

— Transverse

— Oblique

Open
(Compound)

Comminuted

FIGURE 38-6 Types of fractures

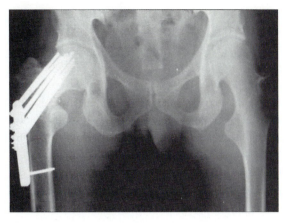

FIGURE 38-7 Fractured bones are held in place with plates, pins, and screws.

- Closely observing the uncasted areas of the extremities, such as the fingers and toes, for signs of decreased circulation. Report coldness, cyanosis, swelling, increased pain, or numbness immediately.
- Closely observing skin areas around the cast edges for signs of irritation (Figure 38-8). Rough edges should be covered with adhesive strips to prevent skin irritation.

Recall the following key of reportables when checking the patient:

- C = color
- M = motion
- E = edema
- T = temperature

Special Care After Cast Is Dry. After the cast has completely dried:

- Turn the patient to the noncasted side. This is particularly important in moving a patient with a body cast (**spica cast**) because turning to the casted side may crack the cast.
- Always support the cast when turning or moving a patient.

Be sure you know how to operate each bed and attachment before attempting care. In many facilities, an RN must be present when the bed is turned. Know and follow the policy of your facility.

Care of Patients with Casts. Two types of cast materials are commonly used:

1. Plaster of Paris, which can take up to 48 hours to dry completely
2. Fiberglass, which dries very rapidly

Cast material is wet when it is applied. During the drying period, the cast gives off heat. Special care for the newly casted patient includes:

- Supporting the cast and body in good alignment with pillows covered by cloth pillowcases, and keeping the cast uncovered.
- Turning the patient frequently to permit air circulation to all parts of the cast. Maintain support. Use palm of hand, not fingers, to support the wet cast.

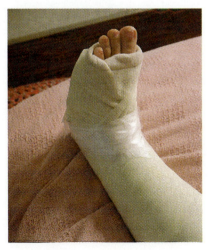

FIGURE 38-8 Carefully and frequently check skin areas around the edges of the cast for signs of irritation.

- Encourage use of an overhead bar, known as a **trapeze**, to assist the patient in helping herself (Figure 38-9).
- Tape edges of casts to prevent pressure and abrasive areas, if edges were not covered when the cast was applied.
- Use plastic to protect cast edges that are near the genitals and buttocks, to help prevent soiling during toileting.

Care of Patients in Traction. Traction is designed to pull two body areas slightly apart to:

- relieve pressure.
- help tightly contracted (spasmodic) muscles relax.
- keep them in proper position as healing takes place.

Traction is of two types:

- Skin traction, where traction is applied to the skin or outside of the body (Figure 38-10)
- Skeletal traction, where traction is applied through the skin to the bone

Traction is applied by attaching weights to a part of the body above or below the area to be treated. The patient's body weight serves as **countertraction** by pulling in the direction opposite to the traction. Belts, head halters, or tapes may be applied to the patient's skin to hold the traction. Traction may be applied continuously or intermittently.

Skeletal traction (Figure 38-11) uses tongs or pins placed into bones with weights applied to the tongs or pins. Skeletal traction is always continuous once applied. The weights for skeletal traction must not be lifted or removed until the traction is to be discontinued.

When patients are in traction:

- Do not disturb the weights or permit them to swing, drop, or rest on any surface.
- Keep the patient in good alignment. Make sure that the body is acting properly as countertraction by keeping the head of the bed low.

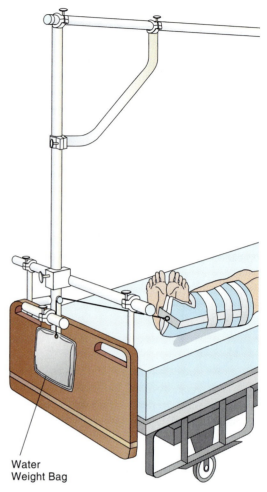

Water
Weight Bag

FIGURE 38-10 Buck's traction is an example of skin traction sometimes used for a fractured hip.

- Check under head halters or pelvic belts for areas of pressure or irritation.
- Make sure straps of halters and belts are smooth, straight, and properly secured.
- Keep bed covers off ropes and pulleys.

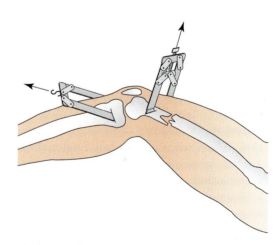

FIGURE 38-11 Skeletal traction immobilizes a body part by attaching weights directly to the patient's bones with pins, screws, wires, or tongs.

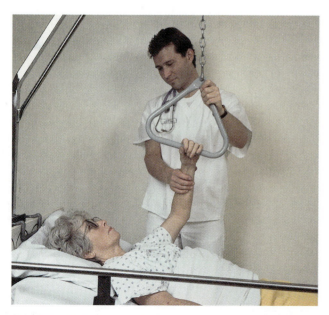

FIGURE 38-9 The overhead trapeze greatly assists in patient care.

Not all patients remain in traction continually. If **pelvic belt traction** (Figure 38-12), or **cervical traction** with a head halter (Figure 38-13), is to be discontinued, take the following steps:

● Slowly raise the weights to the bed. Avoid abrupt or jerking movements, as this may cause the patient pain. If two sets of weights are being used, raise them at the same time and rate.

● Remove the weight holder and weights from the connection with the halter or belt and place them on the floor. Remove the head halter or pelvic belt.

● To reapply traction, reverse the procedure.

● Remember never to jerk or drop the weights quickly or lower them unevenly. Always apply weights smoothly to avoid causing the patient pain.

Bedmaking. Bedmaking for orthopedic patients varies according to the type of traction.

● Two half sheets are often used in place of a large sheet for the bottom.

● Bottom linens may be changed from top to bottom rather than side to side.

● The top linen is arranged according to the patient's special needs. Half sheets and folded bath blankets can be worked around the traction to keep the patient covered and comfortable.

Fractured Hip

It is common to have patients in your care who have fractured hips. Elderly people are especially at risk for falling and breaking their hips. The fracture may be repaired through a surgical procedure called **open reduction/internal fixation**. This means the surgeon makes an incision, manipulates the fractured bone into alignment, and then inserts a device such as a nail, pin, or rod to hold the ends of the fractured bone in place. If you are assigned to a patient who has had this surgery, you must:

● Know how to position the patient in bed. It is important to avoid adduction and internal and external rotation of the affected hip.

● Know the correct procedure if the patient is allowed to

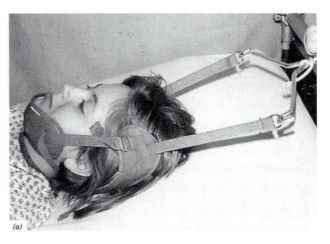

FIGURE 38-13 Cervical traction. *Photo courtesy of Leona A. Mourad*

ambulate. The patient is usually not allowed to bear weight on the affected side for a few weeks after surgery.

Total Hip Arthroplasty. **Total hip arthroplasty** (**THA**), or insertion of a hip prosthesis (artificial body part), is a common procedure. This surgery is done because the patient:

● has fractured a hip and the bone cannot be set by traditional methods, or

● has degenerative arthritis that has caused the hip joint to deteriorate

The patient's hip joint is surgically removed and a metal and plastic ball and socket are inserted (Figure 38-14). There are specific body positions that the patient must avoid to prevent damage to the new joint.

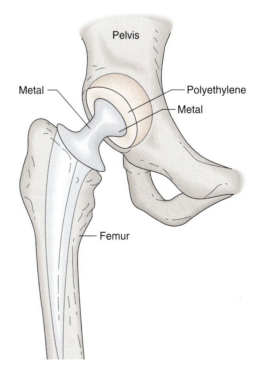

Pelvis

Metal — — Polyethylene

— Metal

— Femur

FIGURE 38-14 Hip prosthesis (total hip arthroplasty) replaces the ball of the femur and the socket.

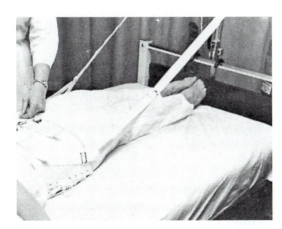

FIGURE 38-12 Pelvic belt traction

GUIDELINES *for*

Caring for Patients with THA

The patient should **not**:

- Flex the hip more than 90 degrees (Figure 38-15A).
- Cross the affected leg over the midline of the body, whether in bed or sitting in a chair (Figure 38-15B).
- Internally rotate the hip on the affected side (Figure 38-15C).

Never do passive range-of-motion exercises on a joint that has had surgery, unless you are specifically instructed to do so—and then only if you have been given instructions as to which actions can safely be performed.

The patient will have limited weight bearing on the affected leg for several days or weeks after surgery.

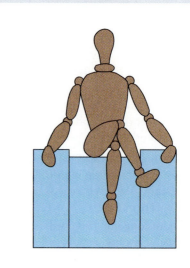

FIGURE 38-15B The patient with a new hip prosthesis should never cross the affected leg over the midline of the body.

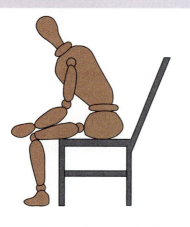

FIGURE 38-15A The patient with a new hip prosthesis should never flex the affected hip more than 90 degrees.

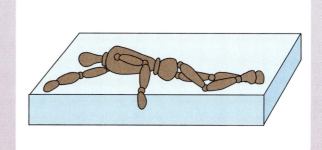

FIGURE 38-15C The patient with a new hip prosthesis should never internally rotate the hip on the affected side.

Ruptured or Slipped Disc

It is possible for a disc to bulge (slip) out of place or for the soft center to rupture. In either case, pressure is placed on the spinal nerves (Figure 38-16). Depending on which disc is injured, the patient may experience, in different parts of the body:

- Pain
- Numbness
- Tingling
- Weakness of one or more muscles

Treatment. Treatment attempts to relieve pressure on the nerve roots. Three techniques are employed:

1. Traction.

2. Surgery to remove the protruding portion of the disc (**laminectomy**). The surgery sometimes includes a fixation (**fusion**) of the vertebral bones.

3. Injections of an enzyme called **chymopapain**. The enzyme, which dissolves the herniated material, is injected into the ruptured disc area while the patient is in the operating room. When the patient returns from surgery, he is given routine postoperative follow-up. The major side effect is the possibility of an anaphylactic reaction (severe hypersensitivity reaction). Because this usually occurs rather rapidly after injection, you would probably not witness it, as the patient would still be in surgery or recovery. However, the reaction can occur several weeks later. Some patients need further surgery to remove disc pieces to relieve pain.

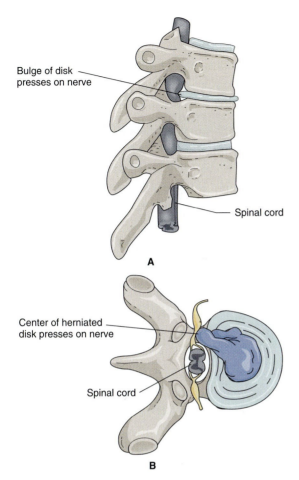

Bulge of disk presses on nerve

Spinal cord

A

Center of herniated disk presses on nerve

Spinal cord

B

FIGURE 38-16 A. Uneven pressure causes the disc to bulge, putting pressure on the nerve root (slipped disc). B. A herniated (ruptured) disc puts pressure on the nerve root as its gel-like center oozes backward.

Lower Extremity Amputation

You may care for patients who have had one or both legs surgically removed (amputated). A leg may have to undergo **amputation** because of circulatory problems, a malignancy, or an accident in which the leg was severely damaged.

It is common for people to experience **phantom pain** after the removal of a limb. Patients with phantom pain may feel pain or tingling where the limb used to be. These feelings may persist for months. The pain is real, although it is difficult to explain.

When you are positioning a patient who has had an amputation of the lower extremities, remember:

- Avoid abduction and flexion of the patient's hip—because the weight of the lower leg is not there, the hip on the affected side will quickly become contracted if flexion is allowed.

- If the patient has a below-the-knee amputation (BKA), avoid flexion of the knee so that a contracture does not form.

After the surgery, the patient will either have the stump wrapped with elastic bandage or will wear a stump shrinker. It is important that these be on at all times except during the bath. It is the nurse's responsibility to apply either of these

items. If you notice that the bandage or shrinker is loose or needs to be reapplied, notify the nurse. The purpose of these items is to make sure that the stump heals in the appropriate shape.

If you bathe a patient with an amputation:

- Gently wash the stump with soap and warm water, rinse well, and pat dry.

- Observe the stump for:
  - redness
  - swelling
  - drainage from the incision
  - open areas in the incision or anywhere else on the stump.

After an amputation, some patients are fitted with an artificial leg (prosthesis). They have to learn how to walk and sit when the prosthesis is worn. A prosthesis is custom-made for the person who will be wearing it. A special health care professional measures the patient and makes the prosthesis. The physical therapist teaches the patient how to apply the prosthesis and how to use it. If you are responsible for helping a patient put on a prosthesis, be sure you know how to attach and secure it, because each device is different.

Various types of materials are used to make prostheses. They need to be cleaned regularly, and the method of cleaning depends on what materials were used to make the prosthesis.

RANGE OF MOTION

To remain healthy, the musculoskeletal system must be exercised. When exercises are not carried out:

- joints become stiff and deformities (contractures) can develop.

- muscles atrophy (shrink) and lose strength.

- bones lose minerals.

- general body circulation is slowed.

Range-of-motion (**ROM**) exercises are routinely carried out by the patient (active) or the staff (passive) to avoid these complications.

The nurse will instruct you as to the type or limitation of range-of-motion exercises to be done. These exercises are usually done during or after the bath and before the bed is made. They may be carried out at other times as well.

When you are assigned to carry out ROM:

- Check with the nurse for specific instructions or limitations.

- Never exercise a joint to the point of pain.

- Perform each exercise five times, or more if ordered.

- Stop the exercise if pain or discomfort develops, and report to the nurse.

- Support each joint above and below the joint being exercised. Provide support *at* the joints to prevent pressure on the muscles.

- Note that special corrective exercises are performed by the physical therapist.

PROCEDURE   94   OBRA

PERFORMING RANGE-OF-MOTION EXERCISES (PASSIVE)

Note: *This procedure may be carried out as an independent procedure or as part of the bath. Repeat each action five times. ROM is described here as an independent procedure.*

Caution: *Passive range of motion that involves the neck is usually carried out by a physical therapist or a registered nurse. Patients who can exercise this area themselves are encouraged to do so. Check your facility policy regarding ROM neck exercises.*

1. Carry out each beginning procedure action.

2. Assemble equipment:
   - bath blanket

3. Position patient on back close to you.

4. Adjust the bath blanket to keep patient covered as much as possible.

5. Supporting the elbow and wrist, exercise shoulder joint nearest you as follows:

   a. Bring the entire arm out at right angle to the body (horizontal abduction) (Figures 38-17A and B).

   b. Return the arm to a position parallel to the body (horizontal adduction).

6. a. With arm parallel to the body, roll entire arm toward body (internal rotation of shoulder).

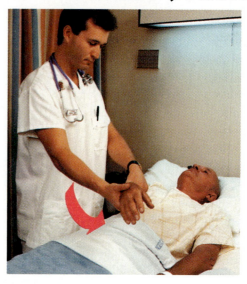

FIGURE 38-17B Return the arm to the side of the body.

   b. Maintaining the parallel position, roll entire arm away from body (external rotation of shoulder).

7. With shoulder in abduction, flex elbow and raise entire arm over head (shoulder flexion) (Figure 38-18).

8. With arm parallel to body (palm up—**supination**), flex and extend elbow (Figures 38-19A and B).

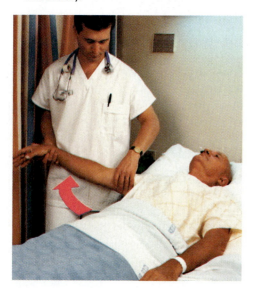

FIGURE 38-17A Shoulder abduction and adduction. Supporting the elbow and wrist, bring the entire arm out at a right angle from the body.

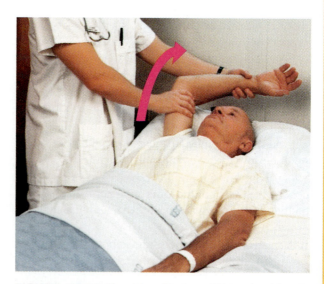

FIGURE 38-18 Shoulder flexion. With shoulder in abduction, flex elbow and raise entire arm over head.

continues

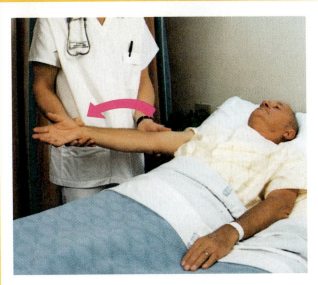

FIGURE 38-19A Elbow extension and flexion. Supporting the upper arm and wrist, straighten elbow.

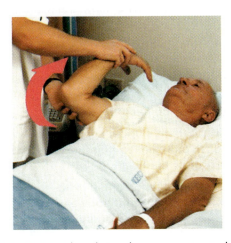

FIGURE 38-19B Then bring lower arm toward upper arm.

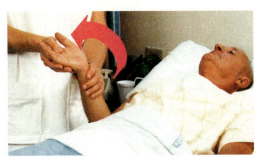

FIGURE 38-20A Wrist extension and flexion. Supporting arm above wrist and hand, straighten wrist.

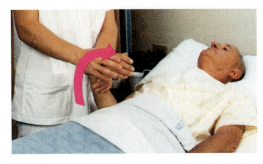

FIGURE 38-20B Place hand over patient's hand while supporting wrist and bend wrist.

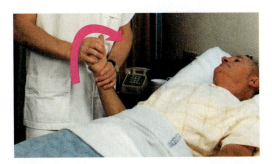

FIGURE 38-21A Finger flexion. Supporting wrist with one hand, cover patient's fingers and curl them to make a fist.

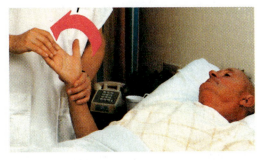

FIGURE 38-21B Finger extension. Slip your fingers over patient's flexed fingers and straighten fingers.

9. Flex and extend wrist (Figures 38-20A and B). Flex and extend each finger joint (Figures 38-21A and B).

10. Move each finger, in turn, away from the middle finger (abduction) (Figure 38-22A) and toward the middle finger (adduction) (Figure 38-22B).

11. Abduct the thumb by moving it toward the extended fingers (Figure 38-23).

12. Touch the thumb to the base of the little finger, then to each fingertip (opposition) (Figure 38-24).

continues

PROCEDURE **94** *continued*

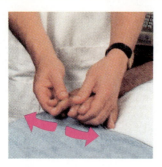

FIGURE 38-22A Abduction of the fingers

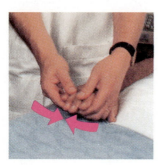

FIGURE 38-22B Adduction of the fingers

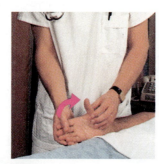

FIGURE 38-23 Abduction and adduction of thumb and fingers. Supporting the hand, draw the thumb toward and away from the extended fingers.

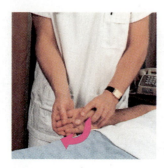

FIGURE 38-24 Thumb opposition. Supporting the hand, touch each finger with the thumb.

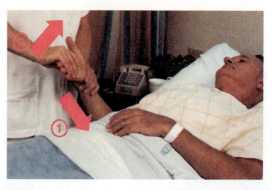

FIGURE 38-25 Wrist inversion (supination) and eversion (pronation). Grasp patient's wrist with one hand and patient's hand with the other and bring wrist toward body and then away from body.

13. Turn hand palm down(**pronation**), then palm up (supination).

14. Grasp patient's wrist with one hand and patient's hand with the other. Bring wrist toward body (**inversion**) and then away from the body (**eversion**) (Figure 38-25).

15. Point hand in supination toward thumb side (**radial deviation**), then toward little-finger side (**ulnar deviation**).

16. Cover patient's upper extremities and body. Expose only the leg being exercised. Face the foot of the bed.

17. Supporting the knee and ankle, move the entire leg away from body center (abduction) and toward the body (adduction) (Figures 38-26A and B).

18. Turn to face bed. Supporting the knee in bent position (flexion), raise the knee toward

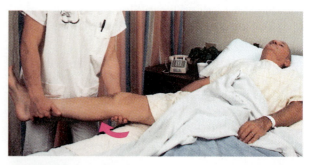

FIGURE 38-26A Abduction of the hip. Supporting patient's knee and ankle, move entire leg away from body center.

continues

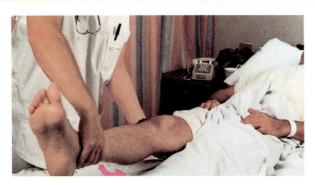

FIGURE 38-26B Adduction of the hip. Supporting leg, return toward center of body.

the pelvis (hip flexion) (Figure 38-27). Straighten the knee (extension) (Figure 38-28), as you lower the leg to the bed.

19. a. Supporting leg at knee and ankle, roll leg in a circular fashion away from body (lateral hip rotation).

b. Continuing to support leg, roll leg in the same fashion toward the body (medial hip rotation).

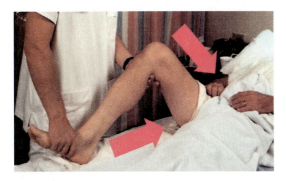

FIGURE 38-27 Hip and knee flexion. Supporting leg, return toward center of body.

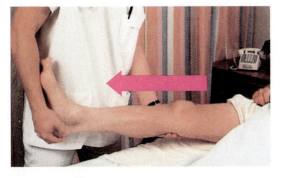

FIGURE 38-28 Knee extension. Supporting knee and ankle, straighten knee.

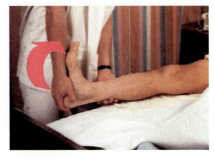

FIGURE 38-29A Ankle flexion. Grasp the patient's heel with one hand using your upper arm to support the foot. Dorsiflex the ankle by bringing the toes and foot toward the knee.

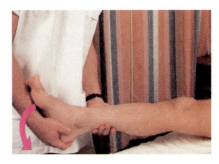

FIGURE 38-29B Plantar flex the ankle by drawing the foot in a downward position.

20. Grasp patient's toes and support ankle. Bring toes toward the knee (dorsiflexion) (Figure 38-29A). Then point toes toward the foot of the bed (plantar flexion) (Figure 38-29B).

Note: The patient may be more comfortable if the knee is slightly flexed during this motion.

21. Gently turn patient's foot inward (inversion) (Figure 38-30) and outward (eversion) (Figure 38-31).

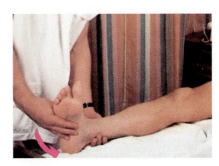

FIGURE 38-30 Foot inversion. Grasp patient's foot and gently turn it inward.

continues

PROCEDURE **94** *continued*

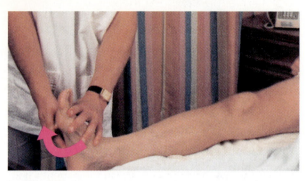

FIGURE 38-31 Foot eversion. Grasp patient's foot and gently turn it outward.

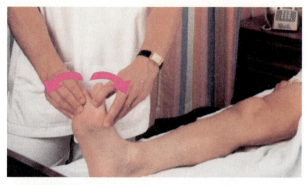

FIGURE 38-32A Toe abduction. Move each toe away from the second toe one at a time.

22. Place your fingers over patient's toes. Bend toes (flexion) and straighten toes (extension).

23. Move each toe away from the second toe (abduction) (Figure 38-32A) and then toward the second toe (adduction) (Figure 38-32B).

24. Cover the leg with the bath blanket. Raise the side rail and move to the opposite side of the bed.

25. Move the patient close to you and repeat steps 5 through 24.

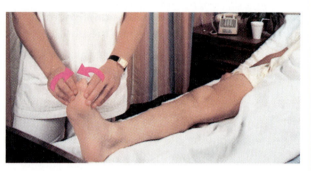

FIGURE 38-32B Toe adduction. Move each toe toward the second toe one at a time.

DIAGNOSTIC TECHNIQUES

Some techniques used to diagnose problems of the musculoskeletal system include:
- Radiographic techniques such as x-ray.
- Electromyography (EMG) test to measure the effectiveness of muscle/nerve interaction.
- Measurements of alkaline and acid phosphatases.
- Bone marrow examination, when a sample of the bone marrow is removed and evaluated.

- CAT scan to check for bone, muscle, and joint conditions.
- Radioisotope scanning, a technique that often can detect early bone and joint changes.
- Arthroscopy for direct visualization of a joint.
- Magnetic resonance imaging (MRI) shows conditions of tissues around bones to help diagnose tumors, ruptured disc between two vertebrae, and other conditions.

REVIEW

A. True/False.

Mark the following true or false by circling T or F.

1. T F Chymopapain is used to treat arthritis.

2. T F If ROM is not carried out faithfully, the patient's future mobility is threatened.

3. T F When carrying out ROM, always support the parts being exercised at the joint.

4. T F The nursing assistant will carry out special corrective exercises.

5. T F Aging is a contributory factor in osteoarthritis.

6. T F When the patient has a painful arthritic joint, it should be exercised vigorously.

7. T F An overbed bar (trapeze) will assist orthopedic patients to move more easily and to help themselves.

8. T F A fracture is any break in a bone.

9. T F Before operating beds or attachments used with orthopedic patients, the nursing assistant must be sure of his or her competency to operate this equipment.

10. T F It only takes a few moments for a cast to dry completely.

11. T F Patients recovering from fractured hips are generally not allowed to bear weight on the affected side for several weeks.

12. T F If a patient has an open reduction/internal fixation for a fractured hip, it means a cast will have been applied.

13. T F Phantom pain after an amputation is imaginary and of no concern to caregivers.

14. T F The nursing assistant is responsible for teaching patients with prostheses how to use them.

15. T F It is important to prevent contractures after an amputation.

B. Matching.

Choose the correct word from Column II to match each phrase in Column I.

Column I	Column II
16. _____ correct position	**a.** arthritis
17. _____ small fluid-filled sacs found around joints	**b.** spica
	c. closed
18. _____ name given to a cast covering hips and one or both legs	**d.** bursae
	e. simple
19. _____ fracture where bone breaks through skin	**f.** alignment
	g. open
20. _____ inflammation of joints	

C. Multiple Choice.

Select the one best answer for each question.

21. When assigned to perform ROM, you should
   a. exercise every joint.
   b. exercise joints to the point of pain.
   c. check with the nurse for any limitations before starting.
   d. perform each exercise four times.

22. A greenstick fracture
   a. occurs mainly in children.
   b. fragments the bone.
   c. occurs mainly in the elderly.
   d. none of these.

23. While a leg cast is drying,
   a. cover it tightly so moisture will not be lost.
   b. maintaining general alignment is not important.
   c. carefully observe the extremities for circulation.
   d. use only fingertips to handle the cast.

24. When caring for the patient in traction,
   a. maintain proper alignment.
   b. lift the weights rapidly.
   c. allow weights to rest on the floor.
   d. allow the patient's feet to press against the footboard.

25. Your patient has a ruptured disc. You should note and report
   a. tingling.
   b. paralysis.
   c. numbness.
   d. all of these.

Nursing Assistant Challenge.

You are assigned to care for Mrs. Nellie Goldstein, 62 years old, who had a total hip arthroplasty two days ago. She will be starting rehabilitation today and will continue her therapy as an outpatient after she is discharged in three more days. Mrs. Goldstein is a very active person and is eager to be "up and going."

26. What restrictions do you need to be aware of when taking care of Mrs. Goldstein?

Endocrine System

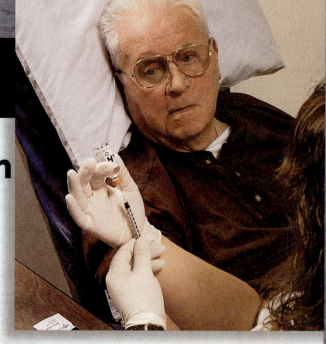

As a result of this unit, you will be able to:

- Spell and define terms.
- Review the location and functions of the endocrine system.
- List five specific diagnostic tests associated with conditions of the endocrine system.
- Describe some common diseases of the endocrine system.

- Recognize the signs and symptoms of hypoglycemia and hyperglycemia.
- Describe nursing assistant actions related to the care of patients with disorders of the endocrine system.
- Perform blood tests for glucose levels if facility policy permits.
- Perform the following procedure:
  - Procedure 95 Testing Urine for Acetone: Ketostix® Strip Test

VOCABULARY

Learn the meaning and the correct spelling of the following words and phrases:

acetone	hypercalcemia	islets of Langerhans	polydipsia
Addison's disease	hyperglycemia	ketosis	polyphagia
adrenal glands	hypersecretion	morbidity	polyuria
assimilate	hyperthyroidism	mortality	progesterone
Cushing's syndrome	hypertrophy	non–insulin-dependent	scrotum
diabetes mellitus	hypoglycemia	diabetes mellitus	simple goiter
endocrine glands	hyposecretion	(NIDDM)	sperm
estrogen	hypothyroidism	ovaries	testes
glucagon	insulin	ovum	testosterone
glucose	insulin-dependent	parathormone	tetany
glycogen	diabetes mellitus	parathyroid gland	thyrocalcitonin
glycosuria	(IDDM)	pineal body	thyroid gland
gonads	iodine	pituitary gland	thyroxine
hormones			

STRUCTURE AND FUNCTION

The **endocrine glands** (Figure 39-1):

- secrete hormones.
- control body activities and growth.
- are found as distinct glands or clusters of cells.
- are subject to disease that can result in **hyposecretion** (underproduction) or **hypersecretion** (overproduction) of hormones.

Hormones are chemicals that regulate the body's activities.

Pituitary Gland

Because it controls most of the other glands, the **pituitary gland** is called the master gland.

The pituitary gland has two portions called *lobes*. Each of the lobes secretes more than one hormone.

1. The anterior lobe secretes:
   - STH (somatotropic hormone)—a growth hormone that stimulates the growth of long bones
   - TSH (thyroid-stimulating hormone)—stimulates the thyroid gland
   - FSH (follicle-stimulating hormone)—promotes growth of the ovarian follicle in which the egg develops during the menstrual cycle
   - ACTH (adrenocorticotropic hormone)—stimulates production by the adrenal gland
   - LH (luteinizing hormone)—in females, helps stimulate ovulation during the menstrual cycle
   - ICSH (interstitial cell-stimulating hormone)—stimulates the male testes
   - Lactogenic hormone (LTH)—stimulates milk production in pregnant women

2. The posterior lobe secretes:
   - ADH (antidiuretic hormone)—acts on kidneys to prevent excess water loss
   - Pitocin (oxytocin)—stimulates uterine contractions during childbirth

Pineal Body

The **pineal body** is a small gland that is also located in the skull beneath the brain. Very little is known about this gland. It is thought to be related somehow to sexual growth, because it tends to get smaller at maturity. It produces:

- Glomerulotropin, which influences the adrenal gland

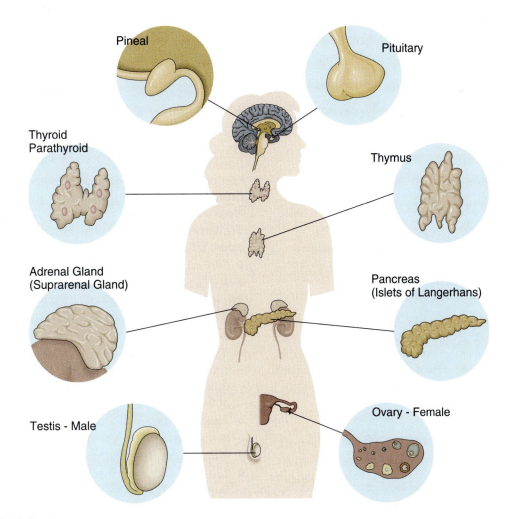

FIGURE 39-1 Endocrine system

- Serotonin, which acts in the brain
- Melatonin, which keeps sexual maturity from occurring too early

Adrenal Glands

There are two **adrenal glands**. Each gland is located on top of one of the two kidneys. Each gland has two distinct portions that secrete separate hormones.

1. The adrenal medulla (inside) produces norepinephrine (noradrenalin) and epinephrine (adrenalin), which stimulate the body to produce energy quickly during an emergency.
2. The adrenal cortex (outside) produces:
   - Glucocorticoids—elevate blood sugar levels and control the response of the body to stress and inflammation. They also depress inflammation.
   - Mineral corticoids—manage sodium and potassium levels.
   - Gonadocorticoids—influence both male and female sex hormones.

Gonads

The term **gonads** refers to the male and female sex glands. The female gonads (two **ovaries**):

- Are located within the pelvic cavity on either side of the uterus.
- Produce two hormones, **estrogen** and **progesterone**. These hormones are responsible for the development of female characteristics such as:
  - Breast development
  - Pubic and axillary hair
  - Onset and regulation of menstruation
  - Pregnancy

The male gonads (two **testes**):

- Are located on the outside of the body in a pouch called the **scrotum**.
- Produce the hormone **testosterone**. This hormone is responsible for secondary male characteristics such as:
  - Muscular development
  - Deepening voice
  - Hair growth

The male and female gonads also produce special cells—in the female, the **ovum** and in the male, the **sperm**. These cells unite during fertilization to form the embryo that becomes a new human being.

Thyroid Gland

The **thyroid gland** has two lobes and is found in the neck, anterior to the larynx. Hormones secreted by this gland are thyroxine and thyrocalcitonin. **Thyroxine** regulates metabolism. **Iodine** is an important component of this hormone. **Thyrocalcitonin** regulates calcium and phosphorus levels.

Parathyroid Glands

The tiny **parathyroid glands** are embedded in the posterior thyroid gland. The hormone they manufacture is called parathormone. **Parathormone** helps control the body's use of two minerals, calcium and phosphorus. Insufficient amounts of calcium result in severe muscle spasms or tetany. Untreated tetany can lead to death.

Islets of Langerhans

The **islets of Langerhans** are small groups of cells found within the pancreas. These cells produce two hormones: insulin and glucagon. **Insulin** lowers blood sugar. **Glucagon** elevates blood sugar.

COMMON CONDITIONS OF THE THYROID GLAND

The thyroid gland may secrete too much or not enough hormones. Either situation is treatable. If not treated, severe illness or death will occur.

Hyperthyroidism

Hyperthyroidism, or overactivity of the thyroid gland, results in production of too much thyroxine (hypersecretion). The person shows:

- Irritability and restlessness
- Nervousness
- Rapid pulse
- Increased appetite
- Weight loss
- Sensitivity

Nursing Assistant Actions. When caring for these patients, the nursing assistant must be understanding and have patience. The room should be kept quiet and cool. The patient's increased nutritional needs should be met with foods that are liked.

Treatment. Treatment of hyperthyroidism is designed to reduce the level of thyroxine through:

- Surgical thyroidectomy
- Radiation to reduce the number of functional cells

Thyroidectomy. It may be necessary to treat hyperthyroidism with surgery. You may be assigned to assist in the postoperative care. Following surgery:

- The patient is placed in a semi-Fowler's position, with neck and shoulders well supported. Remember at all times to support the back of the neck. Hyperextension of the neck may damage the operative site.
- Assist with oxygen, if ordered, using all oxygen precautions.
- Give routine postoperative care.
- Check for and report the following:
  - Any signs of bleeding (this may drain toward the back of the neck). The pillows behind the patient should be checked, as well as the dressings.

— Signs of respiratory distress.

— Inability of the patient to speak. Initial hoarseness is common, but any increase should be reported.

— Greatly elevated temperature and pulse, pronounced apprehension, or irritability.

— Numbness, tingling, or muscular spasm (tetany) of the extremities.

Hypothyroidism

Hypothyroidism results in an undersecretion of thyroxine. Recall that iodine is an essential component of thyroxine. A lack of iodine in the diet can result in low thyroxine production.

- The condition is called simple goiter.
- The thyroid gland enlarges (hypertrophies).
- Secretions produced have low thyroxine content.

Hypothyroidism can usually be successfully managed with thyroxine replacement.

COMMON CONDITIONS OF THE PARATHYROID GLANDS

Parathormone, secreted by the parathyroids, regulates the levels of electrolytes, calcium, and phosphates. Hypersecretion of this hormone results in:

- Excessively high levels of blood calcium (hypercalcemia)
- Developmental of renal calculi (kidney stones)
- Loss of bone calcium

Hypersecretion is usually caused by tumors. Tumors can be treated by surgical removal.

Hyposecretion can lead to:

- Abnormal muscle-nerve interaction
- Severe muscle spasm (tetany)

This can be an emergency situation, requiring management of the muscle spasms and administration of calcium. In the chronic state, calcium replacements and increased dietary calcium are prescribed.

COMMON CONDITIONS OF THE ADRENAL GLANDS

The adrenal gland secretions regulate:

- Development and maintenance of sexual characteristics
- Carbohydrate, fat, and protein metabolism
- Fluid balance
- Electrolyte levels of sodium and potassium

Hypersecretion results in Cushing's syndrome, which is characterized by:

- Weakness due to loss of body protein
- Increased blood sugar levels (hyperglycemia)
- Edema
- Hypertension

- Loss of potassium and retention of sodium
- Masculinization of a female

Therapy is primarily surgical and supportive.

Hyposecretion results in Addison's disease, which is characterized by:

- Loss of sodium and retention of potassium
- Abnormally low blood sugar (hypoglycemia)
- Dehydration
- Low stress tolerance

Addison's disease is treated by hormone replacement therapy and techniques to combat dehydration.

DIABETES MELLITUS

The United States has the highest rate of diabetic morbidity (illness) and mortality (death) in the world. Each year 250,000 new cases of diabetes mellitus are added to the more than 4 million known cases. Many new cases are discovered during routine physical examinations. In addition, it is estimated that millions more people are unaware that they are diabetics.

Although forms of the condition can appear at any age, it is more common in the middle and later years. About 80% of all diabetics are over 40 years of age. As many as 5% of those over age 65 require treatment.

The incidence of diabetes mellitus increases as people age. In the elderly, the disease:

- Is much more stable and predictable than in the young.
- Has fewer incidents of ketosis (diabetic coma) or insulin shock. When insulin shock or diabetic coma does occur in the elderly, either can be severe, resulting in heart attacks or strokes.
- May not require insulin for management. Less than half of the elderly patients with diabetes require insulin.

These statistics tell us that many of our patients will have this condition.

The reason why diabetes develops is not fully understood. Factors that seem to play a role in the incidence of diabetes are:

- Heredity
- Obesity
- Age
- Infectious agents
- Autoimmune reactions

All diabetics should wear or carry a Medic Alert® identification so that proper and immediate care can be provided in an emergency. It is also recommended that the diabetic carry food that provides a quick source of carbohydrates.

Disease Mechanism

In diabetes, the normal metabolism of fats, carbohydrates, and proteins is unbalanced. Normally, when carbohydrates are absorbed into the bloodstream, the blood sugar (glucose) level rises. The pancreas responds to an increase of glucose by secreting more insulin. *Insulin* is the hormone primarily responsible for:

- Lowering the blood sugar level by allowing glucose to cross the cell membrane.
- Increasing the oxidation of glucose by the tissues.
- Stimulating the conversion of glucose to glycogen by the liver. Glycogen is a storage form of energy.
- Decreasing glucose production from amino acids.
- Stimulating glucose formation into fat for storage.

In diabetes, there is insufficient insulin for these metabolic functions.

- Glucose cannot be properly utilized for energy.
- Fats and proteins are incompletely broken down. This leads to an accumulation of ketone bodies, in the forms of acetone and other acids, in the blood.
- The excess glucose is eliminated, along with water and salts, through the kidneys. This causes dehydration and electrolyte imbalance.
- The characteristic symptoms of excessive thirst, hunger, and increased urination are directly related to the loss of fluids, electrolytes, and sugar.

Types of Diabetes Mellitus

Diabetes mellitus is typed and named according to the need for insulin. Examples are insulin-dependent diabetes mellitus (IDDM) and non–insulin-dependent diabetes (NIDDM). Either form of diabetes may occur at any age. However, IDDM appears more commonly in the young and NIDDM is more common in older people.

Insulin-dependent diabetes mellitus (IDDM) (Type I) first appears in youth and in those under 40 years of age. The disease tends to be severe and unpredictable. It always requires insulin. Typical signs and symptoms are:

- Polyuria (excessive urination)
- Polydipsia (thirst)
- Polyphagia (hunger)
- Glycosuria (sugar in the urine)

Non–insulin-dependent diabetes mellitus (NIDDM) (Type II) is sometimes known as old-age diabetes or ketosis-resistant diabetes. It usually begins in later years. It is 10 times more common than the juvenile form. About half of the patients show obvious signs (as listed above). The rest show less well-defined symptoms. These may include:

- Easy fatigue
- Skin infections
- Slow healing
- Itching
- Pruritus vulvae (itching of the vulva)
- Burning on urination
- Pain in fingers and toes
- Vision changes
- Obesity

Often only one or two symptoms are apparent in the elderly person. The older person may:

- complain of constant fatigue.
- have a skin lesion that takes an unusually long time to heal.
- experience vision changes that may be mistakenly attributed to general aging.

Care of the diabetic is directed toward maintaining a normal blood glucose level so that complications may be prevented. To regulate blood glucose, the diabetic person must:

- eat a healthful, well-balanced diet as prescribed by the physician.
- exercise regularly in a manner appropriate for the person's age and ability.
- use insulin or oral antidiabetic agents correctly if ordered by the physician.

For some persons this may require life-style changes. Nurses and dieticians are responsible for teaching patients who are newly diagnosed with diabetes how to care for themselves. People with diabetes who are knowledgeable about the disease and who are willing to manage their lives accordingly can live happily and productively (Figure 39-2).

Diet

Diet is an important part of diabetic treatment. Physicians do not fully agree as to how strictly a diet must be followed by all patients.

- Weight reduction is favored.
- Weight reduction alone may be sufficient to bring the condition under control in NIDDM.

The Exchange Systems. The diabetic exchange system of foods was formulated by a committee with representatives from the American Diabetic Association and the

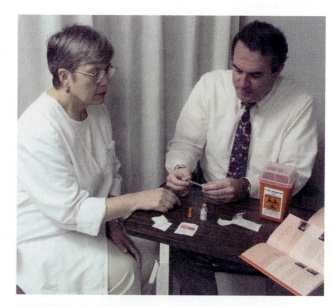

FIGURE 39-2 A patient who is newly diagnosed with diabetes mellitus is taught how to manage the disease by the nurse.

diabetic branch of the U.S. Public Health Service. The use of food lists based on the exchange system has simplified the task of measuring food by weight. Measurements can now be made using a standard 8-ounce measuring cup, teaspoon, and tablespoon.

Exercise

Exercise is an important part of the overall treatment. The amount and type of exercise the patient routinely engages in is balanced by the food intake and insulin or hypoglycemic drug requirements.

Hypoglycemic Drugs

Diabetes mellitus is treated by one of two main drug groups. One is administered subcutaneously. The other is given orally.

At present, there are several types of insulin. They vary in their:

- Speed of action
- Duration
- Potency or strength

Insulin is:

- Administered by the nurse. The nurse rotates the administration sites.
- Given by injection.
- Increasingly given through use of an insulin pump. The insulin pump delivers a prescribed amount of insulin on a regular basis into the patient's body.
- Used to treat IDDM.
- Persons living at home are taught to administer their own insulin.

Note: When insulin is self-administered, it is important to report any missed injections or signs of infection around the administration site.

Hypoglycemic drugs are:

- Administered by the nurse.
- Given by mouth.
- Used to treat NIDDM.

Complications

Long-standing diabetes mellitus is often complicated by:

- Diabetic retinopathy (eye disease)
- Renal disease
- Circulatory impairments that often result in gangrene (Figure 39-3) and amputation
- Poor healing
- Diabetic coma
- Insulin shock (hypoglycemia)

Hypoglycemia (Low Blood Sugar)

Hypoglycemia occurs when the blood glucose level is below normal. It:

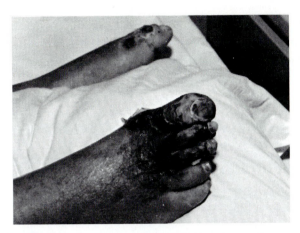

FIGURE 39-3 Gangrene of the toes and feet will require amputation.

- May occur rapidly.
- Occurs far less commonly when oral antidiabetic agents are given.
- Is referred to as insulin reaction or insulin shock when due to an overdose of insulin.

Hypoglycemia can be brought on by:

- Skipping meals
- Unusual activity
- Stress
- Vomiting
- Diarrhea
- Omission of planned snack or meals
- Interaction of drugs
- Too much insulin

Signs and Symptoms. The signs and symptoms of hypoglycemia include:

- Shallow, rapid respiration
- Rapid pulse
- Hunger
- Pale, moist skin
- Excitement and nervousness

If the patient is awake and alert, treatment includes intake of orange juice, milk, or another easily absorbed carbohydrate such as hard candy. If the patient is unconscious, the physician or nurse may give glucagon, which causes a rapid elevation of blood sugar.

Hyperglycemia (High Blood Sugar)

Hyperglycemia (diabetic coma) or ketosis:

- Occurs when there is insufficient insulin for metabolic needs.
- Is less apt to occur in NIDDM.
- Usually develops slowly, sometimes over a 24-hour period.
- May be seen as confusion, drowsiness, or a slow slippage into coma in a patient who is confined to bed.

Hyperglycemia may be brought on by:

- Stress
- Illness such as infection
- Dehydration
- Injury
- Forgotten medication
- Intake of too much food

Signs and Symptoms. The signs and symptoms of diabetic coma include:

- Early headache, drowsiness, or confusion
- Sweet, fruity odor to the breath
- Deep breathing
- Full, bounding pulse
- Low blood pressure
- Nausea or vomiting
- Flushed, dry, hot skin

Treatment includes administration of insulin, fluids, and electrolytes.

Other Complications

Persons with diabetes should have regular health monitoring so that complications may be detected early and treated promptly. Health monitoring should include:

- Eye examinations by an ophthalmologist for early detection of diabetic retinopathy, which can lead to impaired vision and eventually blindness
- Urinalysis and other urological examinations to evaluate the condition of the kidneys.
- Cardiac evaluation; monitoring of heart action and blood pressure.
- Circulatory evaluation
- Care and treatment of any wounds.

Nursing Assistant Responsibilities

- Know the signs of insulin shock and diabetic coma.
- Be alert for the signs of diabetic coma or insulin shock and report them immediately to the nurse.
- Know the storage location of orange juice or other easily **assimilated** (absorbed) sources of carbohydrates.
- Keep easily assimilated carbohydrates, such as orange juice, crackers, hard candy, or Karo syrup, available if caring for the diabetic patient at home.
- Make sure you serve the patient proper trays of food.
- Do not give extra nourishments without special permission.
- Keep a record of the food consumed, on the patient's chart.
- Report uneaten meals to the nurse (Figure 39-4).
- Give special attention to care of the diabetic patient's feet.
  - Wash daily, carefully drying between toes.
  - Inspect feet closely for any breaks or signs of irritation.

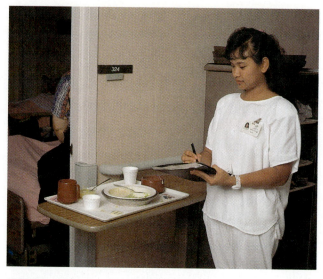

FIGURE 39-4 The amount and type of food consumed by a patient with diabetes mellitus must be carefully observed and recorded.

- Report any abnormalities to the nurse.
- Do not allow moisture to collect between toes.
- The toenails of a diabetic should be cut only by a podiatrist, a specialist who is trained in foot care.
- Shoes and stockings should be clean, free of holes, and fit well. Anything that might injure the feet or interfere with the circulation must be avoided.
- Do not allow the patient to go barefoot.

DIAGNOSTIC TECHNIQUES

Techniques used to diagnose problems of the endocrine system include:

- Blood analysis for hormone levels
- Urine analysis for hormone levels
- Radioisotope scanning for thyroid disease
- Radioactive iodine uptake for thyroid function
- Basal metabolic rate (BMR) to measure the speed of oxygen uptake

BLOOD GLUCOSE MONITORING

Blood glucose monitoring is a procedure taught to diabetic patients so that they may closely monitor and record their blood glucose levels. The physician uses this record to determine the amount of insulin or oral hypoglycemics the patient needs. If the patient is hospitalized or admitted to a long-term care facility, the procedure is continued by the nurses. Nursing assistants are not usually expected to perform this procedure.

You may however, be expected to test the patient's urine for acetone. **Acetone** is a substance that accumulates in the body when the blood glucose is out of balance. A simple urine test detects the presence of acetone.

TESTING URINE FOR ACETONE: KETOSTIX® STRIP TEST

📝 *Note:* *If the results of the blood glucose tests are above normal, the nurse may request the urine be tested for acetone.*

1. Carry out each beginning procedure action.
2. Assemble equipment:
   - disposable gloves
   - Ketostix® reagent strips
   - sample of freshly voided urine in container
3. Put on disposable gloves.
4. Remove one test strip from bottle and recap bottle.
5. Dip one end of the test strip (the end with the reagent areas) into the urine (Figure 39-5).

6. Remove and hold strip horizontally.
7. Fifteen seconds later, compare the strip with the color chart on the bottle label (Figure 39-6). Match it as closely as possible to one of the colors on the chart. Do not touch wet strip to bottle label.
8. Dispose of strip and urine specimen unless orders have been given to save either or both of them.
8. Remove and properly dispose of gloves according to facility policy.
9. Carry out each procedure completion action.

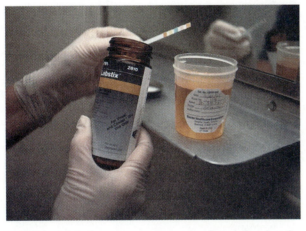

FIGURE 39-5 Remove a test strip from the bottle. Recap bottle. Dip strip into fresh urine sample.

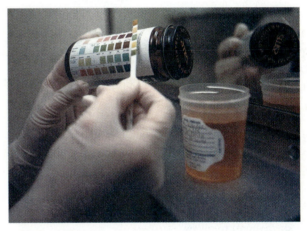

FIGURE 39-6 Compare strip with color chart on bottle to determine results. Do not touch wet strip to label of bottle

REVIEW

A. True/False.

Mark the following true or false by circling T or F.

1. T F The person with polyphagia has a high urine output.
2. T F The morbidity rate for diabetes mellitus is very high.
3. T F Glucose is another name for blood sugar.
4. T F The person with hyperthyroidism is slow moving and lethargic.
5. T F Hyperthyroidism causes people to lose weight.

6. T F You should keep the room of a patient with hyperthyroidism quite warm.
7. T F Obesity may play a role in the incidence of diabetes mellitus.
8. T F If the patient with IDDM appears drowsy and confused, you should suspect the possibility of ketosis.
9. T F Foot care is especially important for the diabetic patient.
10. T F Disposable gloves should be worn when testing urine for sugar.

B. Matching.

Choose the correct item from Column II to match each phrase in Column I.

Column I

11. _____ internal secretion produced by glands
12. _____ diabetic coma
13. _____ illness rate
14. _____ excess thirst
15. _____ sugar in the urine
16. _____ produces hormones
17. _____ excess hunger
18. _____ death rate
19. _____ blood sugar
20. _____ overweight

Column II

a. polydipsia
b. polyphagia
c. polyuria
d. glycosuria
e. endocrine gland
f. hormone
g. ketosis
h. mortality rate
i. morbidity rate
j. obesity
k. glycogen
l. NIDDM
m. insulin shock
n. glucose

C. Multiple Choice.

Select the one best answer for each question.

21. Your patient has had a thyroidectomy. You should
    a. keep the patient flat in bed.
    b. watch for and report signs of respiratory distress.
    c. carry out ROM exercises immediately.
    d. position the patient in a left Sims' position.

22. Lack of iodine in the diet can result in
    a. hypothyroidism.
    b. hyperthyroidism.
    c. diabetes mellitus.
    d. ketosis.

23. The pituitary gland is responsible for secreting hormones that
    a. stimulate ovulation during the menstrual cycle.
    b. manage sodium and potassium levels.
    c. control calcium and phosphorus.
    d. regulate blood sugar.

24. Your patient is an insulin-dependent diabetic. You know this
    a. is a stable form of the disease.
    b. affects older persons.
    c. requires hypoglycemic drugs.
    d. is a less stable form of the disease.

25. Insulin is an important hormone because it
    a. lowers blood sugar.
    b. raises blood sugar.
    c. stimulates the conversion of glycogen to glucose.
    d. breaks fat down to form glucose.

D. Nursing Assistant Challenge.

You are assigned to two patients who both have diabetes. Sally Sakowski is 29 years old and has had diabetes for 10 years. She is considered to be IDDM. Ruth Young is 72 years old and has just been diagnosed with NIDDM. Although these patients both have the same diagnosis, there may be many differences in their signs, symptoms, and problems. Consider these questions:

26. What differences would you see in the signs and symptoms experienced by these two women?

27. What differences would you expect in their treatment?

28. Knowing the difference in their ages, how would you expect the disease to affect the life-style of each woman?

29. Hypoglycemia and hyperglycemia may be a complication for either patient. List the differences in the signs and symptoms of both complications.

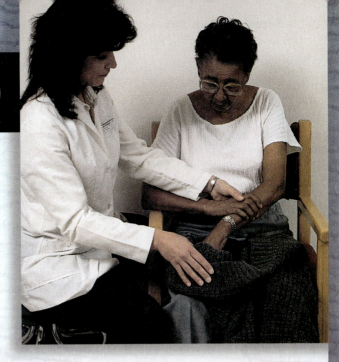

U N I T **40**

Nervous System

As a result of this unit, you will be able to:
- Spell and define terms.
- State the location and functions of the organs of the nervous system.
- List five diagnostic tests used to determine conditions of the nervous system.
- Describe eight common conditions of the nervous system.
- Describe nursing assistant actions related to the care of patients with conditions of the nervous system.
- Explain the proper care, handling, and insertion of an artificial eye.

- Explain the proper care, handling, and insertion of a hearing aid.
- Demonstrate the following procedures:
  — Procedure 96 Caring for Eye Socket and Artificial Eye
  — Procedure 97 Applying a Behind-the-Ear Hearing Aid
  — Procedure 98 Removing a Behind-the-Ear Hearing Aid
  — Procedure 99 Applying and Removing an In-the-Ear Hearing Aid

VOCABULARY

Learn the meaning and the correct spelling of the following words and phrases:

akinesia	convulsion	macular degeneration	pupil
aphasia	cornea	meninges	quadriplegia
aura	dendrite	meningitis	receptive aphasia
axon	emotional lability	multiple sclerosis	retinal degeneration
brain attack	epilepsy	nerve	semicircular canal
brain stem	eustachian tube	neuron	spatial-perceptual deficit
cataract	expressive aphasia	neurotransmitter	status epilepticus
cerebellum	global aphasia	nystagmus	stroke
cerebrospinal fluid (CSF)	grand mal seizure	ossicle	synapse
cerebrovascular accident (CVA)	hemianopsia	otitis media	transient ischemic attack (TIA)
	hemiplegia	otosclerosis	
cerebrum	intention tremor	paralysis	tremor
cochlea	intracranial pressure	paraplegia	tympanic membrane
cognitive impairment	iris	Parkinson's disease	unilateral neglect
conjunctiva	lacrimal gland	petit mal seizure	vertigo
	Lhermitte's sign	position sense	

STRUCTURE AND FUNCTION

The nervous system controls and coordinates all body activities, including the production of hormones. Special parts of the nervous system are concerned with maintaining normal day-to-day functions. Other parts act during emergency situations. Still others control voluntary activities. Neurological conditions require highly specialized nursing care. You will assist with the less technical aspects of that care.

Neurons

Cells of the nervous system are called **neurons** (Figure 40-1A). They are specialized to conduct electriclike

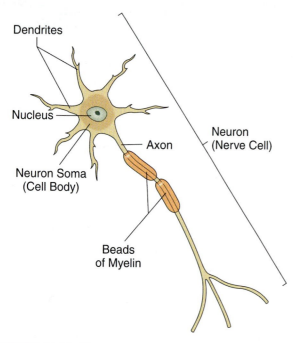

FIGURE 40-1A The neuron

impulses. The neuron has extensions called **axons** and **dendrites**. Impulses enter the neuron only through the dendrites and leave only through the axon.

Although neurons do not actually touch each other, the axon of one neuron lies close to the dendrites of many other neurons. In this way, impulses may follow many different routes. The space between the axon of one cell and the dendrites of others is called a **synapse**. Axons and dendrites in the periphery are covered with *myelin*, which acts as insulation.

Neurotransmitters

Neurotransmitters are chemicals that enable messages (nerve impulses) to pass from one cell to another (Figure 40-1B). If the chemicals are not produced in the right amounts, the message pathway becomes confused or blocked.

Nerves

Some axons and dendrites are long. Others are short. Axons and dendrites of many neurons are found in bundles. The bundles are held together by connective tissue. These bundles resemble telephone cables and are called **nerves**. The cell bodies of the axons and dendrites in these nerves may be found far from the ends of the nerves in clusters called *ganglia*.

Sensory nerves are made up of dendrites. They carry sensations to the brain and spinal cord from the various body parts. Feeling is lost when these nerve impulses are interrupted. Motor nerves carry impulses from the brain and spinal cord to muscles that cause body activity. Paralysis or loss of function occurs when these nerves are damaged.

For easier study, the nervous system can be divided into two parts: the central nervous system (CNS) and the peripheral nervous system (PNS). The CNS is composed of the brain and spinal cord (Figure 40-2). The PNS is composed of the 12 pairs of cranial nerves and 31 pairs of spinal nerves that reach throughout the body (Figure 40-3). Remember,

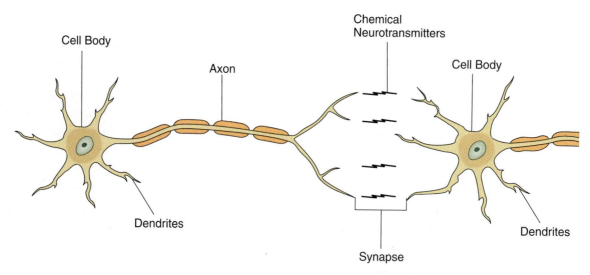

FIGURE 40-1B Chemicals called neurotransmitters help pass the nerve message across the synapse from one neuron to the next.

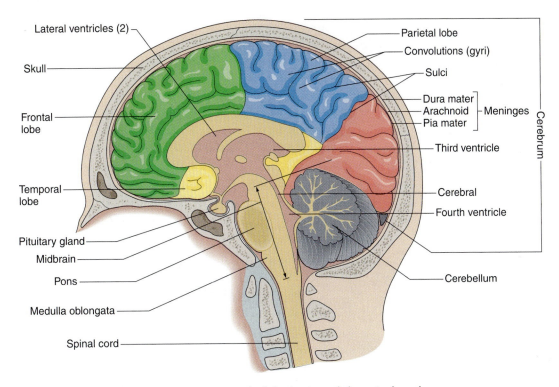

FIGURE 40-2 The central nervous system is composed of the brain and the spinal cord.

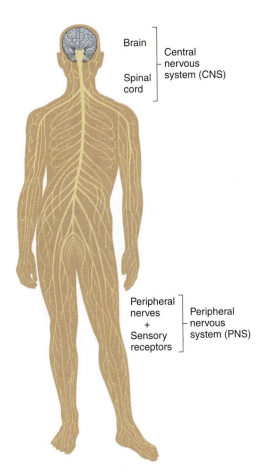

FIGURE 40-3 The peripheral nervous system connects the central nervous system to the various structures of the body. Messages are relayed from these structures back to the brain through the spinal cord.

though, that the nervous system is one interwoven system, a complex of millions of neurons.

The Central Nervous System

The brain and spinal cord are:

● Surrounded by bone

● Protected by membranes called *meninges*

● Cushioned by cerebrospinal fluid (CSF)

The brain and spinal cord are a continuous structure found within the skull and spinal canal. The spinal cord is about 17 inches long. It ends just above the small of the back. Nerves extend from the brain and the spinal cord.

The Brain

The brain (encephalon) is a large, soft mass of nerve tissue contained within the cranium. It is composed of gray matter and white matter. Gray matter consists principally of nerve-cell bodies. White matter consists of nerve cells that form connections between various parts of the brain.

The brain can be further subdivided into the:

● Cerebrum—The largest portion of the brain. The outer portion is formed in folds known as convolutions and separated into lobes. The lobes take their names from the skull bones that surround them (Figure 40-4).

   – The outer portion, the cerebral cortex, is composed of cell bodies and appears gray.

   – The inner portion is composed of axons and dendrites and so appears white.

   – All mental activities—thinking, voluntary movements, interpreting sensations and emotions—are

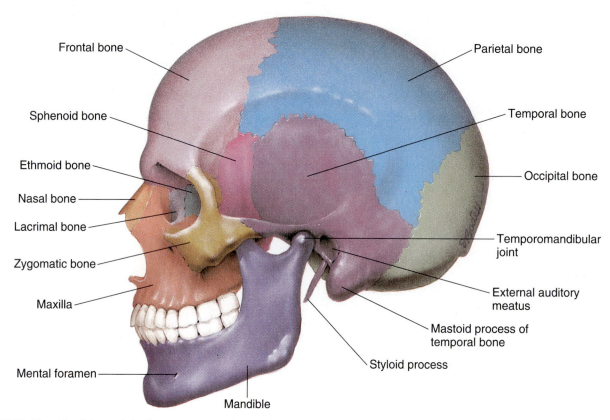

FIGURE 40-4 The lobes of the brain are named according to the skull bones.

carried out by cerebral cells (Figure 40-5). Certain activities are centered in each lobe.

— In general, the right side of the cerebrum interprets for and controls the left side of the body and vice versa.

● **Cerebellum**—Found beneath the occipital lobe of the cerebrum. It too has an outer layer of gray cell bodies. This portion of the brain coordinates muscular activities and balance.

● **Brain stem**—The midbrain, pons, and medulla are in the brain stem. They are composed mainly of axons and dendrites. These fibers serve as connecting pathways between the control centers in the cerebrum and cerebellum and the spinal cord. Control centers are found within the brain stem for involuntary movements of such vital organs as the:

— Heart
— Blood vessels
— Lungs
— Stomach
— Intestines

The Spinal Cord

The spinal cord (Figure 40-6) extends from the medulla to the second lumbar vertebra in the spinal canal, which is above the small of the back, a distance of about 17 inches.

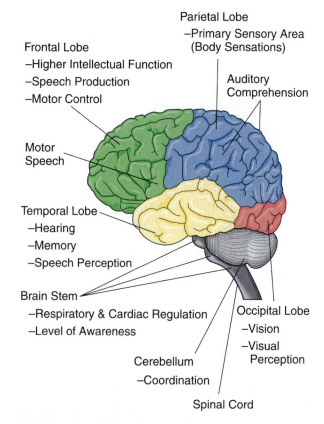

FIGURE 40-5 Each lobe of the brain is responsible for a different function.

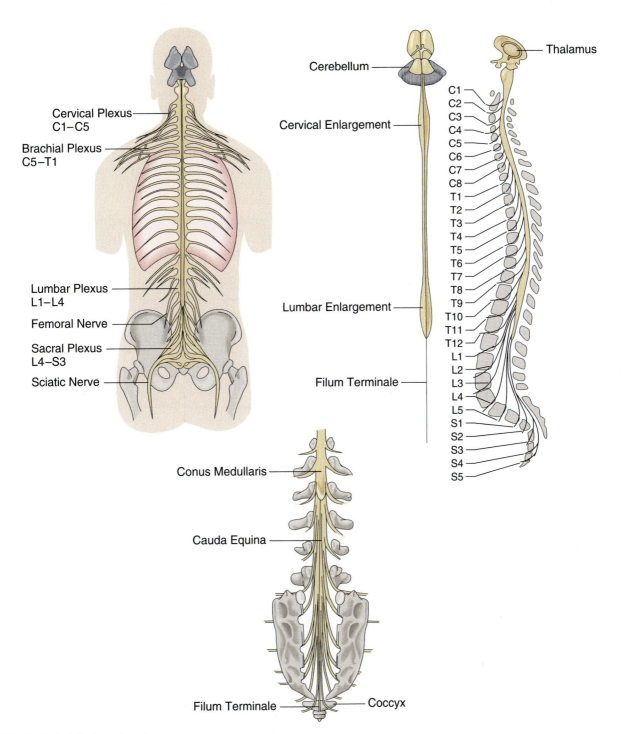

FIGURE 40-6 Spinal cord and nerves

Nerves entering and leaving the spinal cord carry impulses to and from the control centers. Certain reflex activities performed without conscious thought are controlled within the cord. Pulling your hand away from something hot is an example of this type of reflex activity (Figure 40-7).

The Meninges

Three membranes called meninges surround both the brain and the spinal cord. They are the dura mater, the arachnoid mater, and the pia mater.

The dura mater is the tough outer covering. The arachnoid mater is the middle, loosely structured layer. It is filled with cerebrospinal fluid. The pia mater is the innermost, delicate layer. It is very vascular (contains many blood vessels) and clings to the brain, spinal cord, and nerve roots.

Cerebrospinal Fluid

Ventricles are cavities within the cerebrum that are lined with highly vascular tissue. These tissues produce cerebrospinal fluid (CSF), which flows around the brain and the spinal

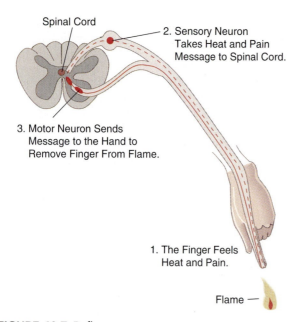

FIGURE 40-7 Reflex arc

cord. The cerebrospinal fluid bathes the central nervous system as tissue fluid and cushions it against shock and possible injury.

Special Relationships: The Autonomic Nervous System

The phrase *autonomic nervous system (ANS)* refers to special pathways that travel in cranial and spinal nerves (Figure 40-8). The control center is in the brain stem. The pathways begin in the CNS and reach out to the glands, smooth muscle walls of organs, and heart.

The autonomic nervous system consists of two parts: sympathetic fibers and parasympathetic fibers. Sympathetic fibers stimulate activities that prepare the body to deal with emergency situations. It is called the mechanism of "fight or flight." Parasympathetic fibers control the usual functions of moderate heartbeat, digestion, elimination, respiration, and glandular activity.

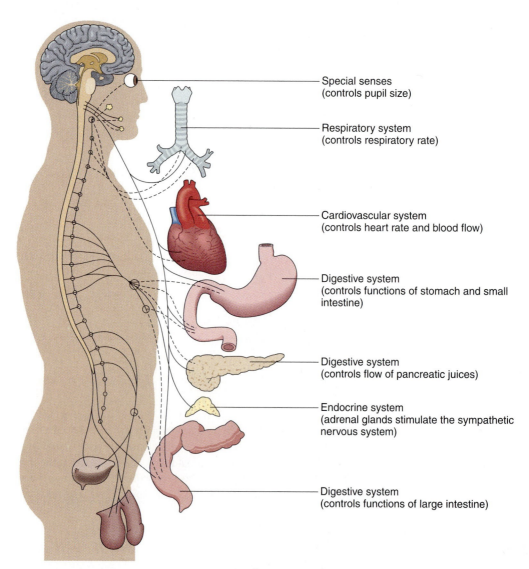

FIGURE 40-8 Autonomic nervous system

Sensory Receptors

The ends of the dendrites carrying sensations to the central nervous system are found throughout the body.

- Some begin in joints and bring information about body positions to the brain.
- Others in the skin carry sensations of pain, heat, pressure, and cold.
- Those in the nose carry the sense of smell.
- The dendrites in the tongue carry the sense of taste.

Sensory dendrites also receive stimulation through two very special end organs, the eye and the ear. All of these structures are called sensory receptors because they carry information about the outside world to the brain. The brain interprets and processes the information.

The Eye

The eye (Figures 40-9A and B) is a hollow ball filled with two liquids called the *aqueous humor* and the *vitreous humor*. The wall of the eye is made up of three layers:

- The sclera: A tough, white outer coat that is protective. The cornea is the transparent portion in the front. Light rays pass through the cornea into the eye.
- The choroid: The nutritive layer found beneath the sclera. The choroid nourishes the eye tissues through its large number of blood vessels.
- The retina: The innermost layer is made up of neurons that are sensitive to light. The neurons join together and their axons leave the eye as the optic nerve. The two nerves cross beneath the brain and carry their impulses to the occipital lobe of the cerebrum to let us know what we are seeing.

Seeing. We see as light enters the eye through the cornea. The amount of light entering the eye is controlled by the iris. The iris is the colored portion of the eye. It is found behind the cornea. Fluid between the cornea and iris helps to bend the light rays and bring them to focus on the retina. The opening in the iris is called the pupil. The pupil appears black because there is no light behind it. Directly behind the iris is the lens. Small muscles pull on either side of the lens to change its shape. The changing shape of the lens makes it possible for us to adjust the range of our vision from far to near or from near to far.

The eye is:

- Held within the bony socket by muscles that can change its position.
- Covered by a mucous membrane, called the conjunctiva. The conjunctiva lines the eyelids and covers the eye.

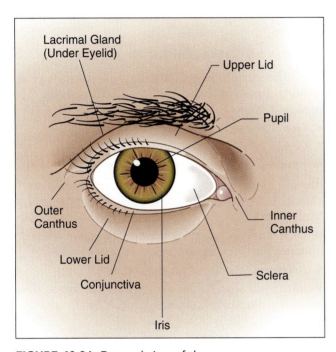

FIGURE 40-9A External view of the eye

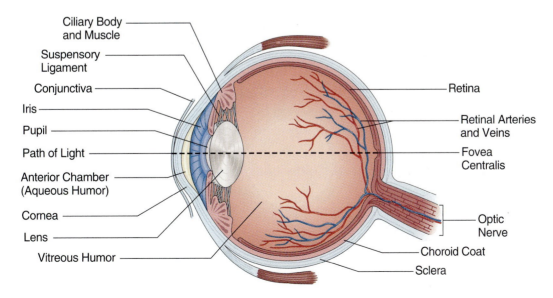

FIGURE 40-9B Internal view of the eye

- Protected by the eyelids and eyelashes. Tears are manufactured by the lacrimal glands found beneath the lateral side of the upper lid. Tears protect the eye as they wash across the eye, keeping it moist, and then drain into the nasal cavity.

The Ear

Just as the eye is sensitive to light, the ear is sensitive to sound (Figure 40-10). The ear functions in hearing and equilibrium (balance). The ear has three parts: the outer ear, the middle ear, and the inner ear. The outer ear consists of the visible external structure known as the pinna and a canal, which directs sound waves toward the middle ear. At the end of the canal is the eardrum, or tympanic membrane. Sound waves cause the eardrum to vibrate.

The middle ear is made up of three tiny bones called ossicles. The ossicles form a chain across the middle ear from the tympanic membrane to an opening in the inner ear. These bones are known as the:

- Incus or anvil
- Malleus or hammer
- Stapes or stirrup

Small tubes, called the eustachian tubes, lead from the nasopharynx into the middle ear to equalize pressure on either side of the eardrum. Sound waves pushing against the tympanic membrane cause the ossicles to vibrate and push against the opening of the inner ear. This motion starts fluid moving in the inner ear.

The inner ear is a very complex structure. It has two main parts: the cochlea and three semicircular canals. The cochlea looks somewhat like a coiled snail shell. Within the cochlea are the tiny dendrites of the hearing or auditory nerve. Fluid covers the dendrites. When the fluid is set in motion by the vibration of the middle ear bones, it stimulates the dendrites with sound sensations. The auditory nerves, one from each ear, carry the sensations to the temporal lobe of the cerebrum to let us know what we are hearing.

The three semicircular canals also contain liquid and nerve endings. When these nerve endings are stimulated, impulses about the position of the head are sent to the brain. This helps us keep our balance.

COMMON CONDITIONS

The nervous system usually remains healthy. However, injury or disease to the brain, spinal cord, or nerves requires appropriate treatment.

Increased Intracranial Pressure

The structures within the skull normally exert a certain amount of pressure, called the intracranial pressure. The pressure is due to:

- Nervous tissue
- Cerebrospinal fluid
- Blood flowing through cerebral vessels

Any change in the size or amount of these components changes the pressure. Increased intracranial pressure can result from:

- Head injury. Bleeding from damaged blood vessels and edema puts pressure on the delicate nervous tissue.
- Inflammation or infection plus edema.
- Intracranial bleeding due to ruptured blood vessels. This is called a cerebrovascular accident (CVA).

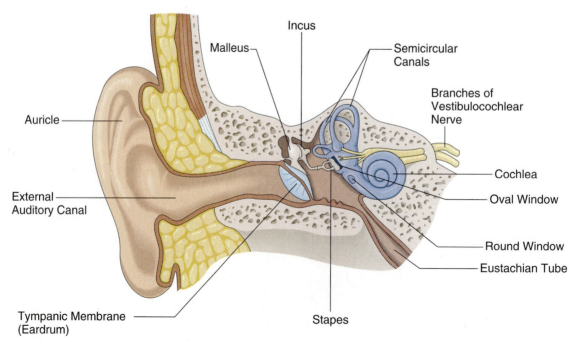

Incus

Malleus

Semicircular Canals

Branches of Vestibulocochlear Nerve

Auricle

Cochlea

Oval Window

External Auditory Canal

Round Window

Eustachian Tube

Tympanic Membrane (Eardrum)

Stapes

FIGURE 40-10 Internal view of the ear

- Toxins.
- High temperature.
- Blockage of the normal flow of cerebrospinal fluid.
- Tumors.

Signs and Symptoms. Indications of increased intracranial pressure include:

- Alteration in pupil size and response to light. In the normal eye, the pupil becomes smaller when a flashlight is directed at each eye. The equality of the pupils and their ability to react to light is an important observation when a head injury occurs.
- Headache.
- Vomiting.
- Loss of consciousness and sensation.
- Paralysis—loss of voluntary motor control.
- Convulsions (seizures)—uncontrolled muscular contractions that are often violent.

How long all or part of the symptoms remain depends on the extent and cause of damage to the brain cells. Remember also that paralysis is not always accompanied by sensory loss.

Specific Nursing Care. Patients who are acutely ill with head injuries or increased intracranial pressure require skilled nursing care (Figure 40-11). The nurse is responsible for monitoring the patient's:

- Level of consciousness
- Degree of orientation to time and place
- Reaction to pain and stimuli
- Vital signs

If you note any change in the patient's response or behavior as you are assisting in care, bring it to the nurse's attention immediately. Changes that might be very significant include:

- Incontinence
- Uncontrolled body movements
- Disorientation
- Deepening or lessening in the level of consciousness

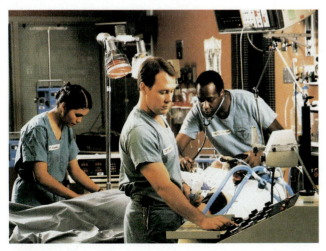

FIGURE 40-11 Critical care nursing. "Be All You Can Be." *Courtesy United States government, as represented by the Secretary of the Army.*

- Dizziness
- Vomiting
- Alterations in speech

Once improved, the patient may be moved from a critical unit to an intermediate unit. From there, the patient may go to a long-term care facility for a possibly long period of convalescence. The patient may require extensive rehabilitation to regain functional skills. The nursing measures first established in the critical care unit must be maintained throughout this extended period.

Loss of sensation and decreased mobility make these patients more prone to pressure sores, infection, and contractures. You must continue to:

- Give special skin care.
- Carry out range-of-motion exercises.
- Check skin over pressure points frequently.
- Change the patient's position regularly.
- Report early signs of infection.
- Monitor elimination. Loss of muscle tone and inactivity may lead to constipation and impaction.
- Check drainage tubes such as indwelling catheters. They must receive careful attention.
- Provide reality orientation as needed.
- Be alert to any signs of mood changes and plan extra time to provide essential support. Patients recovering from these illnesses often experience anxiety and depression.
- Keep a careful check on vital signs of any patient with a head injury. A special record (neurosurgical watch) may be kept for recording all observations (Figure 40-12).

Transient Ischemic Attack

A transient ischemic attack (TIA) is a temporary period of diminished blood flow to the brain. The attack comes on rapidly and may last from 2 to 15 minutes or for as long as 24 hours. Symptoms are similar to those of a stroke but are temporary and reversible. Transient ischemic attacks may occur once or several times in a lifetime. Persons experiencing TIAs are at risk for eventually suffering a stroke.

Stroke

A stroke is also called a cerebrovascular accident (CVA) or brain attack. It affects the vascular system and the nervous system. The complete or partial loss of blood flow to the brain tissue is frequently a complication of atherosclerosis or brain hemorrhage. Causes of CVA include:

- Vascular occlusion due to a thrombus, atherosclerotic plaques, or emboli that obstruct the flow of blood
- Intracranial bleeding as blood vessels rupture, releasing blood into the brain tissue

Remember, most nerve pathways cross. Therefore, damage on one side of the brain results in signs and symptoms on the opposite side of the body. Symptoms vary depending on the extent of interference with the circulation and on the area

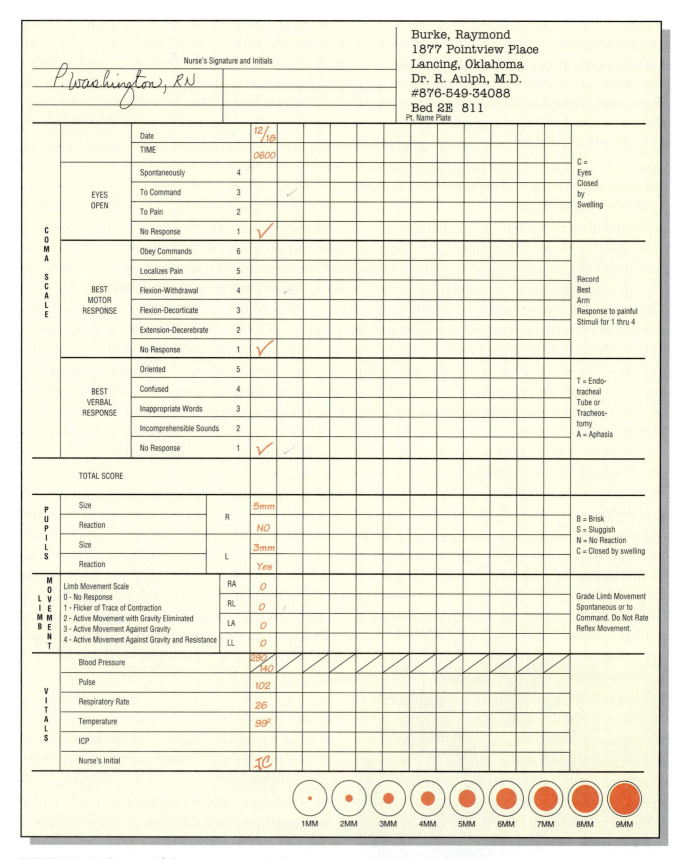

				12/18										
		Date		12/18										C = Eyes Closed by Swelling
		TIME		0600										
C O M A S C A L E	EYES OPEN	Spontaneously	4											
		To Command	3		✓									
		To Pain	2											
		No Response	1	✓										
	BEST MOTOR RESPONSE	Obey Commands	6											Record Best Arm Response to painful Stimuli for 1 thru 4
		Localizes Pain	5											
		Flexion-Withdrawal	4		✓									
		Flexion-Decorticate	3											
		Extension-Decerebrate	2											
		No Response	1	✓										
	BEST VERBAL RESPONSE	Oriented	5											T = Endo- tracheal Tube or Tracheos- tomy A = Aphasia
		Confused	4											
		Inappropriate Words	3											
		Incomprehensible Sounds	2											
		No Response	1	✓	✓									
		TOTAL SCORE												
P U P I L S		Size	R	5mm										B = Brisk S = Sluggish N = No Reaction C = Closed by swelling
		Reaction		NO										
		Size	L	3mm										
		Reaction		Yes										
L I M B M O V E M E N T	Limb Movement Scale 0 - No Response 1 - Flicker of Trace of Contraction 2 - Active Movement with Gravity Eliminated 3 - Active Movement Against Gravity 4 - Active Movement Against Gravity and Resistance		RA	0										Grade Limb Movement Spontaneous or to Command. Do Not Rate Reflex Movement.
			RL	0	∕									
			LA	0										
			LL	0										
V I T A L S		Blood Pressure		290/140										
		Pulse		102										
		Respiratory Rate		26										
		Temperature		99²										
		ICP												
		Nurse's Initial		IC										

Nurse's Signature and Initials

P. Washington, RN

Burke, Raymond
1877 Pointview Place
Lancing, Oklahoma
Dr. R. Aulph, M.D.
#876-549-34088
Bed 2E 811
Pt. Name Plate

1MM 2MM 3MM 4MM 5MM 6MM 7MM 8MM 9MM

FIGURE 40-12 This type of documentation is made on patients with neurological trauma.

and amount of tissue damaged. Patients with damage to the right side of the brain will exhibit:

- Paralysis on the left side of the body (left **hemiplegia**).
- **Spatial-perceptual deficits**. This means it is difficult to distinguish right from left and up from down. The world may appear "tilted" to the person with right-brain damage. The patient will have problems propelling a wheelchair, setting down items, and carrying out the activities of daily living.
- Change in personality. The individual with right brain damage becomes very quick and impulsive.

If the left side of the brain is damaged, you will note:

- Paralysis on the right side of the body (right hemiplegia) (Figure 40-13).
- **Aphasia**—an inability to express or understand speech.
- Change in personality. The individual becomes very cautious, anxious, and slow to complete tasks.

Other symptoms may be present with either right- or left-brain damage. These include:

- Sensory-perceptual deficits
  - Loss of **position sense**. The person cannot tell, for example, where an affected foot is or what position it is in without looking at it.
  - The inability to identify common objects such as a comb, a fork, a pencil, or a glass.
  - The inability to use common objects. The patient may know what an item is, such as a fork, but be unable to pick it up and use it. This is not a result of paralysis but is due to brain damage.
- **Unilateral neglect**. The patient ignores the paralyzed side of the body. For example, the affected arm may hang over the side of the wheelchair without the patient realizing where the arm is.
- **Hemianopsia**. This is impaired vision. Both eyes have only half vision. For example, if the patient has left hemiplegia, the left half of both eyes is blind (Figure 40-14).
- **Emotional lability**. Patients who have had a stroke may start to cry or laugh for no apparent reason. They have very little control over this and may be embarrassed.
- **Cognitive impairments**. There may be changes in the patient's intellectual function. This may affect memory, judgment, and problem-solving abilities.

Nursing Care. The goals of poststroke care include:

1. Maintaining the skills and abilities that the patient has left.
2. Preventing complications caused by immobility:
   - Contractures
   - Pressure ulcers
   - Pneumonia
   - Blood clots
3. Helping the patient regain functional abilities:
   - Activities of daily living (Figure 40-15)
   - Bowel and bladder control
   - Mobility
   - Communication skills

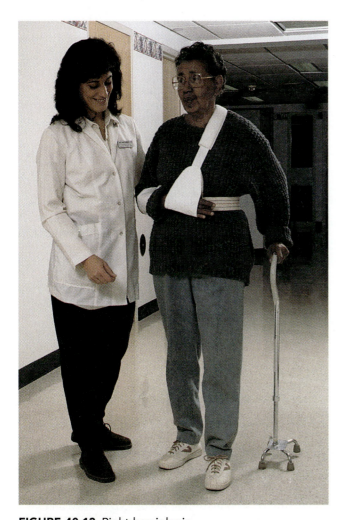

FIGURE 40-13 Right hemiplegia

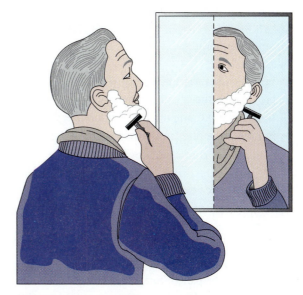

FIGURE 40-14 Hemianopsia is a common problem after a stroke.

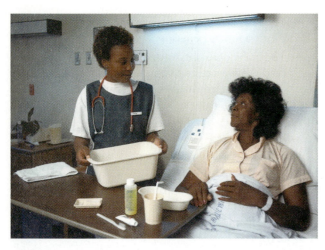

FIGURE 40-15 The patient who has had a stroke may need to relearn how to do the activities of daily living.

During Recovery. Recovery from a stroke is often a very frustrating experience for the patient. Caregivers must be patient. In your approach to the patient, remember two things:

1. The patient has more than enough frustration for the two of you, so be careful not to let yours show. The last thing the patient needs is your silent reinforcement of his helplessness.

2. It is well known that the degree and speed of recovery are directly related, in most cases, to the patience and encouragement of the caregivers with whom the patient has close contact.

Other interventions during recovery include:

- Physical therapy to increase independent mobility: bed movement, getting to the side of the bed, standing by the side of the bed, transferring out of bed and into a chair, and ambulation.
- Occupational therapy to regain the ability to perform the activities of daily living, such as bathing, grooming, dressing, and eating, with little or no assistance.
- Speech therapy to regain or to learn different methods of communication.
- Nursing care to:
  — Implement bowel and bladder training programs or providing catheter care if necessary
  — Implement pressure ulcer prevention programs
  — Reinforce the programs provided by the therapists
- Care to prevent contractures by:
  — Positioning the patient appropriately and changing positions at least every two hours
  — Performing passive range-of-motion exercises as directed
  — Applying splints or braces as ordered

All staff can help with rehabilitation efforts by:

- Encouraging the patient to communicate
- Maintaining a positive and supportive attitude at all times

- Providing only the assistance that the patient needs
- Following approaches consistently as outlined in the patient's care plan

Convalescence is often long. The nursing care is demanding, requiring much patience and understanding.

Aphasia

Stroke victims often suffer from aphasia or language impairment. They have difficulty forming thoughts or expressing them in coherent ways. This is extremely frustrating and frightening for the patient and family.

- **Receptive aphasia** means that the person cannot comprehend communication.
- **Expressive aphasia** means that the person cannot properly form thoughts or express them coherently.
- **Global aphasia** means that the person has lost all language abilities.

Review Unit 7 for guidelines for communicating with patients with aphasia.

Parkinson's Disease

Parkinson's disease is believed to be caused by not having enough neurotransmitters (dopamine) in the brain stem and cerebellum. The symptoms are progressive over many years. Some people will show minor changes. Others will have much more obvious symptoms.

Signs and Symptoms. Signs and symptoms of Parkinson's disease include:

- **Tremors** (uncontrolled trembling). Tremors of the hands commonly affect the fingers and thumb in such a way that an affected person will appear to be rolling a small object (such as a pill) between them. These tremors occur frequently. They usually begin in the fingers, then involve the entire hand and arm, and finally affect an entire side of the body. Starting on one side, the tremors eventually involve both sides of the body. Tremors are more evident when the person is inactive. A typical posture of a patient suffering from Parkinson's disease is shown in Figure 40-16.
- Muscular rigidity (loss of flexibility). The muscular rigidity is more evident when the patient is inactive. It seems to be lessened when the person sleeps or engages in activities such as walking or other exercises that require large-muscle involvement. The rigidity makes the person with Parkinson's disease more prone to falls and injury.
- **Akinesia** (difficulty and slowness in carrying out voluntary muscular activities). Persons with advanced Parkinson's typically have:
  — A shuffling manner of walking
  — Difficulty starting the process of walking
  — Difficulty stopping smoothly once walking has started
  — Affected speech, causing words to be slurred and poorly spoken (enunciated)

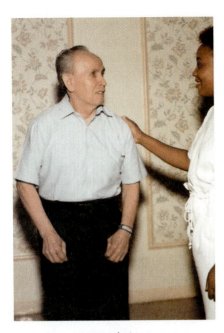

Ventral view

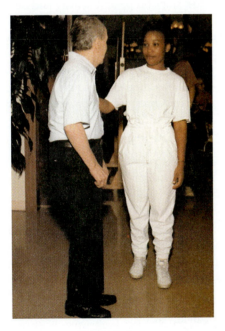

Lateral view

FIGURE 40-16 Note the typical posture from a front and lateral view of the patient with Parkinson's disease.

— Facial muscles that lose expressiveness and emotional response
- Loss of autonomic nervous control. Because of loss of autonomic nervous control, persons with Parkinson's may:
  — drool.
  — become incontinent.
  — become constipated.
  — retain urine.

- Mood swings and gradual behavioral changes. A patient may appear up and positive one moment, and then be depressed the next. The depression tends to be progressive. Personality and behavioral changes may occur that cause psychotic breakdowns and dementia in later stages.

Treatment. The treatment consists of:

- Surgery for some younger persons
- Drug therapy
- Therapy to limit the muscular rigidity and to meet the basic physical and emotional needs

Nursing Care. Nursing care of the person with Parkinson's disease includes:

- Maintaining a calm environment. Symptoms are more intense when the patient is under stress.
- Assisting and supervising the activities of daily living. For example, directing food into the mouth and then keeping it there to be chewed and swallowed is very difficult for many persons with Parkinson's disease.
- Providing emotional support and encouragement.
- Carrying out a program of general and specific exercises.
- Providing protection for patients with dementia.

Multiple Sclerosis

Multiple sclerosis (**MS**) generally occurs in young adults. It is the result of the loss of insulation (myelin) around central nervous system nerve fibers. This interferes with the ability of the nerve fibers to function.

The cause of MS is unknown. Many individuals live the usual life span even though they have this chronic condition. The symptoms are variable and may not be the same for all individuals. Symptoms may include:

- Loss of sensation with regard to temperature, pain, and touch
- Feelings of numbness and tingling
- **Vertigo** (a spinning or dizzy sensation)
- **Lhermitte's sign** (a tingling, shock-like sensation that passes down the arms or spine when the neck is flexed)

Problems with vision occur in almost half of the people who have MS. The problem may be temporary or permanent. Vision symptoms may include:

- Blurriness, color blindness, or difficulty seeing objects in bright light
- Double vision
- **Nystagmus** (jerky eye movements)

Mobility is usually affected:

- Pain in the legs that disappears with rest
- **Paraplegia** (paralysis of both legs) and **quadriplegia** (paralysis of all four extremities) in advanced cases
- Spasticity of muscles
- **Intention tremor** (shaking of the hands that gets worse as the individual tries to touch or pick up an object)

In severe MS, speech is affected because of the weakness of the muscles in the chest, face, and lips. The speech may be slow, with poor articulation. The mind usually remains alert. Incontinence of bowel and bladder are common in advanced cases.

One of the most disabling features of MS is fatigue. The fatigue is very real and is not psychological.

MS may follow one of four courses:

- *Benign course:* mild attacks with long periods of no symptoms.
- *Exacerbating-remitting:* Severe attacks (exacerbations) followed by periods of partial or complete recovery (remissions). Often the periods of exacerbation get longer and more severe with shorter periods of remission.
- *Slowly progressive:* slow, steady deterioration.
- *Rapidly progressive:* deterioration is rapid and progressive and may be life-threatening.

Nursing Care. Nursing care of the patient with multiple sclerosis includes:

1. Implement pressure ulcer prevention program.
2. Implement contracture prevention programs through consistent changes of position and passive range-of-motion exercises. Apply splints correctly, if ordered.
3. Pay careful attention to catheter care if patient has an indwelling catheter, to prevent bladder infections.
4. Encourage independence. Follow instructions of nurse or the therapists for specific techniques to use.
5. Help the patient maintain a balanced schedule of rest and activity.
6. Provide emotional support and encouragement.

Treatment. There is no known way to stop the progression of the disease. Treatment consists of maintaining functional ability as long as possible through general health practices and physical therapy.

Seizure Disorder (Epilepsy)

Seizure disorder (convulsions, epilepsy) involves recurrent, transient attacks of disturbed brain function. It is characterized by various forms of convulsions called *seizures.* Not all seizures are alike. A seizure occurs when one or more of the following is present:

- An altered state of consciousness, which may be momentary or prolonged
- Convulsive uncontrolled movements
- Disturbances of feeling or behavior

Seizures may develop:

- congenitally, associated with a difficult birth.
- following a head injury.
- as a result of increased intracranial pressure.
- as a result of lesions of the brain such as tumors.
- as a result of cerebrovascular accidents.
- as a result of high fever, especially in infants and children.

Some persons experience an aura just before the seizure occurs. An aura involves one of the senses. The person may smell an unusual odor or hear a sound. The aura is usually consistent and remains the same each time it is experienced. For some people the aura serves as a warning so the person can get to a safe place. Other people may not remember the aura.

Seizure activity is classified as follows:

- Partial seizures
  - There may or may not be loss of consciousness.
  - Seizures generally begin in one part of the body and involve only one side of the body.
- Generalized seizures (Figure 40-17)
  - These include grand mal seizures. There is bilateral generalized motor movement and muscular rigidity. Consciousness is lost and special awareness may or may not precede convulsive movements. The sensory awareness or aura may be in the form of lights, sounds, or aromas and is part of the seizure.
  - Petit mal seizures are characterized by momentary loss of muscle tone. They may involve temporary erratic behavior without awareness. For example, the individual stops his present activity and carries out an unrelated repetitive activity for a few moments. Then he returns to the original activity with no awareness of the interruption.
- Status epilepticus is a condition in which one convulsive seizure follows another so rapidly that the person does not regain consciousness between them. It is a very serious condition.

Nursing Care During Seizures. The main nursing focus during a seizure is to:

- Prevent injury by:
  - Staying with the person
  - Assisting the person to lie down, if there is time
  - Making no attempt to restrain the person's movements or to put anything in her mouth
  - Moving away any object the person might hit, to protect the person from injuring herself
  - Placing a pillow under the person's head
- Maintain an airway by:
  - Loosening clothing, particularly around the neck
  - Turning the person's head to one side so that saliva or vomitus drains out
  - Opening an airway, if necessary, by lifting the person's shoulders and allowing the head to tilt back

If you find a person who is having a seizure:

- Do not leave the person.
- Do not move the person.
- Maintain an airway.
- Ring or call for assistance.
- Protect the person from self-inflicted injury.
- Watch the person carefully.
- Apply standard precautions when caring for a patient with seizure activity. There is a high probability of con-

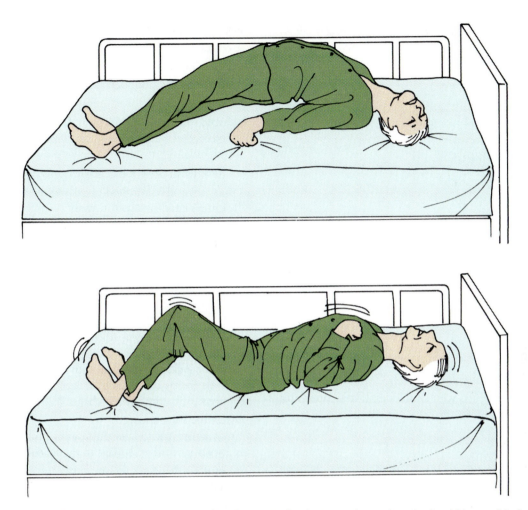

FIGURE 40-17 Generalized grand mal seizures involve the entire body. Note that side rails should be padded and up during a seizure. The side rails are down in the figure for clarity of the view.

tact with blood, body fluids, secretions, and excretions during the care of this patient.

Observation of the patient should be made during and following the seizure. Breathing should be carefully monitored. Ring for assistance, if possible, but do not leave the patient alone. As much as possible, protect the patient from injuring herself during the seizure.

Spinal Cord Injuries

Injuries to the spinal cord result in loss of function and sensation below the level of the injury. These patients are particularly prone to contractures and pressure ulcers. Special terms have been given to the conditions resulting from such injury:

- Quadriplegia—both arms and legs are paralyzed (paralyzed from the neck area down)
- Paraplegia—lower part of the body is paralyzed

Responsibilities of the Nursing Assistant. Spinal cord injury patients need long-term nursing care, which includes:

- Listening. Many persons with spinal cord injury are

taught to give directions to caregivers who are doing for the person what the individual cannot do for himself.

- A consistently calm and patient approach, because the loss of sensory and motor functions often makes self-care difficult.
- Acceptance of the patient's expressions of anger, fear, and depression, as well as clumsy attempts at self-care. Remember that the patient's ability to think is not necessarily impaired. Frustration is even greater because these patients can no longer will their actions.
- Careful skin care, because:
  - Incontinence not only causes the patient embarrassment and discomfort but also makes the skin prone to breakdown
  - The lack of nervous stimulation decreases circulation to the skin
  - Pain and pressure cannot be felt
- Attention to elimination needs. For example, suppositories may be given daily. A catheter may be inserted into the bladder, so catheter and drainage care will be needed. Special pads within plastic incontinence pants may also be used.

- Constant care to prevent contractures. This care involves:
  - Regular turning
  - Proper positioning
  - ROM exercises
- Proper attention and care to prevent:
  - Respiratory infections
  - Urinary tract infections
  - Pressure ulcers

Meningitis

Meningitis is an inflammation of the meninges. It is usually caused by microorganisms.

The signs and symptoms of meningitis are:

- Headache
- Nausea
- Stiffness of the neck
- Seizures
- Chills
- Elevated temperature

This condition is treated with antibiotics. If it is communicable, droplet precautions are used.

Cataracts

Cataracts cause the normally clear lens of the eye to become cloudy. The cloudy (opaque) lens will not allow light rays to pass through. Therefore, the person is no longer able to see.

Treatment. Removal or replacement of the lens permits light rays to enter the eye. Sight is then restored. The lens is needed to adjust vision to different distances. When the lens is removed, glasses must be worn to compensate for the loss. In selected patients, it may be possible to insert an intraocular lens at the time of surgery.

Cataract surgery is performed under local anesthesia. The surgery is performed either as an outpatient procedure or in a day surgery center. The patient is admitted to the center in the morning and remains for one to two hours after the surgery, or until vital signs are stable.

Nursing Care. Nursing care of the cataract patient includes:

- Routine postoperative care related to the specific anesthesia used.
- Relief of pain. Be sure to report discomfort, *especially* any sharp pain in the involved eye.
- Positioning the patient on the noninvolved side or back with the head of the bed slightly elevated.
- Being sure all needed items, such as signal cords, are within easy reach.
- Assisting with all activities, to minimize strain.
- Encouraging the patient not to move rapidly, bend over, or cough. This might cause strain.
- Checking the dressing and reporting drainage to the nurse.

- Taking extra precautions if the patient is confused or restless.
- Checking vital signs until stable.

Orders regarding postoperative activity usually include:

- Protecting the eye for the first four weeks.
- Avoid straining activities such as bending over, lifting objects that weigh more than 20 pounds, or strenuous coughing.
- No water in the eye for the first three weeks.
- Removing crusts around eyelashes with antibiotic ointment and/or a cotton swab.
- Using eyedrops as directed.
- Not sleeping on the operative side.
- Informing the physician if there is an increase in pain or loss of vision.

Retinal Degeneration

Breakdown of the retina, known as retinal degeneration or macular degeneration, occurs over a period of months or years. The incidence increases with age. Central vision is progressively lost as the macula (area of acute central vision) is damaged. Subretinal hemorrhages lead to scarring of this important area.

Early treatment with laser therapy can seal the tiny capillaries to prevent further damage to the macula.

Vision Impairment

Cataracts, glaucoma, retinal degeneration, eye infections, and other eye conditions, such as ocular tumors, can cause blindness. Persons who are legally blind may still have partial vision. The degree of visual limitation must be considered when giving care. It is also important to consider the patient's attitude to the limitations. Adjustment to blindness is both a physical and an emotional process.

Allow the blind or nearly blind person the opportunity to do as much as possible in personal care and other activities. Many blind people are capable and independent. In fact, most blind people do well with minimal help and support once they are fully oriented to their surroundings.

Review Unit 7 for guidelines for working with visually impaired persons.

Artificial Eye

Situations such as severe injury to the eye or untreatable cancer may require the surgical removal of an eye. An eye prosthesis (artificial eye) is usually inserted after the surgery. The care plan should provide information if the patient has an artificial eye. It is necessary to clean the eye socket and artificial eye on a regular basis (see Procedure 96).

Otitis Media

Otitis media is an infection of the middle ear. Infections of the nose and throat can move along the eustachian tube to the middle ear, causing inflammation of the middle ear.

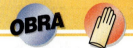

PROCEDURE 96

CARING FOR EYE SOCKET AND ARTIFICIAL EYE

1. Carry out each beginning procedure action.

2. Assemble equipment:
   - eye cup or clean denture cup
   - small plastic bag
   - 4 to 6 cotton balls
   - 2 4 × 4 gauze pads
   - emesis basin with lukewarm water
   - disposable gloves
   - towel

3. Place patient in supine position, if tolerated. Place towel across patient's chest.

4. Put on disposable gloves.

5. Moisten cotton balls in lukewarm water in emesis basin.

   a. Ask patient to close eyes.

   b. Wipe upper lid of affected eye from inner corner of eye to outer edge. Repeat with a clean cotton ball until area is clean and free of mucus.

6. Dispose of cotton balls in plastic bag.

7. Place a 4 × 4 gauze pad in the bottom of the eye cup or denture cup.

8. Remove the artificial eye:

   a. Gently pull down lower eyelid with thumb. Open upper lid with your index finger.

   b. Grasp the artificial eye as it comes out of the eye socket and place it on the gauze in the cup.

9. Use clean cotton balls moistened with water or solution as ordered and clean the empty eye socket. Dry gently with clean, dry cotton balls. Use a new cotton ball for each wipe.

10. Carry cup with artificial eye to sink. Fill sink one-third full with lukewarm water.

11. Wash the eye under lukewarm running water. Use gauze if necessary to loosen and remove any accumulation from eye.

12. Rinse the eye and place it on a dry 4 × 4 gauze pad. (Do not dry artificial eye.)

13. Discard water in eye cup and rinse cup.

14. Remove gloves. Wash hands. Carry artificial eye to patient's bedside.

15. Explain to patient what you are going to do. Put on clean gloves.

16. Insert artificial eye into eye socket:

    a. Position notched edge toward patient's nose.

    b. Lift upper lid with your index finger. Insert eye in eye socket with your other hand. The eye should slip into the socket. Press down gently on lower eyelid so it slips over eye.

17. Carry out each procedure completion action.

Fluid and pus form within the middle ear. This may result in fusion (locking) of the middle ear bones. Increased pressure may cause the eardrum to rupture. Both conditions decrease the ability to transmit sound waves. This condition, which is rare in adults, is common in children.

Antibiotics are usually given. A surgical opening (myringotomy) is sometimes made in the eardrum to drain the pus. Small tubes may be inserted for drainage.

Otosclerosis

Otosclerosis is a progressive form of deafness of unknown cause. The process involves the growth of new, abnormal bone in the bony labyrinth. This growth prevents the stapes from vibrating properly.

Hearing is improved by the use of a hearing aid. Surgery (stapedectomy) removes the excess bone and replaces it with a prosthesis.

Hearing Impairment

Some of your patients will be hard of hearing or completely deaf. A hearing aid (Figure 40-18) will sometimes improve

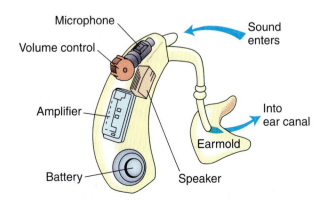

FIGURE 40-18 Parts of the hearing aid

GUIDELINES *for*

Caring for a Hearing Aid

- Store hearing aids at room temperature when not being worn. Temperature extremes can damage hearing aids. They should not be worn for more than a few minutes in very cold weather. Avoid exposing them to hair dryers.
- Keep hearing aids dry. If an aid is worn accidentally in the shower, ask the nurse how to dry it. Never try to dry the aid with a hair dryer.
- Store extra batteries in a cool, dry place. Remove batteries from the hearing aid at night or open the battery compartment. This allows any moisture to evaporate.
- Keep hearing aids safe. They break easily if dropped on a hard surface.
- Remove the hearing aid if hair spray is being used, as the spray may cause damage.
- Turn the hearing aid off when not in use. Turn the aid off before removing it.
- Wipe in-the-ear aids daily with a dry tissue.
- Check regularly to make sure the opening of the aid or earmold is free of wax. In-the-ear types come with a cleaning tool. This should be used only by someone who has been instructed how to use it.

GUIDELINES *for*

Troubleshooting Hearing Aids

If the aid is not producing sound, before inserting it in the patient's ear:

- Check to make sure the "+" (positive) side of the battery is next to the "+" inside the hearing aid battery case or compartment.
- Try a new battery—the old one may be dead.
- Check the earmold to see if it is plugged with wax.
- Make sure the hearing aid is set on "M" (microphone), not "T" (telephone switch).

If the hearing aid is making squealing sounds:

- Determine if the earmold fits properly. It should be completely in the ear. If it does not fit well, report it to the nurse.
- Check the volume on the aid. If it is too high, turn it down until the squealing stops.
- Check the plastic tubing on a behind-the-ear aid. If it is cracked or split, it must be replaced.

Review Unit 7 for guidelines for working with hearing-impaired persons.

Caring for Hearing Aids

A hearing aid is a delicate and expensive prosthesis. It requires safe handling and regular care.

the patient's level of hearing and comprehension. (Refer to Procedures 97 to 99.) Lip reading or sign language may be needed to communicate.

PROCEDURE 97

APPLYING A BEHIND-THE-EAR HEARING AID

1. Carry out each beginning procedure action.

2. Assemble equipment:
   - hearing aid

3. Check the appliance to be sure batteries are working and tubing is not cracked (Figure 40-19).

4. Check to make sure the hearing aid is off or the volume is turned to its lowest level.

5. Check patient's ear for wax buildup or any abnormalities.

> **Note:** *If the patient complains that the hearing aid hurts or does not fit properly, it may need to be refitted; the ear structure changes with age. Report this to the nurse.*

6. Handle the aid carefully.
   - Do not drop it.
   - Do not allow it to get wet.
   - Store it carefully with the switch in the off position when it is not in use. Some aids should have batteries removed when being stored.

continues

PROCEDURE **97** *continued*

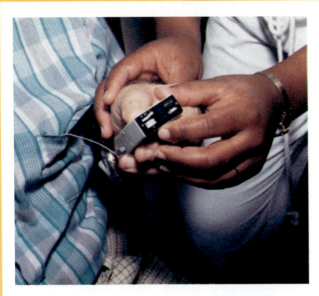
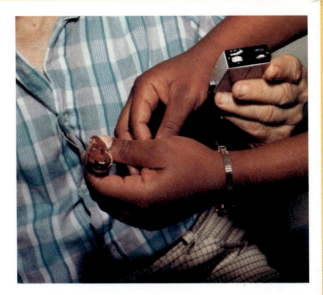

FIGURE 40-19 Check the appliance to be sure batteries are working and tubing is not cracked.

7. Hand the aid to patient so that you support the appliance as the patient inserts the earmold into the ear canal.

Alternate Actions:

8. Place the hearing aid over patient's ear, allowing the earmold to hang free.

9. Adjust the hearing aid behind patient's ear.

10. Grasp the earmold and gently insert the tapered end into the ear canal.

11. Gently twist the earmold into the curve of the ear, pushing upward and inward on the bottom of the earmold, while pulling on the ear lobe with the other hand.

12. Turn on control switch and adjust volume to a comfortable level.

13. Carry out each procedure completion action.

PROCEDURE **98**

REMOVING A BEHIND-THE-EAR HEARING AID

1. Carry out each beginning procedure action.

2. Explain to patient what you plan to do.

3. Turn off the hearing aid.

4. Loosen the outer portion of the earmold by gently pulling on the upper part of the ear.

5. Lift the earmold upward and outward.

6. Make sure on-off switch is in off position. Store hearing aid in a safe area.

7. Carry out each procedure completion action.

PROCEDURE   99

APPLYING AND REMOVING AN IN-THE-EAR HEARING AID

Applying the Hearing Aid

1. Carry out each beginning procedure action.

2. Assist patient into a comfortable position, with head turned so that the ear needing the hearing aid is closest to you.

3. Turn the hearing aid off and turn the volume down.

4. Make sure you insert the aid in the correct ear.

   a. Grasp the earmold and gently insert the tapered end into the ear canal (Figure 40-20).

   b. Gently twist the earmold into the curve of the ear while gently pulling on the ear lobe with the other hand. The hearing aid should fit snugly but comfortably, flush with the ear.

5. Turn on the control switch. To adjust the volume, talk to patient as you increase the volume. Stop when patient can hear you.

Removing the Hearing Aid

1. Wash hands and explain to patient what you plan to do.

2. Turn off the hearing aid.

3. Loosen the outer portion of the earmold by gently pulling on the upper part of the ear.

4. Lift earmold upward and outward.

5. Store in safe area. Either remove batteries and store in safe place or open compartment.

6. Carry out each procedure completion action.

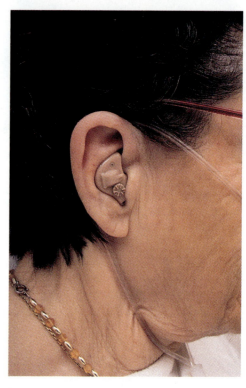

FIGURE 40-20 Gently insert the tapered end of an in-the-ear aid into the ear canal.

DIAGNOSTIC TECHNIQUES

Numerous tests and techniques help physicians diagnose problems of the nervous system. Diagnostic tests include:

- Magnetic resonance imaging (MRI)
- Computerized axial tomography (CAT) scan
- Electroencephalogram (EEG) to measure electrical activity of the brain
- Myelogram, which introduces a traceable dye into the central nervous system
- Tonometry to measure intraocular pressure
- Audiometry to evaluate hearing
- Spinal puncture

Spinal Puncture

Spinal or lumbar punctures are done to withdraw cerebrospinal fluid for examination or to introduce medication or anesthetic into the spinal column. The physician inserts a long, sterile needle between the lumbar vertebrae into the fluid-filled space between the arachnoid mater and pia mater. The pressure of the cerebrospinal fluid is measured. A sample is withdrawn and placed in a sterile test tube. This test may be performed in the patient's room with nurses or nursing assistants helping with the procedure. The patient is placed in a position that will make it easier for the needle to enter the spinal column. It is important that the patient not move during the procedure. The patient may be placed in a lateral position:

- The patient is placed on the side facing away from the physician.
- The knees are drawn up to the abdomen with head bent down on the chest.
- The arms are comfortably flexed (Figure 40-21).

The patient may also be placed in a sitting position (Figure 40-22):

- The patient is seated on the edge of the bed facing away from the physician.
- The shoulders are hunched forward.
- The patient may lean on an overbed table for support.
- It is important for someone to steady the table to prevent the patient from falling.

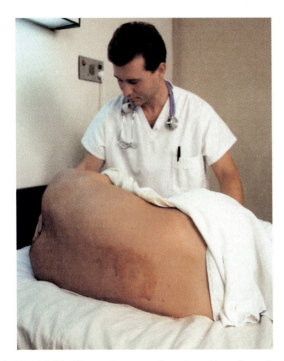

FIGURE 40-21 The patient may be placed in a flexed position for a cerebrospinal puncture.

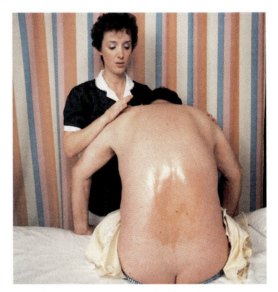

FIGURE 40-22 An alternate position for cerebrospinal puncture

REVIEW

A. True/False.

Mark the following true or false by circling T or F.

1. T F The patient with right-brain damage will not be able to speak.

2. T F If a patient has aphasia, it is not necessary to speak to him because he cannot understand anyway.

3. T F The patient suffering from CVA will need assistance in carrying out ROM.

4. T F Hemiplegia is a paralysis on one side of the body.

5. T F The patient with Parkinson's disease characteristically has a "pill-rolling" tremor to the hands.

6. T F Status epilepticus is a serious condition.

7. T F The Parkinson's disease patient often has mood swings.

8. T F The person with quadriplegia is paralyzed on the left side only.

9. T F Fluid may be withdrawn from the spinal canal for examination.

B. Multiple Choice.

Select the one best answer for each question.

10. The brain and spinal cord make up the
    a. central nervous system.
    b. peripheral nervous system.
    c. sensory organs.
    d. all of these.

11. Neurotransmitters are
    a. neurons.
    b. special nerves.
    c. chemicals that help pass messages from one cell to another.
    d. brain cells.

12. The brain stem controls
    a. voluntary movement.
    b. thinking.
    c. vital functions of the body.
    d. emotions.

13. When the lens of the eye becomes cloudy and impairs vision, it is called
    a. glaucoma.
    b. macular degeneration.
    c. diabetic retinopathy.
    d. cataract.

14. Hearing aids should be kept
    a. at room temperature.
    b. dry.
    c. free of wax.
    d. all of these.

15. Persons with Parkinson's disease generally have
    a. tremors.
    b. rigidity.
    c. slowness of movement.
    d. all of these.

16. A person who has had a stroke on the left side of the brain will
    a. have left hemiplegia.
    b. become quick and impulsive.
    c. have aphasia.
    d. all of these.

17. The person who has had a stroke on the right side of the brain will
    a. have left hemiplegia.
    b. have aphasia.
    c. become slow, anxious, and cautious.
    d. all of these.

18. Patients with stroke
    a. need proper positioning to prevent contractures.
    b. need passive range-of-motion exercises at least twice a day.
    c. should be encouraged to do as much as possible.
    d. all of these.

19. Multiple sclerosis occurs because
    a. the myelin sheath of the neuron is damaged.
    b. of a hemorrhage in the brain.
    c. of a lack of a certain neurotransmitter.
    d. of muscle damage.

20. Patients with multiple sclerosis may experience
    a. loss of sensation to temperature, pain, and touch.
    b. visual impairments.
    c. tremors.
    d. all of these.

21. Increased intracranial pressure can develop from
    a. head injuries.
    b. infections.
    c. CVAs.
    d. all of these.

22. If you are assisting in the care of a patient with a head injury, you should note and report
    a. disorientation.
    b. alterations in speech.
    c. changes in levels of consciousness.
    d. all of these.

23. You come into a room and find a patient having a seizure. You should
    a. leave and find help.
    b. restrain the patient's movements.
    c. raise the foot of the bed.
    d. remove any object the patient might hit.

C. Matching.

Choose the correct item from Column II to match each phrase in Column I.

Column I

24. _____ uncontrolled trembling
25. _____ CVA
26. _____ difficulty and slowness in carrying out voluntary muscular activities
27. _____ language impairment
28. _____ convulsion
29. _____ aura
30. _____ nystagmus

Column II

a. akinesia
b. aphasia
c. tremors
d. seizure
e. sclera
f. stroke
g. involuntary movement of the eye seen in multiple sclerosis
h. sensation experienced by some persons just before having a seizure

D. Nursing Assistant Challenge.

You are assigned to care for Mr. Johnson, who has had a stroke. You learn from his care plan that he has right hemiplegia and aphasia. Consider these questions:

31. From this information, you know that which part of Mr. Johnson's brain was affected by the stroke?

32. What does right hemiplegia mean?

33. What will you expect from Mr. Johnson's attempts to communicate verbally?

34. What complications is he at risk for? What can you do to prevent these complications?

35. What observations might you make that would indicate cognitive impairment?

Gastrointestinal System

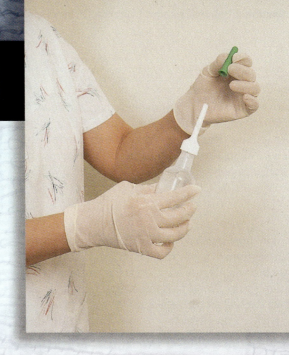

As a result of this unit, you will be able to:

- Spell and define terms.
- Review the location and functions of the organs of the gastrointestinal system.
- List specific diagnostic tests associated with disorders of the gastrointestinal system.
- Describe some common disorders of the gastrointestinal system.
- Describe nursing assistant actions related to the care of patients with disorders of the gastrointestinal system.

- Identify different types of enemas and state their purpose.
- Demonstrate the following procedures:
  - Procedure 100 Collecting a Stool Specimen
  - Procedure 101 Giving a Soap Solution Enema
  - Procedure 102 Giving a Commercially Prepared Enema
  - Procedure 103 Inserting a Rectal Suppository
  - Procedure 104 Inserting a Rectal Tube and Flatus Bag

Learn the meaning and the correct spelling of the following words and phrases:

bile	duodenal resection	herniorrhaphy	peristalsis
bolus	duodenal ulcer	hydrochloric acid (HCl)	proctoscopy
cholecystectomy	enema	ileostomy	pyloric sphincter
cholecystitis	fecal	impaction	sigmoidoscopy
cholelithiasis	flatus	incarcerated	stool
chyme	gastrectomy	(strangulated) hernia	suppository
colon	gastric resection	nasogastric tube (NG	ulcer
colostomy	gastric ulcer	tube)	ulcerative colitis
constipation	gastroscopy	occult blood	urgency
defecation	hernia	pepsin	

INTRODUCTION

The digestive tract extends from the mouth to the anus. It receives the help of the teeth, tongue, salivary glands, liver, gallbladder, and pancreas in breaking food into simpler substances. These substances are used by the body cells to carry on their work of supplying nutrition and eliminating wastes.

STRUCTURE AND FUNCTION

The gastrointestinal system is also called the GI or digestive tract. It extends from the mouth to the anus and is lined with mucous membrane (Figure 41-1). The organs along the length of this system change food into simple forms that can pass through the walls of the small intestine and into the circulatory system. The circulatory system then carries the nutrients to the body cells. The gastrointestinal system includes the:

- Mouth, teeth, tongue, salivary glands
- Pharynx
- Esophagus (gullet)
- Stomach
- Small intestine
- Liver, gallbladder, pancreas
- Large intestine

In the digestive system:

- proteins are changed to amino acids.
- carbohydrates are changed to simple sugars like glucose.
- fats are changed to fatty acids and glycerol.

These changes are brought about by mechanical action and chemicals called *enzymes*. The nondigestible portions of what we eat are moved along the intestines and are finally excreted from the body as feces. Several organs contribute to the digestive process and many disease conditions affect them.

Mouth

In the mouth (Figure 41-2), food is chewed so it can be swallowed easily. The digestive process begins with the help of the:

- Tongue—a skeletal muscle that is covered by tastebuds. The tongue pushes the food between the teeth to be broken up. It assists in mastication (chewing). It propels the food backward toward the pharynx to assist in swallowing. It also aids in speech formation.
- Salivary glands—secrete saliva containing a digestive enzyme called salivary amylase.
  — Salivary amylase begins carbohydrate digestion
  — 1 1/2 quarts of saliva are secreted daily
  — Saliva moistens food to help in swallowing
- Teeth—mechanically break up the food into smaller particles, forming a **bolus** of food. The bolus is then swallowed. There are two natural sets of teeth. The first set (deciduous or temporary) numbers 20. The second set (permanent) numbers 32 and gradually replaces the deciduous set.
- Pharynx—allows the passage of both food and air. It leads to the esophagus.
- Esophagus—a tube 10 to 12 inches long that carries the food to the stomach. Strong muscular contractions called *peristaltic waves* move the food along the tract. These waves begin in the esophagus and continue throughout the intestinal tract.

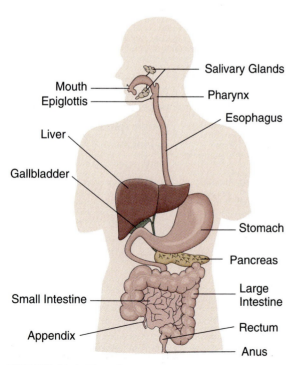

FIGURE 41-1 Digestive system

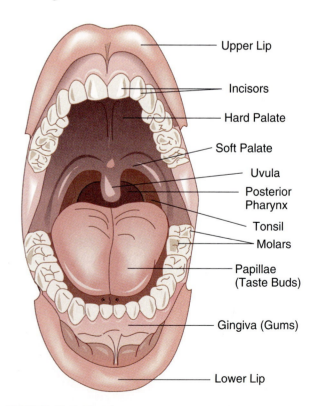

FIGURE 41-2 Mouth

The Stomach

The stomach

- Is a hollow, muscular, J-shaped organ
- Is found in the peritoneal cavity
- Is two-thirds to the left of the midline
- Is just below the diaphragm
- Has circular muscles at either end that hold the food while it is thoroughly mixed with digestive enzymes
- Begins the chemical process of digestion
- Holds the food between 3 to 4 hours

The stomach has three parts:

1. Fundus—the area above the entrance of the esophagus
2. Body—holds the food
3. Pylorus—the long, narrowly tapered distal end that connects with the small intestines. The muscle guarding this exit point is called the **pyloric sphincter**. Sometimes in babies this muscle is so tight (pyloric stenosis) that milk cannot get through and the muscle must be cut surgically.

The stomach cells produce gastric juice, which contains:

- Proteolytic enzyme (**pepsin**) to begin protein breakdown
- Hydrochloric acid (HCl)
- Intrinsic factor, needed for the absorption of vitamin B_{12}

The Intestines

When food leaves the stomach, it is in a semiliquid form called **chyme**. Chyme enters the small intestine, where any undigested nutrients are broken down by intestinal and pancreatic enzymes and bile from the liver.

Materials continue to be moved through the intestines by waves of **peristalsis**. Food digestion is completed in the small intestine. Most of the nutrients and food the body needs are absorbed into the bloodstream through the walls of the small intestine.

The small intestine is about 20 feet long. It coils within the peritoneum. There are three main portions:

1. The duodenum—about 12 inches long. Has an opening in the back to receive the bile and pancreatic secretions.
2. The jejunum—about 8 feet long.
3. The ileum—the last 12 to 13 feet. Terminates in the ileocecal valve and is connected to the large intestine. The ileocecal valve prevents food from traveling backward into the small intestine.

The large intestine (colon) is 4 1/2 feet long. It is divided into several sections:

- Cecum
- Ascending colon
- Transverse colon
- Descending colon
- Sigmoid colon
- Rectum
- Anus

No digestive enzymes are secreted in the colon. The colon is the place where:

- Some vitamins are absorbed into the circulatory system.
- More complex carbohydrates are acted upon by bacteria.
- Much of the remaining water is absorbed through the walls of the large intestine, changing wastes to a more solid form. In this way, the large intestine helps to maintain the water balance of the body.

Peristalsis continues to move waste through the large intestine until it reaches the rectum. When a certain amount has been collected in the rectum, it is eliminated as feces through the anus. This process is called **defecation**.

The Appendix

The appendix is located in the lower right quadrant, attached to the cecum. Its function is not known. When it becomes inflamed, the condition is called *appendicitis.*

Liver and Gallbladder

The liver is a large gland that has four lobes. It is located just beneath the right diaphragm. It carries on numerous metabolic functions. For example, the liver helps control the amount of protein and sugar in the blood by changing and storing excess amounts. It produces blood proteins such as prothrombin and fibrinogen, which are important factors in the blood clotting process. The liver also produces bile, which is carried directly to the small intestine for use in digestion or to the gallbladder for storage. Bile prepares (emulsifies) fats for digestion.

The gallbladder is a small hollow sac that is attached to the underside of the liver. It holds about two ounces of bile that it receives from the liver. It releases bile into the small intestine to help digest a fatty meal. The presence of bile in the digestive tract gives solid wastes their usual brown color.

The Pancreas

The pancreas is a glandular organ that produces both exocrine secretions (digestive enzymes) and endocrine secretions (insulin and glucagon). It extends from behind the stomach into the curve of the duodenum. It manufactures pancreatic juice. The pancreatic juice is sent into the duodenum to aid in the digestion of foods. The pancreas also produces insulin and glucagon. Both insulin and glucagon are sent directly into the bloodstream.

COMMON CONDITIONS

The tubelike mucus membrane structure of the alimentary canal lends itself to the possibility of malignancies, ulcerations, obstructions, and herniations.

Malignancy

Malignancies (cancers) of the gastrointestinal tract are very common. The symptoms they cause depend on their location. Among the symptoms are:

- Obstruction. The blocking of the passageway is sometimes the first major indication of a long-growing tumor.

- Indigestion.
- Vomiting.
- Constipation.
- Changes in the shape of the stool (bowel movement).
- Flatus (gas).
- Blood in the stool.

Treatment. Malignancies of the intestinal tract are usually treated surgically by removing the affected part. For example:

- Esophagectomy—removal of the esophagus
- Subtotal gastrectomy—removal of part of the stomach
- Colectomy (bowel resection)—removal of a part of the colon (large intestine).
- Colostomy—creation of an artificial opening in the abdominal wall and bringing a section of the colon to it for the elimination of feces
- Ileostomy—creation of an artificial opening in the abdominal wall and bringing a section of ileum through it for the elimination of waste

Ulcerations

An ulcer (sore or tissue breakdown) can occur anywhere along the digestive tract. Common places are the:

- Colon—ulcerative colitis. In colitis, malnutrition and dehydration are brought about by loss of fluids in frequent, watery, offensive-smelling stools with mucus and pus.
- Stomach—gastric ulcer.
- Duodenum—duodenal ulcer.

Treatment. Treatment of ulcerative colitis includes:

- Medication to slow peristalsis (the wave-like contractions of the intestines) and reduce patient anxiety.
- Modification of diet to include high protein, high calories, and low residue. The low-residue diet is one in which the foods are almost completely digested. There is little waste with this type of diet.
- Medication (steroids) to reduce inflammation.
- Antibiotics to control infection by the microorganism *H. pylori.*

Patients with gastric or duodenal ulcers have periodic burning pain about two hours after eating. Most patients improve when they are placed on a diet in which foods that cause distress are not served. Medications are given to neutralize the hydrochloric acid (HCl), to coat the stomach, and to decrease anxiety. It is sometimes necessary to remove part of the stomach (gastrectomy or gastric resection) or duodenum (duodenal resection). Following such surgery, the patient is:

- Placed on NPO. Special mouth care is therefore needed.
- Placed on gastrointestinal drainage. A nasogastric tube (NG tube) (Figure 41-3) is inserted through the patient's nose and into the stomach. The tube is attached to a drainage bottle. Additional tubes are inserted into the intestinal tract. Be careful not to dis-

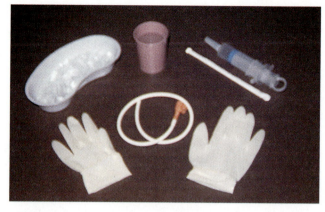

FIGURE 41-3 Materials for nasogastric tube insertion

turb the tubes. Check frequently to ensure that the drainage is not blocked. If drainage becomes blocked, report it to your supervisor at once. The type and amount of drainage are noted and recorded.

Hernias

A hernia results when a structure such as the intestine pushes through a weakened area in a normally restraining wall. The danger of such abnormal protrusions is that some of the protruding tissue can become trapped in the weakened area. Circulation then becomes limited so that the tissue is in danger of dying. This is called an incarcerated (strangulated) hernia.

Frequent sites of herniation are:

- Groin area (inguinal hernia)
- Near the umbilicus (umbilical hernia)
- Through a poorly healed incision (incisional hernia)
- Through the diaphragm (hiatal hernia)

Hernias are usually repaired surgically with a herniorrhaphy.

Gallbladder Conditions

Two common conditions affecting the gallbladder are:

- Cholecystitis—an inflammation of the gallbladder.
- Cholelithiasis—the formation of stones in the gallbladder. The stones may obstruct the flow of bile (fluid that aids digestion), giving rise to signs and symptoms such as:
  - Indigestion
  - Pain
  - Jaundice (yellow discoloration of the skin and whites of the eyes)

Treatment. Cholecystitis and cholelithiasis may be treated by:

- Low-fat diet.
- Surgery to remove the gallbladder and stones. This surgical procedure is called a cholecystectomy.
- Laser therapy to break up the stones.

Drains are often placed in the operative areas. Large amounts of yellowish-green drainage may be expected.

In addition to routine postoperative care:

- Position the patient in a semi-Fowler's position.
- Do not disturb drains.
- If you notice fresh blood on the dressing, increased jaundice, or dark urine, report it immediately to your team leader.

Fecal Incontinence and Constipation

Fecal incontinence is less common than urinary incontinence and is more easily controlled. Bowel retraining aims at establishing continence and preventing impaction.

An **impaction** is the most serious form of constipation and results when the fecal mass loses so much water that it is dry and hard and impossible to eliminate. The dried waste acts as an irritant to the bowel. Mucus tends to dissolve the outer part of the mass, which then drains from the bowel as diarrhea. Whenever there are frequent, small amounts of diarrhea, report this to the nurse, who will check the patient for fecal impaction.

- When retraining is not possible, a fecal incontinence collector may be used (Figure 41-4).

DRAINABLE FECAL INCONTINENCE COLLECTOR WITH FLEXTEND SKIN BARRIER

Preparation and Application

1. Turn patient on one side, bending the upper knee up towards the chest.
2. Clean and dry the perineal area thoroughly.
3. If necessary, trim the skin barrier to fit the perineal area.
   - For females with a narrow perineal bridge, the skin barrier should be cut to fit.
   - Follow the cutting guide, leaving as much of the skin barrier as possible. The barrier should not cover the labia or the vaginal opening.
4. Remove the release paper.
5. Fold the skin barrier in half.
6. Separate the buttocks.
7. Position the pre-cut hole over the anus. Do not enlarge pre-cut hole.
8. Apply and press firmly.
   - Apply barrier to perineal area first, pressing firmly, holding for thirty seconds to allow it to adhere properly.
9. To empty, open drain cap and direct the stool into an appropriate receptacle. For best results, connect to a bedside drainage collector.
10. To remove, gently ease the barrier from the patient's skin, using fabric tab.

Preparation and Application

- Remove oily substances of powders from the skin which interferes with skin barrier adhesion.
- Skin gel wipes on skin may decrease wear time.
- DO NOT cut the barrier opening.
- Trim excess hair with scissors, DO NOT use a razor.

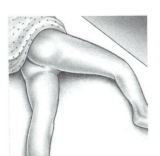

1. Position patient on side.

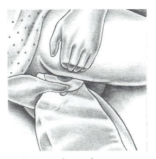

2. Clean and dry skin.

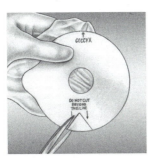

3. Trim barrier, if needed.

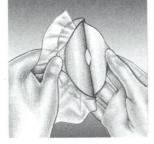

4. Remove release paper.

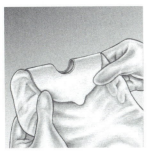

5. Fold barrier.

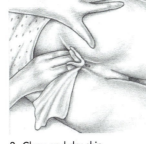

6. Separate buttocks.

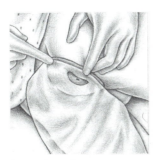

7. Position collector.

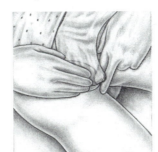

8. Press and seal barrier.

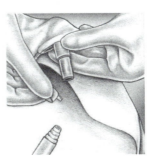

9. Connect to bedside collector.

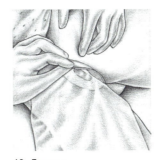

10. Remove.

FIGURE 41-4 Fecal incontinence collection system. *Permission to reproduce this copyrighted material has been granted by the owner, Hollister Incorporated, Libertyville, IL*

PROCEDURE   100

COLLECTING A STOOL SPECIMEN

1. Carry out each beginning procedure action.

2. Assemble equipment:
   - disposable gloves
   - bedpan and cover or collection container
   - specimen container and cover
   - biohazard specimen transport bag
   - label, including:
     - patient's full name
     - room number
     - date and time of collection
     - physician's name
     - examination to be performed
     - other information required
   - toilet tissue
   - tongue depressors
   - basin

3. Wash hands and put on disposable gloves.

4. Uncover container used to collect bowel movement (bedpan or commode receptacle). (If toilet insert is used, specimen will be collected from insert.) If patient is incontinent of feces, use tongue depressors to obtain specimen from bed linens, diaper, or protective padding. A specimen may also be obtained from a fecal incontinence collection bag when it is changed.

5. Following defecation, patient washes hands. Fill basin with water at 105°F. Assist patient if needed. If patient is incontinent, carefully clean and dry area around anus. Change bed linens as needed.

6. Take container with bowel movement to the bathroom. Use tongue blades to remove specimen and place in specimen container (Figure 41-5). Do not contaminate the outside of the specimen container or the cover. If possible, take a sample (about 1 teaspoon) from each part of the specimen.

7. Empty collection container into toilet. Clean or dispose of collection container according to facility policy. If patient was incontinent, dispose of soiled brief or padding as biohazardous waste. Place soiled linen in proper hamper.

8. Remove and dispose of gloves according to facility policy.

9. Wash your hands.

10. Cover container and attach completed label. Make sure cover is on container tightly. Place container in biohazard transport bag.

11. Take or send specimen to laboratory promptly. (Stool specimens are never refrigerated.)

12. Carry out each procedure completion action.

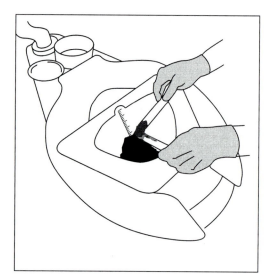

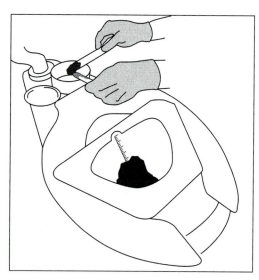

FIGURE 41-5 Use tongue depressors to transfer the stool specimen from the collection container to the specimen container.

- The cause of constipation (difficult defecation) is not always evident. Certainly improper diet, lack of exercise, and inaccessibility of the toilet are contributing factors.

Stool Specimens

A specimen of stool is a sample of fecal material (solid body waste or bowel movement) collected in a special container. (See Procedure 100.) The specimen is then sent to the laboratory for examination. In the laboratory, stool may be examined for:

- Pathogenic microorganisms (germs)
- Parasites
- Occult blood (hidden blood or blood that cannot be seen by the naked eye)
- Chemical analysis

The following advanced procedures are included in Unit 47:

- Testing for Occult Blood Using Hemoccult® and Developer
- Testing for Occult Blood Using Hematest® Reagent Tablets

SPECIAL DIAGNOSTIC TESTS

Some techniques used to diagnose problems of the gastrointestinal system include:

- Gastrointestinal (GI) series—a liquid called barium is either swallowed (upper GI series) or given as an enema (lower GI series). X-rays are then taken.
- Direct visualization procedures:
  - Proctoscopy—visualization of the rectum
  - Sigmoidoscopy—visualization of the sigmoid colon
  - Gastroscopy—visualization of the stomach

In preparation for the tests, the entire GI tract must be emptied before the x-rays.

- No food is permitted for eight hours or longer.
- Enemas are given before the series until only the clear liquid returns.
- Laxatives are given the night before the test.

Cholecystogram (Gallbladder Series)

A gallbladder (GB) series is an x-ray examination similar to the GI series except that the dye tablets are swallowed. Orders for preparing patients for this test vary. Cleansing enemas are frequently ordered. A special diet may also be required beforehand.

Ultrasonography

Ultrasound is very high frequency sound that cannot be heard. When concentrated in a beam and directed at body organs and tissues, the ultrasound moves at different speeds through the tissues, because of the varying tissue density. This permits a picture to be made of the tissues being examined. Ultrasonography is the use of sound to produce an image of an organ or tissue.

ENEMAS

A cleansing enema is the technique of introducing fluid into the rectum to remove feces and flatus (gas) from the colon and rectum. (Refer to Procedures 101 and 102.) Enemas are given:

- to aid illumination during x-rays.
- before surgery.
- before testing.
- during bowel retraining programs.
- to relieve constipation and impaction.
- to instill drugs.

The fluids often used for enemas are:

- Soap solution (SSE)
- Salt solution (saline)
- Tap water (TWE)
- Phosphosoda

These solutions create a feeling of urgency in the patient's bowel. Solutions are expelled a short time after they are given. Urgency is the term used to describe the need to empty the bowel. When enemas are given in preparation for diagnostic x-rays or to instill drugs, the fluid is retained as long as possible.

General Considerations

Some general considerations to keep in mind are:

- If the patient is to get up following the enema and use the bathroom, make sure the bathroom is available and not in use before giving the enema.
- When possible, the enema should be given before the patient's bath or before breakfast.
- Do not give an enema within an hour following a meal.
- You must have a physician's order for an enema.

Position

The best position for the patient to receive an enema is in the left Sims' position. Fluid flows into the bowel more easily when the patient is in this position. The left Sims' position and several alternative positions are shown in Figure 41-6.

At times, the enema may have to be administered with the patient on the bedpan in the supine position. The supine position can be used if the patient is unable to hold the fluid or to assume Sims' position.

- The patient's knees are flexed and separated.
- An orthopedic (fracture) bedpan is more comfortable than a regular bedpan. It may have to be padded when the patient is very thin.

Some patients may not be able to hold the enema fluid. For this reason, disposable gloves are worn when administering an enema.

Disposable Enema Units

Disposable enema units are available to give:

- Soap solution enema

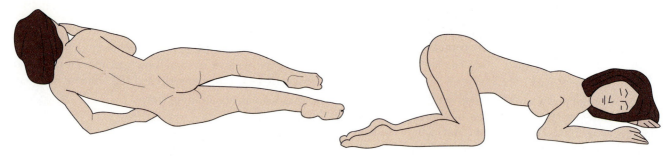

Sims' (left-lateral) Position

Knee-Chest Position

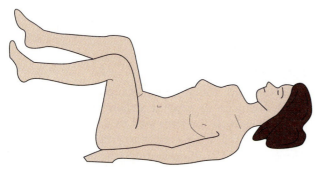

Position for Self-Administration

Child's Position

FIGURE 41-6 Alternative positions for enema administration. *Courtesy of C.B. Fleet Co., Inc.*

- Commercially prepared enema
- Phosphosoda enema
- Oil-retention enema

Administration of disposable enemas is simple. Time is saved in preparing and cleaning the equipment. The techniques for using reusable equipment for oil-retention or soap solution enemas are the same. The procedures when using a prepackaged prepared solution follow.

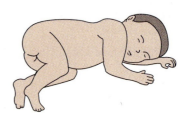

PROCEDURE 101

GIVING A SOAP SOLUTION ENEMA

1. Carry out each beginning procedure action.
2. Assemble equipment:
   - disposable gloves
   - disposable enema equipment, consisting of a plastic container, tubing with rectal tube, clamp, and lubricant (equipment is commercially available as a kit)
   - bedpan and cover
   - bed protector
   - toilet tissue
   - bath blanket
   - castile soap packet
   - towel, soap, basin
3. In the utility room:
   a. Connect tubing to solution container (Figure 41-7A).

continues

PROCEDURE **101** *continued*

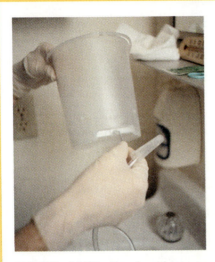

FIGURE 41-7A Attach tubing to container.

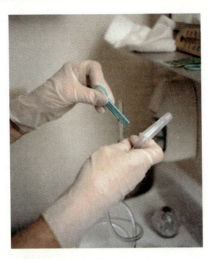

FIGURE 41-7B Slip clamp over tubing.

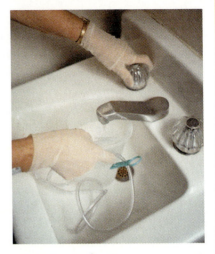

FIGURE 41-7C Fill container with warm water.

b. Adjust clamp on tubing and snap shut (Figure 41-7B).

c. Fill container with warm water (105°F) to the 1,000-mL line (500 mL for children) (Figures 41-7C and D).

d. Open packet of liquid soap and put the soap in the water (Figure 41-7E).

e. Using the tip of the tubing, mix the solution (mix gently so that no suds form) or rotate the bag to mix. Do not shake.

f. Run a small amount of solution through tube to eliminate air and warm the tube

(Figure 41-7F). Clamp the tubing (Figure 41-7G).

4. Place chair at the foot of the bed and cover with a bed protector. Place the bedpan on it.

5. Elevate bed to comfortable working height. Be sure opposite side rail is up and secure for safety.

6. Cover patient with a bath blanket and fanfold linen to foot of bed.

7. Wash hands and put on gloves.

8. Place bed protector under buttocks.

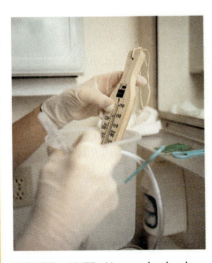

FIGURE 41-7D Use a bath thermometer to be sure temperature of water is about 105°F.

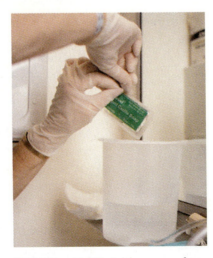

FIGURE 41-7E Add soap from packet.

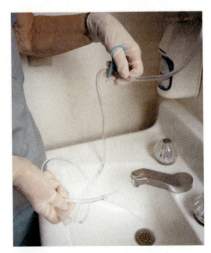

FIGURE 41-7F Let a small amount of water flow through the tube to expel air.

continues

PROCEDURE   101   continued

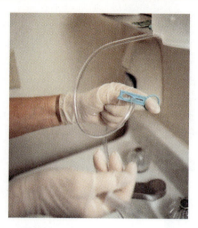

FIGURE 41-7G Clamp the tubing.

9. Help patient turn to left side and flex knees.

10. Place container of solution on chair so tubing will reach patient.

11. Adjust bath blanket to expose anal area.

12. Expose anus by raising upper buttock.

13. Lubricate tip of tube. Patient should breathe deeply and bear down as tube is inserted, to relax the anal sphincter. Insert tube 2 to 4 inches into the anus.

14. Never force the tube. If tube cannot be inserted easily, get help. There may be a tumor or a mass of feces blocking the bowel. The mass of feces is known as an *impaction*.

15. Open the clamp and raise the container 12 inches above the level of the anus so that the fluid flows in slowly (Figure 41-7H).

• Ask patient to take deep breaths to relax the abdomen.

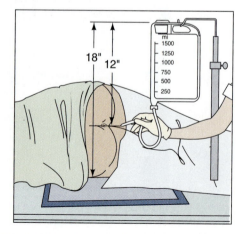

FIGURE 41-7H Raise container above level of anus so fluid flow is unobstructed.

• If patient complains of cramping, clamp the tube and wait until cramping stops. Then open the tubing to continue fluid flow.

16. Clamp the tubing before container is completely empty.

17. Tell patient to hold breath while upper buttock is raised and tube is gently withdrawn.

18. Wrap tubing in paper towel. Put it in the disposable container.

19. Place patient on bedpan or assist to bathroom.

20. Using a paper towel, so your glove does not contaminate the control or crank, raise the head of the bed to a comfortable height if patient is on the bedpan. Raise side rail for safety if bed is left in the higher horizontal position.

21. Place toilet tissue and signal cord within reach of patient. If patient is in bathroom, stay nearby. Caution patient not to flush toilet.

22. Discard disposable materials as biohazardous waste, according to facility policy.

23. Remove gloves and discard according to facility policy. Wash hands.

24. Return to bedside. Wash hands and put on gloves.

25. Remove bedpan. Place it on a bed protector on chair and cover.

26. Cleanse the anal area.

27. Remove the bed protector and discard according to facility policy.

28. Remove gloves and wash hands.

29. Give patient soap, water, and towel to wash and dry hands.

30. Replace top bedding and remove bath blanket.

31. Put on gloves. Take bedpan to bathroom. Dispose of contents according to facility policy or, using a paper towel, flush toilet.

32. Remove gloves and dispose of according to facility policy.

33. Wash hands.

34. Air the room and leave room in order.

35. Unscreen unit.

36. Clean and replace all other equipment used according to facility policy.

37. Carry out each procedure completion action.

Giving an Enema with a Commercially Prepared Chemical Enema Solution

Commercially prepared enemas are convenient to administer and more comfortable for the patient. The enema may be either an oil-retention enema or a phosphosoda enema and is following by a cleansing (soap solution) enema.

- The solution is already measured and ready to use.
- A small amount of fluid will remain in the container after administration.
- The solution in a phosphosoda enema draws fluid from the body to stimulate peristalsis.
- The oil-retention enema solution softens the feces, making them easier to expel.
- The amount of solution administered is about 4 ounces.
- The tip of the container is pre-lubricated.
- The enema solution is in an easy-to-handle plastic container.
- The solution is sometimes used at room temperature.
- You may be asked to warm the solution by placing the container in warm water before administration. Check with the nurse regarding your facility's policy.

PROCEDURE **102**

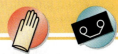

GIVING A COMMERCIALLY PREPARED ENEMA

Note: This procedure may be followed when giving an oil-retention or a phosphosoda enema.

1. Carry out each beginning procedure action.
2. Assemble equipment:
   - disposable gloves
   - disposable pre-packaged enema
   - bedpan and cover
   - bed protector
   - pan of warm water (if enema solution is to be warmed)
3. Open package and remove plastic container with enema solution. Place solution container in warm water (if it is to be warmed).
4. Lower head of bed to horizontal position and elevate bed to comfortable working height. Raise side rail on opposite side of bed for safety.
5. Put on gloves.
6. Place bedpan and cover on the chair close at hand.
7. Assist patient to turn to the left side and flex the right leg.
8. Place bed protector under patient.
9. Expose only patient's buttocks by drawing the bedding upward in one hand.
10. Remove the cover from the enema tip (Figure 41-8). Gently squeeze to make sure tip is undamaged (patent).
11. Separate buttocks, exposing anus, and ask patient to breathe deeply and bear down slightly.

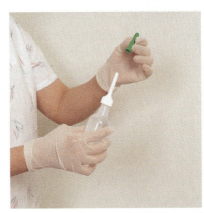

FIGURE 41-8 Remove cover from pre-lubricated tip of container.

12. Insert lubricated enema tip 2 inches into the rectum.
13. Squeeze the plastic container slowly from the bottom of the container until all fluid has entered patient's body (Figure 41-9).

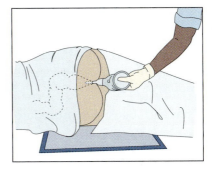

FIGURE 41-9 Squeeze bottle from bottom until all the liquid has gone into the rectum.

continues

PROCEDURE 102 *continued*

14. Remove the tip from patient and place the container in the box. Encourage patient to hold the solution as long as possible.

15. Remove gloves and dispose of properly. Wash hands.

16. Discard the used enema as biohazard waste.

17. Provide privacy. This enema should be retained for 20 minutes. Give patient the call signal and leave.

18. When patient feels the urge to defecate, lower bed and assist patient to the bathroom or commode, or position patient on the bedpan.

19. Raise the head of the bed to a comfortable height if patient is on the bedpan.

20. Place toilet tissue and signal cord within reach of patient. Raise side rail for safety if bed is left in high position. If patient is in bathroom, stay nearby. Caution patient not to flush toilet.

21. Return to patient when signaled. Wash hands. Lower nearest side rail if up. Put on gloves.

22. Remove bedpan and place on bed protector on chair. Observe contents of bedpan. Cover bedpan.

23. Clean anal area of patient, if required.

24. If the patient has used commode or toilet:
    a. Clean anal area if required.
    b. Observe contents of commode or toilet.
    c. Flush toilet using paper towel, or cover commode.
    d. Remove gloves and discard according to facility policy. Assist patient into bed.

25. Put on gloves. Take bedpan or commode container and equipment to the bathroom. Dispose of contents according to facility policy.

26. Remove and dispose of gloves properly. Wash your hands.

27. Give patient soap, water, and a towel to wash hands. Return equipment. Leave side rails down unless needed for safety and leave bed in low position.

28. Carry out each procedure completion action.

Rectal Suppositories

Rectal **suppositories** are used to stimulate bowel evacuation or to administer medication. Medicinal suppositories must be inserted by the nurse. You may be asked to insert the type of suppository that softens stool and promotes elimination.

(See Procedure 103.) Check your facility policy to be sure this is a nursing assistant function. The suppository must be placed beyond the rectal sphincter (circular muscle that controls the anal opening) and against the bowel wall so it can melt and lubricate the rectum.

PROCEDURE 103

INSERTING A RECTAL SUPPOSITORY

 Note: *Be sure this is a nursing assistant procedure at your facility.*

1. Carry out each beginning procedure action.

2. Assemble equipment:
   - disposable gloves
   - suppository as ordered
   - toilet tissue
   - bedpan and cover, if needed
   - lubricant
   - bed protector

3. Wash hands and put on gloves.

4. Help patient turn on the left side and flex

continues

PROCEDURE 103 *continued*

the right leg. Place bed protector under hips.

5. Adjust bed linen to expose buttocks only.

6. Unwrap suppository.

7. With left hand, separate the buttocks, exposing the anus.

8. Apply a small amount of lubricant to anus and to the suppository and insert the suppository. Suppository must be inserted deeply enough to enter the rectum beyond the sphincter (approximately 2 inches) (Figure 41-10).

9. Encourage patient to take deep breaths and relax (until the need to defecate is felt in 5 to 20 minutes).

10. Remove gloves and dispose of properly. Wash hands.

11. Adjust the bedding and help patient to assume a comfortable position.

12. Place call bell near patient's hand, but check every 5 minutes.

13. Wash hands and put on gloves.

14. Assist patient to bathroom or commode, or position patient on bedpan.

15. Provide privacy. Once patient is finished, assist with hygiene if necessary.

16. Observe results and note any unusual characteristics of stool. If stool is unusual, save and report to nurse.

17. Dispose of stool and clean equipment according to facility policy. Store equipment as required.

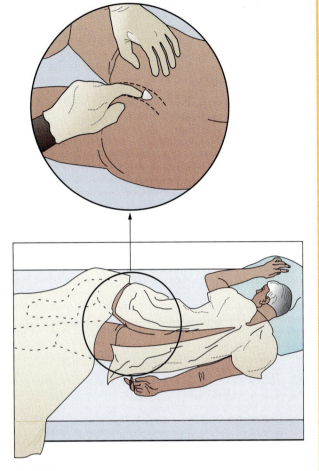

FIGURE 41-10 Lubricate anus and insert suppository beyond the rectal sphincter muscle.

18. Remove and dispose of gloves according to facility policy. Wash hands.

19. Carry out each procedure completion action.

Rectal Tube and Flatus Bag

The rectal tube is used to reduce flatus (gas) in the bowel. Placing a rectal tube into the rectum provides a passageway for the gas to escape. Flatus distends the intestines, causing pain and stress on incisions.

You can assist the patient as follows:

- Encourage activity.
- Promote regularity.
- Accept the expulsion of gas as a natural body function. Do not contribute to the patient's embarrassment.

- Use flatus-reducing procedures when ordered.
- Insert a rectal tube with flatus bag if ordered. (Remember that your facility policies must state that nursing assistants can perform this procedure.) (See Procedure 104.)

The disposable tube is used once in a 24-hour period for no more than 20 minutes.

- Relief may occur as soon as the tube is inserted.
- Check the amount of abdominal distention (stretching).
- Question the patient about the amount of relief.

PROCEDURE **104**

INSERTING A RECTAL TUBE AND FLATUS BAG

1. Carry out each beginning procedure action.

2. Assemble equipment:
   - disposable gloves
   - disposable rectal tube and flatus bag
   - bed protector
   - lubricant
   - tissue
   - tape
   - paper towel

3. Identify patient and screen unit. Explain what you plan to do.

4. Lower the head of the bed to horizontal position.

5. Wash hands and put on gloves.

6. Assist patient to turn to the left side and flex the right leg. Place bed protector under hips.

7. Adjust bed linen to expose only patient's buttocks.

8. Lubricate tip of rectal tube.

9. Separate buttocks, exposing anus, and ask patient to breathe deeply and bear down gently.

10. Insert lubricated tip or rectal tube 2 to 4 inches.

11. Secure rectal tube in place with small piece of hypoallergenic adhesive (Figure 41-11).

12. Remove gloves and dispose of properly. Wash hands.

13. Adjust bedding and make patient comfortable. Leave unit neat and tidy. Place signal cord within reach of patient.

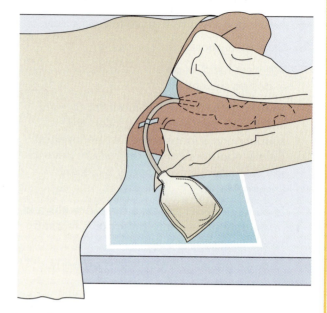

FIGURE 41-11 Secure rectal tube with flatus bag in place using a small amount of hypoallergenic tape

14. Return to unit in 20 minutes. Wash your hands.

15. Put on gloves.

16. Gently remove rectal tube and place on paper towel.

17. Clean area around anus as needed.

18. Dispose of wrapped rectal tube and bag according to facility policy.

19. Remove and dispose of gloves according to facility policy. Wash hands.

20. Carry out each procedure completion action.

REVIEW

A. True/False.

Mark the following true or false by circling T or F.

1. T F A herniorrhaphy is the surgery performed when there is bowel malignancy.

2. T F The drainage from a new cholecystectomy patient is normally yellowish-green.

3. T F The patient is placed on the left side, if possible, for the administration of an enema.

4. T F When administering an enema using a pre-packaged chemical solution, approximately 4 ounces are given.

5. T F Be sure the bathroom is free before giving an enema.

6. T F A flatus tube is used to reduce abdominal distention from gas.

7. T F A physician's order is needed before an enema can be given.

8. T F When giving a soap solution enema, approximately 2,000 mL are used.

9. T F Gastric ulcers are located in the esophagus.

B. Matching.

Choose the correct word from Column II to match each word or phrase in Column I.

Column I	Column II
10. ___ gas	**a.** stool
11. ___ yellow discoloration of skin	**b.** flatus
12. ___ large bowel	**c.** cholelithiasis
13. ___ feces	**d.** cyanosis
14. ___ gallstones	**e.** cholecystectomy
	f. colon
	g. jaundice

C. Multiple Choice.

Select the one best answer for each question.

15. Signs of possible gastrointestinal malignancy might be
    a. good appetite.
    b. change in stool color.
    c. weight gain.
    d. pallor.

16. Your patient has just returned from surgery for gallstones. She will be most comfortable in the
    a. dorsal recumbent position.
    b. lithotomy position.
    c. semi-Fowler's position.
    d. left Sims' position.

17. Enemas are given before
    a. surgery.
    b. delivery.

c. testing.
d. all of these.

18. The oil-retention enema is usually
    a. preceded by a soap solution enema.
    b. retained one hour.
    c. followed by a soap solution enema.
    d. given in the semi-Fowler's position.

19. Urgency is a term that means
    a. need to urinate.
    b. need to empty the bowel.
    c. pain from flatus.
    d. need to vomit.

D. Completion.

Complete the statements in the spaces provided.

20. The enema given to soften feces is known as ____.

21. The purpose of a soapsuds enema is to ____.

E. Nursing Assistant Challenge.

Mr. Rayburn has been admitted with a provisional diagnosis of gastric ulcers. He had been complaining of a burning sensation in his stomach halfway between meal times. He is scheduled for an upper GI series at 8 AM in the morning. Answer the following questions regarding Mr. Rayburn and his care.

22. What acid is naturally found in Mr. Rayburn's stomach? ____.

23. Before the GI series, will it be all right to serve Mr. Rayburn breakfast in the morning? ____.

24. What procedure will you be asked to carry out before the test? ____.

25. Will Mr. Rayburn swallow the barium or will he be given a barium enema? ____.

26. Will x-rays be taken? ____.

Urinary System

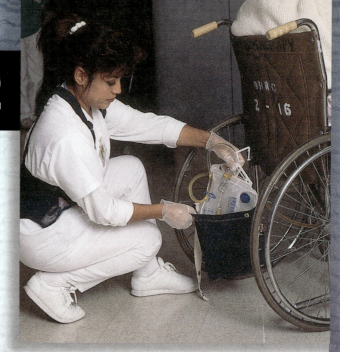

OBJECTIVES

As a result of this unit, you will be able to:

- Spell and define terms.
- Review the location and function of the urinary system.
- List five diagnostic tests associated with conditions of the urinary system.
- Describe some common diseases of the urinary system.
- Describe nursing assistant actions related to the care of patients with urinary system diseases and conditions.
- Demonstrate the following procedures:
  - Procedure 105 Collecting a Routine Urine Specimen
  - Procedure 106 Collecting a Clean-Catch Urine Specimen
  - Procedure 107 Collecting a Fresh Fractional Urine Specimen
  - Procedure 108 Collecting a 24-Hour Urine Specimen
  - Procedure 109 Testing Urine with the Hema-Combistix®
  - Procedure 110 Routine Drainage Check
  - Procedure 111 Giving Indwelling Catheter Care
  - Procedure 112 Emptying a Urinary Drainage Unit
  - Procedure 113 Disconnecting the Catheter
  - Procedure 114 Applying a Condom for Urinary Drainage
  - Procedure 115 Connecting a Catheter to a Leg Bag
  - Procedure 116 Emptying a Leg Bag

VOCABULARY

Learn the meaning and the correct spelling of the following words and phrases:

Bowman's capsule	glomerulus	nephritis	suppression
catheter	hematuria	nephron	ureter
condom	hydronephrosis	pelvis	urethra
cortex	indwelling catheter	pyelogram	urinalysis
cystitis	intravenous pyelogram	renal calculi	urinary bladder
cystoscopy	(IVP)	renal colic	urinary incontinence
dialysis	kidney	retention	urinary meatus
dysuria	lithotripsy	retrograde pyelogram	void
Foley catheter	medulla		

INTRODUCTION

The urinary system consists of the kidneys, ureters, bladder, and urethra. The functions that this system performs are vital. It:

- excretes liquid wastes.
- manages blood chemistry.
- manages fluid balance.

Because the chemistry of the blood and urine reflect the chemistry of the cells, many tests are performed on urine specimens. It is important that urine samples be obtained and preserved properly.

STRUCTURE AND FUNCTION

The urinary system is shown in Figure 42-1. As the name implies, the organs of this system produce urine—liquid waste—that is excreted from the body. The urinary system also helps to control the vital water and salt balance of the body. Inability to secrete urine by the kidneys is known as **suppression**. Inability to excrete urine that has been produced by the kidneys is called **retention**. The organs of this system include:

- **Kidneys**: Organs that produce the urine.
- **Ureters**: Tubes that carry the urine from the kidneys to the urinary bladder. These tubes are 10 to 12 inches long and about 1/4-inch wide.
- **Urinary bladder**: Holds the urine until expelled. The urge to urinate (micturate or void) occurs when 200 to 300 mL of urine are in the bladder, although the bladder can hold more urine than this.
- **Urethra**: The tube that carries the urine to the outside. The female urethra is about 1-1/2 inches long. The male urethra is about 8 inches long. The opening to the outside is called the external **urinary meatus**. The meatus is guarded by a round sphincter muscle that relaxes to release the urine.

The Kidneys

The two bean-shaped kidneys are located behind the peritoneum. They are held in place by capsules of fat. Each kidney weighs about 5 ounces. The outer portion of the kidney is called the **cortex**. This area produces the urine. The middle area is known as the **medulla**. It is a series of tubes that drain the urine from the cortex. The **pelvis** of the kidney receives the urine and directs it to the ureter.

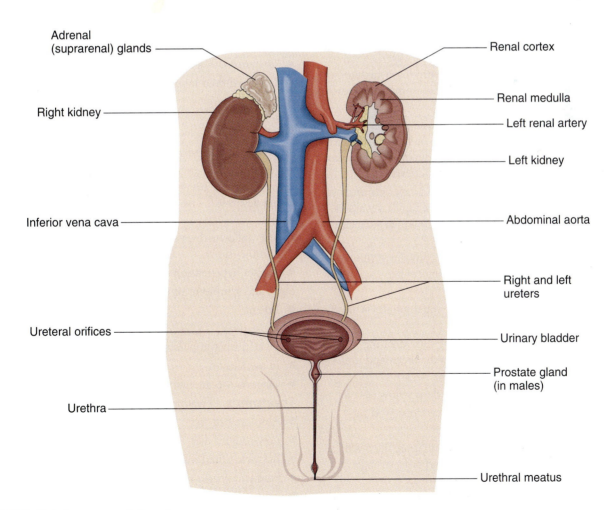

FIGURE 42-1 Structures of the urinary system

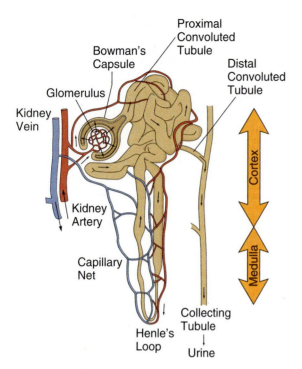

FIGURE 42-2 Nephron and related structures. Small arrows indicate the flow of blood through the nephron. The urine produced by the nephron flows through the collecting tubule.

Urine Production. The renal arteries carry blood to each kidney. Their many branches pass through the medulla to the cortex. In the cortex, urine is produced in filtering units called **nephrons** (Figure 42-2). It is estimated that each kidney contains 1 million nephrons.

Blood arriving at the kidneys carries waste products such as acids and salts. These waste products must be eliminated from the body. Urine is a liquid waste solution containing water and dissolved substances. In the kidneys:

- Waste products, helpful products, and large quantities of water are passed (filtered) through the capillary walls of the **glomerulus** (capillary bed) into **Bowman's capsule**, forming a liquid called *filtrate*.
- The filtrate moves slowly along the convoluted tubules where some water and helpful substances like sugar are reabsorbed into the blood.
- The liquid remaining in the convoluted tubules is urine, which contains wastes.
- The urine passes into the collecting tubules of the medulla, then out of the kidney to the ureter and into the urinary bladder.
- Normal urine is acidic and pale to deep yellow in color.
- Dilute urine has more water and fewer dissolved substances, so it is white to pale yellow.
- Concentrated urine has less water and more dissolved substances, so it is darker in color and has a stronger odor.
- The amount of urine produced depends on the amount of intake and various physical conditions. Inadequate

water intake leading to dehydration results in a small amount of concentrated urine.

The substances in the urine provide good information about the chemistry of the body and how well it is functioning. Tests are frequently performed on the urine (**urinalysis**).

COMMON CONDITIONS

Common conditions affecting the urinary system include inflammations due to ascending or descending infections and obstructions to the normal flow of fluids through the tube structure.

Cystitis

Cystitis, or inflammation of the urinary bladder, is fairly common. It is particularly common in women because of the shortness of the female urethra. Signs and symptoms of cystitis include:

- Frequent urination
- **Hematuria** (blood in the urine)
- **Dysuria** (painful urination and/or burning upon urination)
- Bladder spasm

Treatment. Treatment is aimed at relieving the symptoms and eliminating the cause. Treatment includes:

- Sitz baths
- Rest
- Bacteriostatic agents
- Increased fluid intake
- Antibiotics

Nephritis

Nephritis means inflammation of the kidney. Nephritis:

- May follow an attack of infectious disease or may result from general arteriosclerosis. In either case, kidney cells are destroyed. This results in decreased urine production.
- May follow a disease course that is acute (rapid) or chronic (slow).
- Causes hypertension and edema.

Signs and symptoms of nephritis are:

- Edema
- Hematuria
- Proteinuria (protein in urine)
- Hypertension
- Oliguria (occasionally) (decreased urination)

Treatment. Treatment includes:

- Absolute bed rest
- Low-sodium diet
- Restricted fluid intake, at times
- Frequent checks on vital signs
- Accurate intake and output (I/O) measurement
- Steroid medication in some cases

If both kidneys are involved, the patient will require regular dialysis until the diseased kidneys can be replaced with a healthy kidney (kidney transplant). **Dialysis** is the process of removing the waste products from the blood with a hemodialysis machine, commonly called an artificial kidney.

Many patients on dialysis receive treatment in a hospital dialysis unit or in special outpatient dialysis centers. Other patients receive dialysis at home, using portable dialysis machines. The patient's overall physical condition is an important factor in determining if home dialysis is an option.

Renal Calculi

Renal calculi are kidney stones. They can cause obstructions when they become lodged in the urinary passageways.

There may be no sign of the development of renal calculi until some obstruction develops. Then:

- The pain is sudden and intense. It is called **renal colic**.
- Calculi may be passed in the urine.
- As stones pass along the tract, tissue damage may occur, resulting in hematuria (blood in the urine).

Treatment. The goal of treatment is to relieve the blockage and eliminate the stones.

- Encouraging fluids increases urine output. This helps to move the stones along the tract.
- All urine must be strained through gauze or filter paper, which is inspected for stones before it is discarded (Figure 42-3). Stones that are found can be analyzed. With information from the stones, the diet can sometimes be changed to make the formation of stones less likely.

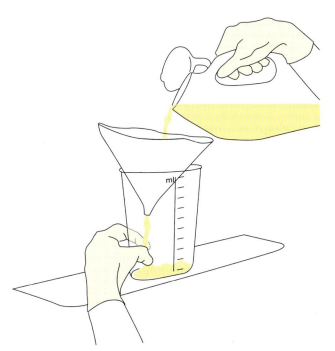

FIGURE 42-3 The urine can be strained through filter paper to retrieve kidney stones that are excreted through the bladder.

- When it is impossible for the patient to pass the stones, surgery may be necessary. This type of surgery can be done by passing a cystoscope through the urethra or through a surgical incision. With the cystoscope, the physician is able to see inside the bladder and locate stones. The stones may then be crushed so they can be flushed out in the urine.
- At other times, the stones can be reached and removed only through a surgical incision. When a surgical incision is made, the patient usually returns from surgery with two drainage tubes in place. One tube is inserted in the urinary bladder. The other tube is inserted in the ureter or kidney.
  - The nurse will see that proper drainage is established.
  - In addition to routine postoperative care, you must check frequently to be sure the drainage is not blocked by kinks in the tubes or by the patient's body lying on the tubes.
  - The amount and type of drainage from each area should be carefully noted.
- **Lithotripsy** is a technique that uses carefully directed sound waves to crush the stones without the need for any surgical incision. The patient receiving this form of treatment is usually in the hospital less than 24 hours.

Hydronephrosis

Hydronephrosis results from accumulation of fluid within the kidney. The increasing amount of urine causes pressure on the kidney cells. As a result, kidney cells are destroyed. The fluid accumulates in the kidney because something is blocking its flow. The flow may be blocked by:

- Renal calculi
- Kinking or twisting of the ureters
- Tumors, especially benign prostatic hypertrophy
- Distended bladder

Symptoms may be acute and similar to those of renal calculi, or they may occur so gradually that they go unnoticed until much damage has been done.

Treatment. The condition is treated by draining the urine above the blockage to relieve pressure and then correcting the cause.

RESPONSIBILITIES OF THE NURSING ASSISTANT

Be sure you understand the orders for each individual patient before you assist in nursing care. Orders regarding positioning, drainage, and activity for urological (urinary) patients vary.

There are some important measures that will apply to most urinary patients in your care:

- Accurately measure intake and output (Figure 42-4).
- Promptly report signs and symptoms of:
  - Bleeding
  - Chilling

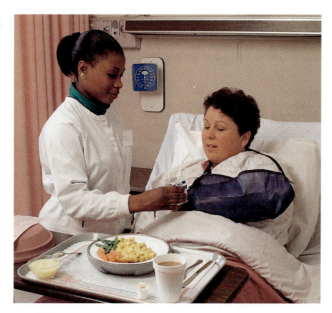

FIGURE 42-4 Once the patient is finished, carefully measure the amount of fluid consumed and mark the amount on the I/O chart.

— Elevated temperature
— Reduced output
— Increased edema
— Pain
- Properly care for urinary drainage.
- Know the proper steps to take for forcing fluids and for limiting fluids.
- When assisting with urination, collecting a urine sample, or recording I/O, note and report the following:
  — Amount of urine
  — Color of urine
  — Odor of urine
  — Presence and type of sediment

URINARY INCONTINENCE

Urinary incontinence (loss of control of urination) may be due to one or a combination of factors. It is not unusual to find more than one factor present at the same time.

- Any interruption of cerebral control can lead to incontinence, including stroke, brain damage that destroys the control centers or pathways, confusion and decreased awareness due to general cerebral degeneration, or aphasia leading to the patient's inability to communicate to others the need for help.

- Incontinence may occur simply because the patient is unable to reach the proper facilities in time. The condition may be related to fecal impaction. Fecal impaction acts as a mechanical obstruction, causing the urine to be retained. The incontinence in this case is actually overflow. Perhaps the most common reason for incontinence is infection. Inflammation irritates sensory nerve

---

GUIDELINES for

Caring for the Patient with Incontinence

Nursing assistant responsibilities include:
- Assisting patients who need help to toilet regularly.
- Answering call lights promptly.
- Always being courteous and patient when assisting patients with toileting.
- Maintaining a positive attitude when changing soiled garments and bed linen and never being critical.
- Performing good perineal care and being sure skin is clean and dry.
- Checking the skin for signs of irritation whenever toileting or bathing a patient or performing perineal care.
- Giving special attention to patients who are confused or forgetful, because they may be unable to clearly state their need for assistance.
- Changing wet linen immediately. This limits discomfort and embarrassment of the patient. Prolonged exposure of the skin to urine is a major cause of skin breakdown. In addition, pathogens grow rapidly on the warmth and moisture and can quickly move upward through the urinary tract, causing life-threatening infection.
- Helping the patient become continent. Little reference should be made to the temporary incontinence. Nursing assistants can do much to give emotional support and reassurance to patients who are incontinent.

---

endings in the bladder. Mucosal and bladder contractions are increased, causing the incontinence.

- Incontinence may be temporary, lasting only a few days. For example, after a period of illness, continence may improve as the patient becomes more able to respond to the environment. Attention to the underlying causes and the temporary use of incontinence pads may be all that is needed. Every effort should be made to help the patient become continent as soon as possible, with little reference to the temporary incontinence. You can do much to give emotional support and reassurance to the patient.

- Incontinence of an established nature continues even though the patient is ambulatory. This is a more difficult, but still not impossible, form of incontinence to treat. Drugs are sometimes used to achieve bladder control. Retraining may also be needed.

DIAGNOSTIC TESTS

Techniques used to diagnose problems of the urinary tract include:

- Magnetic resonance imaging (MRI)
- CAT scan
- Urinalysis—one common method of learning about the condition of the kidneys is to examine and test the urine.
- Cystoscopy—a test usually performed during surgery. It enables the physician to look inside the bladder. An instrument called a cystoscope is inserted through the urethra. Following this examination, frequency of urination is to be expected, but heavy bleeding or a complaint of sharp, intense pain should be reported at once.
- Pyelogram—an x-ray examination of the urinary tract, similar to the GB and GI series. The dye may be given intravenously (intravenous pyelogram or IVP) or inserted during cystoscopy (retrograde pyelogram) through the urethra. Preparation of the patient usually includes cleansing enemas. Satisfactory results of the x-ray examination are largely based on proper patient preparation.
- Blood chemistry tests
  - Blood urea nitrogen (BUN)
  - Creatinine

Urine Specimens

Routine Urine Specimen. Urinalysis is the most common laboratory test. The specimen is usually taken when the patient first **voids** (urinates) in the morning. (See Procedures 105 to 107.) Properties of fresh urine begin to change after 15 minutes. Therefore, it is important that you immediately take the sample to the laboratory or refrigerate it until delivery can be made.

PROCEDURE **105**

COLLECTING A ROUTINE URINE SPECIMEN

1. Carry out each beginning procedure action.
2. Assemble equipment:
   - disposable gloves
   - bedpan/urinal
   - bed protector
   - sterile specimen container and cover
   - label, including:
     - patient's full name
     - room number
     - facility identification
     - date and time of collection
     - physician's name
     - examination to be done
     - other information requested or required
   - graduate pitcher
   - laboratory requisition slip, properly filled out
   - biohazard specimen transport bag
3. Completely fill out the label of the specimen container.
4. Wash hands and put on disposable gloves.
5. If patient cannot ambulate, offer bedpan or urinal.
6. Instruct the patient not to discard toilet tissue in the pan with the urine. Provide a small plastic bag in which to place the soiled tissue.
7. After patient has voided, cover pan and place on bed protector on chair. Offer wash water to patient.
8. If patient can ambulate to bathroom, place specimen collector in toilet.
9. Assist patient to bathroom. Ask patient to void into specimen collector. Instruct patient to discard soiled toilet tissue in plastic bag provided. Tissue must not be placed in collector.
10. Provide privacy.
11. Put on gloves. Remove specimen collector from toilet. If patient is on I/O, note amount of urine (Figure 42-5). If patient used bedpan, pour urine into graduate to measure. Note amount. Remove gloves and discard according to facility policy. Wash hands.
12. Remove cap from specimen container, and place it (inside up) on shelf or other flat surface in bathroom or utility room. Do not touch inside of cap or container.

continues

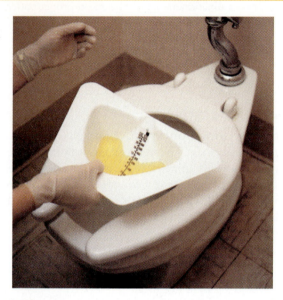

FIGURE 42-5 Remove specimen collector from toilet. Note amount of voiding if patient is on I/O.

13. Put on gloves. Carefully pour about 120 mL urine into specimen container from collector (Figure 42-6).

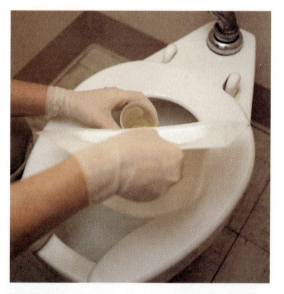

FIGURE 42-6 Carefully pour specimen from collector into container.

14. Remove and discard gloves according to facility policy.
15. Wash your hands.
16. Place cap on specimen container. Do not contaminate outside of container. Attach completed label to container (Figure 42-7). Place specimen container in biohazard specimen transport bag and attach laboratory requisition slip (Figure 42-8).
17. Carry out each procedure completion action.
18. Follow facility policy for transporting specimen to laboratory.

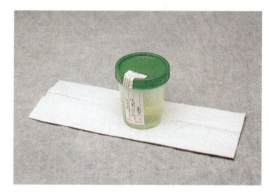

FIGURE 42-7 After specimen is placed in container and cap is put on, place label on container.

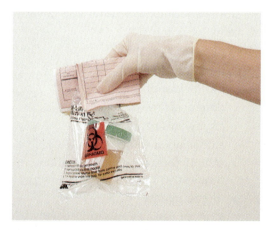

FIGURE 42-8 The properly labeled specimen container is placed in a biohazard specimen transport bag and a laboratory requisition is attached.

PROCEDURE 106

COLLECTING A CLEAN-CATCH URINE SPECIMEN

1. Carry out each beginning procedure action.

2. Assemble equipment:
   - disposable gloves
   - sterile specimen container and cover
   - label for container, with:
     - patient's full name
     - room number
     - facility identification
     - date and time of collection
     - physician's name
     - type of specimen test to be performed
     - any other information requested
   - gauze squares or cotton
   - antiseptic solution
   - laboratory requisition slip, properly filled out
   - biohazard specimen transport bag

3. Wash hands and put on disposable gloves.

4. Wash patient's genital area properly or instruct patient to do so. If soiled due to incontinence, perform perineal care.

   a. *For female patients:*

      i. Using the gauze or cotton and the antiseptic solution, cleanse the outer folds of the vulva (folds are also called *labia* or *lips*) from front to back. Use a separate cotton/gauze square for each side. Discard the gauze/cotton in plastic bag.

      ii. Cleanse the inner folds of the vulva with two pieces of gauze and antiseptic solution, again from front to back. Discard gauze/cotton in plastic bag.

      iii. Cleanse the middle, innermost area (meatus or urinary opening) in the same manner. Discard the gauze/cotton in plastic bag.

      iv. Keep the labia separated so that the folds do not fall back and cover the meatus.

   b. *For male patients:*

      i. Using the gauze/cotton and the antiseptic solution, cleanse the tip of the penis from the urinary meatus down, using a circular motion.

      ii. Discard gauze/cotton in plastic bag.

5. Instruct the patient to void, allowing the first part of the urine to escape. Then:

   a. Catch the urine stream that follows in the sterile specimen container.

   b. Allow the last portion of the urine stream to escape.

   Note: If the patient's I/O is being monitored, or if the amount of urine passed must be measured, catch the first and last part of the urine in a bedpan, urinal, or specimen collection container.

6. Place the sterile cap on the urine container immediately to prevent contamination of the urine specimen.

7. Allow patient to wash hands.

8. With the cap securely tightened, wash the outside of the specimen container. Dry the container.

9. Remove and dispose of gloves according to facility policy.

10. Wash your hands.

11. Attach completed label to the container and place specimen in the transport bag.

12. Carry out procedure completion actions.

13. Follow facility policy for transporting specimen to laboratory.

PROCEDURE   107

COLLECTING A FRESH FRACTIONAL URINE SPECIMEN

1. Carry out each beginning procedure action.

2. Assemble equipment:
   - disposable gloves
   - two specimen containers
   - urinal or bedpan
   - completed labels for specimen containers
   - testing materials if urine testing is to be performed (Ketostix)
   - small plastic bag for used toilet tissue
   - biohazard bag
   - laboratory requisition slip, properly filled out

3. About one hour before testing is to be done, wash your hands and take equipment to bedside. Instruct patient that two samples will be taken: an initial sample now and a smaller sample in about one hour or less.

4. Screen unit and offer bedpan or urinal (patient may be assisted to the commode, if permitted).

5. Put on disposable gloves.

6. Encourage patient to empty bladder.

7. Do not permit tissue to be placed in receptacle. Place in plastic bag and discard.

8. Take receptacle to bathroom or utility room.

9. Pour sample into one specimen container.

Test this sample in case patient fails to void second specimen.

10. Make a note of the test result but do not officially record it. Discard after testing. This reading will be used only if second sample is not obtained.

11. Clean equipment according to facility policy and return to the proper area. Measure and record urine if patient is on I/O.

12. Remove and dispose of gloves according to facility policy.

13. Wash your hands.

14. Offer wash water for patient to wash his or her hands.

15. If permitted, encourage patient to drink water. Be sure to record intake on I/O sheet.

16. Tell patient when you will return for the second sample. Return to patient's unit at the proper time.

17. Wash your hands and identify patient. Explain what you plan to do, and how patient can help.

18. Repeat steps 4 to 14.

19. Place second specimen in protective biohazard bag and attach requisition for transport.

20. Carry out each procedure completion action.

Catheterized Urine Specimen. When a urine specimen is needed that is free of contamination from organisms found in areas near the urinary meatus (opening), the specimen may be collected by inserting a sterile tube (**catheter**). The nurse will perform this procedure.

Twenty-Four Hour Specimen. If a 24-hour urine specimen is ordered, all urine excreted by the patient in a 24-hour period is collected and saved. (See Procedure 108.) A 24-hour urine specimen requires that the patient start the 24-hour time period with an empty bladder. For this reason, the first specimen is discarded.

- All urine is saved in a large, carefully labeled container that is supplied by the laboratory and may contain a preservative.

- The container is usually surrounded by ice. If the patient has an indwelling catheter, place the catheter bag in a container surrounded by ice. Empty the bag into the container supplied by the laboratory.

- The patient is asked to void. This first urine is discarded so that the bladder is empty at the time the test begins.

- All other urine is saved, including that voided as the test time finishes.

- No toilet tissue should be allowed to enter the container.

- If you or the patient forget to save a specimen during the test period, report it immediately to the nurse. The test must be discontinued and started again for another 24 hours.

Remember to put on disposable gloves and remove and dispose of them properly each time you collect a specimen.

Urine Testing

The HemaCombistix® is used to test for the presence of protein, blood, and glucose, and for pH (acidity) of urine. See Procedure 109.

PROCEDURE 108

COLLECTING A 24-HOUR URINE SPECIMEN

1. Carry out each beginning procedure action.

2. Assemble equipment:
   - disposable gloves
   - 24-hour specimen container (supplied by health care facility)
   - label
   - bedpan, urinal, or commode, or specimen collector for toilet
   - sign for patient's bed
   - biohazard bag

3. Label the container with:
   - patient's name
   - room number
   - test ordered
   - type of specimen
   - time started
   - time ended
   - date
   - physician's name

4. Emphasize to patient the necessity of saving all urine passed.

5. Place the specimen collection container in the bathroom in a pan of ice (Figures 42-9A and B). The ice will keep the specimen cool for 24 hours.

6. Put on disposable gloves.

7. Allow the patient to void.

   a. Assist with the bedpan or urinal as needed.

   b. Measure the amount of urine passed if the patient's I/O is being monitored.

   c. Discard the urine specimen.

   d. Note the date and time of voiding. This time will mark the start of the 24-hour collection.

8. Place a sign on patient's bed to alert other health care team members that a 24-hour urine specimen is being collected. (The sign may read: *Save all urine—24-hour specimen.*)

9. From this time on, for a period of 24 hours, all urine voided is added to the specimen container (Figure 42-9C). The container is kept on ice when not in use. Check facility policy regarding handling of the specimen container.

10. At the end of the 24-hour period:

    a. Put on disposable gloves.

    b. Ask patient to void one last time.

    c. Add this urine to the specimen container.

11. Remove sign from patient's bed. Check container label for accuracy and completeness. Attach the appropriate requisition slip.

12. Remove and dispose of gloves according to facility policy.

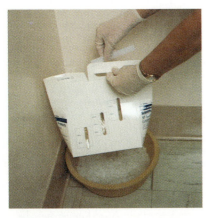

FIGURE 42-9A Place the 24-hour specimen container in patient's bathroom. A plastic fastener holds the top secure. Place specimen container in pan of ice.

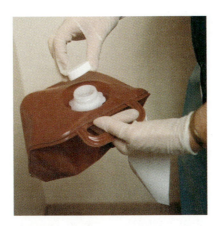

FIGURE 42-9B Some facilities use plastic containers with screw tops when collecting a 24-hour specimen.

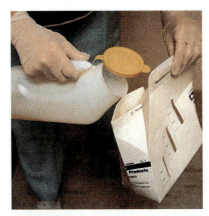

FIGURE 42-9C Open mouth of container wide to avoid spilling specimen.

continues

PROCEDURE 108 *continued*

13. Place specimen in protective biohazard bag for transport.

14. Carry out each procedure completion action.

15. Clean and replace all equipment used, according to facility policy.

16. Follow facility policy for transporting specimen to laboratory.

PROCEDURE 109

TESTING URINE WITH THE HEMACOMBISTIX®

1. Assemble equipment:
   - disposable gloves
   - bottle containing HemaCombistix® reagent strips
   - fresh sample of urine

2. Wash hands and put on gloves.

3. Take reagent strips and sample to bathroom.

4. Remove cap and place on table top side down.

5. Shake bottle gently until reagent strips protrude from end.

6. Remove one reagent strip. Do not touch test areas of strip with fingers. Be sure your gloves are dry.

7. Dip reagent end of strip in fresh, well-mixed urine—remove immediately.

8. Tap edge of strip against container to remove excess urine.

9. Compare reagent side of test areas with corresponding color charts on the bottle (Figure 42-10) at the time intervals specified (Table 42-1).

10. Remove and dispose of gloves according to facility policy. Wash hands.

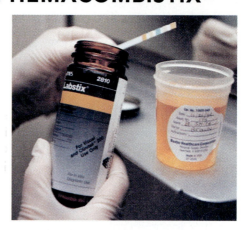

FIGURE 42-10 HemaCombistix® results

TABLE 42-1 HEMACOMBISTIX® RESULTS		
Test	**Reaction Time**	**Results**
Blood	30 sec.	Light blue green to deep blue
Glucose	10–30 sec.	Light blue to dark brown
Protein	Immediately	Yellow to green
pH	Immediately	Orange to blue

RENAL DIALYSIS

As a result of disease or trauma, the kidneys may not be able to carry out their life-sustaining function of filtering impurities from the blood. In this case, mechanical dialysis is substituted to remove wastes from the blood.

Patients requiring this treatment usually have tubing permanently placed in the arm to make it easier to connect to the dialysis machine. The graft attaches to an artery and a vein to provide ready access to the blood circulatory system. When not in use, the tubing from the artery and the tubing from the vein are joined.

 Note: The nursing assistant should never use the arm with a graft to measure blood pressure.

When dialysis is performed, the two sections of tubing are separated and attached to the dialysis machine. Blood passes from the artery to the machine, where impurities are filtered out. The blood is then returned to the patient's vein by way of the graft. The process takes six to eight hours. It is usually performed two to three times per week. Patients with chronic renal failure may be maintained in this manner for some time, often for more than one year.

Sometimes a compatible kidney can be obtained from a donor and transplanted into the person suffering from renal failure. If the kidney is not rejected, it will take on the life-sustaining role of the original kidneys.

URINARY DRAINAGE

Many patients with urinary problems will be on urinary drainage.

- Urine is drained from the bladder through a tube called a *catheter.*
- French catheters or straight catheters (Figure 42-11A) are hollow tubes. They are usually made of soft rubber or plastic. These catheters are used to drain the bladder. They do not remain in the bladder.
- Foley catheters (Figure 42-11B) have a balloon surrounding the neck. The balloon is inflated after the catheter is introduced into the bladder. This is known as an indwelling or retention catheter.

The insertion of a catheter is a sterile procedure. It is performed by the nurse or physician. Closed urinary drainage systems (Figure 42-12) protect the patient from infection.

You have definite responsibilities when patients have urinary drainage:

- Apply the principles of standard precautions.
- Keep the urinary meatus clean.
- Wash the area around the meatus daily with a solution approved by your facility.
- Check regularly for signs of irritation or urinary discomfort and report them to the nurse.
- Secure the tubing so that there is no strain on the catheter or tubing. A catheter strap should be applied to the leg to secure the tubing.

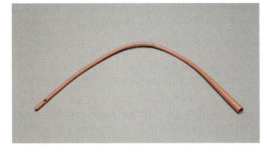

FIGURE 42-11A A straight catheter

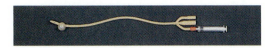

FIGURE 42-11B A three-way Foley catheter with inflated balloon.

- Maintain the drainage bag below the level of the bladder.
- Clamp and unclamp the catheter tubing at specific times. The clamping allows the bladder to fill, stimulating muscle tone.
- Do not open the closed system.
- Make sure the tubing is not kinked or obstructed. Never attach it to the side rail.
- Ensure that the collection bag does not touch the floor.
- Measure the amount of drainage in the collection bag at the end of each shift, note the character of the urine, and report and record the information. (See Procedure 112.)
- Check the entire drainage setup each time care is given and at the beginning and end of your shift (see Procedure 110).
- Report changes in the character or quantity of urine.

Catheter Care

Once the Foley catheter is inserted, the urinary meatus must be kept clean and free of secretions. The area around the meatus is washed daily with a solution approved by your facility or with soap and water. In some facilities, this procedure may be performed on each shift. This care is called indwelling catheter care.

Indwelling catheter care may be performed during routine morning care, as part of perineal care, or as a separate procedure (see Procedure 111). Report signs of irritation or complaints of discomfort, and changes in the character or quantity of drainage.

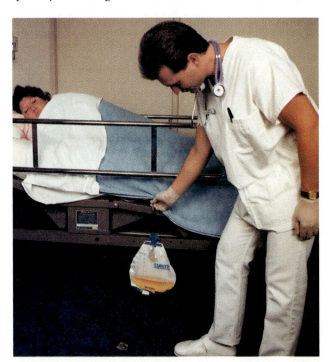

FIGURE 42-12 The closed drainage system carries the urine directly from the patient to the container. There is less danger of infection to the patient using this type of closed system.

PROCEDURE 110

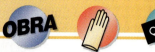

ROUTINE DRAINAGE CHECK

1. Carry out each beginning procedure action.
2. Wash hands. Put on gloves.
3. Raise bedding to observe tubing.
4. Check condition of catheter and meatus.
5. Keep drainage tubing coiled on bed so there is a direct drop to the collection bag (Figure 42-13).
6. Collection bag height must be lower than patient's hips.
7. Keep end of drainage tube above urine level in bag.
8. Be sure drainage bag is attached to bed frame (not side rail).
9. Note color and character and flow of urine.
10. Measure urine using proper technique.

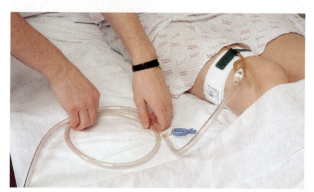

FIGURE 42-13 Check that the tubing is coiled on the bed.

11. Remove gloves and discard according to facility policy.
12. Carry out each procedure completion action.

PROCEDURE 111

GIVING INDWELLING CATHETER CARE

1. Carry out each beginning procedure action.
2. Assemble equipment:
   - disposable gloves
   - bed protector
   - bath blanket
   - plastic bag for disposables
   - daily catheter care kit (if available)
   - washcloth, towel, basin, and soap if kit is unavailable
   - antiseptic solution
   - sterile applicators
   - tape
3. Elevate bed to comfortable working height. Be sure opposite side rail is up and secure. Position patient on back, with legs separated and knees bent, if permitted.
4. Cover patient with bath blanket and fanfold bedding to foot of bed.
5. Ask patient to raise hips. Place bed protector underneath patient.
6. Position bath blanket so that only genitals will be exposed.
7. Arrange catheter care kit and plastic bag on overbed table. Open kit.
8. Wash hands and put on gloves and draw drape back.
9. *For the male patient:*
   - Gently grasp penis and draw foreskin back, if not circumcised (Figure 42-14).
   - Using a new applicator dipped in antiseptic solution for each stroke, cleanse the glans from the meatus toward the shaft for approximately 4 inches.
   - After each stroke, dispose of used applicator in plastic bag.
   - **Alternate action:** Clean around the catheter first and then around the meatus

continues

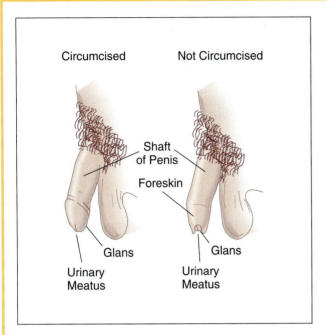

Circumcised   Not Circumcised

Shaft
of Penis

Foreskin

Glans   Glans

Urinary   Urinary
Meatus   Meatus

FIGURE 42-14 Comparison of circumcised and uncircumcised penis

and glans. Wash with soap and water using a circular motion. Dry in the same manner. Make sure to return the foreskin (if not circumcised) to its proper position.

For the female patient:

- Separate the labia.
- Using a new applicator dipped in antiseptic for each stroke, cleanse from front to back.
- After each stroke, dispose of used applicator in plastic bag.
- **Alternate action:** Using a clean cloth, soap, and water, clean labia majora from front to back. Repeat, cleaning labia minora, and then wash meatus. Clean catheter down about 4 inches. Dry carefully.

10. Remove gloves and discard in plastic bag. Wash hands.

11. Check catheter to be sure it is secured properly to the leg (see Figure 42-13). Readjust Velcro® strap for slack, if needed. If a Velcro® strap is not available, use tape (Figure 42-15).

12. Check to be sure tubing is coiled on bed and hangs straight down into drainage container. Empty bag and measure contents, if necessary. Do not raise bag above level of patient's hips.

13. Replace bedding and remove bath blanket.

14. Fold bath blanket and store or put in linen hamper.

15. Lower bed. Adjust side rails for safety.

16. Carry out each procedure completion action.

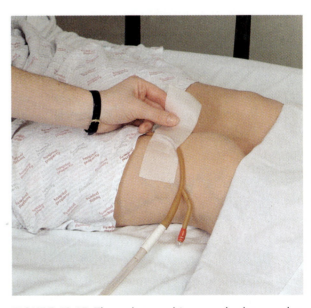

FIGURE 42-15 The catheter tubing can also be taped to the thigh using hypoallergenic tape.

PROCEDURE   112

EMPTYING A URINARY DRAINAGE UNIT

1. Carry out each beginning procedure action.

2. Assemble equipment:
   - disposable gloves
   - graduated container
   - sterile cap or sterile 4 × 4 pad (needed if container has no bottom drain tube)
   - antiseptic wipes

3. Wash hands and put on gloves.

4. Place paper towel on the floor under the drainage bag. Place a graduate on paper towel under drain of collection bag.

5. Remove drain from holder (Figure 42-16) and open. Allow the urine to drain into the graduate, using aseptic technique. Do not allow the tip of the tubing to touch the sides of the graduate.

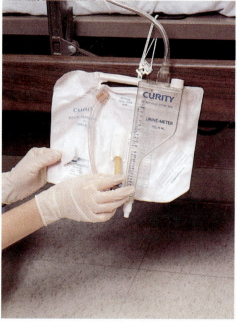

FIGURE 42-17 Return drain to the holder without contaminating the end.

6. Close the drain and replace it in the holder (Figure 42-17). If accidental contamination occurs, wipe the drain tip with antiseptic wipe before returning it to the holder. Dispose of antiseptic wipe in plastic bag.

7. Pick up paper towel, touching top surface only, and discard.

8. Check position of drainage tube.

9. Take graduate to bathroom and empty it.

10. Wash and dry graduate and store it according to facility policy.

11. Record amount of urine and note character.

12. Remove gloves and discard according to facility policy.

13. Carry out each procedure completion action.

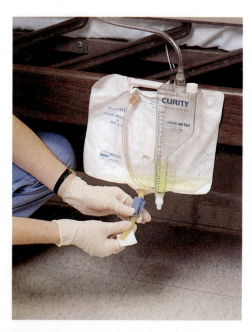

FIGURE 42-16 Remove drain from holder; be careful not to touch the tip.

Ambulating with a Catheter

When patients are ambulatory or using a geri-chair or wheel-chair, you must be careful about the placement of the urinary drainage bag. Remember that the drainage bag must always be lower than the bladder so the urine cannot flow back into the bladder. The bag may be secured to the patient's leg or clothing when the patient ambulates.

When the patient is seated in a wheelchair, the tubing should run below and under the wheelchair so the drainage bag can be secured to the wheelchair back. The drainage bag or tubing must never touch the floor.

At times, the catheter may be disconnected to make ambulation easier. However, there is always the danger of contamination.

Infection Risk

You must follow the procedure for disconnecting the catheter carefully. The patient who has an indwelling catheter is at risk for infection. There are several sites where infection can enter the drainage system (Figure 42-18):

- Urinary meatus, where the catheter is inserted
- Connection between the catheter and drainage tube
- Connection between the drainage bag and drainage tubing
- Opening used to empty the drainage bag

Disconnecting the Catheter

It is preferable never to disconnect the drainage setup, but at times it is necessary. If sterile caps and plugs are available, they should be used. If not, the disconnected ends must be protected with sterile gauze sponges. (See Procedure 113.)

External Drainage Systems (Male)

External urinary drainage systems are preferred for male patients who require long periods of urinary drainage. In external drainage, a catheter is not inserted in the urethra. Thus, there is less danger of infection. A condom (sheath) is connected or some other type of external drainage appliance is applied to the penis (see Procedure 114). The condom is attached to drainage tubing and a collection bag. The condom is removed every 24 hours and the penis is washed and dried. Different types of drainage systems are available. Urine may be collected in a bag that hangs from the bed or wheelchair or in a bag attached to the patient's leg.

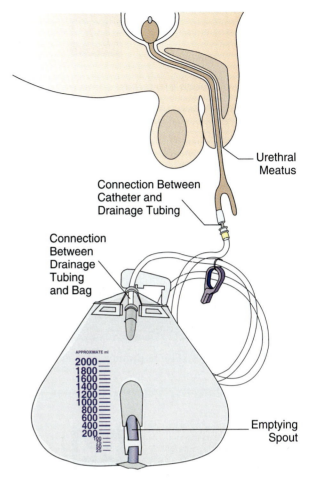

Urethral Meatus

Connection Between Catheter and Drainage Tubing

Connection Between Drainage Tubing and Bag

APPROXIMATE ml
2000
1800
1600
1400
1200
1000
800
600
400
200

Emptying Spout

FIGURE 42-18 Special care must be taken to protect the possible sites of contamination in the closed urinary drainage system.

PROCEDURE **113**

DISCONNECTING THE CATHETER

1. Carry out each beginning procedure action.

2. Assemble equipment:
   - disposable gloves
   - antiseptic wipes
   - gauze sponges
   - sterile caps/plugs
   - clamps

3. Wash hands and put on gloves.

4. Clamp the catheter.

5. Disconnect the catheter and drainage tubing. Do not put the ends down or allow them to

touch anything. If accidental contamination occurs, wipe the ends with antiseptic wipes before inserting plug or placing cap. Dispose of antiseptic wipes in plastic bag.

6. Insert a sterile plug in the end of the catheter. Place a sterile cap over the exposed end of the drainage tube (Figure 42-19).

7. Secure the drainage tube to the bed frame so that it will not touch the floor.

8. Remove and dispose of gloves according to facility policy. Wash hands.

continues

PROCEDURE **113** *continued*

9. Carry out each procedure completion action.

📝 ***Note:*** *Reverse the procedure to reconnect the catheter. If you find an unprotected, disconnected tube in the bed or on the floor, do not reconnect it. Report it at once.*

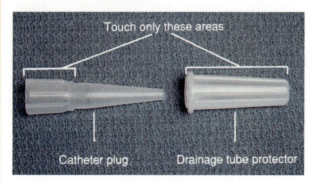

Touch only these areas

Catheter plug   Drainage tube protector

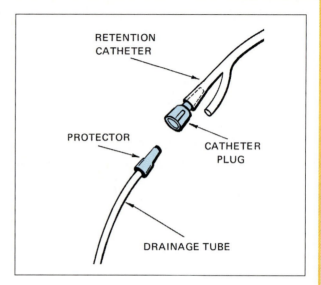

RETENTION CATHETER

PROTECTOR

CATHETER PLUG

DRAINAGE TUBE

FIGURE 42-19 (Left) Sterile catheter plug and protective cap (Right) Plug and protective cap in place

PROCEDURE **114**

APPLYING A CONDOM FOR URINARY DRAINAGE

1. Carry out each beginning procedure action.

2. Assemble equipment:
   - disposable gloves
   - basin of warm water
   - washcloth
   - towel
   - condom with drainage tip
   - bed protector
   - bath blanket
   - towel

3. Arrange equipment on overbed table.

4. Raise bed to comfortable working height. Be sure opposite side rail is up and secure for safety.

5. Lower side rail on the side where you will be working.

6. Cover patient with bath blanket and fanfold bedding to foot of bed.

7. Wash hands and put on gloves.

8. Place bed protector under patient's hips.

9. Adjust bath blanket to expose genitals only.

10. Carefully wash and dry penis. Observe for signs of irritation. Check to be sure condom has "ready stick" surface.

11. Apply condom and drainage tip to penis by placing condom at top of penis and rolling toward base of penis. Leave space between drainage tip and glans of penis to prevent irritation (Figure 42-20). If patient is not circumcised, be sure that foreskin is in normal position.

12. Apply tape provided with condom to secure it to the penis (Figure 42-21).

13. The condom is now ready to be connected to drainage tubing leading to a collection bag.

14. Remove gloves and discard according to facility policy.

15. Wash hands.

16. Adjust bedding and remove bath blanket. Fold bath blanket and store in room or place in laundry hamper.

continues

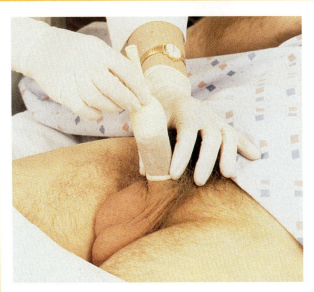

FIGURE 42-20 When condom is placed on penis, leave room between the drainage tip and the glans of the penis to prevent irritation. Roll condom to base of penis.

17. Lower bed. Adjust side rails for safety.

18. Carry out procedure completion actions.

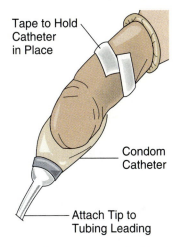

Tape to Hold Catheter in Place

Condom Catheter

Attach Tip to Tubing Leading

FIGURE 42-21 Correctly applied and secured condom ready to be attached to tubing leading to drainage bag

Leg Bag Drainage

Some patients find it easier to ambulate when urine drainage is collected in a leg bag instead of the larger urinary drainage bag. (See Procedure 115.) The leg bag is held to the patient's leg by Velcro® straps around either the thigh or the lower leg (Figure 42-22). Points to keep in mind when patients use a leg bag are:

- The leg bag is smaller and must be emptied more often (see Procedure 116).
- The bag must be placed so there is a straight drop down from the catheter.
- Tension on the catheter tubing must be minimal.
- Care must be taken not to introduce germs when connecting and disconnecting the bag and catheter.

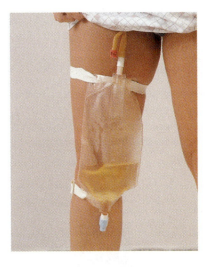

FIGURE 42-22 The leg bag is held in place by adjustable straps. Because it is smaller than the standard drainage bag, it must be emptied more often.

CONNECTING A CATHETER TO A LEG BAG

 Note: *Always check with the nurse before using a leg bag.*

1. Carry out beginning procedure actions.

2. Assemble equipment:

- disposable gloves
- antiseptic wipes
- leg bag and tubing
- emesis basin

continues

PROCEDURE 115 *continued*

- bed protector
- sterile cap/plug
- clamp

3. Wash hands and put on gloves.

4. Place bed protector under the connection between catheter and drainage tube.

5. Clamp the catheter.

6. Disconnect the catheter and drainage tubing. Do not put them down or allow them to touch anything.

7. Insert a sterile plug in the end of the catheter. Place a sterile cap over the exposed end of the drainage tube.

 Note: If accidental contamination occurs, wipe the area with antiseptic wipes before inserting sterile plug or replacing sterile cap over exposed end of drainage tubing. Dispose of antiseptic wipes in plastic bag.

8. Secure the drainage tube to the bed frame. The drainage tube must not touch the floor.

9. Remove catheter plug.

10. Insert the end of the leg bag tubing into the catheter (Figure 42-23).

11. Release the catheter clamp.

12. Secure the leg bag with Velcro® straps to the patient's leg so there is no tension on the tubing. Be sure there is a straight drop down from the catheter to the bag for urine flow. Check for leakage.

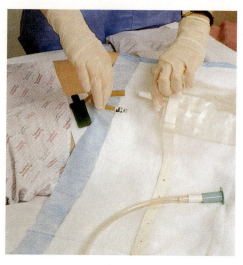

FIGURE 42-23 Connecting leg bag to catheter tubing. Do not let the catheter tubing touch anything that could contaminate it. Note that the tubing to the drainage bag is covered with a sterile cap to protect it until it is reconnected to the catheter.

13. Remove bed protector and discard.

14. Remove gloves and discard according to facility policy. Wash hands.

15. Assist patient to get out of bed. The single-use leg bag should be discarded in a biohazardous waste container.

16. Carry out procedure completion actions.

Note: To reconnect the regular drainage bag, reverse the procedure.

PROCEDURE 116

EMPTYING A LEG BAG

1. Carry out beginning procedure actions.

2. Assemble equipment:
   - disposable gloves
   - antiseptic wipes
   - emesis basin
   - graduate pitcher
   - paper towels

3. Position patient safely.

4. Wash hands and put on gloves.

5. Release Velcro® straps holding leg bag so it can be moved away from leg.

6. Place paper towel on floor under drainage outlet of leg bag.

7. Place graduate on paper towel under drainage outlet.

continues

PROCEDURE 116 *continued*

8. Remove cap, being careful not to touch tip. Drain urine into the graduate. Do not put the cap down and do not touch the inside of the cap. If accidental contamination occurs, wipe the area with antiseptic wipes before replacing cap. Dispose of antiseptic wipes in a plastic bag.

9. Wipe drainage outlet with an antiseptic wipe and replace cap.

10. Refasten Velcro® straps to secure drainage bag to leg.
11. Make sure patient is comfortable and safe.
12. Discard paper towel.
13. Measure urine and note amount, if required.
14. Discard urine. Clean graduate and store.
15. Remove gloves and discard according to facility policy.
16. Carry out each procedure completion action

REVIEW

A. True/False.

Mark the following true or false by circling T or F.

1. T F Insertion of a sterile catheter into the urinary bladder is a routine nursing assistant task.
2. T F Gloves should be worn when emptying a urine collection bag.
3. T F It is preferable never to disconnect a urinary drainage setup.
4. T F The pain associated with kidney stones is referred to as renal colic.
5. T F If you find an unprotected, disconnected catheter on the floor, you should reconnect it immediately.
6. T F The hemodialysis machine takes the place of nonfunctioning kidneys.
7. T F Forcing fluids encourages increased output, which is important in treating kidney stones.
8. T F A catheter with an inflatable balloon is called a French catheter.
9. T F French catheters are indwelling catheters.
10. T F Cystitis is a fairly common problem for women.

B. Matching.

Choose the correct term from Column II to match each phrase in Column I.

Column I

11. ___F___ indwelling catheter
12. ___e___ inability to expel formed urine
13. ___a___ urinate
14. ___c___ inflammation of the bladder
15. ___b___ blood in the urine

Column II

a. void
b. hematuria
c. cystitis
d. retention
e. dysuria
f. Foley catheter
g. suppression

C. Multiple Choice.

Select the one best answer for each question.

16. Your patient has a diagnosis of nephritis. Your care will include
    a. keeping the patient very active.
    b. serving a high-sodium diet.
    c. measuring I/O accurately.
    d. eliminating vital sign measurements so the patient can rest more.

17. Your patient has renal calculi. Included in your care will be
    a. saving all urine.
    b. straining urine.
    c. limiting fluids.
    d. inserting a catheter.

18. A common cause of hydronephrosis is
    a. renal calculi.
    b. twisting of the ureter.
    c. tumors.
    d. all of these.

19. Important signs and symptoms to note when there is a diagnosis involving the urinary system include
    a. chilling.
    b. pain.
    c. temperature evaluation.
    d. all of these.

20. Indwelling catheter care is:
    a. performed once each week.
    b. performed during A.M. care.
    c. safely omitted as long as the patient is in bed.
    d. none of these.

D. Completion.

Complete the following statements.

21. The nursing assistant who finds a disconnected catheter in the bed should _____.

22. A routine check of a patient on urinary drainage should include _____.

E. Nursing Assistant Challenge.

Mr. Starkman is 68 years of age. An external urinary condom is to be applied. Answer the following regarding his care while the condom is being applied.

23. You should wear gloves to apply the condom. _____ (yes) (no)

24. The condom should be applied by _____ of the penis. (pulling it up toward the tip) (rolling it down toward the base)

25. When applying the condom, you should _____ space between the drainage tip and the glans of the penis. (leave) (not leave)

Reproductive System

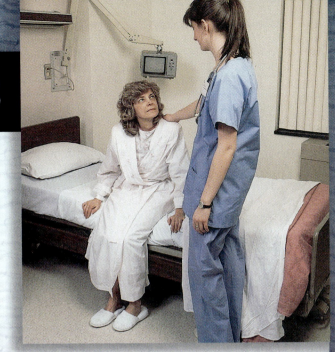

As a result of this unit, you will be able to:

- Spell and define terms.
- Review the location and functions of the organs of the male and female reproductive systems.
- List six diagnostic tests associated with conditions of the male and female reproductive systems.
- Describe some common disorders and conditions of the male reproductive system.
- Describe some common disorders and conditions of the female reproductive system.

- Describe nursing assistant actions related to the care of patients with conditions and diseases of the reproductive system.
- State the nursing precautions required for patients who have sexually transmitted diseases.
- Demonstrate the following procedures:
  - Procedure 117 Breast Self-Examination
  - Procedure 118 Giving a Nonsterile Vaginal Douche

VOCABULARY

Learn the meaning and the correct spelling of the following words and phrases:

amenorrhea
benign prostatic hypertrophy
biopsy
chancre
chlamydia
climacteric
clitoris
colporrhaphy
Cowper's glands
cystocele
dilatation and curettage (D & C)
douche
dysmenorrhea
ejaculatory duct
endometrium

epididymis
fallopian tubes
genitalia
gonorrhea
hemorrhoid
herpes simplex II
hysterectomy
labia majora
labia minora
leukorrhea
lumpectomy
mammogram
mastectomy
menopause
menorrhagia
menstruation
metrorrhagia

oophorectomy
orchiectomy
ovary
oviduct
ovulation
ovum
panhysterectomy
Pap smear
pelvic inflammatory disease (PID)
penis
prostatectomy
prostate gland
puberty
radical mastectomy
rectocele

salpingectomy
seminal vesicles
sexually transmitted disease (STD)
simple mastectomy
sperm
sterility
syphilis
testes
trichomonas vaginitis
uterus
vagina
vas deferens
venereal warts
vulva
vulvovaginitis

STRUCTURE AND FUNCTION

Both the male and female reproductive organs have dual functions. They:

1. Produce reproductive cells. The male produces **sperm**. The female produces the **ovum**.
2. Produce hormones that are responsible for sex characteristics.
   a. Males produce testosterone.
   b. Females produce estrogen and progesterone.

In the reproductive process, the:

- male and female engage in sexual intercourse.
- male ejaculates (propels) the sperm and the seminal fluid in which they swim into the female vagina.
- sperm and egg meet in the female fallopian tube. One sperm penetrates the egg and conception takes place.
- baby (fetus) develops in the uterus until birth.
- female breasts (mammary glands) produce milk to nourish the newborn.

The Male Reproductive Organs: Structure and Function

The male organs (Figure 43-1) include the:

- **Testes**: Two glandular organs located in the scrotum. The testes produce sperm and the hormone testosterone.

- **Epididymis**: A 20-foot-long coiled tube located on the top and back of each testis. The epididymis stores the sperm and allows them to mature.
- **Vas deferens**: A tube that leads from the epididymis. It carries the sperm upward into the pelvic cavity to the seminal vesicles during ejaculation. The vas deferens is accompanied by nerves and blood vessels. Together, they form the spermatic cord.
- **Seminal vesicles**: Located behind the bladder. They receive and store the sperm from the vas deferens. They contribute nutrients to the seminal fluid. The small ejaculator duct leads from the seminal vesicles to the urethra just below the prostate gland.
- **Ejaculatory duct**: Carries the fluid produced in the seminal vesicles. Fluids are added as the sperm are propelled forward. The sperm and fluid form the seminal fluid or ejaculate. The fluid contains nutrients and other substances needed by the sperm.
- **Prostate gland**: Found just below the urinary bladder surrounding the urethra. It secretes a fluid that increases the ability of the sperm to move in the seminal fluid. Enlargement of the prostate gland may prevent urine from passing through the urethra. This is a fairly common occurrence in older men.
- **Cowper's glands**: Two small glands located beside the urethra. They produce mucus for lubrication.

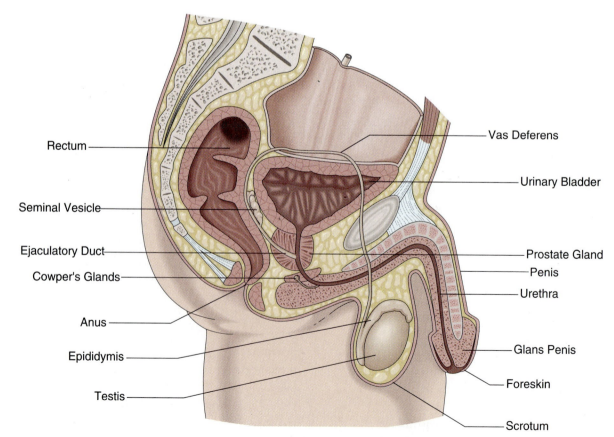

FIGURE 43-1 Cross-sectional view of the male reproductive system

- **Penis**: Composed of special tissue that can become filled with blood, making the organ enlarge and become stiffened so that it may enter the vagina to deposit seminal fluid. Loose-fitting skin (the prepuce or foreskin) covers the penis.

The male urethra passes through the penis and serves two purposes. It carries:

- Reproductive fluid during intercourse
- Urine during voiding

The two activities cannot occur at the same time because they are under the control of different parts of the nervous system.

The Female Reproductive Organs: Structure and Function

The external female structures (**genitalia**) (Figure 43-2) include the:

- **Vulva**: Made up of two liplike structures, the **labia majora** and **labia minora**. When the labia are separated, other external structures may be seen.
- **Clitoris**: A very sensitive structure found just behind the juncture of the labia minora. It functions during sexual stimulation to begin the rhythmic series of contractions associated with female climax (orgasm).
- **Urinary meatus**: The opening of the urethra to the outside.
- **Vaginal meatus**: The opening to the vagina or birth canal.

The Internal Female Structures

The internal female reproductive organs (Figures 43-3 and 43-4) include the following structures.

- **Ovaries**: Two small glands, found on either side of the uterus, at the ends of the oviducts (fallopian tubes) in the pelvis. They produce two hormones, estrogen and progesterone, and the egg (ovum). The eggs are contained in many little sacs called follicles. About once

each month, a follicle matures and releases an ovum. The ovum makes its way into one of the four-inch oviducts. This process is called **ovulation**. The cells of the follicles that are left produce progesterone. The progesterone causes changes within the uterus, readying it for the possibility of receiving a fertilized ovum.

- **Fallopian tubes** (**oviducts**): Two tubes, approximately four inches long, that serve as a pathway between the ovary and uterus. The sperm and egg meet in the tubes. Fertilization takes place here.
- **Uterus**: A hollow, pear-shaped organ. Its walls are made up of involuntary muscles. It is lined with special tissue called **endometrium**. The uterus has three main parts: the fundus, body, and cervix. The body and the fundus can stretch enough to hold a fetus, the amniotic sac, and the afterbirth (placenta). The cervix extends into the vagina. During labor, the cervix opens up to allow the baby to be delivered.
- **Vagina**: Found between the urinary bladder and the rectum. Its muscular walls are capable of much stretching. It is lined with mucous membrane. Two glands known as Bartholin's glands are found on either side of the external vaginal opening. They provide lubrication.

Menstruation and Ovulation

The menstrual cycle (female sexual cycle) begins at **puberty**. Puberty occurs in girls between the ages of 9 and 17. The cycle varies in length, usually between 25 and 30 days. The average is 28 days, which is why it is considered a monthly cycle.

During the menstrual cycle, a mature egg, or ovum (plural, ova):

- is released from one of the ovaries.
- travels from the ovary to one of the fallopian tubes.
- may be fertilized by a male sperm.

At the same time that the ovum is being matured and expelled from the ovary (ovulation), the lining of the uterus (endometrium) is being built up and made ready to receive

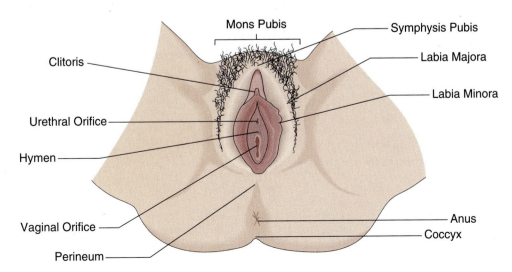

FIGURE 43-2 External female reproductive organs

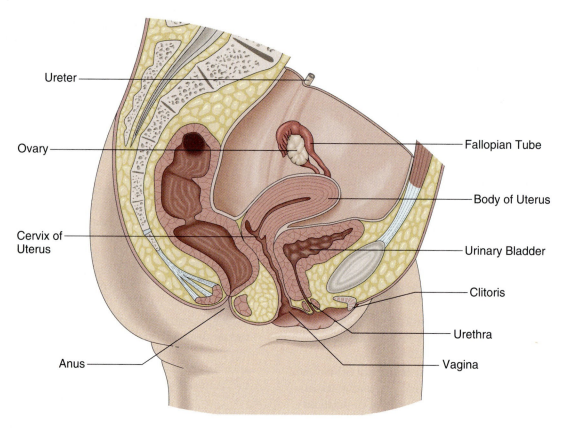

FIGURE 43-3 Female internal reproductive organs (lateral view)

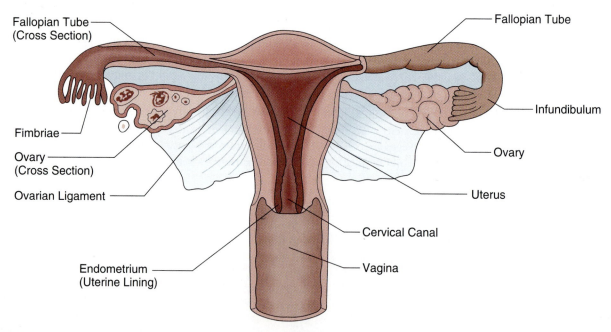

FIGURE 43-4 Female internal reproductive organs (anterior view)

the fertilized ovum. If fertilization does not occur, the endometrium is no longer needed, so it is carried out of the body as the menstrual flow. This process is known as **menstruation**.

Unlike the sperm cells, all the special cells that will become the ova exist when a woman is born. When the last ova are released, the menstrual cycle ceases and **menopause** begins.

Menopause

As women age, the menstrual cycle becomes irregular and gradually ceases altogether. This is called the menopause, or **climacteric**, or change of life.

Menopause usually occurs around the age of 55 and involves a natural series of changes that stops the menstrual cycle. These changes are not abrupt, but usually take place over a period of years. Because ova are no longer being matured and released, pregnancy cannot occur.

Some women may undergo menopause earlier in life after surgical removal of the uterus.

CONDITIONS OF THE MALE REPRODUCTIVE ORGANS

The male organs are subject to the same kinds of disease processes that affect other body parts. Examples of these conditions are tumors and infections. A very common problem experienced by many men involves the prostate gland.

Prostate Conditions

Benign prostatic (of the prostate gland) **hypertrophy**:

- is an enlargement of the prostate gland without tumor development.
- causes narrowing of the urethra, which passes through the center of the prostate gland.
- can cause sufficient enlargement to cause urinary retention.
- is noncancerous.

Signs and symptoms of prostate conditions include difficulty in starting the stream of urine or in emptying the bladder completely.

Treatment. Various surgical approaches are used to remove all or part of the prostate gland (**prostatectomy**) to relieve urinary retention.

- Transurethral prostatectomy (TURP)—only enough of the gland is removed, working from inside the urethra, to permit urine to pass.
- Perineal prostatectomy—the entire gland is removed through surgical incisions in the perineum.
- Suprapubic prostatectomy—an incision is made just above the pubis and part of the gland is removed.

Male patients are likely to be disturbed by the necessity of prostate surgery. Men often fear that they will not be able to have sexual intercourse after a prostatectomy. They feel that their manhood is threatened.

Postsurgical Care. In addition to routine postoperative care, the prostatectomy patient:

- will have a Foley catheter in place following the surgery.
- may have a suprapubic drain through the suprapubic incision.
- may have a perineal drain in the perineal incision.

The nursing assistant should:

- Wear personal protective equipment and apply the principles of standard precautions if contact with blood, body fluids, mucous membranes, or nonintact skin is likely.
- Be careful the tubes do not become twisted, stressed, or dislodged when positioning the patient.
- Carefully note the amount and color of drainage from all areas.
- Report at once any sudden increase in bright redness or the appearance of clots that seem to block the tube.
- Report to the nurse if dressings become wet with urinary drainage.
- Be patient and understanding of the patient's emotional stress.
- Refer questions about possible sexual limitation to the nurse so that the patient may be provided with accurate information and support.

At times, it will be necessary to irrigate (wash out) the drainage tubes. This is a sterile procedure that will be carried out by the nurse or physician.

Cancer of the Testes

Cancer of the testes is seen commonly today. It may require the removal of the testicles (**orchiectomy**). This procedure is performed when there is testicular malignancy. When an early diagnosis is made, treatment can be started early. Orchiectomy can then be avoided.

Testicular self-examination is an important way to locate lumps or changes in the testes. This procedure should be performed by all adult males:

- At least once each month
- During a warm shower so the scrotum will be relaxed
- With soapy fingers
- By palpating each testis between the fingers and thumb

CONDITIONS OF THE FEMALE REPRODUCTIVE ORGANS

Like the male organs, female reproductive organs are subject to disease processes, including tumors and infections.

Rectocele and Cystocele

Rectoceles and cystoceles are hernias. They usually occur at the same time.

- **Rectoceles** are a weakening of the wall shared between the vagina and rectum. These hernias frequently cause constipation and **hemorrhoids** (varicose veins of the rectum).
- **Cystoceles** are a weakening of the muscles between the bladder and vagina. Cystoceles cause urinary incontinence.

Treatment and Nursing Care. A surgical procedure called **colporrhaphy** tightens the vaginal walls.

In addition to routine postsurgical care, you may assist in:

- Applying ice packs
- Giving sitz baths
- Giving vaginal douches (irrigations) (see Procedure 118)
- Checking carefully for signs of excessive bleeding or foul discharge

Vulvovaginitis

Vulvovaginitis is most often caused by a fungal infection caused by *Candida albicans*.

- There is a thick, white, cheesy vaginal discharge.
- Inflammation and itching are intense.
- Douches are not given for this condition.
- Special drugs and creams are prescribed to fight the infection.

Tumors of Uterus and Ovaries

Benign and malignant tumors of the uterus and ovaries are frequent. Malignancies of the cervix are very common. The cure rate is very high if treated in time.

The most common indications of tumors of the uterus and ovaries are changes in the menstrual flow, such as:

- Menorrhagia (excessive flow)
- Amenorrhea (lack of menstrual flow)
- Dysmenorrhea (difficult or painful menstrual flow)
- Metrorrhagia (bleeding at completely irregular intervals)

Treatment. Several different types of procedures may be performed to treat tumors of the female reproductive tract, including chemotherapy, radiation, and surgery. Some surgical procedures are:

- Total hysterectomy—removal of the entire uterus, including the cervix.
- Oophorectomy—removal of an ovary. In younger women, at least a portion of the ovary is left to continue hormone production whenever possible.
- Salpingectomy—removal of a fallopian tube.
- Panhysterectomy—removal of the uterus and both ovaries and tubes. The surgical approach may be abdominal or vaginal. If a panhysterectomy is performed, the patient experiences surgically induced menopause. The more uncomfortable symptoms are usually relieved with hormone supplements.

Postoperative Care. In addition to the usual postoperative care, the care following a hysterectomy will include:

- caring for catheter drainage.
- possibly caring for a nasogastric tube, which may be in place to relieve abdominal distention and nausea.
- giving special attention to maintaining good circulation, because slowing of the blood supply to the pelvis may result in clot formation.
- introducing fluids and foods gradually after the initial nausea subsides.
- carefully observing the patient for low back pain.

- monitoring urine output and bleeding.
- checking both the abdominal incisional area and the vagina for presence and type of drainage.

Tumors of the Breast

Tumors, both benign and malignant, are commonly found in the breasts. Signs and symptoms of breast tumors include:

- Painless lump or mass
- Nipple discharge
- Retraction of nipple
- Scaly skin around nipple
- Dimpling of the skin
- Enlarged lymph nodes

Treatment. Mastectomy means removal of the breast. All or part of the breast tissue may be removed in a mastectomy.

- A simple mastectomy removes the breast tissue only.
- A radical mastectomy includes the breast tissue, underlying muscles, and the glands in the axillary area. This procedure is not performed as often as it was previously.
- A lumpectomy removes the abnormal tissue and only a small amount of the breast tissue.

Any form of mastectomy requires a great deal of psychological adjustment for the patient. There is the fear of disfigurement and the fear of loss of femininity. Many excellent breast forms are now available to restore the outward physical appearance of the mastectomy patient. Breast implants are another way of restoring the physical form of the breast. There are also support groups to aid in the psychological adjustment.

Postoperative Care. In addition to routine postoperative care, you will:

- Wear personal protective equipment and apply the principles of standard precautions if contact with blood, body fluids, mucous membranes, or nonintact skin is likely.
- Realize that because a large amount of blood can be lost during a mastectomy, transfusions are likely to be ordered. Monitor a blood transfusion as you would monitor an intravenous infusion.
- Check pressure dressings frequently for signs of excess bleeding.
- Check the bed linen, because blood may drain to the back of the dressing.
- Report immediately numbness or swelling in the arm of the operative side.
- Be ready to offer support; walking may be difficult for the patient, who may feel unbalanced.
- Offer your fullest emotional support.
- Assist the patient in rehabilitative exercises.
- Refer questions about disfigurement and loss of femininity to the nurse, who will see that the patient is provided with accurate information and support.

SEXUALLY TRANSMITTED DISEASE (STD)

Sexually transmitted diseases (**STDs**) affect both men and women. Although most sexually transmitted diseases can be treated and cured, patients do not develop immunity to repeated infections. It is possible to transmit the organisms causing STDs from:

- Mucous membrane to mucous membrane, such as from genitals to mouth or genitals
- Mucous membrane to skin, such as genitals to hands
- Skin to mucous membrane, such as hands to genitals

Using standard precautions correctly will protect the nursing assistant from contracting these diseases when caring for patients.

Any disease that is transmitted mainly in this way is a STD. There are many sexually transmitted diseases. Some are seen more commonly than others. It is important to realize that patients may:

- not always be aware that they have been infected.
- be too embarrassed to tell you about the problem.
- not realize the serious damage these infectious diseases can do to the body.

The most common sexually transmitted diseases are gonorrhea, herpes simplex II, and syphilis. Other sexually transmitted diseases are caused by chlamydia, human papilloma virus, HIV, and the trichomonas parasite.

Trichomonas Vaginitis

Trichomonas vaginitis is caused by a parasite, the *Trichomonas vaginalis.* This condition:

- is sexually transmitted.
- may affect the male reproductive tract with no signs and symptoms.
- in females, causes a large amount of white, foul-smelling vaginal discharge called **leukorrhea.**
- can be controlled with medication.
- requires that both sex partners receive treatment.

Gonorrhea

Gonorrhea is a serious STD caused by the bacterium *Neisseria gonorrheae.* The disease causes an acute inflammation. In the male:

- Greenish-yellow discharge appears from the penis within two to five days after contact.
- There is burning on urination.
- The disease can spread throughout the reproductive tract, causing **sterility** (inability to reproduce).

In the female:

- 80% may have no signs or symptoms for quite a while. Thus, it is possible to spread the disease before becoming aware of being infected.

- **Pelvic inflammatory disease** (**PID**) can lead to formation of abscesses and sterility.

It is important for all sex partners to be treated with antibiotics. When a pregnant woman has gonorrhea, her baby's eyes may be permanently damaged if they are contaminated by the disease during birth. As a preventive measure, all babies' eyes are routinely treated with silver nitrate drops or antibiotics shortly after birth.

Syphilis

Syphilis is caused by the microorganism *Treponema pallidum.* Both sexes show the same effects of the disease. If untreated, this disease passes through three stages.

1. First stage—a sore (**chancre**) develops within 90 days of exposure. The chancre heals without treatment. Because it is not painful, it may go entirely unnoticed.

2. Second stage—may be accompanied by a rash, sore throat, or other mild symptoms suggestive of a viral infection. Again, the signs and symptoms disappear without treatment. The disease is infectious during the first and second stages and may be transmitted to a sexual partner. By this time, the microorganisms have gained entrance into vital organs such as the heart, liver, brain, and spinal cord.

3. Third stage—permanent damage is done to vital organs, though the damage may not appear for many years.

An additional danger of syphilis during pregnancy is that the microorganism can attack the fetus, causing it to die or be seriously deformed.

Herpes

Herpes simplex II (genital herpes) is an infectious disease caused by the herpes simplex virus. It is transmitted primarily through direct sexual contact. The person who has herpes:

- may develop red, blister-like sores on the reproductive organs.
- has sores that are associated with a burning sensation.
- usually has sores that heal in about two weeks.
- must remember that the fluid in the blisters is infectious.
- may transmit (shed) organisms even when an outbreak is not present.

People with the herpes infection may have only one episode or may have repeated attacks. In many cases, repeated attacks are milder. In addition to the local discomfort:

- There seems to be a greater incidence of cancer of the cervix and miscarriages among female sufferers than among women who do not have this condition.
- Newborn children can be infected when the mother gives birth.
- The mother with an active case of herpes simplex II is usually delivered by cesarean section.

Treatment reduces the discomfort and degree of communicability. There is no cure at the present time.

Venereal Warts

Venereal warts are caused by a virus.

- Lesions develop on the genitals, on both skin and mucous membranes.
- The warts are cauliflower-shaped, raised, and darkened.
- They may be removed by ointments or surgery but often recur.
- They may cause discomfort during intercourse and may cause bleeding when dislodged.
- Warts predispose the patient to development of cancerous changes.
- Venereal warts are one of the most rapidly growing forms of STD.

Chlamydia Infection

Chlamydia are small infectious organisms that can invade mucous membranes of the body. These organisms can be:

- Introduced into the eyes, infecting the conjunctiva. This causes inflammation (conjunctivitis) and a more serious condition called trachoma. Trachoma can lead to blindness.
- Sexually transmitted; this commonly causes infections of the reproductive tract.
- The cause of serious pelvic inflammatory disease (PID), with scarring and even systemic infections. The scarring can result in sterility.
- Responsible for signs and symptoms similar to those of gonorrhea, except that the discharge is usually yellow to whitish in color.
- Treated with antibiotics.

Patients with pelvic infections are usually checked for gonorrhea. If they are found negative for gonorrhea, they are frequently diagnosed as having nongonorrheal urethritis (NGU) or nonspecified urethritis (NSU), because many different organisms may cause the infection. However, chlamydia organisms are the most common cause.

Acquired Immune Deficiency Syndrome (AIDS)

AIDS is a viral disease. It is transmitted primarily through direct contact with the bodily secretions of an infected person. Therefore, it can be transmitted through direct sexual contact. A complete discussion of this disease is found in Unit 11.

DIAGNOSTIC TESTS

Techniques used to diagnose problems of the reproductive system include:

- Cultures for microorganisms.
- Urinalysis for hormone levels.
- **Pap smear**—test using cells from the cervix to detect possible cancer of the cervix. The test:
  - is painless.

- can be performed in the physician's office during the routine pelvic examination.
  - should be done regularly.
- **Dilatation and curettage (D & C)**—a surgical procedure used to help diagnose conditions of the uterus, including tumors. In a D & C, the opening of the cervix is stretched open (dilated) and the uterus is scraped with a surgical instrument known as a curette.
- **Biopsy** (examining a sample of living tissue) is used to make a diagnosis. The biopsy sample is obtained through a needle. The procedure may be performed in the physician's office or in the hospital.
- Blood tests for cancer of the prostate.
- MRI and CT scans to help define the presence and extent of tumors.
- Cystoscopy—used to evaluate prostate conditions.
- Self-examination.
  Breast self-examination should be performed:
  - by all adult females (see Procedure 117).
  - each month on the last day of the menstrual flow.
  - on one selected day of the month, after menopause.
  - Faithfully in a routine manner.
  Testicular self-examination should be performed:
  - by all adult males.
  - at least once each month.
  - during a warm shower so the scrotum will be relaxed.
  - with soapy fingers.
  - by palpating each testis between the fingers and thumb.
- Mammography—x-rays of the breasts. A **mammogram**:
  - can identify the presence of tumors up to two years before the tumor can be felt during self-examination.
  - Should be performed when the woman is between the ages of 35 and 40 years, to provide a baseline evaluation.
  - Thereafter, should be performed every one to two years until age 50.
  - Should be performed yearly after age 50.

VAGINAL DOUCHE

A vaginal **douche** is an irrigation of the vagina with fluid or medication. It is done by physician's order.

A vaginal douche requires standard precautions. When a douche is given to administer medications, it is given by the nurse. Other douches may be given by the nursing assistant if it is the policy of the facility. Be sure to check. Vaginal douches are given to:

- Remove odor or foul discharge
- Stop bleeding
- Relieve inflammation and pain
- Neutralize vaginal secretions
- Disinfect the vagina
- Cleanse the vagina before surgery or examination
- Administer antiseptic drugs

BREAST SELF-EXAMINATION

1. Disrobe above the waist and stand or sit in front of a mirror. Observe breasts for changes in shape or size (Figure 43-5A).

 Note: Some women prefer to perform breast self-examination standing in the shower.

2. Raise arms above your head and clasp hands (Figure 43-5B). Press inward with hands while observing breasts. Note any "dimpling" of the breast tissue.

3. Fold a small towel.

4. Lie on the bed with the towel under your right shoulder.

5. Flex right arm and bring it over your head.

6. With the fingers of the left hand, examine the right breast (Figure 43-5C).

   - Use fingertips.
   - Use a rolling motion.
   - Start at the nipple and work around the entire breast so that all tissue is examined (Figure 43-5D).

7. Examine the right axilla in the same way.

8. Repeat the procedure with the opposite breast and axilla.

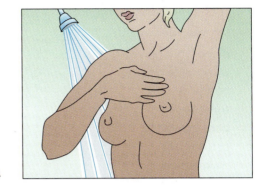

A

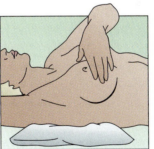

B

C

Finger pads

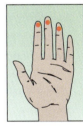

D

FIGURE 43-5 Breast self-examination. Each breast is examined systematically. A. With the fingers flat, check for a knot, lump, or thickening. B. Raise your arms and compare breast shape. C. Lie down with a small pillow under the shoulder and one arm behind the head. Check again for any knot, lump, or thickening. Move fingers in a circular motion, inward toward the nipple. Use pads of fingers. D. Direction of motion of fingers over breast during examination. *Courtesy of The American Cancer Society*

PROCEDURE 118

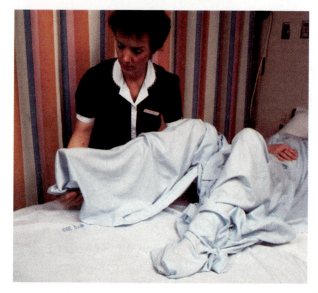

GIVING A NONSTERILE VAGINAL DOUCHE

1. Carry out each beginning procedure action.

2. Assemble equipment:
   - disposable gloves
   - disposable douche
   - bed protector
   - toilet tissue
   - bath blanket
   - cotton balls
   - disinfectant
   - cup
   - irrigating standard
   - bedpan and cover
   - plastic bag

3. Pour a small amount of the specified disinfecting solution over the cotton balls in the cup.

4. Measure water in douche container. Temperature should be about 105°F. Add powder or solution as ordered.

5. Hang douche bag on standard. Close clamp on tubing. Leave protector on sterile tip.

6. Place a bed protector on chair and assemble equipment where it can be easily reached. Screen unit.

7. Elevate bed to comfortable working height and put up side rails for safety.

8. Wash hands and put on gloves. Lower side rail on working side.

9. Assist patient into the dorsal recumbent position.

10. Place bed protector beneath patient's buttocks.

11. Remove the perineal pad (if used) from front to back and discard in plastic bag.

12. Drape patient with bath blanket (Figure 43-6). Fanfold top bedding to foot of bed.

13. Place bedpan under patient and ask her to void.

14. Cleanse perineum.
    - Use one cotton ball with disinfectant for each stroke.
    - Cleanse from vulva toward anus.
    - Cleanse labia majora first.

FIGURE 43-6 Drape the patient.

- Expose labia minora with thumb and forefinger and cleanse.
- Give special attention to folds.
- Discard cotton balls in plastic bag.

15. Open clamp to expel air. Remove protector from sterile tip of disposable douche.

16. Allow small amount of solution to flow over inner thigh and then over vulva. Do not touch vulva with nozzle.

17. Allow solution to continue to flow and insert nozzle slowly and gently into the vagina with an upward and backward movement for about 3 inches (Figure 43-7).

18. Rotate nozzle from side to side as solution flows.

19. When all solution has been given, remove nozzle slowly and clamp tubing.

20. Have patient sit up on bedpan to allow all solution to return.

21. Remove douche bag from standard and place on bed protector.

22. Dry perineum with tissue. Discard tissue in bedpan.

23. Cover bedpan and place on bed protector on chair.

continues

PROCEDURE 118 *continued*

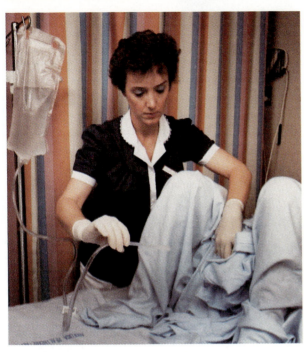

FIGURE 43-7 Insert the nozzle slowly and gently.

24. Have patient turn on side. Dry buttocks with tissue.

25. Place clean pad over vulva from front to back. Do not touch inside of pad.

26. Remove bed protector and bath blanket. Replace with top bedding.

27. Observe contents of bedpan. Note character and amount of discharge, if any. Discard contents of bedpan according to facility policy. Care for equipment according to facility policy. Remove gloves and dispose of them according to facility policy. Wash hands.

28. Carry out each procedure completion action.

REVIEW

A. True/False.

Mark the following true or false by circling T or F.

1. T F D & C is a surgical procedure that can help establish a diagnosis related to the female reproductive system.

2. T F Following a panhysterectomy, you should check the patient for increased bleeding.

3. T F Salpingectomy means removal of the ovaries.

4. T F Foul-smelling leukorrhea is associated with the condition called trichomonas vaginitis.

5. T F The female with gonorrhea may not know she has been infected with the disease.

6. T F Untreated gonorrhea passes through three stages.

7. T F Syphilis presents an additional danger that is caused by a bacterium.

8. T F AIDS may be sexually transmitted.

9. T F The discharge in gonorrhea is white in color and very irritating.

B. Matching.

Choose the correct term from Column II to match each phrase in Column I.

Column I

10. ___c___ inability to reproduce

11. ___f___ inflammation of the vagina

12. ___a___ painful menstruation

13. ___b___ removal of a breast

14. ___d___ whitish discharge

Column II

a. dysmenorrhea

b. mastectomy

c. circumcision

d. leukorrhea

e. sterility

f. vaginitis

C. Multiple Choice.

Select the one best answer for each question.

15. You are to give a nonsterile douche. You will remember to

   a. place the patient in a high Fowler's position.

   b. use a solution with a temperature of about 115°F.

   c. insert the nozzle about 3 inches into the vagina.

   d. allow the nozzle to touch the vulva.

16. Breast self-examination should be performed
   a. daily.
   b. weekly.
   c. monthly.
   d. yearly.

17. Your patient has just returned from a suprapubic prostatectomy. You know that
   a. there will be no incision.
   b. there will be a Foley catheter drain.
   c. there will be a suprapubic drain.
   d. both b and c.

18. Testicular self-examination should be
   a. done once each month.
   b. performed in a warm shower.
   c. performed with soapy fingers.
   d. all of these.

D. Completion.

Complete the following statements.

19. The type of precautions to be used when caring for patients with STD is _____.

20. Women over the age of 50 should have a mammogram _____.

21. Breast self-examination should be performed _____.

E. Nursing Assistant Challenge.

Mrs. Forstein is 39 and has been admitted for a large pelvic mass. Her doctor suspects that she has a large tumor in her left ovary. She has experienced menorrhagia, dysmenorrhea, and pelvic pain. She is scheduled for an oophorectomy after tests are complete.

Briefly answer the following questions:

22. How else might you have described her menorrhagia and dysmenorrhea?

23. Does the doctor plan to remove the entire uterus, including the cervix?

24. What type of pain would be very significant following surgery?

25. What two areas would you check for drainage?

26. Why is it so important to maintain good circulation postoperatively?

12

Expanded Role of the Nursing Assistant

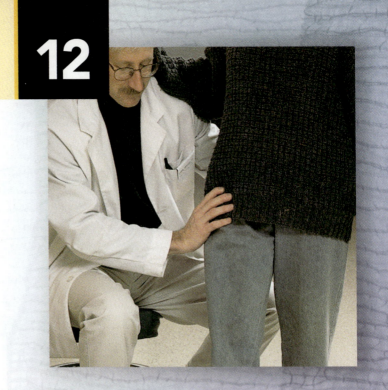

UNIT 44
Rehabilitation and Restorative Services

UNIT 45
Obstetrical Patient and Neonate

UNIT 46
Pediatric Patient

UNIT 47
Special Advanced Procedures

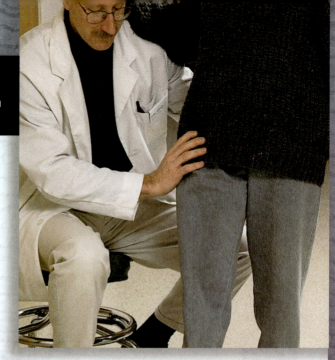

UNIT 44

Rehabilitation and Restorative Services

OBJECTIVES

As a result of this unit, you will be able to:

- Spell and define terms.
- Describe the differences between rehabilitation and restorative care.
- List five members of the interdisciplinary team.
- Describe the role of the nursing assistant in rehabilitation.
- Describe the principles of rehabilitation.
- List the elements of successful rehabilitation/restorative care.
- List six complications resulting from inactivity.
- Describe four perceptual deficits.
- Describe four approaches used for restorative programs.
- Describe the guidelines for implementing restorative programs.

VOCABULARY

Learn the meaning and the correct spelling of the following words and phrases:

activities of daily living (ADLs)	disability	mobility skills	rehabilitation
adaptive device	disuse osteoporosis	perceptual deficit	restorative
atrophy	geriatric	physiatrist	self-care deficit
	handicap		

INTRODUCTION TO REHABILITATION AND RESTORATIVE CARE

The term **rehabilitation** refers to a process in which the patient is assisted to reach an optimal level of ability. That means we are concerned with helping the patient be the best that he or she can be; physically, mentally, and emotionally. Rehabilitation and restorative care are similar processes, but there are some differences:

- Rehabilitation is usually more aggressive and intense than restorative care (Figure 44-1). Therapies are planned for a period of several weeks. Restorative care is a slower process; it may be planned for weeks or months or go on indefinitely.

- Rehabilitation requires the skills of many disciplines, including nursing and various therapies. **Restorative** care is basically a nursing responsibility with consultation from the therapists.

- Rehabilitation services may be provided in a general acute care hospital, in a rehabilitation center, in the skilled care facility, in a subacute care unit, or in the patient's home. Most restorative care is given in a skilled care facility or in the patient's home.

- OBRA regulations require that restorative services be provided to patients in skilled care facilities. Nursing assistants in these facilities must have the knowledge and skills to participate in this process.

The goals of both rehabilitation and restorative care are to:

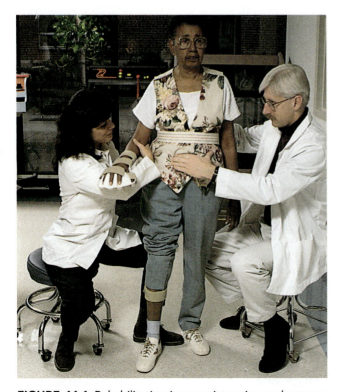

FIGURE 44-1 Rehabilitation is more intensive and aggressive than restorative care.

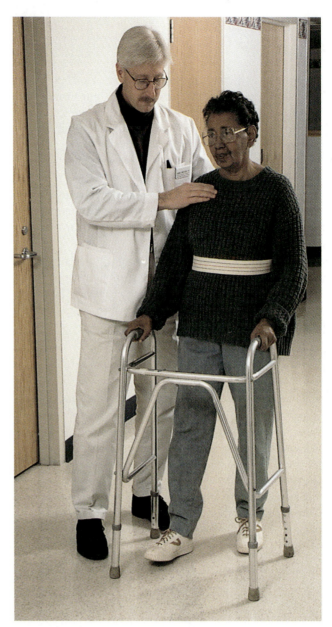

FIGURE 44-2 Increasing mobility skills is a goal of both rehabilitation and restorative care.

- Increase the patient's physical abilities. This may include **mobility skills** (Figure 44-2) and the ability to carry out **activities of daily living** (**ADLs**). Activities of daily living include the tasks that we learn as children and do throughout life. These tasks include: bathing, oral care, hair and nail care, dressing and undressing, eating, toileting, and mobility.

- Prevent complications such as pressure sores and contractures.

- Maintain the patient's current abilities.

- Help the patient adapt to limitations imposed by a disability.

- Increase the patient's quality of life.

The information in this unit applies to both rehabilitation and restorative care.

REASONS FOR REHABILITATION/ RESTORATIVE CARE

A person may need rehabilitation because of a **disability**. A disability exists when the person has an impairment that affects the ability to perform an activity that a person of that age would normally be able to do. Adults, for example, are able to dress and undress independently. If a person is unable to do this because of a disease or injury, a disability exists. A disability may be temporary or permanent.

A **handicap** exists if the disability limits or prevents the person from fulfilling a role that is normal for that person. This might include such functions as holding a job, managing a household, and raising a family.

If a disability is permanent, such as quadriplegia (paralysis from the neck down) from a spinal cord injury, it is unrealistic to expect that rehabilitation will enable the patient to walk again. In these situations, the interdisciplinary team will teach the patient to:

- adapt to the present circumstances.
- assume responsibility for personal well-being by directing others who give the care.
- use adaptive devices to increase independence.

Impairments or disabilities result from trauma or disease. Disorders of the musculoskeletal system, such as amputation (Figure 44-3) of an extremity or arthritis, may require rehabilitation. Stroke, spinal cord injury, and brain injuries are examples of nervous system disorders that will benefit from rehabilitation. A patient who has been in bed for a long time because of a serious illness such as heart disease may require rehabilitation for reconditioning or to restore the individual to a previous level of ability.

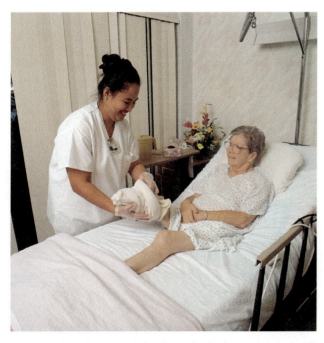

FIGURE 44-3 Patients who have had an amputation will benefit from rehabilitation.

THE INTERDISCIPLINARY HEALTH CARE TEAM

Physicians who specialize in rehabilitation are called **physiatrists**. Nurses and nursing assistants who work in rehabilitation receive additional training and education. Many other disciplines may be involved in the rehabilitation process. For instance, a person who has had a stroke may receive:

- physical therapy to learn how to walk again.
- occupational therapy to relearn the activities of daily living.
- speech therapy to learn new communication methods.
- nursing services for bowel and bladder training, prevention of pressure ulcers, and other complications.
- psychological support to adapt to the sudden changes brought about by the stroke.
- social services to plan for the impending discharge.

Each discipline has specific responsibilities, but all disciplines work together with the patient and family to resolve problems and to plan care.

There are many subspecialties in rehabilitation. Health care professionals may choose to work in **geriatric** (care of the elderly) or pediatric rehabilitation (Figure 44-4). Others may specialize in the care of patients with strokes, spinal cord injuries, brain injuries, amputations, or arthritis.

The Role of the Nursing Assistant in Rehabilitation

The nursing assistant who works in rehabilitation will assist the nurses with

- procedures to prevent complications: passive range-of-motion exercises and positioning.
- mobility skills: transfers and ambulation.
- bathing and personal care procedures.
- bowel and bladder training programs.
- maintaining the patient's nutritional status.
- programs to increase the patient's independence.

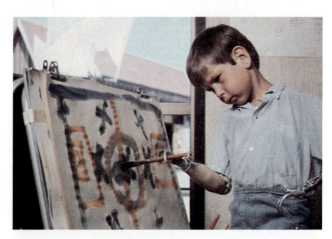

FIGURE 44-4 Pediatric rehabilitation is a specialized field. *Photo courtesy of the March of Dimes—Birth Defects Foundation*

PRINCIPLES OF REHABILITATION

Four principles form the foundation for successful rehabilitation or restorative care.

- *Treatment begins as soon as possible.*

  This means that plans for maintaining or increasing abilities begin as soon as the patient's condition is stable. For example, if a patient has had a stroke, passive exercises and positioning techniques are initiated in the critical care unit to prevent contractures, pressure ulcers, and other complications that would prohibit or delay rehabilitation.

- *Stress the patient's ability, not disability.*

  Care providers must think in terms of what the patient can do, not what the patient cannot do. The patient's strengths are used to help in adapting to any limitations. A *strength* refers to anything the patient is able to do. Perhaps a patient whose dominant hand is paralyzed cannot use that hand to feed himself, but instead of having nursing staff feed him, he can be taught to use the other, stronger hand.

- *Activity strengthens and inactivity weakens.*

  Complications result from physical and mental inactivity. These can cause further disability or even be life-threatening. A rehabilitation or restorative plan of care always includes approaches and goals for both physical and mental activity.

- *Treat the whole person.*

  When we are giving care to patients, we are not concerned only with their physical well-being. We also must attend to their emotional and mental health needs (Figure 44-5). An angry or depressed patient will not be able to concentrate on the work involved in rehabilitation.

We must also work with the patients' families. They directly influence the emotional and mental health of the patients.

The elements of successful rehabilitation/restorative care require that members of the team:

- have a positive attitude about the patients and their capabilities.
- have confidence in their own abilities as caregivers.
- be willing to learn from other care providers, patients, and their families.
- use problem-solving skills in place of unproductive coping methods.
- use all available tools and resources to give effective care.
- work with other staff as team members.
- realize that ideal working situations seldom exist, but strive to bring ideal and real closer together.
- continually learn and acquire new skills by participating in educational programs.
- accept the need for change to improve the quality of care for all patients.

COMPLICATIONS FROM INACTIVITY

People with disabilities may be unable to move about at will. The inactivity or immobility can result in numerous complications affecting body systems:

1. Musculoskeletal system.
   - Muscles become weak and **atrophy** (decrease in size and strength).
   - Contractures can form, making any movement impossible. A contracture (Figure 44-6) occurs when a joint is in a permanent state of flexion.
   - **Disuse osteoporosis** develops. This means that calcium drains from the bones, causing them to become brittle. Fractures can occur even without trauma.
2. Integumentary system.
   - Pressure sores develop over pressure areas.

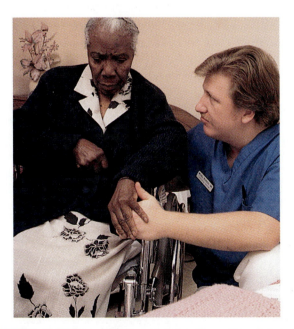

FIGURE 44-5 The patient's mental and emotional state is as important as her physical condition.

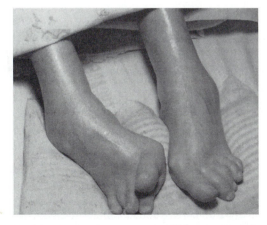

FIGURE 44-6 Contractures can result from immobility.

3. Cardiovascular system.
   – The heart takes longer to return to a normal pace after activity.
   – Blood does not circulate as efficiently. This can lead to thrombus (blood clot) and embolus (a blood clot that moves through the circulatory system).
4. Respiratory system.
   – The lungs do not expand. Secretions collect in the lungs and cause pneumonia.
   – Respiratory tract infections are more common.
5. Gastrointestinal system.
   – Appetite decreases, causing weight loss.
   – The risk of pressure sores increases with weight loss and lack of nutrition.
   – Peristalsis slows down, causing indigestion and constipation.
6. Urinary system.
   – The bladder does not empty completely. This increases the risk of bladder infection.
   – Incontinence can result from inability to get to the bathroom.
   – Urinary stones may develop from calcium in the bloodstream resulting from osteoporosis.
7. Psychosocial reaction.
   – Depression can occur from physical and mental inactivity.
   – Inactivity and lack of sensory stimulation can cause disorientation.

Activities of Daily Living

One purpose of restorative care is to increase the patient's physical abilities. This includes mobility skills and the ability to carry out activities of daily living.

These tasks or skills are taught to us as children. Healthy adults do these tasks automatically. If the patient cannot complete any or all of the ADLs, a **self-care deficit** exists. Adults may have self-care deficits because of:

- Diseases such as multiple sclerosis, arthritis, Parkinson's disease, or Alzheimer's disease
- Injuries causing damage to the extremities, brain, or spinal cord
- Vision impairment
- Emotional illness

Deficits are caused by problems that limit the patient's ability to do self-care. Examples of these problems are:

- Decreased strength
- Lack of endurance
- Limited range of motion
- Depression
- Disorientation
- Perceptual deficits

There are many types of **perceptual deficits**. These usually occur because of damage to the brain from disease or injury. Here are some examples of perceptual deficits:

- An inability to organize a task. ADLs cannot be completed unless the individual is able to prepare for the task, get the necessary items together, and then do it.
- An inability to sequence a task. When putting on clothing, for example, a slip must go on before the dress and socks before shoes.
- Lack of judgment. This deficit may be noted if a patient puts on a wool coat in hot weather (when appropriate clothing is available).
- An inability to identify common objects, such as eating utensils and grooming items (*agnosia*). The patient may try to use a fork to comb her hair, for example.
- An inability to use common items (*apraxia*). The patient may be able to identify the item but be unable to use it (even though there is no physical reason such as paralysis).
- An inability to initiate a task.

Patients with self-care deficits are evaluated by therapists and nurses. The results of evaluation will determine whether a patient's functional (physical) abilities can be increased. In other words, can the interdisciplinary team help this person to relearn an activity of daily living? This is discussed with the patient and the family.

RESTORATIVE PROGRAMS

If the patient has the potential to relearn an ADL and is motivated to try, a restorative program is planned. These programs are sometimes called retraining programs or ADL programs.

When the patient is unable to do any of the ADLs independently, it is generally best to concentrate on just one at a time. The first step is to find out what the patient wants to work on first. The interdisciplinary team then works with the patient and family to plan the process. They will:

- Establish goals. Each ADL consists of several steps, as shown in Table 44-1. The patient will not be able to do all steps right away. Some patients may never be able to do all of the steps. Goals, therefore, are very small. For example, if the patient is in a restorative program for eating, the first goal may be to hold a glass and take a drink from it. All goals are functional. Instead of saying the patient will walk 30 feet, the goal will state: "Patient will walk to the dining room for breakfast."
- Plan approaches. The approaches include the techniques and procedures carried out by the interdisciplinary team. The approaches are planned to help the patient relearn the ADL.

Approaches Used in Restorative Programs

Which approach to use should be indicated on the care plan. It is important that the same approach be used consistently.

- *Setup.* Patients with self-care deficits are not able to set up or prepare for activities of daily living. You may need

TABLE 44-1 FUNCTIONAL STEPS OF ACTIVITIES OF DAILY LIVING	
Bathing	• Gets to tub/sink/shower • Regulates water flow and temperature • Washes/rinses upper body • Washes/rinses lower body • Dries body
Dressing/Undressing	• Obtains/selects clothing • Puts on/takes off slipover top • Puts on/takes off cardigan-style top • Manages buttons, snaps, ties, zippers • Puts on/takes off skirt/pants • Buckles belt • Puts on shoes/socks
Eating	• Gets to table • Uses spoon, fork, knife appropriately • Opens/pours • Brings food to mouth • Chews, swallows • Uses napkin
Toileting	• Gets to commode/toilet • Manipulates clothing • Sits on toilet • Eliminates in toilet • Cleans self • Flushes toilet • Gets clothing back in place • Washes hands
Mobility	• Gets self to side of bed • Maintains upright position • Comes to standing position • Places self in position to sit in chair • Locks wheelchair brakes • Turns body to sit • Lowers self into chair • Propels wheelchair • Repositions self in chair • Raises self from chair • Places self in position to sit on edge of bed • Walks alone/with assistance • Uses assistive device

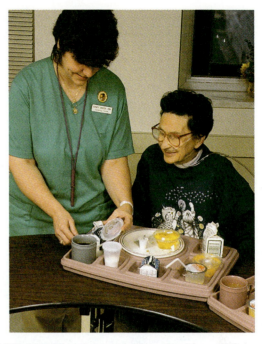

FIGURE 44-7 This patient is able to feed herself if the nursing assistant provides a tray setup.

to provide the setup (Figure 44-7). Example for bathing: collect all needed items, prepare the bath tub or shower, help the patient into the tub or shower.

● *Verbal cues.* The care provider uses short, simple phrases to prompt the patient. Example: give the patient a prepared washcloth and then say, "Please wash your face" (Figure 44-8).

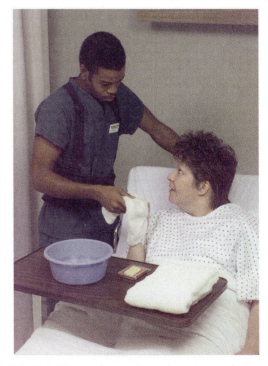

FIGURE 44-8 This nursing assistant is using verbal cues to assist the patient.

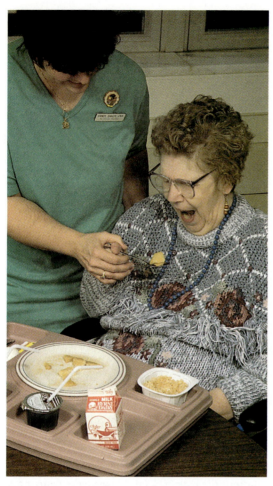

FIGURE 44-9 Hand-over-hand techniques are another approach used to help patients gain independence.

- *Hand-over-hand techniques.* Example for eating program: Place a glass in the patient's hand. Place your hand over the patient's hand. Guide the glass to the patient's mouth (Figure 44-9).
- *Demonstration.* Act out what you want the patient to do. Example: Before giving the patient a toothbrush, make the motions of brushing your teeth with the toothbrush (Figure 44-10).

Adaptive devices are sometimes used to simplify an ADL. **Adaptive devices** are ordinary items that have been modified for use by patients with various types of problems.

Not all patients are candidates for restorative programs. For those who are not, the goals are to prevent complications and maintain remaining abilities as long as possible. Some patients reach the point where even maintenance is difficult. We are then basically concerned with preventing complications.

The Restorative Environment

All patients benefit from living in an environment that attempts to improve the quality of life. The interdisciplinary team can help promote this environment:

- Give the patient a sense of control and opportunities to make decisions.

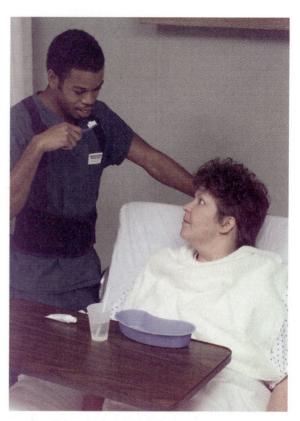

FIGURE 44-10 Demonstrating an activity of daily living helps the patient understand the instructions.

- Remember that mental and physical activity are essential to the patient's well-being.
- Encourage and assist patients to be well dressed and well groomed.
- Use touch freely in appropriate ways with patients.

GUIDELINES *for*

Implementing Restorative Programs

- Know why the patient has the self-care deficit.
- Keep your directions simple but not childish.
- Avoid distractions. Do the ADL in a private area.
- Be consistent. Read the care plan and follow the specific directions each time you work with the patient.
- Use adaptive devices consistently and correctly.
- Do not show impatience. Be encouraging and give praise.
- Treat the patient with dignity at all times.
- Realize that the patient's progress may be uneven and inconsistent.

- Provide cues for orientation throughout the building.
- Respect the patients' identity, individuality, and privacy at all times.
- Respect and understand the patient's sexuality and need for intimacy.

- Give patients opportunities to help others.
- Encourage and assist patients to remain a part of the community.
- Create an environment that is safe, serene, and colorful.

REVIEW

A. True/False.

Mark the following true or false by circling T or F.

1. T F Rehabilitation services are provided only in special hospitals.

2. T F OBRA regulations require that restorative services be provided to patients in skilled care facilities.

3. T F Rehabilitation and restorative services both strive to prevent complications.

4. T F Persons with disabilities will never recover their lost skills.

5. T F All persons with disabilities are considered to be handicapped.

B. Multiple Choice.

Select the one best answer for each question.

6. A patient with a permanent disability is
   a. taught to adapt to the present circumstances.
   b. not a good candidate for rehabilitation.
   c. given much sympathy.
   d. encouraged to be helpless.

7. Disabilities may result from
   a. arthritis.
   b. stroke.
   c. spinal cord injury.
   d. all of these.

8. A patient who is unable to communicate verbally will be treated by a
   a. physical therapist.
   b. occupational therapist.
   c. nursing assistant.
   d. speech and language therapist.

9. Physical inactivity can cause
   a. pressure ulcers.
   b. contractures.
   c. blood clots.
   d. all of these.

10. Agnosia is a perceptual deficit in which the patient cannot
    a. organize a task.
    b. identify common items.
    c. sequence a task.
    d. initiate a task.

11. Adaptive devices are
    a. inappropriate for patients receiving rehabilitation.
    b. used by nursing assistants to feed patients.
    c. ordinary items modified for use by patients with self-care deficits.
    d. used only by occupational therapists.

12. Placing your hand over the patient's hand to guide the patient's actions is an approach called
    a. giving verbal cues.
    b. demonstration.
    c. hand-over-hand technique.
    d. setting up.

C. Completion.

Complete the statements by choosing the correct word from the following list.

activities of daily living
atrophy
contracture
disability
disuse osteoporosis
embolus
geriatric
handicap
mobility skills
physiatrist
rehabilitation
self-care deficit
verbal cues

13. The process used to help a patient reach an optimal level of ability is ____.

14. Ambulation and transfers are examples of ____.

15. Dressing and undressing are examples of ____.

16. An impairment that affects the ability to perform an activity that a person of that age would normally be able to do is called a/an _____.

17. When the impairment limits or prevents the person from fulfilling a role that is normal for that person, a/an _____ exists.

18. A person who chooses to work with rehabilitation of the elderly is specializing in _____ rehabilitation.

19. A physician who specializes in rehabilitation is called a/an _____.

20. A/An _____ occurs when a joint is in a permanent state of flexion.

21. _____ occurs when a muscle shrinks and loses strength.

22. Physical inactivity can cause calcium to drain from the bones, resulting in _____.

23. A/An _____ is a blood clot that moves through the circulatory system.

24. A/An _____ exists when an adult cannot complete one or more activities of daily living.

25. Using short, simple phrases to prompt the patient to complete an activity of daily living is called _____.

D. Nursing Assistant Challenge.

You are working as a nursing assistant in the rehabilitation unit of a subacute care section of a skilled nursing facility. Think about what you have learned in this unit and answer the following questions:

26. What types of patients will you see?

27. What kinds of disabilities will the patients have?

28. What may be the cause of the self-care deficits experienced by your patients?

29. What kinds of problems can limit a patient's ability to do self-care?

30. What are the differences between rehabilitation and restorative care?

31. What are the responsibilities of the nursing assistant when giving restorative care?

The Obstetrical Patient and Neonate

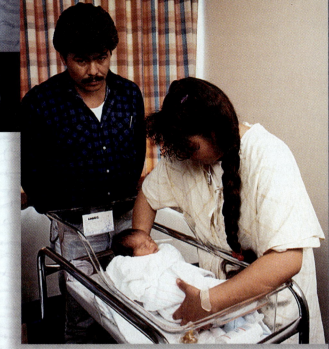

📋 **Notice to the Reader:** By state law, you may not be permitted to perform some of the advanced procedures discussed in this section. Consult with your instructor or supervisor to be sure you know your legal responsibilities. Do not perform or assist in any procedure you are not permitted by law to do.

OBJECTIVES

As a result of this unit, you will be able to:

- Spell and define terms.
- Assist in the prenatal care of the normal pregnant woman.
- List reportable observations of patients in the prenatal period.
- Assist in care of the normal postpartum patient.
- Properly change a perineal pad.

- Recognize reportable observations of patients in the postpartum period.
- Recognize reportable signs and symptoms of urine retention in the postpartum patient.
- Assist in care of the normal newborn.
- Demonstrate three methods of safely holding a baby.
- Assist in carrying out the discharge procedures for mother and infant.

VOCABULARY

Learn the meaning and the correct spelling of the following words and phrases:

amniocentesis	engagement	involution	postpartum
amniotic fluid	episiotomy	isolette	prenatal
amniotic sac	expulsion stage	labor	quickening
Apgar score	fetal monitor	lactation	rooming-in
cesarean	fetoscopy	lochia	status
circumcision	fetus	neonate	trimester
colostrum	foreskin	obstetrical	ultrasound
dilation stage	fundus	placenta	umbilical cord
efface	gestational age	placental stage	vaginal examination
endoscope			

INTRODUCTION

When a baby is ready to be born, it is normally upside down in the mother's uterus with its head toward the birth canal (Figure 45-1). Before the baby is born, it is known as a fetus. It is surrounded by a membranous bag called an amniotic sac. The fetus floats in a liquid called amniotic fluid.

The fetus gets nourishment from the mother through the umbilical cord. The umbilical cord is attached to the fetus and the placenta (afterbirth). The placenta is attached to the wall of the mother's uterus.

After the baby is born and separated from the umbilical cord, the placenta, amniotic sac, and remaining cord are expelled as the afterbirth. After a period of time, the mother's uterus, or womb, which was greatly stretched to accommodate the pregnancy, will return to its normal size and shape.

There are three phases of pregnancy:

- Prenatal (before birth)
- Labor and delivery
- Postpartum (after birth)

The nursing assistant, who is specially trained, helps provide care and support throughout each phase.

PRENATAL CARE

The care of the mother begins in the prenatal period, when she first learns she is pregnant. You may meet her as you work in a doctor's office or in an obstetrical (pregnancy) clinic.

A normal pregnancy lasts about 280 days and is divided into trimesters (3 months). Each trimester is noted by specific signs and symptoms:

First trimester (1 through 12 weeks)

- Absence of menstrual period
- Nausea and vomiting (usually in the morning)
- Swelling and tenderness of breasts
- Frequent urination
- Constipation
- Positive pregnancy test within 7 to 10 days after conception
- Softening of uterus and cervix, and bluish color of vagina noted by examiner
- Increased vaginal secretions

Second trimester (13 through 27 weeks)

- Weight gain
- Abdominal enlargement
- Stretch marks may be noted on abdominal skin
- Breast enlargement–colostrum may be noted at about 20 weeks
- Hemorrhoids may be noted
- Uterus and fetus enlargement noted by examiner— mother will feel quickening (movements of fetus) about the 20th week

Third trimester (28th through 40th week)

- Mother feels occasional painless uterine contractions (the contractions are strengthening the uterus for labor)
- Uterus and fetus increase in size; this may cause indigestion, insomnia, and shortness of breath
- Mother may have backaches related to posture changes due to weight of fetus
- Edema of ankles may be present
- Varicose veins may appear

The care of the mother throughout pregnancy is important to ensure the birth of a healthy baby. The first trimester is an especially critical time. During the first three months, the fetus is very susceptible to the negative effects of tobacco, alcohol, caffeine, and other drugs, as well as to viruses and bacteria. Exposure to any of these may cause physical and/or mental harm to the developing fetus.

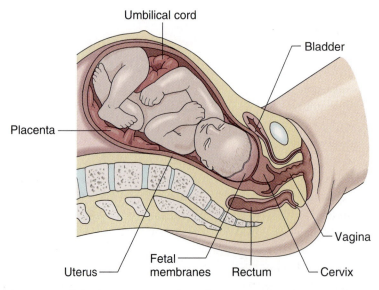

FIGURE 45-1 The usual position of the fetus at term. This is known as a head (vertex) presentation.

The pregnant woman is usually advised to visit the physician, nurse practitioner, or midwife at least once a month during the first trimester. During the first visit, the examiner will complete a very thorough history and physical examination, which will include:

- Routine information: age, occupation (to determine exposure to any hazards), education, race (some genetic diseases such as sickle cell anemia are found only in certain races), religion (this may have an impact on the mother's health care practices)
- History of menstruation, contraception, pregnancies
- Medical and family history
- Nutritional status
- Examination of fetus

Visits become more frequent as the pregnancy progresses. Routine procedures during the visits include:

- Weighing the mother
- Taking the blood pressure and pulse
- Urine testing
- Counseling and teaching the mother about diet, lifestyle, and signs and symptoms that she should report to the physician
- Palpating the abdomen to check fetal size
- Listening for fetal heart tones

You should call anything unusual to the attention of the nurse. Examples of items to report are:

- Complaints of persistent headache
- Elevated blood pressure
- Vaginal bleeding
- Complaints of dizziness
- Swelling of the hands and feet

PREPARATION FOR BIRTH

Both parents are encouraged to participate fully in the birth of their baby. Special training for the birth begins in the prenatal period. It prepares the parents to participate in the birthing process. Many parents choose to participate in natural childbirth. This technique of birthing:

- allows the mother to be awake and fully participate in the birth.
- encourages the father or an alternative support person to act as coach for the mother.
- necessitates little, if any, pain-controlling medication. One of the most popular of these methods is called the Lamaze method.

Training Classes

In birth training classes:

- The father or some other person learns to act as a coach for the mother.
- The mother learns ways of cooperating with her body during labor and delivery, using special breathing and relaxation techniques.

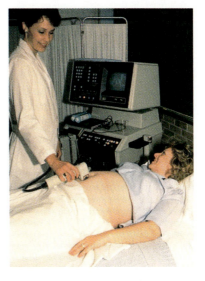

FIGURE 45-2 The ultrasound test is used to check normal fetal development and detect defects in the structure of fetal organs. *Courtesy of Jackson Community College, Jackson, MI*

- The couple sees films of the birth process.
- Vaginal and cesarean deliveries are discussed.
- There are opportunities to ask questions of a trained professional.

PRENATAL TESTING

Congenital abnormalities (those present at birth) can sometimes be identified through prenatal testing. Testing methods include:

- **Ultrasound**—a technique of using sound waves to identify **gestational age** (time of development) and defects in the structure of fetal organs (Figure 45-2).
- **Amniocentesis**—a procedure in which a sterile needle is inserted into the fetal sac and cells are withdrawn for examination. Some genetic defects may be identified in this way.
- **Fetoscopy**—a direct visualization of the fetus in the uterus through a small visualization instrument (**endoscope**). Blood abnormalities may also be identified from samples of the fetal blood that is withdrawn.

LABOR AND DELIVERY

At the end of 40 weeks (within 2 weeks more or less), the signs of impending **labor** will be noted:

- **Engagement** or lightening (the fetus moves downward—sometimes referred to as "dropping")
- Mucous plug is expelled from cervix
- Dilation of cervix begins
- Amniotic membranes may rupture just before actual labor begins, or may rupture during labor
- Uterine contractions begin
  - Irregular at first
  - Stronger, more regular, and closer together as labor progresses

The mother is told during her pregnancy when she should go to the hospital.

Dilation

The **dilation** (opening) **stage** begins with the first regular uterine contractions. It ends when the cervix is fully dilated or opened. This may take 18 to 24 hours in a first pregnancy. As the labor progresses, the cervix also thins (**effaces**) so that the fetus may move downward into the birth canal and out of the mother's body. The degree of dilation at any given time is measured by the nurse or physician. The nurse or physician places a gloved finger in the patient's vagina and measures (approximately) the size of the cervical opening. This procedure is called **vaginal examination**.

Relief of Discomfort

Drugs may be given to the mother in the labor and delivery phase to reduce pain. Three approaches are frequently employed for a vaginal delivery:

1. Epidural—this is the most common technique. The anesthetic drug is introduced into the epidural space around the spinal cord. Because the drug is not introduced into the cerebrospinal fluid, its effect is more localized in the reproductive organs. The patient's legs can move, but they are weak. Women who are pregnant for the first time may be given this relief when they have reached 5 to 6 cm cervical dilation. Women who have had more than one pregnancy may have it started at 3 to 4 cm dilation without slowing the progress of labor. Controlled introduction of drugs through the epidural route offers relief throughout the delivery. Patients receiving epidural pain relief must be carefully monitored for changes in pulse and blood pressure. Report a drop in blood pressure to the nurse at once.

2. Regional caudal block—this technique introduces the anesthetic drug into the cerebrospinal fluid. It affects a somewhat larger area, but the legs can still move. This form of relief is commonly known as a *saddle block.* This is usually given in the delivery room.

3. Pudendal block—this technique specifically blocks the function of the nerves in the perineum. This medication is usually administered in the delivery room.

When any of these procedures is used, the patient will not feel an episiotomy or its repair, but she will still be able to move her legs. The type of pain relief given to the mother during labor and delivery determines the postpartum care she will receive.

Fetal Monitors

In many hospitals, a **fetal monitor** (instrument to check the well-being of the baby during labor) (Figure 45-3) is attached either to the mother's abdomen or to the baby's head.

Expulsion

Expulsion stage is the period extending from the point of full cervical dilation until the baby is delivered. This may be 1 to 2 hours or more.

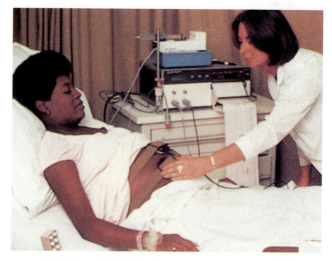

FIGURE 45-3 The fetal monitor allows the staff to evaluate the infant's condition during labor. *Courtesy of Memorial Medical Center of Long Beach, CA*

The baby moves down the birth canal. The mother is encouraged to help the process by "bearing down" with her abdominal muscles with each contraction. Figures 45-4 and 45-5 show the baby being assisted in delivery and rotated as the shoulders are presented.

During delivery, it may be necessary to enlarge the vaginal opening. This is done by making a cut in the perineum. The cut is called an **episiotomy**. The episiotomy is sutured (sewn up) after delivery.

Forceps may be used at this stage to assist in delivery of the head. Once delivered, the baby is held head down to clear the respiratory tract. The baby is then usually placed on the mother's abdomen while the cord is clamped and cut. In addition:

- An Apgar score is determined.
- The mother is encouraged to hold her newborn, now called a **neonate**, to establish emotional bonding. This is done even when the baby is delivered by cesarean section.

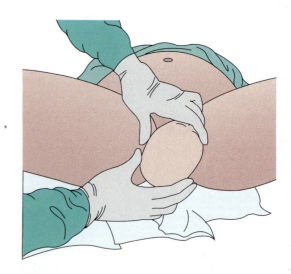

FIGURE 45-4 The baby's head emerges.

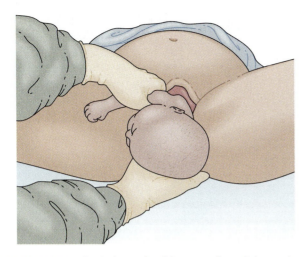

FIGURE 45-5 The baby's shoulders are then delivered.

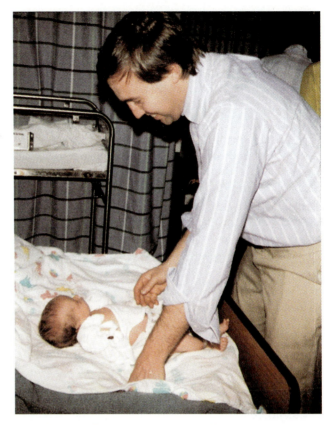

FIGURE 45-6 Fathers are encouraged to participate in the care of the newborn.

Placental Stage

The placental stage lasts from delivery of the baby through the delivery of the placenta. This is a short period. The placenta is usually delivered within an hour of the delivery of the baby.

In this stage, the placenta separates from the wall of the uterus. Uterine contractions push it downward and out through the birth canal. After delivery of the placenta:

- If an episiotomy was needed, it is repaired.
- The mother's uterus is checked for firmness. Drugs may be given to help it contract to control bleeding.
- Both mother and child are identified with name tags before being separated.
- The baby is footprinted along with the mother's thumbprint.
- The baby's eyes are treated to prevent infection.

In most hospitals today, the labor, delivery, and postpartum (period after delivery) care are all carried out in the same room. Keeping the newborn in the same room with the mother is called rooming-in. The baby can be taken to the nursery if the mother has complications or is unable to rest with the baby in the room. The usual length of stay for the new mother and baby is about two days unless there are complications. After the mother has recovered from anesthesia and any medications that were given during labor, she is encouraged to do as much self-care as possible. She is allowed to get out of bed soon after delivery if there are no complications.

The father or another supportive person who has attended the prenatal classes with the pregnant woman is encouraged to participate in the labor, delivery, and care (Figure 45-6) of the newborn. The baby's siblings, grandparents, and other family members are allowed to visit during the postpartum period and to hold and love the baby (Figure 45-7). Many hospitals serve the new parents a special, private meal the evening before discharge.

In the last several years there has been a trend toward

- making the delivery a family affair.
- having the delivery take place at home or in a homelike environment.
- continuing to provide for the safety of both mother and infant.

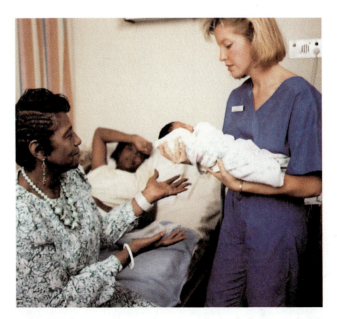

FIGURE 45-7 Family members are allowed to visit, to hold, and to love the newborn.

CESAREAN BIRTH

Cesarean section is another way of delivering a baby. The baby is delivered through an incision in the abdomen rather than through the birth canal. Between 20 and 30% of all births in the United States are made in this way.

A spinal anesthetic is administered before the surgery. This type of procedure introduces the drugs into the cerebrospinal fluid and blocks sensation from the upper abdomen down to the toes. Until the anesthetic wears off, the patient will not be able either to feel or move her legs.

After the delivery, the mother sometimes is given a general anesthetic that allows her to sleep during the rest of the procedure.

Cesarean deliveries may be performed when there is:

- Fetal distress
- A preterm infant
- Breech (nonhead first) presentation
- Prolonged rupture of the membranes
- Prolapsed cord
- Genital herpes
- Premature separation of the placenta
- Placenta previa
- Dysfunctional labor

The incision in the abdominal wall may be:

- Vertical, along the midplane
- Transverse, across the lowest and narrowest part of the abdomen (bikini cut)

The mother's coach or partner is encouraged to be in the operative area to offer emotional support while the cesarean is being done. The same basic activities are carried out in the operating room as are followed after a vaginal delivery.

After the surgery is complete, the baby is usually admitted to the nursery (Figure 45-8). The mother is moved to the

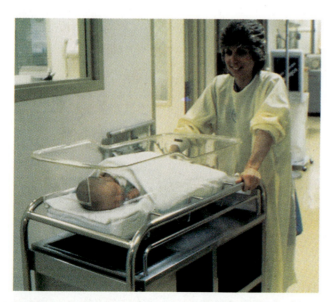

FIGURE 45-8 Babies are transported in their own bassinets from delivery room to newborn nursery. *Courtesy of Memorial Medical Center of Long Beach, CA*

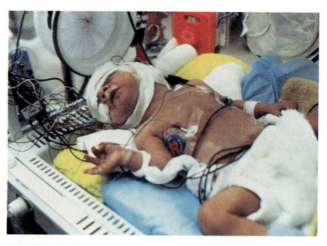

FIGURE 45-9 This baby has been moved to a neonatal intensive care unit following a cesarean delivery. The eyes are covered to protect them. *Courtesy of Memorial Medical Center of Long Beach, CA*

recovery room for immediate post-anesthesia care. If the infant is in distress, it will be taken to the neonatal intensive care unit (Figure 45-9).

POSTPARTUM CARE

You may be assigned to assist in caring for the mother during the postpartum period.

With other team members, you will assist the mother from the stretcher into bed. A protective pad (Chux) may be placed under the patient's buttocks.

Always wear gloves and follow standard precautions when caring for the postpartum patient. There is a high probability of contact with blood, mucous membranes, urine, and breast milk. All of these body fluids are considered potentially infectious.

Anesthesia

If an anesthetic was used, follow the procedures for postoperative care of surgical patients, which were covered in Unit 28.

- Keep the patient flat on her back.
- Make sure the patient has a fresh gown and clean bed linen.
- Check blood pressure, pulse, and respirations as ordered until the patient is stable.
- Continue to monitor vital signs every 4 hours for 24 hours.
- If the patient complains of being cold, an extra blanket may provide comfort. If the patient does not become comfortable, inform the nurse.

Drainage

Carefully check the condition of the perineum and the perineal pad for the amount and color of drainage.

- When removing the pad, always lift it away from the body from front to back.

- Red vaginal discharge, called lochia, is expected. The amount of discharge and any clotting should be reported.

Initially, the lochia is bright red and moderate in amount. Over the next week, the lochia will lessen and become pink to pink-brown in color. A discharge that is yellowish-white or brown may continue for 1 to 3 weeks after delivery and then stop. Note and report:

- Signs of tenderness
- Signs of inflammation
- Presence of an episiotomy

The Uterus

The size and firmness of the uterus should be checked and reported. A soft and enlarging uterus indicates excessive bleeding.

Massaging. The top of the uterus, the fundus, is massaged in a circular fashion while the opposite hand is held against the pubic bone. Massaging the fundus stimulates the uterine muscles to contract, firming the uterus.

Measuring Height of Uterus. The level of the fundus is measured by placing the fingers lengthwise across the abdomen between the fundus and the navel. On the first postpartal day, the level of the fundus is usually at the umbilicus or one to two fingers'-width below.

Cramping. As the uterus begins to return to its normal size (involution), the patient may experience strong uterine contractions or cramps. Cramping may also be associated with breast feeding. This is normal, but be sure to report any complaints of pain to your team leader, who can administer medication for relief.

Voiding

The new mother should be encouraged to void within the first 6 to 8 hours after the delivery. Check carefully for signs of urine retention. These include:

- A uterus that is unusually high or pushed to one side
- Swelling just above the pubis
- Complaints of urgency (the need to void), but with voidings of 200 mL or less

Be sure to report:

- Signs of possible urine retention immediately, so the patient's recovery will not be impeded
- Any inability to void within the first 8 hours postpartum
- Voidings of less than 100 mL

This is important because a full bladder can cause postpartum hemorrhage.

TOILETING AND PERINEAL CARE

The mother may be:

- Provided with a squeezable bottle filled with warm tap water.

- Instructed to rinse the genitals and perineum after voiding or defecating.
- Instructed to gently pat, not wipe, the perineal area containing the stitches with tissue or special medicated pads—once only, from front to back. The tissue is discarded in the toilet.
- Taught to wash her hands before applying a fresh perineal pad.
- Taught not to touch the inside of the perineal pad.

If the perineum is very uncomfortable:

- Specially medicated pads may be used for cleansing. The procedure is always the same—front to back and discard.
- Anesthetic sprays may be ordered.
- Ice packs may be used to reduce edema and give comfort.

Patients should be cautioned to apply anesthetics and ointments after cleansing.

Sitting may be uncomfortable when an episiotomy has been performed. Instruct the mother to squeeze her buttocks together and hold them in this position until she is seated upright. This reduces tension on the suture line.

BREAST CARE

The mother's first milk is called colostrum. The colostrum:

- Is watery.
- Carries protective antibodies to the child.
- Usually begins to flow about 12 hours after delivery. Lactation, the flow of milk, does not begin until the second or third postpartum day.

Keeping the breasts clean is especially important when the mother is planning to breast-feed her baby.

- The mother's hands and nipples should be washed just prior to feeding the baby.
- During the shower, the mother should wash the breasts, using a circular motion from the nipples outward.
- Creams are sometimes used between feedings to help the nipples remain supple.
- Breast pads absorb milk leakage. They should be changed frequently.
- The breasts should be supported by a well-fitted brassiere.

Even if the mother chooses not to breast-feed, the breasts should be washed daily with soap and water. The breasts should also be supported continuously by a well-fitted brassiere. Medication to suppress milk production is sometimes ordered.

When delivery is uncomplicated, mothers and healthy newborns do not stay in the hospital very long. They are usually able to go home within two days.

NEONATAL CARE

After the newborn is admitted to the nursery, some procedures not carried out in the delivery room are completed.

The physician or nurse will examine the baby and make an evaluation of the baby's condition, or **status**.

Apgar Scoring

The **Apgar score** is an evaluation of the neonate. It is made at one minute and five minutes after birth. The areas evaluated are:

- Heart rate
- Respiratory effort
- Muscle tone
- Reflex, irritability
- Color

A number value is applied to each assessment and recorded on a special form. For example, the neonate who has a heart rate of less than 100 bpm, has slow respirations, offers slight resistance to limb extension, has a weak cry, and is pale and cyanotic would be rated as follows:

Heart rate	1
Respiratory effort	1
Muscle tone	1
Reflex, irritability	1
Color	0
Total	4

Totals indicate the infant's condition. A score of 7 to 10 indicates that the infant is in good condition. A score of 4 to 6 indicates a fair condition. A score of 0 to 4 indicates a poor condition.

In the nursery the baby's vital signs are determined. Measurements of length and weight are also taken.

When the newborn's status becomes stable:

- If the eyes were not treated with silver nitrate drops or antibiotics in the delivery room, or the footprints were not taken (Figure 45-10), these procedures are done at this time.
- The baby is cleaned. Sometimes an admission bath using an antiseptic soap or oil is administered, but pro-

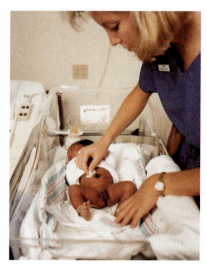

FIGURE 45-11 The area around the cord is carefully cleaned with a solution prescribed by the facility.

cedures for bathing newborns vary from hospital to hospital. In some hospitals, the bath is omitted and the cheesy material known as *vernix caseosa* is allowed to remain on the skin. The area around the umbilical cord is carefully cleaned with a solution prescribed by the facility (Figure 45-11).

- The baby must be kept warm because a newborn's temperature has not yet stabilized. The baby is dressed according to facility policy. A stockinette cap is placed on the head because much body heat can be lost through this surface (Figure 45-12).
- The baby is placed in a crib or **isolette** (Figure 45-13).
- Feeding is not usually started for 12 hours after birth. During these hours, the baby is monitored and observed carefully for successful, independent life. After 12 hours, the baby is either taken to breast or started on feedings of glucose and water. Babies whose mothers are unable to feed will be fed in the nursery.
- Male babies may be circumcised before discharge. In **circumcision**, the excess tissue (**foreskin**) is cut from the tip of the penis. This procedure is no longer performed routinely. However, the procedure is still routinely performed on male babies whose parents are members of Orthodox Jewish congregations.
- Babies who are jaundiced may have their eyes protected and be placed under a special light (bili light) to help clear the levels of bilirubin in the skin.

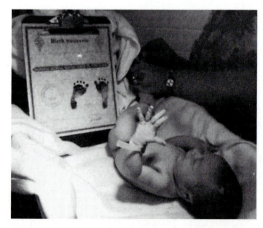

FIGURE 45-10 Footprinting is done in the delivery room or nursery. The baby's identification band is placed on the baby immediately after birth and matches the mother's identification band.

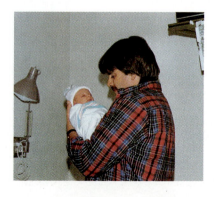

FIGURE 45-12 Caps are placed on the babies' heads to preserve body heat.

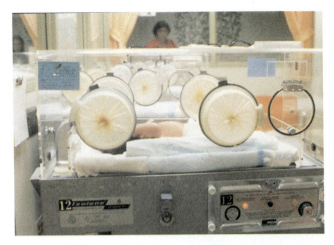

FIGURE 45-13 Babies may be cared for in isolettes that provide a controlled environment. *Courtesy of Memorial Medical Center of Long Beach, CA*

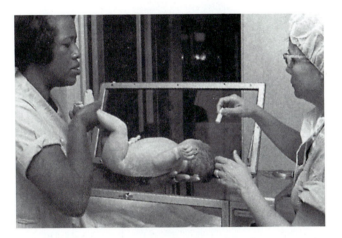

FIGURE 45-14 While grasping the baby's legs securely, slip your other hand under the back to support the head and neck. Note the vernix caseosa on this infant's back.

Handling the Infant

Take care when lifting, carrying, and positioning an infant. Remember to:

- Lift the baby by grasping the legs securely with one hand while slipping the other hand under the baby's back to support the head and neck (Figures 45-14 and 45-15).
- Hold the baby securely.
- Support the head, neck, and back at all times.
- Back through doorways when carrying a baby.
- Never turn your back on an infant when the infant is on an unprotected surface.

PKU Test

The baby's blood is tested to detect the presence of phenylketonuria (PKU) (Figure 45-16). PKU is a congenital, hereditary abnormality. It may lead to mental retardation if undetected and not treated early. In PKU, normal protein digestion is not possible. The disorder cannot be cured, but it can be controlled by a special diet.

Eye Care

This procedure is performed by the nurse. Silver nitrate (AgNO$_3$) in a 1% solution is commonly used, but other medications such as antibiotics may be ordered.

Post-Circumcision Care

The circumcision should be checked each time the diaper is changed and should be a routine part of that care. Observe the incision site for bleeding and report anything unusual. The crib identification should note the new circumcision. A note should also be included on the nursery record as to the condition of the circumcision and first voiding after circumcision.

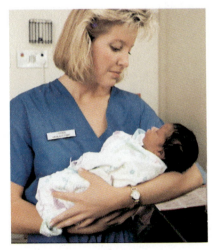
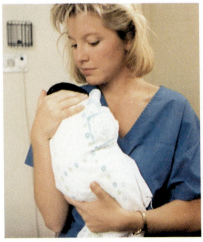
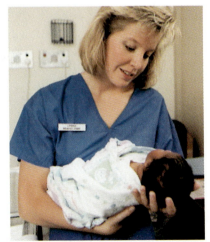

A   B   C

FIGURE 45-15 Techniques for holding a baby: A. Cradle hold B. Shoulder hold C. Football hold

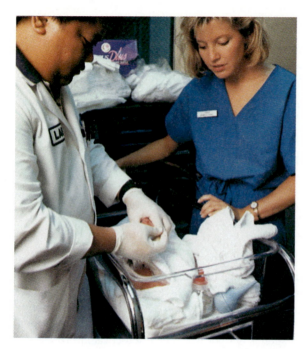

FIGURE 45-16 Blood is drawn from the infant's heel to check for phenylketonuria (PKU). PKU is a congenital, hereditary disorder that can lead to mental retardation if undetected and untreated.

DISCHARGE

To carry out the discharge procedure from a facility:

- Match the baby's identification with the mother's.
- Dress the child in his or her own clothing (Figure 45-17). This may be done in the nursery or in the mother's room.
- Wrap the baby in a blanket, using the technique of "papoosing," as shown in Figures 45-18A through D.
- Check to be sure that the mother has received and understands any special discharge instructions. If not, inform the nurse.

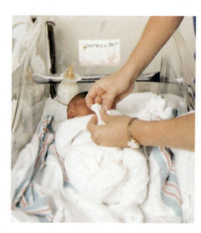

FIGURE 45-17 Dress the infant in his or her own clothing.

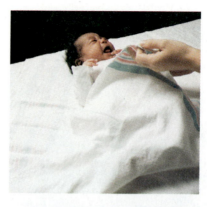

FIGURE 45-18A Place a receiving blanket under the infant so the corners are at the head and feet. Bring the bottom corner up over the infant.

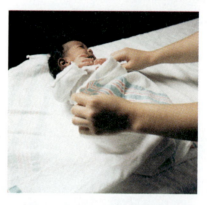

FIGURE 45-18B Bring one side corner of the blanket over the infant.

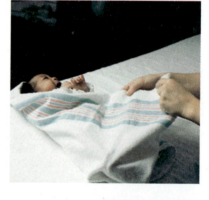

FIGURE 45-18C Then bring the other side corner of the blanket over the infant.

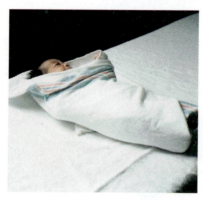

FIGURE 45-18D Tuck the final corner under the infant. The infant is ready to be discharged.

- Check to be sure equipment or needed formula is ready when the parents and newborn are ready to go home (Figure 45-19).
- Transport the mother, carrying her baby, by wheelchair to the discharge area. Stay with them until they leave.

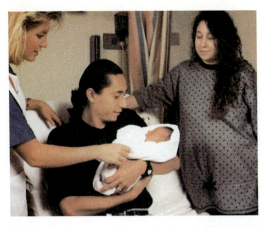

FIGURE 45-19 Parents prepare to leave the hospital with their newborn

- Record discharge information on the charts of both mother and child. Include the condition of each and the time of release.

Home Care

The discharged mother faces many new challenges. It will take approximately six weeks for her reproductive organs to recover. Home care of the mother includes:

- Providing adequate nutrition
- Allowing for sufficient rest
- Attending to proper elimination
- Providing emotional support during any transitory depression
- Providing breast care, if she is nursing the baby

REVIEW

A. True/False.

Mark the following true or false by circling T or F.

1. T F You are responsible for noting and reporting the first postpartal voiding.

2. T F Care of the mother begins in the prenatal period.

3. T F The nurse or physician monitors the progress of labor by performing a vaginal examination.

4. T F Immediate postpartum lochia should be yellowish-white.

5. T F Massaging the cervix stimulates the uterine muscles to contract.

6. T F A congenital abnormality is one that is present at birth.

7. T F Ultrasound is a technique used to examine the baby before birth.

8. T F In the first pregnancy, the period of labor and delivery called expulsion lasts 18 to 24 hours.

9. T F As labor progresses, the uterine cervix becomes more and more tightened.

10. T F The shoulder hold is a safe way to hold and support an infant.

11. T F The first feeding for the newborn is usually given 12 hours after birth.

12. T F The mother's hands and nipples should be washed before she nurses the baby.

B. Matching.

Choose the correct term from Column II to match each phrase in Column I.

Column I	Column II
13. _____ surgery to remove the foreskin	**a.** lochia
	b. umbilical cord
14. _____ maintains an even temperature for the fetus	**c.** fundus
	d. lactation
15. _____ mother's first postpartum breast secretions	**e.** colostrum
	f. circumcision
16. _____ attachment between baby and placenta	**g.** vernix caseosa
	h. isolette
17. _____ vaginal discharge following delivery	**i.** placenta

C. Nursing Assistant Challenge.

You are working in a prenatal clinic for a nurse practitioner. One of the patients is Mrs. McDonnel, who is coming in today for her first appointment. She tells you she has missed two menstrual periods. Answer the following questions.

18. What signs and symptoms do you expect to see today and for the next month or so?

19. Because this is the patient's first visit, what equipment and supplies do you need to have ready for the nurse practitioner?

20. What signs and symptoms will you observe during the second trimester?

21. What signs and symptoms will you observe during the third trimester?

22. Which procedures would be completed at each visit?

23. What statements by the patient would you report immediately?

Pediatric Patient

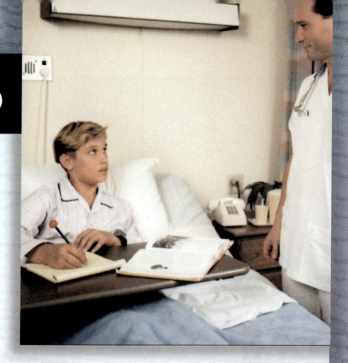

As a result of this unit, you will be able to:

- Spell and define terms.
- Describe the major developmental tasks for each pediatric age group.
- Describe how to foster growth and development for hospitalized pediatric patients.
- Describe how to maintain a safe environment for the pediatric patient.
- Discuss the role of parents and siblings of the hospitalized pediatric patient.
- Demonstrate the following procedures:
  — Procedure 119 Admitting a Pediatric Patient

— Procedure 120 Weighing the Pediatric Patient
— Procedure 121 Changing Crib Linens
— Procedure 122 Changing Crib Linens (Infant in Crib)
— Procedure 123 Measuring Temperature
— Procedure 124 Determining Heart Rate (Pulse)
— Procedure 125 Counting Respiratory Rate
— Procedure 126 Measuring Blood Pressure
— Procedure 127 Bottle-Feeding the Infant
— Procedure 128 Burping (Method A)
— Procedure 129 Burping (Method B)

VOCABULARY

Learn the meaning and the correct spelling of the following words and phrases:

adolescence	developmental	foster parent	legal guardian
adoptive parent	milestones	initiative	regress
autonomy	developmental tasks	legal custody	stepparent
biological parent	family		

INTRODUCTION

Children, like adults, get sick and need hospitalization for diagnosis and treatment of their illnesses. But children are different. They are not just small adults. Children can differ in age, in size, and in developmental level. When you work with children, you will also be working with the people who are most important to them—their parents or those responsible for their upbringing. When a child is sick and hospitalized, the illness affects the entire family. The family is an important part of the child's life regardless of the child's age. When working with pediatric patients, you will need to include the parents in giving care to the child.

In today's society, the words *parents* and *family* can have different meanings. A child may live with one or both parents. The words *biological, adoptive, foster,* and *step* can refer to the various types of parents that may be part or all of a child's family. The terms are defined as follows:

- **Biological parent**—birth (genetic) parent
- **Adoptive parent**—person who has legally assumed responsibility for parenting
- **Foster parent**—person who carries out parenting duties under the authority of a legal agency
- **Stepparent**—person who assumes the parenting role by marrying a birth or adoptive parent

Families may also include combinations of parents. For example, a child may live with a biological father and an adoptive or stepmother. Or a child may live with a single parent, who could be either biological, adoptive, or foster. Other family arrangements may include the child living with a relative while the parent maintains legal custody of the child. **Legal custody** refers to the person who has the right to give consent for hospitalization and for the procedures that may be needed while the child is hospitalized. This person is known as the **legal guardian**. The child may live with someone other than the legal guardian.

The word **family** refers to the household unit in which the child lives. Members of the family may include the parents, siblings (biological, adoptive, or step), and/or other relatives or persons in the household.

As a member of the health care team, it is important for you to identify the child's caretakers as well as the person who has legal custody.

This unit provides guidelines for care of the hospitalized child. The nursing assistant must recognize that hospitalization may interrupt the child's normal growth and development. This is a traumatic time for the child. Suggestions are given to show how the nursing assistant can assist and encourage the child's development during hospitalization.

Safety is an important part of providing care. This unit presents guidelines for creating a safe environment for each pediatric age group. Because families are important, suggestions are also made on creating a family-centered approach to pediatric health care.

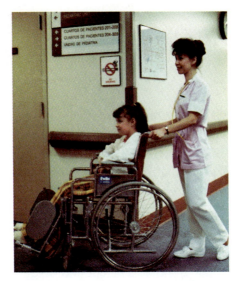

FIGURE 46-1 The nursing assistant transports an older child to the pediatric unit following admission.

PEDIATRIC UNITS

Pediatric units are typically set up in one of two ways:
1. According to specific age groups of children
2. According to the types of patients, such as surgical, orthopedic, cardiac, and so on

You may have the opportunity to work with children in a specific age group, or you may work with children in a variety of age groups. Regardless of the ages of the children, working in pediatrics will offer you many rewards and challenges.

When a child is admitted to the hospital, you may be involved in the admission procedure (Figure 46-1). A nurse will obtain a medical and social history from the parents. Information obtained will include the child's nickname, the ages and names of siblings, the child's likes and dislikes, and normal times and routines for meals, naps, and bedtimes. Any information that will make the child's hospital stay easier is marked in the history. Once the history is complete, you can continue with the admission procedure (see Procedure 119).

In this unit, guidelines are presented for caring for children by age groups. The groups are:
- Infancy (0–1 year)
- Toddler (1–3 years)
- Preschooler (3–6 years)
- School-age (6–12 years)
- Adolescent (13–18 years)

DEVELOPMENTAL TASKS

For each age group, it is expected that the child will have reached a certain developmental level. Each level is characterized by physical and psychological tasks that the average

PROCEDURE **119**

ADMITTING A PEDIATRIC PATIENT

1. Introduce yourself to the child and his parents.
2. Show them all to the child's room and familiarize them with the unit.
3. Explain what you will do.
4. Wash your hands.
5. Place an identification band on the child.
6. Dress the child in his own pajamas or hospital clothing.
7. Obtain the child's height and weight. Record according to hospital policy. (Refer to Procedure 120.)
8. Measure the child's vital signs. (Refer to Procedures 123 through 126.)
9. Obtain a urine specimen. (Refer to Unit 42.)
10. Wash your hands.
11. Assist the physician with examination of the child as necessary.
12. Explain rooming-in and visiting policies to parents.
13. If parents leave, stay with the child to provide comfort.

---

child in the group can perform. If you understand the **developmental tasks** for each age group, it will be easier to find ways to help and encourage the child's development during hospitalization. The approaches suggested here should be personalized for each patient. Some children may appear younger than their stated age due to medical and/or emotional problems. It is also normal for children to **regress** (go backward) when hospitalized.

CARING FOR INFANTS (BIRTH–1 YEAR)

During the first year of life, the normal infant will:
- Double her birth length.
- Triple her birth weight.
- Show progress in gaining mastery over gross motor behavior, beginning with the head and moving down the trunk toward the feet.

The normal infant begins by gaining head control. The infant then progresses to rolling over, sitting up, crawling, and walking. These motor skills generally occur within specific weeks or months of the infant's life. Achievement of these skills is referred to as the infant's **developmental milestones**. These milestones are outlined from birth through two years of age in Table 46–1.

Learning to trust is the primary psychosocial developmental task for the infant. All infants depend on others for all of their basic needs. They depend on others for their survival. How the infant's needs are met lays the foundation for the infant's developing personality.

Normally, the mother is the caregiver and prime source for developing trust. However, when the infant is hospitalized, the hospital caregivers assume the role of substitute mother. A caregiver can continue to develop the infant's trust by responding to her cry and her needs. Trust is fostered by feeding, holding, touching, and talking to the infant (Figure 46-2), in addition to keeping her warm and dry.

It is important for the infant to have consistent mothering. Therefore, it is ideal to have the mother room-in with her infant. If this is not possible, an alternative approach is to use the same caregivers for an infant. This means that every time a nurse or nursing assistant works, he will care for the same infants. Besides being consistent for the infant, it also allows the caregiver to become familiar with the infant as a unique

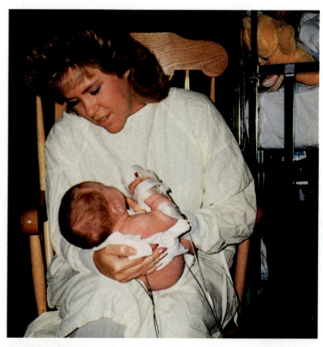

FIGURE 46-2 Hold and talk to the infant to help build trust by the infant. Security and affection are also promoted by this contact.

TABLE 46-1 NORMAL AGE FOR ATTAINMENT OF MAJOR DEVELOPMENTAL MILESTONES

Age	Motor Skill	Language	Adaptive Behavior
4–6 wks.	Head lifted from prone position and turned from side to side	Cries	Smiles
4 mo.	No head lag when pulled to sitting from supine position Tries to grasp large objects	Sounds of pleasure	Smiles, laughs aloud, and shows pleasure re familiar objects or persons
5 mo.	Voluntary grasp with both hands	Primitive sounds: "ah goo"	Smiles at self in mirror
6 mo.	Grasps with one hand Rolls prone to supine Sits with support	Range of sounds greater	Expresses displeasure and food preference
8 mo.	Sits without support Transfers objects from hand to hand Rolls supine to prone	Combines syllables: "baba, dada, mama"	Responds to "No"
10 mo.	Sits well Creeping Stands holding onto support Finger-thumb opposition in picking up small objects		Waves "bye-bye," plays "patty-cake" and "peek-a-boo"
12 mo.	Stands holding onto support Walks with support	Says two or three words with meaning	Understands names of objects Shows interest in pictures
15 mo.	Walks alone	Several intelligible words	Requests by pointing Imitates
18 mo.	Walks up and down stairs holding support Removes clothes	Many intelligible words	Carries out simple commands
2 yrs.	Walks up and down stairs by self Runs	Two- to three-word phrases	Organized play Points to some parts of body

Source: Mary Fran Hazinski, *Nursing Care of the Critically Ill Child* (St. Louis: C.V. Mosby Company, 1984, p. 387).

person. Consistency is especially important when an infant is between six and seven months of age. At this age, the infant normally begins to display a fear of strangers.

Communicating with Infants

Working with infants can be challenging because the infant cannot tell the caregiver in words what he wants or needs. The infant communicates with his cry and body movements. The cry can vary depending on needs. Just as a mother learns to interpret the sound of her infant's cry, the caregiver will also learn to interpret the meanings of the cry by caring for the infant.

Infants respond to voices, faces, and touch. You should talk to the infant (Figure 46-3) whenever you are giving personal care such as bathing, feeding, or holding.

The Waking Hours

When the infant is awake, she needs to explore the environment. Age-appropriate toys are provided so that the infant can continue development while in the hospital. Appropriate toys include colorful mobiles, rattles, and mirrors.

Importance of Families

Siblings of the infant should be allowed to visit while the infant is hospitalized. Toddlers and preschoolers engage in "magical thinking." In other words, they believe that if they wish the infant to be sick, it happens, or if they wish the baby to be gone she won't be back. Therefore, it is important for both toddlers and preschoolers to see their infant sibling. If the mother is rooming-in with the infant, it is also important for toddlers and preschoolers to see and talk to their mother.

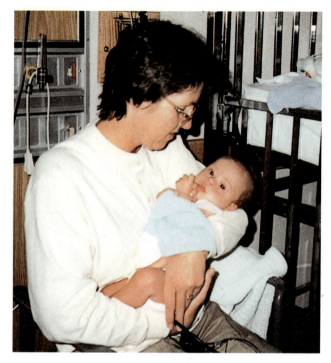

FIGURE 46-3 Talk to the infant or child whenever you give care or when you hold the infant in a quiet moment.

Routine Procedures

When carrying out routine care of the infant, be sure that you hold the infant properly (Figure 46-4). (Refer to Unit 45.)

Before feeding the infant, organize his care so that he can be allowed to digest his food and sleep after he has eaten. You should not move him unnecessarily, as it may cause him to vomit what he has just eaten. In organizing the care, you would weigh him, bathe him, diaper him, and dress him. Then change the crib linens, weigh him, and feed him.

The routine procedures covered here may apply to all pediatric patients. They include:

- Procedure 120—Weighing the pediatric patient (infant and older children)
- Procedure 121—Changing crib linens

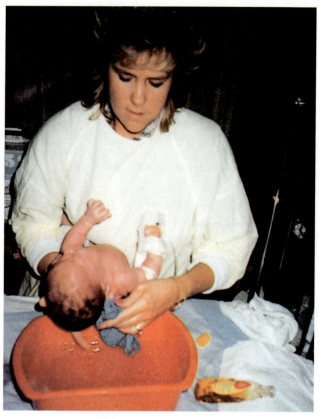

FIGURE 46-4 Hold the infant properly during all care procedures to prevent injury. Note that the nursing assistant supports the infant's head while washing it.

- Procedure 122—Changing crib linens (infant in crib)
- Procedure 123—Measuring temperature (rectal, oral, and axillary)
- Procedure 124—Determining heart rate (pulse)
- Procedure 125—Counting respiratory rate
- Procedure 126—Measuring blood pressure

Weighing the Infant

Routine care includes weighing the infant. This procedure should also be done before feeding.

PROCEDURE 120

WEIGHING THE PEDIATRIC PATIENT

Infant

1. Wash your hands.
2. Place a small sheet or receiving blanket on the scale and balance the scale with the blanket on it.
3. Check infant's previous weight.

4. Check infant's identification band.
5. Remove infant's diaper and shirt.
6. Place infant on the scale, keeping a hand over infant to prevent falling (Figure 46-5).
7. Move the bar to the correct weight until the scale balances.

continues

PROCEDURE **120** *continued*

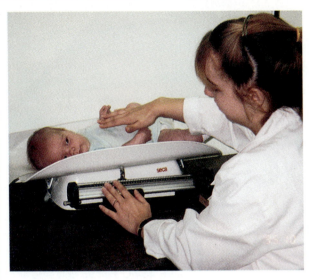

FIGURE 46-5 While keeping one hand slightly over the infant, adjust the scale weights with the other hand.

8. Return infant to the crib. Diaper and dress.
9. Record infant's weight according to hospital policy.
10. Remove the linen from the scale and place in laundry receptacle.
11. Return the scale to its proper storage place.

12. Wash your hands.

Toddler to Adolescent

1. Use an upright scale if child is able to stand. Bring the scale to the bedside, if possible, and balance it.
2. Wash your hands.
3. Check child's identification band.
4. Check child's previous weight.
5. Weigh child in as few clothes as possible. Remove diaper and shoes or slippers.
6. Have child stand on the scale. Move the bar to the correct weight until the scale balances.
7. Record the weight according to hospital policy.
8. Return child to bed.
9. Return the scale to its proper storage place.
10. Wash your hands.

Alternate Action: If the toddler is unable to stand on his own, pick him up and step on the scale. Obtain the combined weight. Put the toddler back in bed, weigh yourself, and subtract your weight from the combined weight. The toddler's weight is the difference in weights.

PROCEDURE **121**

CHANGING CRIB LINENS

1. Wash your hands.
2. Gather supplies:
   - disposable gloves
   - sheet
   - blanket
   - shirt
   - diaper
   - pad

   Do steps 1 and 2 before bathing the infant.
3. When bathing the infant, apply the principles of standard precautions as you would with an adult.

4. After bathing infant, diaper and dress.
5. Place infant in stroller, playpen, or other safe place.
6. Strip linen from crib. Wear gloves if linen is soiled.
7. Remove gloves and discard according to facility policy.
8. Wash your hands.
9. Place clean linen on bed and open sheet, hem side down.
10. Make one side of crib, miter corners top and bottom, and tuck in side (Figure 46-6A).

continues

PROCEDURE **121** *continued*

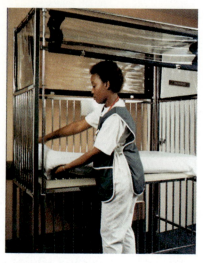

FIGURE 46-6A Make one side of the crib. Miter corners at the top and bottom and tuck under mattress.

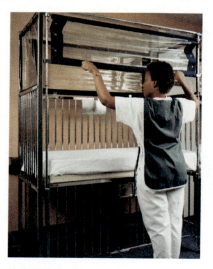

FIGURE 46-6B Pull down crib top.

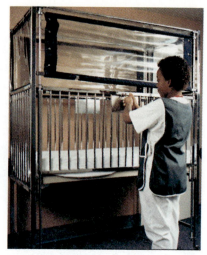

FIGURE 46-6C Pull up crib side and check for security.

11. Pull down crib top (Figure 46-6B). Pull up crib side (Figure 46-6C).

12. Repeat step 10 on opposite side of crib.

13. Place diaper pad on top of sheet, according to hospital policy.

14. Place clean blanket at bottom of bed.

15. Arrange bumper pads around sides of crib.

16. Wash your hands.

17. Return infant to crib, cover with blanket (if appropriate), and pull up crib side.

PROCEDURE **122**

CHANGING CRIB LINENS (INFANT IN CRIB)

1. Wash your hands.
2. Gather linens
   - sheet
   - blanket
   - shirt
   - diaper
   - bathing equipment
   - disposable gloves

   Do steps 1 and 2 before bathing infant.
3. After bathing infant, diaper and dress.
4. Pick up infant and hold in one arm.
5. With free hand, strip old linen off crib. Wear gloves if linen is soiled.
6. Place clean linen on mattress and open sheet, placing hem side down. Place infant on sheet.

7. Place one hand on infant and keep it on infant at all times.

8. Make one side of crib, miter corners top and bottom, and tuck in side.

9. Remove hand from infant and pull up crib side.

10. Go around to other side of crib.

11. Take down crib side, place one hand on infant, and repeat step 8.

12. Place diaper pad under infant and cover with blanket, if appropriate.

13. Arrange bumper pads around crib, if appropriate.

14. Pull up crib side.

15. Wash your hands.

TABLE 46-2 NORMAL VITAL SIGNS

Age	Heart Rate	Respirations	Blood Pressure	
			Systolic	Diastolic
Infants	120–160	30–60	74–100	50–70
Toddlers	90–140	24–40	80–112	50–80
Preschoolers	80–110	22–34	82–110	50–78
School–age	75–100	18–30	84–120	54–80
Adolescents	60–90	12–16	94–140	62–88

Note: Pulse and respiration are taken for a full minute. The apical pulse is used with infants and young children.

Determining Vital Signs

The infant's vital signs must be measured as outlined in the care plan. It is normal for an infant's heart to beat faster than an adult's. The normal ranges of heart rates and respiratory rates for each age group are listed in Table 46-2. An increase in the infant's heart and respiratory rates can be caused by stress (crying, fever, or infection). Therefore, the pulse and respiratory rates should be taken when the infant is quiet, either awake or sleeping.

PROCEDURE 123

MEASURING TEMPERATURE

Temperatures on children five years of age and under are usually taken rectally unless there is a medical reason not to. Axillary temperature can be taken in place of rectal temperatures.

Rectal Temperature

All other vital signs should be measured before the temperature if a rectal temperature is to be measured.

1. Wash your hands and put on gloves.
2. Check patient's identification band.
3. Explain to the parents and child what you are going to do.
4. Inspect thermometer for breaks.
5. Shake down thermometer.
6. Lubricate thermometer.
7. Lay child on his back on bed (Figure 46-7A) or on her stomach across your lap (Figure 46-7B).
8. Insert thermometer 1/2 inch into rectum and hold. Hold child securely and gently so child does not move about.

9. Leave in place for required amount of time (3 to 5 minutes). See your hospital policy.
10. Remove thermometer, wipe off lubricant, and read thermometer.
11. Remove gloves and wash your hands.
12. Record.
13. Report any deviations from normal according to hospital policy.

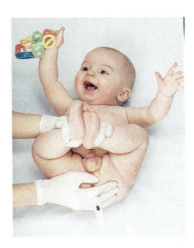

FIGURE 46-7A
Infant in supine position

continues

PROCEDURE **123** *continued*

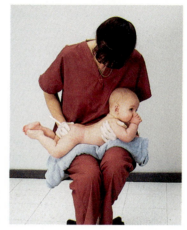

FIGURE 46-7B
Infant in prone position

Oral Temperature

1. Explain to the parents and child what you will be doing.
2. Check patient's identification band.
3. Wash your hands.
4. Inspect thermometer for breaks.
5. Shake down thermometer.
6. Apply gloves.
7. Instruct child to hold the thermometer under his tongue. If child cannot hold the thermometer in his mouth, then obtain either a rectal or an axillary temperature.
8. Leave thermometer under child's tongue for the required amount of time (usually 5 to 8 minutes).

9. Remove and read thermometer.
10. Remove gloves and discard according to facility policy.
11. Wash your hands.
12. Record temperature.
13. Report any deviations from normal according to hospital policy.

Axillary Temperature

1. Explain to the parents and child what you are going to do.
2. Check patient's identification band.
3. Wash your hands.
4. Inspect thermometer for breaks.
5. Shake down thermometer.
6. Place the thermometer in child's armpit.
7. Hold child's arm close to her chest for the required amount of time (10 minutes).
8. Remove thermometer and read.
9. Wash your hands and record temperature value.
10. Report any deviations from normal according to hospital policy.

 Note: *If an electronic thermometer is used, follow the manufacturer's directions supplied with the equipment.*

 Note: *Tympanic thermometers are also used to measure temperature.*

PROCEDURE **124**

DETERMINING HEART RATE (PULSE)

With infants and children, the easiest way to find the heart rate is to place the stethoscope over the heart (Figure 46-8). This is called the apical pulse. It should be done when the child is quiet or at rest because stress and crying can result in a higher than normal reading.

1. Wash your hands.
2. Check patient's identification band.

3. Explain procedure to patient and/or his parents. Clean stethoscope ear pieces and diaphragm with antiseptic wipe and dry. (Allow a child to play with the stethoscope first.)
4. Rub the diaphragm of the stethoscope to warm it so that it will not be cold when placed on infant's chest.

continues

PROCEDURE **124** *continued*

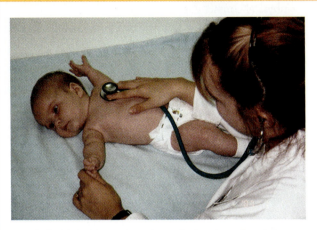

FIGURE 46-8 Measuring the apical pulse of an infant

5. Place the stethoscope over infant's heart and count the number of beats you hear in a minute.

6. Clean stethoscope ear pieces and diaphragm with antiseptic wipe and dry.

7. Wash your hands and record results.

8. Report rates higher or lower than the normal for the appropriate age group according to hospital policy.

📓 **Note:** *The radial pulse can be used for children 6 years and over. The procedure used is the same as for adults. Refer to Procedure 42 in Unit 18.*

PROCEDURE **125**

COUNTING RESPIRATORY RATE

Infants and toddlers use their abdominal muscles for breathing. To count the respiratory rate for this age group, look at the abdomen and chest and count the respirations for a minute.

To obtain the respiratory rate for preschoolers and older children, follow Procedure 44 in Unit 18, as for adults, but count the respirations for a full minute.

PROCEDURE **126**

MEASURING BLOOD PRESSURE

A blood pressure measurement may not always be required for all pediatric patients. If blood pressure is to be recorded, you must have the correct size cuff for the child. The cuff should cover two-thirds of the upper arm.

1. Select the correct cuff size for the patient.

2. Assemble all equipment. Clean stethoscope ear pieces and diaphragm with antiseptic wipe and dry.

3. Wash your hands.

4. Check patient's identification band.

5. Explain the procedure to child, e.g., "This will feel like a tight hug on your arm."

6. Wrap the cuff securely around the upper arm.

7. Feel for the brachial pulse.

8. Place stethoscope ear pieces in ears and place diaphragm near pulse.

9. Pump up cuff until pulse is no longer heard. Release valve and listen for systolic and diastolic sounds.

10. Wash your hands and record results according to hospital policy.

Feeding

Feeding is important to the infant because it satisfies her hunger and sucking needs. Sucking provides the infant with a pleasant sensation, whether she receives food with her sucking or not. The amount of time an infant needs to suckle will vary with each infant. Always provide the infant with the opportunity to suck. This is even more important if the infant cannot eat.

When feeding an infant:

- Hold the infant unless there is a medical reason not to.
- If an infant cannot be held, you should still hold the bottle for her while she eats.
- An infant should never be left in a crib with a bottle propped in his mouth. This is dangerous because the infant could get too much formula at one time, vomit, and choke.
- Holding the infant during a feeding also allows close, physical contact with the person feeding her.
- During feeding and following feeding, the infant should be burped.

Note: If an infant cannot be fed, she should still be held and allowed to suck on a pacifier unless a medical reason prevents removal of the infant from the crib.

Burping

The frequency with which you burp the infant will depend on the infant's age and medical condition. Burping is impor-

---

PROCEDURE   127

BOTTLE-FEEDING THE INFANT

1. Wash your hands.
2. Gather infant's formula and diaper pad, washcloth, or bib.
3. Check infant's identification band.
4. Pick up infant and hold to feed unless there is a medical reason not to.
5. Sit in a chair or rocker.
6. Hold infant in the crook of your arm, with head of infant slightly raised (Figure 46-9).
7. Place a diaper, washcloth, or bib under infant's chin, covering chest.
8. Tip bottle so nipple is filled with formula.
9. Stroke side of infant's cheek closest to you. Infant will automatically turn toward the side stroked and open mouth. Place nipple in infant's mouth.
10. If nipple is in mouth and infant is not sucking, gently lift up under infant's chin to close mouth on nipple.
11. Hold bottle so nipple is filled with formula while infant feeds.
12. Feed infant the ordered amount of formula and burp according to infant's age and hospital policy. (See procedure following.)

    Note: *Bottle-fed infants swallow a lot of air while sucking. Burping is important to remove the air from their stomachs.*

13. If the infant starts to vomit while feeding, remove bottle and turn infant to side with

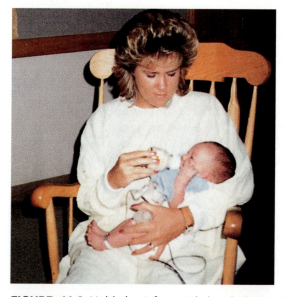

FIGURE 46-9 Hold the infant with head elevated for bottle-feeding. Make sure fluid always fills the nipple of the bottle while the infant sucks.

head lowered to prevent aspiration. Seek help as needed.

14. After feeding, return child to crib and place on back or side.
15. Pull up crib side.
16. Wash your hands.
17. Record amount of formula infant took, according to hospital policy.

tant because bottle-fed infants swallow a lot of air while sucking. The infant can be burped as frequently as after every half-ounce of formula. Older infants can be burped after 1 to 2 ounces during feeding and at the conclusion of feeding. Refer to your hospital policy for the frequency of burping. There are two methods of burping an infant. (See Procedures 128 and 129.)

Breast-Feeding

If the rooming-in or visiting mother is breast-feeding, she should be directed to an area where she can be assured of privacy as well as comfort. As a nursing assistant, you may be responsible for weighing the infant before and after feeding, according to your hospital policy. Refer to the steps for weighing in Procedure 120.

When the infant is returned to his crib after feeding, he should not be placed on his back. Place the infant on his abdomen or on his side. A rolled blanket can be used to keep him on his side. This is done to prevent choking should he spit up or vomit.

Restraints

It is generally not necessary to obtain a physician's order to restrain an infant or a child. The infant or child is considered to be incompetent. Restraints can be used for the child's safety. Restraints are used to protect the child from injury to herself or to others, or to protect the child from injury by equipment used in her care. Any child who is restrained in any way should be freed from the restraints at least once per shift and allowed to exercise the extremities under supervision. Restraints should never be tied to a crib side or bed rail, only to the bed or crib frame.

A *jacket restraint* is a sleeveless cloth garment. It is fitted to the child's chest and crosses in the back, out of the child's reach. It has long straps that can be tied under the mattress or through a chair. When tied this way, the child can move extremities, sit up, lie down in bed, or turn side-to-side without falling.

An *extremity restraint* may be used on the child's arms, hands, legs, or feet. Commercial restraints are available in sheepskin, Velcro, or disposable materials. This restraint is

PROCEDURE 128

BURPING (METHOD A)

1. Place diaper or cloth over your shoulder.
2. Lift infant up to shoulder, holding infant close to your chest (Figure 46-10).
3. Holding infant in place with one hand, use the other hand to gently rub or pat infant's back until infant burps.

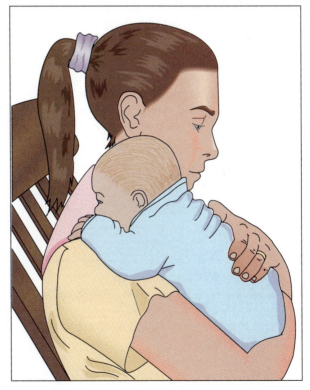

FIGURE 46-10 Burping the infant during and following feeding helps to eliminate air swallowed. Gently rub or pat the infant's back.

PROCEDURE **129**

BURPING (METHOD B)

1. Place diaper, cloth, or bib under infant's chin.

2. Place child in sitting or upright position. Put one hand on infant's chest, supporting infant's weight (Figure 46-11). With the other hand, gently rub or pat infant's back until infant burps.

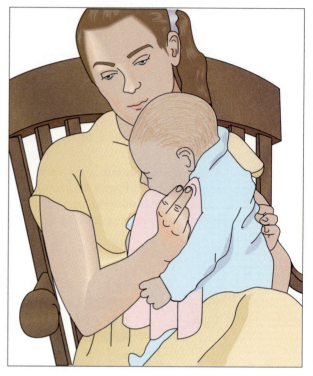

FIGURE 46-11 An alternative method of burping the infant. Remember to place a cloth or bib under the infant's chin.

placed on the child's extremity according to the package directions. The ties are tied to the frame of the crib. For very small infants, the ties may be pinned to the mattress.

GUIDELINES *for*

Ensuring a Safe Environment for Infants

- Always keep crib side rails up.
- Always keep one hand on the infant when the crib side rail is down.
- Use crib bumpers or rolled blankets to prevent injury.
- Never tie balloons or toys to cribs.
- Never use toys with small removable parts or pointed objects.
- Never prop bottles.
- Never tape pacifiers in an infant's mouth.

Summary of Nursing Assistant Tasks and Responsibilities When Caring for Infants

- Maintain a safe environment.
- Provide information to the health team through monitoring of vital signs (temperature, pulse, respiration), weight, intake, and output.
- Provide routine care such as bathing, feeding, and changing.
- Collect and test specimens.
- Assist with treatments, examinations, and procedures.
- Provide warmth, security, and affection.

CARING FOR TODDLERS (1–3 YEARS)

The years between 1 and 3 can be a difficult time for a child to be hospitalized. This is the age when a child is trying to be independent and in control. Between 1-1/2 and 3 years of age, the child:

- Increases motor coordination

- Becomes more verbal
- Becomes more curious about the world

At the same time, her parents are trying to toilet train her. They also are beginning to set limits on her behavior. The developmental task for the toddler is autonomy (independent action).

When caring for the toddler, allow her as much independence and choice as possible (within hospital policy guidelines). Avoid situations that could create a struggle between the caregiver and the child. Expect delays when the toddler is feeding herself or bathing. Be sure to allow the toddler time to do these activities.

The Hospital Environment

When a toddler is hospitalized, it is important to provide an environment that allows as much independence and control as possible while ensuring safety. An example of this is the choice of bed (crib) for the toddler. If a crib is to be used, it should have a top and sides to prevent the child from climbing out and possibly falling (Figure 46-12). If the child has been sleeping in a bed at home, then it is more appropriate to provide a child-sized hospital bed with side rails, if available. Hospital policies vary, so check your hospital policy with reference to toddlers.

If the child is toilet trained, it is important to know the words the child uses for urination and bowel movements. It is also important to know if the child uses a potty chair or the toilet at home. You should try to provide the same arrangement for toileting in the hospital. It is not uncommon for a hospitalized child to regress. You should not be surprised if a toddler

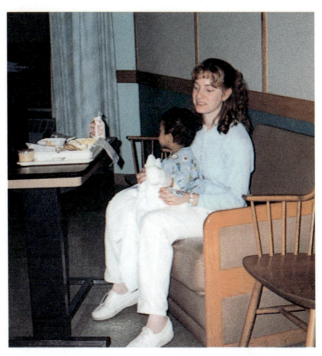

FIGURE 46-13 The nursing assistant can help the toddler with routine activities such as feeding, but it is important to allow the toddler as much independent action as possible. Do not hurry the toddler through mealtimes.

who is toilet trained starts to have "accidents" while in the hospital. Do not scold the child if this happens. The incident should be treated in a matter-of-fact manner. In addition, a hospitalized toddler may ask for a bottle or pacifier. Even though the toddler may have been weaned from them, treat the request as normal. Do not try to reason with the child.

The Toddler's Need for Autonomy

The toddler is learning to be independent. He may want to feed, dress, and wash himself while in the hospital. It will be your responsibility to help the toddler with these activities (Figure 46-13). You should allow him his independence. At the same time, you must keep him safe. For example, when bathing the toddler in the bathtub, you must never leave him alone, even for a minute. Before you put the toddler in the tub, check the temperature of the bath water.

Emotional Reaction to Illness

Another important area in the care of toddlers concerns their feelings of responsibility for their own illnesses. You must stress that the illness is not the toddler's or anyone else's fault.

To overcome anxiety about routine procedures, allow the toddler to handle equipment whenever possible. A few extra minutes spent to familiarize the toddler with the equipment to be used may make the difference between a frightened child and an interested one (Figure 46-14).

The toddler will have a difficult time if separated from the mother. One way to prevent this is to permit the mother to room-in. If this cannot happen, either because a parent cannot stay or hospital policy does not permit it, then parents

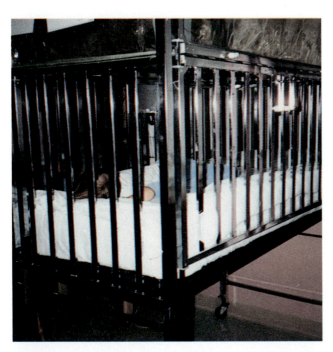

FIGURE 46-12 If the toddler is to use a crib while in the hospital, it should provide a safe environment to protect the toddler from falls. At the same time, it should provide room for freedom of movement (if medical condition permits).

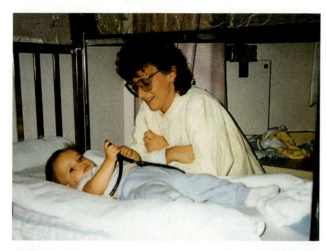

FIGURE 46-14 Allow the toddler to become familiar with equipment used in routine care. This may help relieve anxiety about procedures to be performed. (Crib sides are down only to improve the visibility of the picture.)

should be encouraged to visit frequently. If a parent is not going to stay:

- Reassure the child that she will not be alone.
- Tell her the names of the people who will care for her.
- Encourage each person caring for the toddler to introduce himself when entering the room.
- Whenever possible, the toddler who does not have a parent staying with her should be placed in a room near the nurses' station.
- Encourage parents who cannot visit to call, or you can call the parents so the child can talk to them.

Routine Activities

Routines are important to toddlers. Ask the parents to describe the child's normal day. Try to follow the child's usual schedule as much as possible for eating, naps, toileting, and other activities. Ask the parents about the child's nickname, likes, dislikes, names of siblings and pets, and anything else the parents feel the nursing assistant should know about the child.

Toddlers love to play but, because they have short attention spans, they cannot play with one toy for a long time. Plan a variety of activities to keep the toddler amused. For example:

- Finger painting
- Moving toy cars or trucks
- Coloring
- Handling blocks
- Push-pull toys
- Reading of stories

Educational toys that teach how to dress, button, and zip can also be fun for the toddler. Stethoscopes, masks, and gloves make good hospital toys because they can allow the toddler to work out his fears.

Toddlers will not play together, but they will play near or next to each other.

Temper tantrums can be common with toddlers. If they occur, ignore the tantrum as long as the child cannot hurt herself or others. If a toddler is misbehaving, set limit in a firm, consistent manner.

When working with the toddler, remember that he is trying to be independent. Allow the toddler as much choice as possible. For example, at snack time ask if he wants an apple or a cracker. If no choice can be given, be firm and say what will occur. For example, "It's time to take your nap now." It is best to be truthful and to give simple explanations to toddlers. If the child is having a blood test, tell him just before it happens. It does not do any good to prepare toddlers in advance because they do not have any concept of time. Such advance warning only increases their anxiety.

The toddler has great natural curiosity and loves to explore. It is important to maintain a safe environment in the hospital.

Summary of Nursing Assistant Tasks and Responsibilities When Caring for Toddlers

- Maintain a safe environment.
- Apply standard precautions if contact with blood, body fluids, mucous membranes, or nonintact skin is likely.
- Provide information to the health team through monitoring of vital signs (temperature, pulse, and respiration), weight, intake, and output.
- Supervise and assist with routine care such as bathing, feeding, and dressing.
- Collect and test specimens.

GUIDELINES *for*

Ensuring a Safe Environment for Toddlers

- All poisonous liquids should be kept in a locked container or cabinet.
- All open electrical sockets should have protective covers. Never leave toddlers unattended or unsupervised.
- Never leave toddlers alone in the bathtub or bathroom.
- Keep thermometers out of toddlers' reach.
- Keep crib sides and side rails up when the toddler is in bed.
- Never allow toddlers to play with balloons unless supervised.
- Avoid toys with sharp edges, long strings, or small removable parts.
- Keep doors to stair, kitchen, treatment, and storage areas closed and locked whenever possible.
- Keep doors to linen chutes locked.

- Assist with treatments, examinations, and procedures
- Provide and assist with opportunities for play.
- Provide warmth, security, and affection.
- Promote independence by providing opportunities for choices.

CARING FOR PRESCHOOL CHILDREN (3–6 YEARS)

Developmental Tasks

Between the ages of 3 and 6 years, the child's language, fine motor, and gross motor skills continue to increase with activity. The preschooler continues to develop independence, but the primary developmental task for the age group is initiative (doing things themselves). Children in this age group need to be able to initiate physical and intellectual activities to feel more competent. The preschooler learns her sex role in life by imitating the behavior of the same-sex parent.

The preschooler needs his independence, but he still needs to feel safe and secure. The caregiver must provide the correct balance of independence and control for the preschooler. This is normally the job of the parents, but when the preschooler is hospitalized, you will be considered the caregiver.

Emotional Reactions to Illness

Preschoolers normally have many fears. One fear is that their body parts will be injured or changed. For example, a preschooler may fear that if an adhesive bandage is taken off some of her will "leak out." Preschoolers cannot tell the difference between a "good hurt" and a "bad hurt"; that is, pain from a procedure versus pain from a spanking. Therefore, it is important to use simple, honest explanations when telling the preschooler what to expect.

Fear of the dark, of night time, and of being alone are other normal fears for the preschooler. You can help reduce this fear by leaving a night light on. Another child in the room can also ease his fears. Be sure to leave the call bell within reach. Sitting with him until he falls asleep will also help. Like the toddler, the preschooler can also benefit from having his mother room-in, because he still fears separation.

"Magical thinking" and fantasy are still present in this age group. Therefore, it is important to stress to the preschooler that it is not her fault that she is sick, and that she is not sick because she was bad. The preschooler needs to know that she will return home. She will not be forgotten and left in the hospital. Siblings should be allowed and encouraged to visit. In addition to easing separation from the family, this can also be a way of assuring the child that no one is taking her place at home.

Explaining Procedures

When telling a preschooler what to expect, simple, honest explanations work best. Choose your words carefully because the preschooler takes things literally (exactly as said).

- If surgery is being planned, show and tell the child what parts of his body will be involved in the procedure.
- Preschoolers have a limited concept of time, so when you explain when something will occur, use time references that are familiar to the child (e.g., meal time, nap time, or the time of a favorite TV show). For example, if the child is scheduled for an x-ray in the late morning, tell her that she will have it after breakfast or before lunch.
- Always explain to the preschooler what you are going to do. Do not assume that he will remember what you told him before. The preschooler needs to maintain some control. Therefore, allow him to make as many decisions as possible. Give him the opportunity to make a choice.
- Allow the preschooler to do as much of her own care as she can, to make her feel independent.

Activities

Imagination and fantasy are part of the preschooler's world. Imaginary playmates are normal for the preschooler. These playmates may find their way to the hospital with the child. These playmates can vary in age and sex. They often have different or unusual-sounding names. If the child talks about his imaginary friend, treat it matter-of-factly and listen. However, you need to be realistic. Do not say that you see or hear this playmate. Just say that you know this playmate exists only in the child's imagination.

Play is important for the hospitalized preschooler. Play may give you clues about what the preschooler is thinking. The preschooler is more coordinated and can enjoy activities such as puzzles, coloring, and drawing. The preschooler enjoys imitating roles and playing with other children. Playing house and doctor is especially fun for this age group. Hand puppets are also a good way to talk to preschoolers because they relate easily to the character of the puppet.

You can help the preschooler deal with her hospital stay by maintaining consistency in her schedule and in the limits put

---

GUIDELINES for

Ensuring a Safe Environment for Preschoolers

- Keep toys from cluttering walkways to prevent falls.
- Keep side rails on bed up at night.
- Keep beds in low position.
- Keep doors to kitchen and storage areas closed.
- Keep a night light on.
- Never leave the child unattended in the tub.
- Never allow children to run with popsicles or lollipops in their mouths.

on her behavior. Positive reinforcers such as hugs or stickers should be used as rewards for appropriate behavior.

Summary of Nursing Assistant Tasks and Responsibilities When Caring for Preschoolers

- Maintain a safe environment.
- Apply standard precautions if contact with blood, body fluids, mucous membranes, or nonintact skin is likely.
- Provide information to the health team through monitoring of vital signs (temperature, pulse, and respiration), weight, intake, and output.
- Supervise and assist with routine care such as bathing, feeding, and dressing.
- Collect and test specimens.
- Assist with treatments, examinations, and procedures.
- Provide and assist with opportunities for play.
- Provide warmth, security, and affection.

CARING FOR SCHOOL-AGE CHILDREN (6–12 YEARS)

In general, the school-age years are a time of exceptionally good health (Figure 46-15). School-age children are more active, stronger, and more steady than younger children. They have either had most of the childhood illnesses or have been immunized against them. The most common problems of these times involve the gastrointestinal system (for

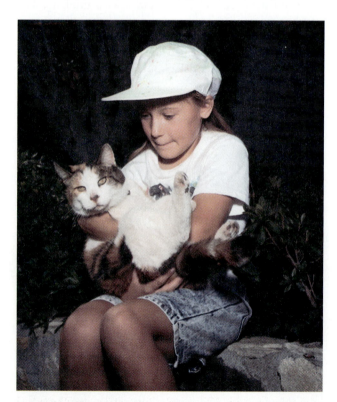

FIGURE 46-15 School-age children tend to be healthier than younger children, but complain mostly of colds and stomach aches.

example, stomach aches) and the respiratory system (for example, colds and coughs).

Developmental Tasks

In this period, the child is striving to achieve a sense of accomplishment through an increasing number of tasks and completion of projects. He also continues to increase control over his environment and his independence. It is important to remember these tasks when caring for the school-age child.

The school-age child's reaction to hospitalization will be significantly different from that of the younger child. The school-age child is better able to handle the stress of illness and hospitalization. In fact, hospitalization presents the school-age child with an opportunity to:

- Explore a new environment
- Meet new friends
- Learn more about her body

Psychosocial Adjustment

Separation from parents will not be as difficult for the school-age child. However, those just entering this period may regress to a preschool level. These children will need their parents' presence.

The school-age child has left the security of home and entered the school system. In school, the child has begun to develop relationships with other children. In the hospital, she may respond more to the separation from her peers than from her parents. It is important to give these children opportunities to communicate with their schoolmates. For example, they can be helped to write letters and make phone calls. When possible, friends can visit.

The older school-age child may welcome the opportunity to be away from his parents. In this situation, the child can test newly developed skills and increase independence. Children of this age group also need privacy—but if the parents are there, they may not get it. Some parents may need to have their child's opposition to their staying explained in this context, because they may think the child is angry with them.

Roommate selection is especially important for this age group. A roommate of approximately the same age will act as a diversion. With a roommate of the same age, the child will be able to continue work on the developmental task of learning to get along with others. Because the school-age child is seeking more independence, she may be reluctant to ask for help even when she needs it. Her feelings may show themselves in different ways, such as:

- Irritability.
- Hostility toward her siblings.
- Other behavior problems. It is important that you, as a caregiver, observe and note these behaviors and bring them to the attention of your supervisor.

Resistance to bedtime may also become a problem during these years. In the hospital, it is important to be aware of the parents' rules and follow them. Learning rules is another developmental task of the school-age years.

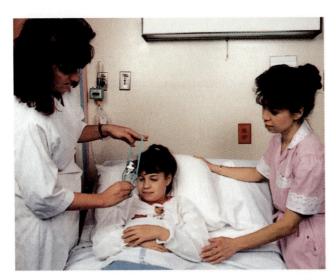

FIGURE 46-16 Explain procedures to the school-age child to give her a feeling of participating in her care.

Adjustment to Illness

Fears or stresses associated with an illness and subsequent hospitalization contribute to the school-age child's feelings of loss of control. By involving the child in her own care, you will help her to be a more cooperative patient (Figure 46-16). Procedures that we routinely do without explanation or without providing options, such as using the bedpan, are particularly upsetting to the school-age child. This child is trying hard to act grown up but is not being given the chance. It is also important for this child's self-esteem that you do not scold him when he does lose control. It is best to just overlook the episode.

The school-age child is able to reason. She also understands the impact of her illness and the potential for disability and death. These children take an active interest in health and enjoy acquiring knowledge. You can help them gain information as well as deal with their fears by explaining all procedures in simple terms. This is also an appropriate age for playing with hospital equipment such as a stethoscope.

Pain is passively accepted by the school-age child. He is able to tell you where his pain is located and what it feels like. This child will hold rigidly still, bite his lip, or clench his fists when in pain, in an effort to keep in control and to act brave. This child does well with distraction during painful procedures. During procedures, you should stay with him whenever possible to talk him through them. This child also tries to postpone all major procedures. For example, when it is time to go to a test, he will need to go to the bathroom. The caregiver needs to put limits on the number of postponements the child is allowed.

Activities

Increased physical and social activities are characteristic of this period. Hospitalization does not usually provide school-age children with adequate diversions. School-age children may also miss the activities of school, although they usually deny this.

You should allow these children time during the day for their own work. This includes school work and visits with friends and other patients. Competitiveness is also characteristic of this period. It adds to the school-age child's need to stay up-to-date with school work. Having the play therapist at the hospital provide appropriate activities will help to reduce the stress the child feels.

Caregivers should encourage the child to take part in her own care as part of her work. Helping to make her bed or clean her room will make her feel useful. She should be held responsible only for tasks that are within her capabilities.

Physically, this child has entered a period of slow, steady growth. Although growth has slowed, it is still important to maintain a balanced diet. School-age children tend to be less picky about what they eat and they are more willing to try new foods.

Summary of Nursing Assistant Tasks and Responsibilities When Caring for School-Age Children

- Maintain a safe environment.
- Apply standard precautions if contact with blood, body fluids, mucous membranes, or nonintact skin is likely.
- Provide information to the health care team through monitoring of vital signs (temperature, pulse, and respiration), weight, intake, and output.
- Supervise and assist with routine care.
- Collect and test specimens.
- Assist with treatments, examinations, and procedures.
- Provide explanations using proper names of body parts, drawings, and books.
- Encourage socialization with other children in the same age group.
- Provide time for school work and tutors.

CARING FOR THE ADOLESCENT (13–18 YEARS)

Adolescence is the transitional period from childhood into adulthood. Like school-age children, adolescents are relatively healthy. The major health problems of this period are usually related to the drastic physical changes that occur during this time, to accidents, to sports injuries, or to chronic and/or permanent disabilities.

Psychosocial Development

Dealing with adolescents is especially difficult for health care providers because:

- The adolescent is developing an identity and becoming increasingly independent.

- Being hospitalized forces the adolescent into a situation where she is now dependent on others to meet her needs. Because of this, it is important to allow the adolescent to make as many of her own decisions as possible. When this is not possible, keep the adolescent involved in the decision-making process.

- Adolescents have a difficult time with authority figures (Figure 46-17). As the caregiver, you will represent authority to this child. You should not get into struggles with the adolescent. Limit the restrictions on them whenever appropriate.

- Adolescents are usually uncooperative. The best approach is to let the adolescent know, in a nonthreatening way, what the rules of the unit are. It is best to do this at the time of his admission. Speak to adolescents as you would to adults. Be as flexible as possible. For example, instead of struggling through the morning trying to get the adolescent up and washed, give him a list of things that have to be accomplished by a certain time. Then allow him the freedom to do things his way and in his order. At the time you decided on, check back with the adolescent to see that the tasks have been completed.

The most important people to adolescents are their friends. A hospital stay makes it more difficult for the adolescent to see friends. It is essential that you:

- allow the adolescent time for visits.
- permit phone calls (Figure 46-18).
- introduce them to other patients their age.

Recognize that adolescents may not want to visit with others if illness has changed their appearance in any way. Body image is important at this age. You can promote a positive image by encouraging the adolescent to continue a normal grooming routine in the hospital. Also encourage the adolescent to wear clothes or her own pajamas. This will make her look and feel better about herself. Use the opportunity to teach good hygiene practices if the hospitalized adolescent does not already practice them. Ask a nurse to help you if you note that this is a problem for your patient.

Keep in mind that the adolescent is very aware of the changes taking place in his body, whether they can be seen or not. It is important to provide the adolescent with privacy. Keep him covered as much as possible during procedures and examinations.

Nutrition and Activity

Adolescents go through a growth spurt. Girls are usually two years ahead of boys. Adequate nutrition and rest continue to be important. In the hospital, the importance of proper eating habits should be stressed to the adolescent. You should:

- Permit the adolescent to continue to make decisions about what and when she will eat, unless it is medically unsafe.

- Recognize that adolescent girls are often on diets. Emotional problems related to weight are common.

- Be aware that adolescents frequently skip breakfast.

The adolescent often stays up late and likes to sleep late in the morning. Sleep requirements are decreased, but a good night's sleep is essential. It is important to explain the routines of the unit and yet provide flexibility for the adolescent. For example, if the television must be turned off at a certain time, the adolescent should be encouraged to find another quiet activity (such as listening to music with headphones) if he does not want to go to sleep. Many hospitals have lounges

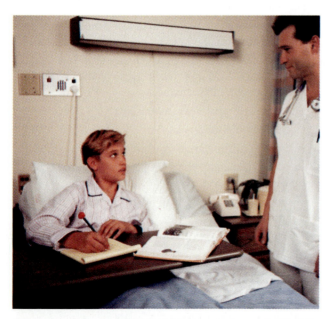

FIGURE 46-17 Adolescent patients sometimes have difficulty with authority figures and may be uncooperative. Be firm and persistent.

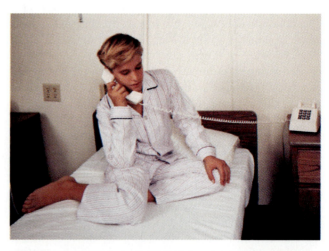

FIGURE 46-18 It is essential that you permit telephone calls so the adolescent can keep in touch with friends

exclusively for the use of this age group, for their own activities and for socializing. Check with your supervisor to find out if there is a specific area for adolescents.

Summary of Nursing Assistant Tasks and Responsibilities When Caring for Adolescents

- Maintain a safe environment.
- Apply standard precautions if contact with blood, body fluids, mucous membranes, or nonintact skin is likely.
- Orient the adolescent to unit and hospital rules.
- Provide information to the health team through monitoring of vital signs (temperature, pulse, and respiration), weight, intake, and output.
- Provide simple explanations to the adolescent.
- Assist with body hygiene to help maintain positive self-image.
- Collect and test specimens.
- Assist with treatment, examinations, and procedures.
- Promote independence. Allow adolescents as much control as possible over schedule of treatments, procedures, and so on.
- Encourage socialization with other adolescents.

GUIDELINES *for*

Ensuring a Safe Environment for Adolescents

- Carefully check all electrical equipment that the adolescent brings to the hospital—radios, hair dryers, and so on—to ensure that it is appropriate and safe to use. Review hospital guidelines regarding use of electrical equipment with the patient.
- Review smoking policies with all adolescents.
- Reinforce to adolescents that alcohol and other drugs are illegal and are not permitted.
- Provide assistance with showers and bathing if the patient is incapacitated or weakened in any way. The adolescent may not ask for assistance.
- Reinforce the use of shoes or slippers to prevent injuries to the feet.
- Remind adolescents to keep staff informed of their whereabouts.
- Keep beds in low position to prevent falls.

REVIEW

A. True/False.

Mark the following true or false by circling T or F.

1. T F It is normal for a child to regress when hospitalized.

2. T F The nursing assistant can foster an infant's sense of trust by keeping him warm and dry.

3. T F The nursing assistant may assume the role of substitute mother.

4. T F Between the ages of 6 and 7 months, the infant loses her fear of strangers.

5. T F Following a feeding, the infant should be encouraged to play.

6. T F Routine weighing of the infant should be carried out right after the 10 A.M. feeding.

7. T F Pulse and respirations should be measured when the child is quiet or asleep.

8. T F The school-age child has an average heart rate of 90 to 140 beats per minute.

9. T F The respiratory rate of the toddler averages 30 to 60 respirations per minute.

10. T F The systolic blood pressure of the child increases with age.

11. T F Preschoolers normally have many fears.

12. T F The preschooler learns his or her sex role in life by imitating the behavior of the opposite-sex parent.

13. T F The most common physical complaints of a school-age child are stomach aches and colds.

14. T F The school-age child would be most comfortable sharing a room with a teenager.

15. T F It is best to overlook the loss of self-control exhibited by the school-age child.

16. T F The best way to measure a pulse rate in an infant or child is the apical method.

17. T F The temperature of a child under 5 years of age should be measured using the rectal method.

18. T F Sucking should be encouraged only when the infant is hungry.

19. T F It is proper to prop a bottle so the infant can eat in his crib if you are very busy.

20. T F After a feeding, the infant should be placed carefully on her back.

21. T F To entertain an infant, tie a bright red balloon to the crib.

22. T F The toddler should be placed in a crib with a top and sides as a safety measure.

23. T F It is permissible to allow a toddler to play unsupervised in a bathtub for a short time before bathing him, as long as the water is warm.

24. T F Adolescents have a difficult time dealing with authority figures.

25. T F Adolescents are particularly sensitive about changes in their body images.

B. Matching.

Choose the correct word from Column II to match each phrase in Column I.

Column I	Column II
26. __d__ physical and psychological achievements	**a.** autonomy
27. __f__ achievement of skills characteristic of a specific age group	**b.** regress
	c. legal guardian
28. __g__ a person married to a biological parent	**d.** developmental tasks
	e. biological parent
29. __b__ to move backward developmentally	**f.** developmental milestone
30. __c__ person who has the right to consent to procedures and hospitalization of a minor	**g.** stepparent
31. __e__ birth parent	
32. __a__ self-determination	

Special Advanced Procedures

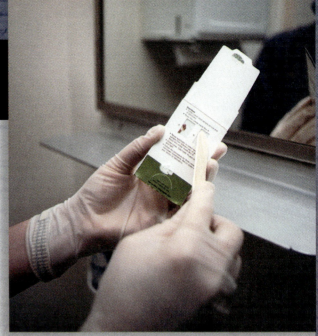

📝 **Notice to the Reader:** By state law, you may not be permitted to perform some of the advanced procedures discussed in this section. Consult with your instructor or supervisor to be sure you know your legal responsibilities. Do not perform or assist in any procedure you are not permitted by law to do.

OBJECTIVES

As a result of this unit—and with advanced training—you will be able to:

- Spell and define terms.
- Demonstrate the following procedures:
  - Procedure 130 Testing for Occult Blood Using Hemoccult® and Developer
  - Procedure 131 Testing for Occult Blood Using Hematest® Reagent Tablets
  - Procedure 132 Collecting a Urine Specimen Through a Drainage Port
  - Procedure 133 Giving Routine Stoma Care (Colostomy)
  - Procedure 134 Routine Care of an Ileostomy (with Patient in Bed)

VOCABULARY

Learn the meaning and the correct spelling of the following words and phrases:

appliance	ileostomy	port	stoma
colostomy	ostomy		

INTRODUCTION

The responsibilities of nursing assistants vary throughout the nation. The scope and type of assignments that are given to nursing assistants are influenced by:

- Basic preparation
- Experience
- Specific advanced training in procedural skills
- Facility policy
- State laws that specify the range of practice of nursing assistants

Important principles to keep in mind are that:

- Some procedures that are considered routine for some workers would not be appropriate or permitted in other situations. Even basic procedures such as bed bathing might be restricted to nurses if the situation or patient conditions warrant such precautions.

- Under no circumstances must it be assumed that because the following procedures are included in this text, they should be assigned to all nursing assistants.
- Each facility has established policies and supervisory practices that are consistent with legal regulations and that ensure competency on the part of the caregiver and safety for the patient/resident.
- These procedures are to be carried out only after adequate practice, with supervision, and only in accord with specific facility policy. Additional information supporting these advanced procedures may be found in the units indicated.

URINE AND STOOL TESTS

Special tests performed on urine and stool samples may be part of your responsibility. Refer to Procedures 130 to 132. Additional information may be found in Units 41 and 42.

PROCEDURE **130**

TESTING FOR OCCULT BLOOD USING HEMOCCULT® AND DEVELOPER

1. Wash your hands and assemble equipment:
   - disposable gloves
   - bedpan with fresh specimen
   - Hemoccult® slide packet
   - Hemoccult® developer
   - tongue blade
   - paper towel
2. Place paper towel on flat surface and open flap of Hemoccult® packet, exposing guaiac paper.
3. Put on gloves.
4. Using a tongue blade, take a small sample of feces and smear on paper area marked *A* (Figure 47-1A).
5. Repeat the procedure, taking fecal sample from a different part of the specimen and making smear in area *B*.
6. Close tab and turn packet over.
7. Open back tab.
8. Apply two drops of Hemoccult® developer directly over each smear (Figure 47-1B). Time reaction.

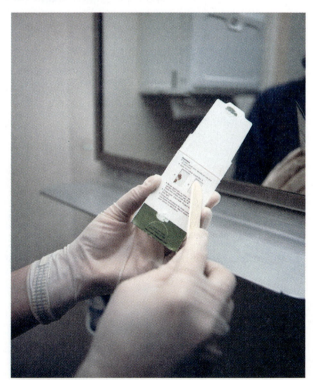

FIGURE 47-1A A small specimen of stool is placed on a special area of the card for an occult blood test.

continues

PROCEDURE 130 *continued*

9. Read results 30 to 60 seconds later.
10. Presence of blood is indicated by a blue discoloration around perimeter of smear.
11. Dispose of specimen.
12. Clean bedpan according to facility policy and dispose of paper towel, packet, and tongue blade.
13. Remove and dispose of gloves according to facility policy. Wash your hands.

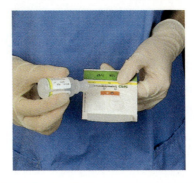

FIGURE 47-1B
Apply drops of Hemoccult® developer on the exposed guaiac paper.

PROCEDURE 131

TESTING FOR OCCULT BLOOD USING HEMATEST® REAGENT TABLETS

1. Wash your hands and assemble equipment:
   - disposable gloves
   - bedpan with fresh specimen
   - Hematest® filter paper
   - glass or porcelain plate
   - Hematest® reagent tablet
   - distilled water
   - dropper
   - tongue blade
2. Place Hematest® filter on a glass or porcelain plate.
3. Put on gloves.
4. Smear a thin streak of fecal material lightly on the filter paper.
5. Place the Hematest® reagent tablet on the smear.

6. Place one drop of distilled water on the Hematest® reagent tablet. Allow 5 to 10 seconds for the water to penetrate the tablet.
7. Then add a second drop so that the water runs down the side of the tablet onto the specimen and filter paper. Gently tap side of plate once or twice to knock water droplets off top of tablet.
8. For up to 2 minutes, observe filter paper for color change.
9. Read reaction. A positive reaction is indicated by a blue halo forming on the paper towel around the smear.
10. Dispose of specimen and equipment per facility policy.
11. Remove and dispose of gloves according to facility policy. Wash your hands.

Collecting a Specimen from a Closed Urinary Drainage System

At some time, it may be necessary to collect a fresh specimen of urine when the patient is on a closed urinary drainage system. Keep in mind that the:

- urine sample must be fresh.
- urine in the bag has accumulated over a period of time.

- specimen may not be taken from the bag.
- specimen must be taken from the catheter.

The procedure to be followed is determined by the type of Foley catheter that is in place. If the catheter has a **port** (opening) for fluid withdrawal, follow Procedure 132. The procedure must be carried out using proper techniques, to avoid introducing infectious organisms into the system.

COLLECTING A URINE SPECIMEN THROUGH A DRAINAGE PORT

1. Carry out each beginning procedure action.
2. Assemble equipment:
   - disposable gloves
   - tube clamp
   - laboratory requisition
   - completed label
   - emesis basin
   - 10-mL syringe
   - specimen cup and lid
   - 21-gauge or 22-gauge needle
   - alcohol wipe
   - bed protector
   - biohazard specimen transport bag
3. Go to bedside half an hour before sample is to be collected.
4. Clamp the drainage tube.
5. Wash your hands. Return to bedside after 30 minutes.
6. Put on gloves.
7. Place bed protector on the bed and place emesis basin on bed protector under the catheter drainage port.
8. Wipe the drainage port with an alcohol wipe (Figure 47-2).
9. Carefully remove the cap on the syringe. Do not contaminate the tip.
10. Attach needle carefully. Do not contaminate the needle tip.

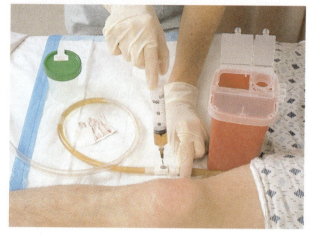

FIGURE 47-3 Draw the specimen into the needle.

11. Open the package with the specimen container. Remove the lid and lay it, inside up, on the bedside stand.
12. Insert the needle into the port and withdraw the specimen (Figure 47-3).
13. Carefully withdraw the needle.
14. Wipe the port with the alcohol wipe.
15. Transfer the urine sample to the specimen container (Figure 47-4).
16. Handling the lid by the top only, cover the container.
17. Remove gloves and dispose of according to facility policy. Wash hands.

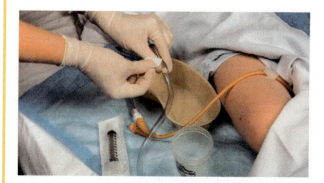

FIGURE 47-2 Wipe the port with an antiseptic wipe or sponge.

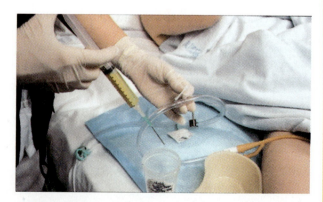

FIGURE 47-4 Transfer the specimen to the container.

continues

PROCEDURE 132 *continued*

18. Remove the catheter clamp.

19. Complete information on label and put label on container. Compare label to the requisition to be sure that the information is complete and accurate.

20. Place specimen container in biohazard transport bag, seal, and attach laboratory requisition (Figure 47-5).

21. Dispose of needle in proper container.

22. Carry out each procedure completion action.

23. Follow instructions for care of the specimen.

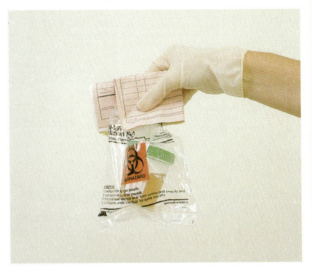

FIGURE 47-5 Place the specimen container in a biohazard specimen transport bag, seal, and attach laboratory requisition.

OSTOMIES

The surgical removal of a section of diseased bowel requires the creation of an artificial opening (ostomy) in the abdominal wall for solid waste elimination.

Care of the Patient with a Colostomy

When the colon is brought through the abdominal wall, the opening is called a colostomy. The mouth of the opening is called a stoma (Figure 47-6). The ostomy may be temporary or permanent. The location of the ostomy (Figure 47-7)

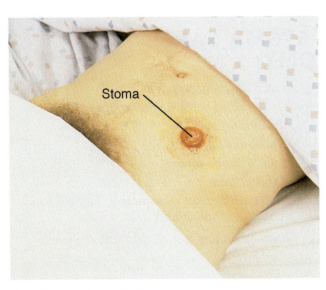

Stoma

FIGURE 47-6 Typical colostomy stoma

determines if the feces are formed, soft and mushy, semi-liquid, or liquid.

The patient with a colostomy does not have normal sphincter control. This means the patient cannot voluntarily control emptying of the bowel in the same manner as emptying through the anus. If the colostomy is located in the bowel where stool is formed, regularity of elimination may be established. As elimination is controlled, the stoma may be covered with a simple dressing between evacuations. Liquid to mushy fecal drainage from a stoma is collected in a disposable drainage pouch, called an appliance, that is attached over the stoma. (Refer to Procedure 133.)

Proper stoma care is required to maintain healthy tissue, because the area around the opening comes into contact with the liquid or semiliquid stool. At the stoma, there may be problems of:

● Leakage

● Odor control

● Irritation of the surrounding area

You can assist the patient who has a colostomy by:

● Keeping the area clean and dry.

● Performing routine stoma care, including removing drainage and/or replacing the appliance if your facility allows you to assist or give this care after you have had special training.

Remember:

● Initial irrigations will be performed by the nurse.

● If the colostomy is to be permanent, patients are taught to carry out the irrigation procedure for themselves.

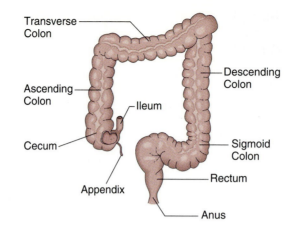

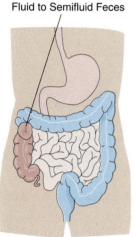
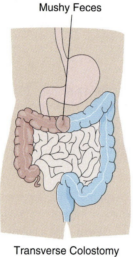
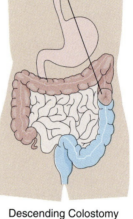
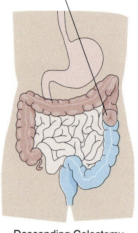
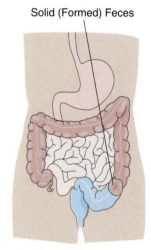

Ascending Colostomy   Transverse Colostomy   Descending Colostomy   Sigmoid Colostomy

FIGURE 47-7 The site of the colostomy determines the character of the feces.

PROCEDURE **133**

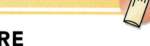

GIVING ROUTINE STOMA CARE (COLOSTOMY)

1. Carry out each beginning procedure action.

2. Assemble equipment:
   - disposable gloves
   - washcloth and towel
   - basin of warm water
   - bed protector
   - bath blanket
   - disposable colostomy bag and belt
   - bedpan
   - skin lotion as directed
   - prescribed solvent and dropper
   - cleansing agent
   - adhesive wafer
   - 4 × 4 gauze square
   - toilet tissue

3. Place bath blanket over patient. Fanfold top bedding to foot of bed.

4. Wash hands and put on disposable gloves.

continues

PROCEDURE **133** *continued*

5. Place bed protector under patient's hips.

6. Place bedpan and cover on bed protector on chair.

7. Remove the soiled disposable stoma bag (appliance) and place in bedpan—note amount and type of drainage.

8. Remove belt that holds stoma bag and save if clean.

9. Gently clean area around stoma with toilet tissue to remove feces and drainage (Figure 47-8). Dispose of tissue in bedpan.

10. Wash area around stoma with soap and water. Rinse thoroughly and dry.

11. If ordered, apply barrier cream lightly around the stoma. Too much lotion may interfere with proper seal of fresh ostomy bag.

12. Position clean belt around patient. Inspect skin under belt for irritation or breakdown.

13. It may be necessary to remove the adhesive wafer. To select the proper size of wafer,

you can use a commercial guide to size the stoma (Figure 47-9).

14. Replace adhesive wafer (Figure 47-10). Place clean ostomy bag over stoma and secure belt.

15. Remove bed protector. Check to be sure bottom bedding is not wet. Change if necessary.

16. Remove gloves and discard according to facility policy. Wash hands.

17. Replace bath blanket with top bedding, making patient comfortable.

18. Using a paper towel to protect hands, gather and cover soiled materials and bedpan. Take to utility room. Dispose of materials according to facility policy.

19. Empty, wash, and dry bedpan. Store according to facility policy.

20. Carry out each procedure completion action.

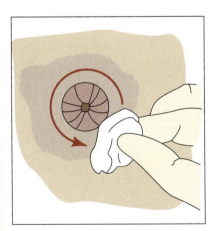

FIGURE 47-8 The area around the stoma is cleaned well but gently and dried before a new appliance is applied.

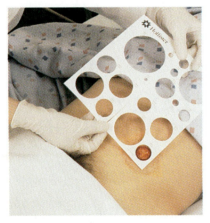

FIGURE 47-9 Check the size of the stoma to be sure the proper size of barrier is used.

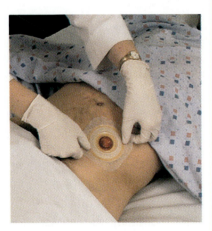

FIGURE 47-10 A new barrier adhesive wafer is applied around the stoma.

Care of the Patient with an Ileostomy

An **ileostomy** is a permanent artificial opening in the ileum (Figure 47-11) that drains through a stoma on the surface of the abdomen. The drainage from the ileum is in liquid form and contains digestive enzymes that are irritating to the skin. (Refer to Procedure 134.)

Considerations for caring for a patient with an ileostomy include:

• The professional nurse cares for the patient with a fresh ileostomy.

• Routine care may be given by nursing assistants.

• The drainage from an ileostomy is very irritating to

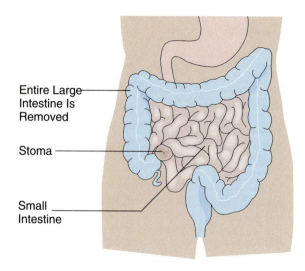

FIGURE 47-11 An ileostomy brings a section of the ileum through the abdominal wall.

the skin, so care of the skin surrounding the stoma is crucial.

- The fit of the ileostomy ring is important so that leakage does not occur. This is true for both the disposable and reusable types of appliances (Figure 47-12).

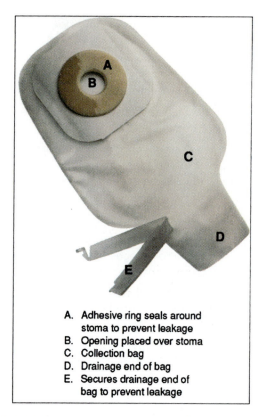

A. Adhesive ring seals around stoma to prevent leakage
B. Opening placed over stoma
C. Collection bag
D. Drainage end of bag
E. Secures drainage end of bag to prevent leakage

FIGURE 47-12 Stoma protector and collection bag. *Courtesy of Hollister Corporation*

PROCEDURE 134

ROUTINE CARE OF AN ILEOSTOMY (WITH PATIENT IN BED)

1. Carry out each beginning procedure action.

2. Assemble equipment:
   - disposable gloves
   - basin of warm water
   - bed protector
   - bath blanket
   - bedpan and cover
   - fresh appliance and belt
   - clamp for appliance
   - prescribed solvent and dropper
   - cotton balls
   - deodorant (if permitted)
   - cleansing agent
   - Karaya ring
   - 4 × 4 gauze squares
   - toilet tissue
   - paper towels

3. Raise opposite side rail for safety. Elevate head of bed and assist patient to turn on side toward you.

4. Replace bedding with bath blanket.

5. Wash hands. Put on disposable gloves.

6. Place bed protector under patient.

7. Place bedpan on bed protector against patient.

8. Place end of ileostomy bag in bedpan. Open clamp and allow to drain (note clamp in Figure 47-12). Note amount and character of drainage.

continues

PROCEDURE 134 *continued*

9. Wipe end of drainage sheath with toilet paper and move out of drainage. Place tissue in bedpan. Cover bedpan.

10. Disconnect belt from appliance and remove from patient. Place on paper towels.

11. With dropper, apply a small amount of solvent around the ring of the appliance. This will loosen it so it can be removed. Wait a few seconds. Do not force the appliance free.

12. Cover stoma with gauze.
    - Carefully inspect skin area around stoma.
    - If the area is irritated or skin is broken, cover patient with bath blanket, raise side rail, and lower bed.
    - Remove gloves and dispose of properly.
    - Wash your hands.
    - Report to the nurse for instructions.
    - Put on fresh gloves before continuing procedure.

13. Remove gauze from stoma and place in paper towels.

14. If appliance is used with a Karaya ring, moisten the ring, allow it to become sticky, and apply it to the stoma. If appliance uses paper-covered adhesive strip around the stoma opening, remove paper and apply around stoma.

15. Clamp appliance bag and apply to ring.

16. Remove gloves and dispose of properly. Wash hands.

17. Adjust clean belt in position around patient and connect it to the appliance.

18. Remove bath blanket and assist patient to wash hands.

19. Wash hands. Put on gloves.

20. Clean patient's bathroom. Wash belt and appliance, if reusable, and allow to dry.

21. Carry out each procedure completion action.

REVIEW

A. True/False.

Mark the following true or false by circling T or F.

1. T F A stool with occult blood will appear bloody.

2. T F The Hemoccult® test is used to determine the presence of bile in the feces.

3. T F Gloves must be used when doing tests on feces or urine.

4. T F The proper amount of time to observe a Hemotest® reagent tablet after placing it on a fecal smear and adding the second drop of water is 5 minutes.

5. T F The drainage tube should be clamped for half an hour before you collect a sample from a drainage port.

6. T F Odor control can be a problem when a patient has an ostomy.

7. T F Drainage from a colostomy is always watery.

8. T F Nursing assistants should follow established policies of their own facilities in carrying out assigned tasks.

9. T F Nursing assistants should not carry out any procedure they have not been taught and for which they have not received supervision.

10. T F It is impossible to safely collect a sample of urine from a closed urinary drainage system.

B. Matching.

Choose the correct term from Column II to match each phrase in Column I.

Column I	Column II
11. _c_ opening	**a.** occult
12. _e_ artificial opening in large intestine	**b.** ileostomy
13. _b_ artificial opening in small intestine	**c.** stoma
14. _a_ hidden	**d.** appliance
15. _d_ drainage pouch	**e.** colostomy
	f. contamination
	g. port

C. Multiple Choice.

Select the one best answer for each question.

16. An artificial opening in the colon is known as a/an
    a. tracheostomy.
    b. colostomy.
    c. ileostomy.
    d. proctostomy.

17. The reaction time for a Hemoccult® test is
    a. 2 to 4 seconds.
    b. 30 to 60 seconds.
    c. 2 to 3 minutes.
    d. 90 to 120 seconds.

18. The port of a closed urinary drainage system should be cleaned before withdrawal with
    a. soap and water.
    b. a paper towel.
    c. antiseptic.
    d. a sterile 4 × 4 gauze pad.

19. During routine care, the area around a colostomy should
    a. never be cleaned.
    b. be covered with petroleum jelly.
    c. be washed with soap and water.
    d. be cleaned with an antiseptic.

20. An ileostomy as compared to a colostomy
    a. has more liquid drainage.
    b. tends to be more irritating.
    c. has drainage containing digestive enzymes.
    d. all of these.

21. You are giving routine stoma care to a patient with a colostomy and find the stoma red and irritated. You should
    a. complete the procedure.
    b. clean the area with alcohol.
    c. apply powder and attach the ostomy bag.
    d. cover the area and notify the nurse.

22. If the skin around an ileostomy stoma is broken, you should
    a. wipe it with alcohol.
    b. wash it with soap and water.
    c. cover it with a 4 × 4 gauze pad.
    d. inform the nurse.

D. Nursing Assistant Challenge.

Mrs. Knight, who is 60 years of age, was in an accident and received a broken right leg and two broken wrists. She has a long-standing colostomy, but because of her injuries cannot provide her own colostomy care. Answer the following questions about her care.

23. Will you need to wear gloves to give her colostomy care? ____

24. What will you use to remove feces from around the stoma? ____

25. What will happen if you apply too much lotion around the stoma? ____

26. How will the ostomy bag be held in place? ____

27. What are the three major problems associated with having a stoma? ____

Response to Basic Emergencies

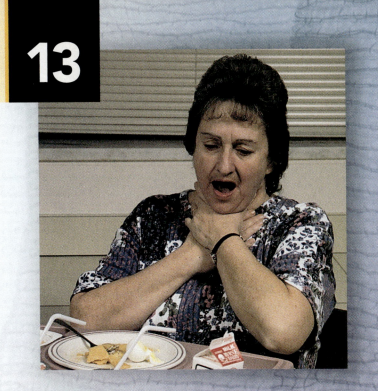

UNIT 48
Response to Basic Emergencies

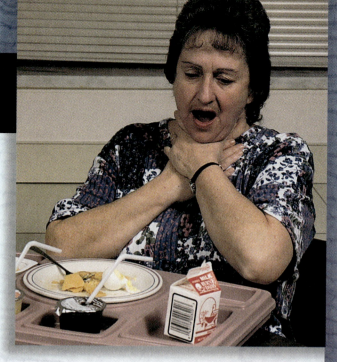

UNIT 48

Response to Basic Emergencies

OBJECTIVES

As a result of this unit, you will be able to:

- Spell and define terms.
- Recognize emergency situations that require urgent care.
- Be able to evaluate situations and determine the sequence of appropriate actions to be taken.
- Recognize the need for CPR.
- Identify the signs, symptoms, and treatment of common emergency situations such as:
  - Fainting
  - Heart attack
  - Bleeding
  - Shock
  - Brain attack (stroke)
  - Seizure
  - Thermal injuries
  - Poisoning
  - Choking
  - Cardiac arrest
- Demonstrate the following procedures:
  - Procedure 135 Adult CPR, One Rescuer
  - Procedure 136 Adult CPR, Two-Person
  - Procedure 137 Heimlich Maneuver—Abdominal Thrusts
  - Procedure 138 Assisting the Adult Who Has an Obstructed Airway and Becomes Unconscious
  - Procedure 139 CPR for Infants
  - Procedure 140 Obstructed Airway: Conscious Infant
  - Procedure 141 Obstructed Airway: Unconscious Infant
  - Procedure 142 CPR for Children, One Rescuer
  - Procedure 143 Child with Foreign Body Airway Obstruction

VOCABULARY

Learn the meaning and the correct spelling of the following words and phrases:

cardiac arrest	emergency care	fracture	shock
cardiopulmonary resuscitation (CPR)	Emergency Medical Services (EMS)	Heimlich maneuver	sprain
dislocation	first aid	hemorrhage	strain
emergency		respiratory arrest	victim

DEALING WITH EMERGENCIES

All emergency situations develop rapidly and unpredictably. Emergency situations can occur at any time to anyone. Examples include:

- Automobile accidents
- Brain attacks (strokes)
- Suddenly feeling weak
- Fainting and falling

An **emergency** is any unexpected situation that requires immediate action and medical attention. In a true emergency, prompt action is needed to prevent further complica-

---

GUIDELINES *for*

Responding to An Emergency

- Always remember the priorities of any emergency as the ABCs:
  - **A**irway: obstructed or unobstructed?
  - **B**reathing: is the victim able to breathe?
  - **C**irculation: is the heart beating, is there bleeding?
- Stay calm. Nothing is accomplished and more problems will result if the people at the scene of the emergency become flustered and agitated. If you are calm, you will be a calming influence on the victim.
- Know what to do to summon immediate help; you need to get the nurse to the scene as soon as possible. Stay with the victim and call out for help. If you are out in the community, tell the closest person to call Emergency Medical Services (EMS).
- Do not move the victim unless the person will be endangered by staying where he is.
- Stay with the victim until the person in charge gives you permission to leave.
- Know your limitations. Be aware of what procedures you are qualified to perform in an emergency. Never attempt to render treatment unless you have received the appropriate training.
- Know the procedures to follow for emergencies. Health care facilities have code names for various emergencies. Know what these are and how to announce a code. If you are out in the community, know the appropriate first aid to apply in emergency situations.
- Know the procedures for activating the **Emergency Medical Services (EMS)** system (Figure 48-1). In most parts of the country, this is done by dialing 911 (Figure 48-2). You will need to:
  - give the address
  - describe what happened (e.g., the person was burned or has had cardiac arrest)
  - the person's name (if you know this information)

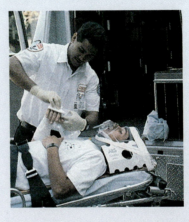

FIGURE 48-1 Know the procedure for activating the EMS system.

- telephone number where call is being made from
- number of persons needing help
- Keep the person warm. Cover with blankets.
- Do not give the person any fluids or food.
- If the person starts to vomit, turn her head to one side to avoid aspiration.
- If the person is conscious, assure him that help has been called and is on the way.
- Protect the person's privacy. Keep other people away from the scene unless they are qualified to assist.
- In all situations, apply standard precautions to prevent exposure to blood, body fluids, mucous membranes, and nonintact skin during the emergency.

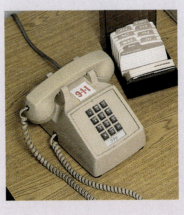

FIGURE 48-2 In most parts of the United States, the EMS system is contacted by dialing 911.

tions and to save the life of the **victim** (person needing help). It is important that you know the signs and symptoms of an emergency and that you be able to take immediate action. The following guidelines are basic actions to remember for any emergency.

BEING PREPARED

While working in the hospital or long-term care facility, you are always close to professional medical help. When you witness an accident away from the medical facility, however, professional help is not always readily available. Whatever course of action you choose, the victim should not be further endangered.

FIRST AID

First aid includes:

- Immediate care for victims of injuries or sudden illness
- Care needed later if medical help is delayed or is not available

First aid will be needed for different conditions in a variety of situations. These conditions can range from the minor to the very severe. When you give first aid, you deal with the:

- Victim's emotional state
- Victim's physical injuries
- Management of the whole accident situation

Persons in life-threatening situations must be given immediate attention. Life-threatening situations include those in which a person:

- Has no airway
- Has stopped breathing
- Is in shock
- Has been poisoned
- Is choking
- Is bleeding profusely

Assessing the Situation

At the scene of an accident, assess the situation and find out the extent of injuries. Quickly determine the number of victims, their potential injuries, and any dangerous factors at the scene.

For example, at the scene of an auto accident, there may be several victims. Some may be trapped in their vehicles, others may be lying on the highway. There may be cars burning and the danger of explosion. In this situation, you must first get yourself and the victims away from further danger.

In the medical facility, unless there is a fire, you usually will be dealing with a single victim. You will be able to focus on the needs of that individual. For example, you might enter a patient's room and find a patient lying on the floor, despite the fact that the bed side rails are up. Make a quick assess-

ment as you signal for help, giving the patient's name and location and describing the scene.

EMERGENCY CARE

Emergency care is care that must be given right away to prevent loss of life.

- Whether you are out in the community or in the health care facility, ask someone nearby to summon help.
- Do not leave people who need urgent care to get help yourself. (Exception—CPR; see CPR directions.)
- As help is on the way, check, in the following order, the:
  - Degree of consciousness
  - Airway/breathing capability
  - Rate of heartbeat
  - Signs of bleeding
  - Signs of shock
- Do not move the person if you do not have to.
- Do not allow the person to get up and walk around.
- Check for other injuries.

CARDIAC ARREST

A person may stop breathing but still have a heartbeat. This is called **respiratory arrest**. If the situation is not reversed, the heart will stop beating. **Cardiac arrest** is the term used when the heart has stopped beating and respirations have ceased. When the heart and lungs are not functioning, blood and oxygen are not circulated to the brain and the rest of the body. The person is clinically dead. Permanent damage to

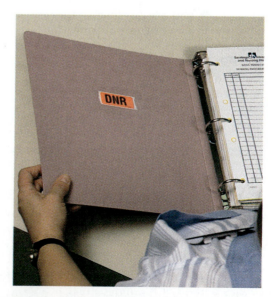

FIGURE 48-3 *DNR* on a patient's chart means that the patient does not wish to be resuscitated in the event of cardiac arrest.

the brain and other organs occurs within 4 to 6 minutes. Indications of cardiac arrest are:

- No response from the victim
- No breathing can be detected
- No pulse

Cardiopulmonary resuscitation (**CPR**) is a procedure used to maintain blood circulation throughout the body until the EMS can respond to the emergency. *You must never perform CPR unless you have completed an approved course, taught by an approved instructor.* The American Heart Association and the American Red Cross both offer such courses in communities across the country. **The information in this book is not intended to take the place of an approved course.** (Refer to Procedures 135 and 136.)

In the health care facility, you must know whether CPR is to be initiated. A patient who is very elderly or who has a terminal illness may not wish to be resuscitated if cardiac arrest occurs. In these cases the physician must write an order "do not resuscitate" (DNR) or "no code" (Figure 48-3). If there is no DNR order, full life support measures are given for cardiac arrest.

PROCEDURE **135**

ADULT CPR, ONE RESCUER

Standard precautions should be followed if at all possible. This means gloves should be worn and a barrier device used. If the victim is bleeding, a gown and mask may also be necessary. These items should be readily available in a health care facility.

Careful assessment is required before CPR is administered.

1. Gently shake the person and ask him, "Are you okay?" Call the victim's name if you know it (Figure 48-4).

2. Call out for help. If someone responds to your call, send her to call the EMS system. If no one responds to your call, call the EMS system yourself and return to the victim as soon as possible.

3. Turn the victim on his back as a unit, supporting the head and back (Figure 48-5). For CPR to be effective, the victim must be lying on his back on a hard surface.

4. Open the airway, using a head-tilt, chin-lift technique (Figure 48-6).

5. Maintain the open airway with the head-tilt, chin-lift technique and place your ear near the victim's mouth. At the same time, observe the victim's chest. You are looking,

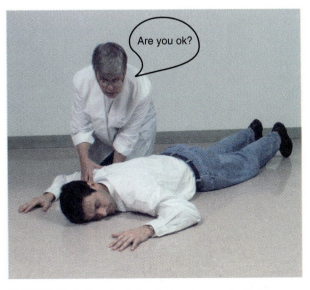

FIGURE 48-4 Gently shake the person and ask "Are you okay?"

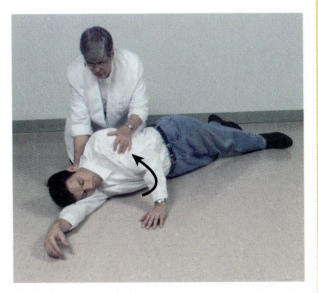

FIGURE 48-5 Support the head and back while turning the victim as a unit.

continues

PROCEDURE **135** *continued*

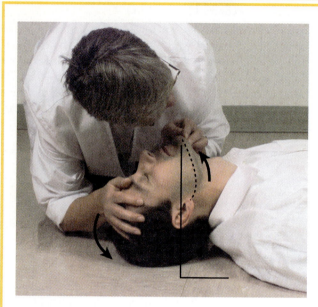

FIGURE 48-6 Use head-tilt, chin-lift technique to open the airway.

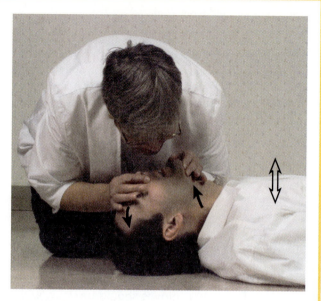

FIGURE 48-8 Seal the victim's nose with your thumb and forefinger and seal the victim's mouth with your mouth or a barrier device.

listening, and feeling for any signs that the victim may be breathing. You should look, listen, and feel for 3 to 5 seconds (Figure 48-7). If victim is breathing, maintain open airway, monitor breathing, call EMS if not done earlier.

6. If there are no signs of breathing, seal the victim's nose with your thumb and forefinger

and seal the victim's mouth, using your mouth or a barrier device (Figure 48-8).

7. Ventilate 2 times, taking 1 1/2 to 2 seconds for each ventilation (Figure 48-9). Allow the chest to deflate between ventilations. Watch the chest rise to determine if enough air is getting through.

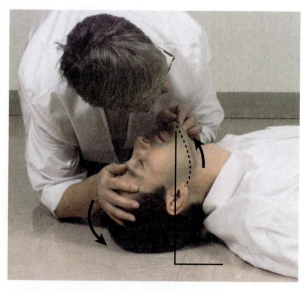

FIGURE 48-7 Take 3 to 5 seconds to look, listen, and feel for breathing.

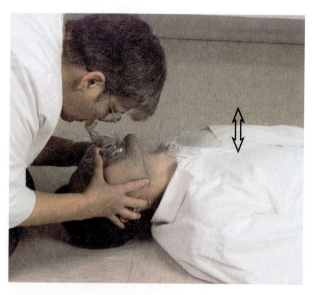

FIGURE 48-9 Take 1 to 1 1/2 seconds for each ventilation.

continues

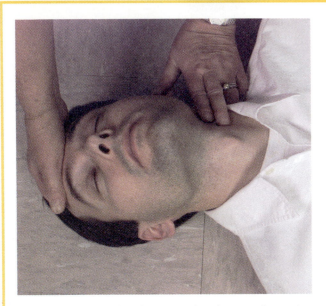

FIGURE 48-10 Take the carotid pulse to determine heart action.

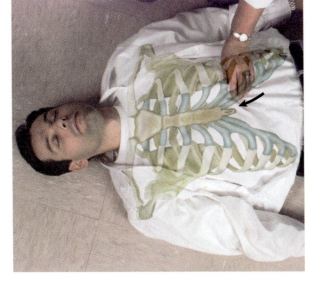

FIGURE 48-11 Determine proper hand placement before beginning compressions.

8. After the ventilations, assess for the presence of a heartbeat. Maintain the open airway, using the head-tilt technique, with one hand. With the other hand, feel for the victim's carotid pulse on the near side of the victim (Figure 48-10). Take 5 to 10 seconds to determine whether there is a pulse. If there is a pulse, but no respirations, continue with ventilations at the rate of 1 every 5 seconds (12 per minute). Continue to check periodically for a pulse.

9. If there is no pulse, begin chest compressions at the ratio of 15 compressions to 2 ventilations. Kneel by the victim's shoulders and determine proper hand placement (Figure 48-11). Your shoulders should be over the victim's sternum. Using correct hand placement and technique, compress the victim's chest 1-1/2 to 2 inches. While doing compressions, you must:

- place your bottom hand over the victim's sternal notch (Figure 48-12).
- place your other hand on top of your bottom hand—only the heel of your bottom hand should be touching the victim's chest (Figures 48-13A, B).
- keep your elbows straight, with your

shoulders directly over the victim's sternum (Figure 48-14).

Compress 1-1/2 to 2 inches each time.

- Maintain hand contact with the victim's chest
- Allow the chest to relax during the upstroke

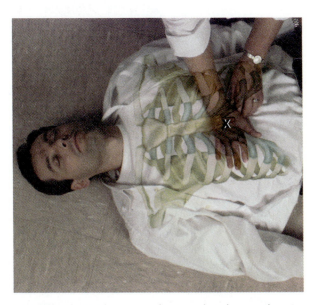

FIGURE 48-12 Place your bottom hand over the victim's sternal notch.

continues

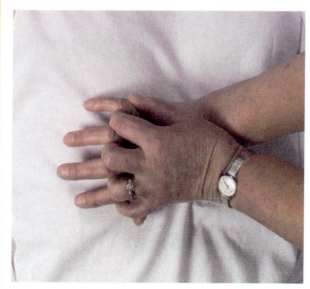

A

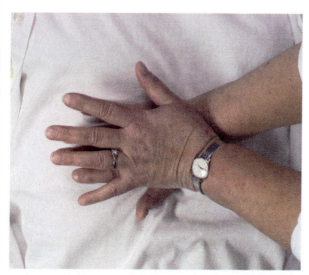

B

FIGURE 48-13 A. Place your other hand on top of your bottom hand. B. Only the heel of your bottom hand should be touching the victim's chest.

- Use a compression rate of 80 to 100 compressions per minute
- Count out loud during compressions: one and, two and, three and, —

10. Do 15 compressions to 2 ventilations per cycle.

11. Do four cycles:

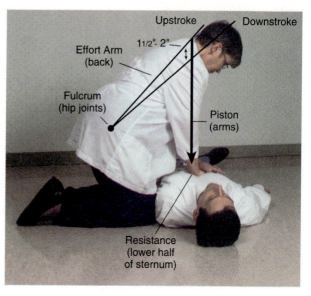

FIGURE 48-14 Keep your elbows straight, with your shoulders directly over the victim's sternum.

- 15 compressions and 2 ventilations for each cycle
- Take 1-1/2 to 2 seconds for each ventilation
- Observe chest rise to check for effectiveness of ventilations
- Use a compression rate of 80 to 100 compressions per minute

12. At the end of four cycles, feel for the carotid pulse for 5 seconds. If there is no pulse, ventilate 2 times.

13. Continue to repeat the cycle of 15 compressions to 2 ventilations. Feel for the carotid pulse every few minutes.

14. If a second rescuer arrives,

- the second rescuer identifies himself, saying, "I know CPR—can I help?"
- the second rescuer does carotid pulse check for 5 seconds.
- the second rescuer does 2 ventilations and continues with one-person CPR as directed in this procedure and the approved training.
- the first rescuer observes the victim's chest during ventilations and does carotid pulse checks during compressions to evaluate the effectiveness of both techniques.

continues

PROCEDURE 135 *continued*

15. If the victim resumes breathing but is unconscious, and if there is no evidence of trauma, place the victim in recovery position on his side (Figure 48-15).

16. If the heart is beating but there is no breathing, continue ventilations at the rate of 1 every 5 seconds or 12 times per minute.

17. If there is no heartbeat and no breathing, continue with chest compressions and ventilations at the ratio of 15 compressions to 2 ventilations.

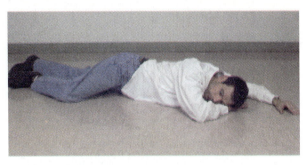

FIGURE 48-15 If the victim is breathing but unconscious, place the victim in recovery position.

PROCEDURE 136

ADULT CPR, TWO-PERSON

The techniques for two-person CPR are exactly the same as for one person. The compression to ventilation rate is 5 compressions to every 1 ventilation. Chest compressions are done at the rate of 80 to 100 per minute. The two rescuers should be on opposite sides of the victim if possible.

1. If CPR is in progress:

   a. The second rescuer comes in after the first rescuer has completed a cycle of 15 compressions and 2 breaths.

   b. One rescuer moves to the victim's head, opens the airway, and checks for the carotid pulse.

   c. The other rescuer finds the correct hand position.

   d. If there is no pulse, the ventilator gives 1 breath and the compressor begins chest compressions, counting "one and, two and, three and, four and, five." At the end of the fifth compression, the compressor pauses to allow the other rescuer to give one ventilation (Figure 48-16).

   e. The cycles continue with periodic pulse checks.

2. If no CPR is in progress and both rescuers arrive on the scene at the same time:

   a. Both rescuers must decide what needs

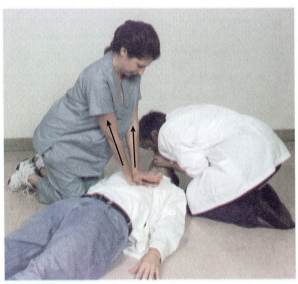

FIGURE 48-16 At the end of the fifth compression, the person doing the compressions pauses to allow the other rescuer to give one ventilation.

to be done, and they must start immediately.

   b. One rescuer calls the EMS system while the other person begins one-rescuer CPR.

   c. One rescuer goes to the head of the victim and

      – determines unresponsiveness

continues

PROCEDURE   136   continued

– positions the victim
– opens the airway
– checks for victim's breathing
– if breathing is absent, says "no breathing" and gives 2 ventilations
– checks for pulse; if no pulse, says "no pulse"

d. Second rescuer (at the same time as first rescuer does above procedure)

– finds location for chest compressions
– places hands in proper position
– initiates external chest compressions after first rescuer says "no pulse"

e. During the cycle, the ventilator should monitor the pulse during compressions and breathing to determine the effectiveness of these procedures.

f. Chest compressions should be stopped for 5 seconds at the end of the first minute and every few minutes thereafter to determine if the victim has resumed spontaneous breathing and circulation.

To Switch Sides

3. When the rescuers are on opposite sides of the victim:

a. The change of positions takes place without interrupting the 5:1 sequence (Figures 48-17A–D).

b. The rescuer performing compressions directs when the switch takes place, at the end of a 5:1 sequence.

– The ventilator gives a breath, assumes the position for compressions, and locates proper hand position.
– The compressor, after the fifth compression, moves to the victim's head and checks the carotid pulse for 5 seconds.
– If no pulse, rescuer at victim's head gives a breath and tells rescuer at chest to continue with CPR.
– If there is a pulse but no breathing, continue with ventilations and monitor the pulse.

4. When the rescuers are on the same side of the victim:

a. The compressor initiates the switch by saying so while continuing chest compressions.

b. The ventilator gives a ventilation after the fifth compression.

c. After the ventilation, the ventilator moves quickly behind and around the compressor and assumes the compressor position.

d. The compressor moves to the victim's head to check pulse and to become the new ventilator.

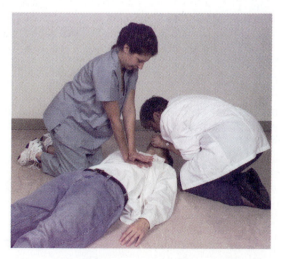

A. Person doing the compressions alerts second rescuer to change position and count to maintain rhythm.

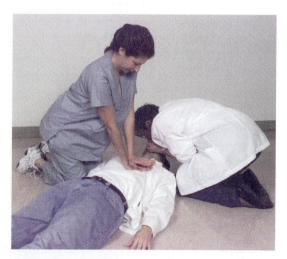

B. Person giving ventilations gives one full breath at the completion of the fifth compression.

FIGURE 48-17 Rescuers can change positions without interrupting the 5:1 sequence of compressions and ventilation.

continues

PROCEDURE **136** *continued*

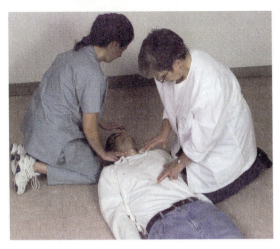

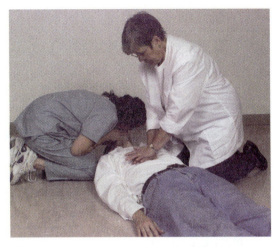

C. Person giving ventilations moves to the victim's chest and finds the compression area after the other rescuer completes the fifth compression. The person who was giving compressions moves to the head and does a pulse and breathing check.

FIGURE 48-17 *continued*

D. The person now giving ventilations gives a breath, and a new cycle of five compressions and one ventilation begins.

e. The new compressor is in position beside the victim's chest, assumes correct hand position, and waits to begin compressions.

f. The new ventilator quickly moves to the victim's head, does a pulse and breathing check, and resumes with correct procedure.

5. Remember, if the victim resumes breathing and the pulse returns, place the victim in the recovery position.

CHOKING

A person chokes when the throat is occluded (closed up or blocked) and air cannot get into the airway. In this situation, you must take quick, decisive action. (Refer to Procedures 137 and 138.)

- The airway can be blocked by accumulation in the back of the throat of:
  - Any foreign body
  - Blood
  - Food
  - Vomitus
- Tilting the head back can sometimes clear the airway, because positioning in this way pulls the tongue forward.
- If the person can speak and is coughing vigorously, do not intervene. Coughing is the most effective way to dislodge materials from the airway. Stay close by and encourage coughing.
- A complete blockage is signaled by the person being unable to speak, high-pitched sounds on inhalation, and grasping the throat in the universal distress signal (Figure 48-18).

- Apply standard precautions, if possible, when assisting a patient who is choking. This involves using gloves and a special mask or face shield during rescue breathing. Know where this equipment is kept and follow your facility policies for use of this equipment in an emergency.

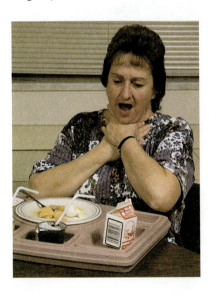

FIGURE 48-18 The distress signal for choking

PROCEDURE 137

HEIMLICH MANEUVER—ABDOMINAL THRUSTS

1. Ask the person if she is choking.

2. If the person starts to cough, wait.

3. If the person cannot speak, cough, or breathe, but is conscious, apply subdiaphragmatic abdominal thrusts (Heimlich maneuver) until the foreign body is expelled.

   a. Stand behind victim and wrap arms around victim's waist.

   b. Clench fist, keeping thumb straight (Figure 48-19A).

   c. Place fist, thumb side in, against abdomen slightly above navel and below tip of xiphoid process.

   d. Grasp clenched fist with opposite hand (Figure 48-19B).

   e. Thrust forcefully with thumb side of fist against midline of abdomen, slightly above navel, inward and upward (Figure 48-19C). Keep your elbows bent and extended away from your body. You do not want to "hug" the victim because the thrust will not be as effective. Be sure you are below the tip of the sternum (xiphoid process).

4. Keep thrusting if object has not been dislodged. If the person begins to cough forcefully, wait.

5. Activate the EMS system.

6. Continue the Heimlich maneuver until obstruction is expelled or victim becomes unconscious. If victim becomes unconscious, place victim in supine position. Proceed with Procedure 138.

Alternative Action: Chest thrusts are used when pressure to the abdomen would be harmful or impossible. Chest thrusts are used if the choking person is in late pregnancy or if the victim is so large you are unable to get your arms around him. Follow steps 1 and 2, then stand behind victim, place arms directly under victim's armpits, and around victim's chest. Place thumb side of fist in middle of breastbone (avoid ribs and xiphoid process). Grab your fist with your other hand and perform thrusts until foreign body is expelled or victim becomes unconscious.

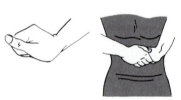

FIGURE 48-19A
Clench fist, keeping thumb straight.

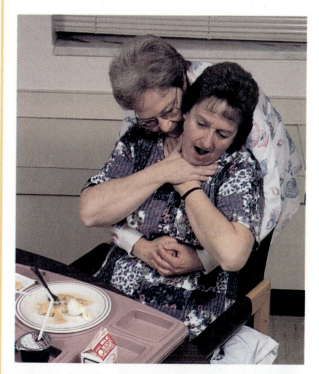

FIGURE 48-19B Grasp clenched fist with opposite hand.

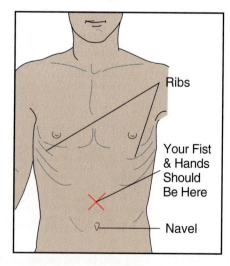

FIGURE 48-19C Thrust forcefully with thumb side of fist against midline of abdomen.

PROCEDURE **138**

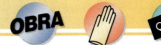

ASSISTING THE ADULT WHO HAS AN OBSTRUCTED AIRWAY AND BECOMES UNCONSCIOUS

1. Activate the EMS system.

2. Apply gloves.

3. Turn victim on back, tip the head back, and check for signs of breathing.

4. If victim is not breathing, give 2 slow breaths through a pocket mask or barrier device (Figure 48-20A). If the air does not go in, reposition the head and try again. If the air still does not go in, begin with 5 abdominal thrusts.

5. Straddle victim's thighs (Figure 48-20B) and administer 5 subdiaphragmatic abdominal thrusts, as follows:

   a. Place the heel of one hand on victim's abdomen slightly above the navel. Hand should be flat with fingers pointing toward victim's head.

   b. Place your other hand in a similar position over the first.

   c. Keep your elbows straight, with your shoulders directly over victim's abdomen.

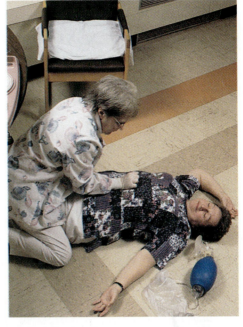

FIGURE 48-20B Straddle the victim's thighs and administer five subdiaphragmatic abdominal thrusts.

Press inward and upward with 5 quick thrusts. Keep hands centered on person's abdomen.

6. To remove a foreign object from the airway, follow these steps:

   a. With victim's face up, grasp the tongue and jaw between thumb and fingers.

   b. Pull upward, opening the mouth and drawing the jaw forward.

   c. Insert index finger of other hand down along in inside of one cheek, toward the base of the tongue.

   d. Bend finger and sweep in from the side with a hooking motion (Figure 48-20C). Do not poke straight in, because that may push the object further down. Use the hooking action, across toward the other cheek, to loosen and remove the object.

   e. Try to bring the foreign object up into the mouth if you can see it.

   f. Be careful not to force the object deeper into the throat.

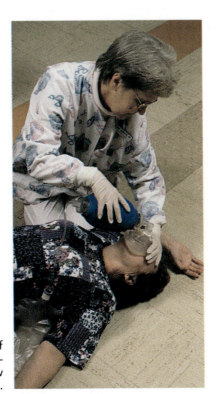

FIGURE 48-20A If victim is not breathing, give two slow breaths.

continues

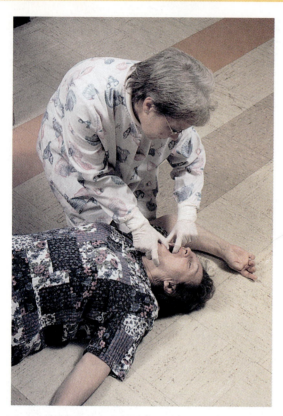

FIGURE 48-20C Open the victim's mouth with tongue-jaw lift method. Sweep deeply into mouth with a bent finger and a hooking motion.

g. If the object can be brought into the mouth, remove it.

7. Try giving breaths through a facemask or ventilation device. If airway is still obstructed, give 5 abdominal thrusts, sweep the mouth, and try to ventilate. Keep repeating these steps until the object moves and the victim can be ventilated or help arrives (EMS).

8. To give chest thrusts, proceed as if you were applying external chest compression, as you learned in your CPR training.

9. Check again for foreign body, using finger-sweep of mouth.

10. After sweeping the mouth, tip the head back, lift the chin, and try to give breaths. If air will not go into the lungs, repeat abdominal thrusts, finger-sweeping, and breaths.

Note: A victim who is given mouth-to-mouth breathing or abdominal thrusts may vomit. Roll a victim who vomits away from you on one side and clean out the mouth with your fingers. Then roll the victim back and continue repeating the sequence of breaths, thrusts, and finger-sweeps.

CPR AND OBSTRUCTED AIRWAY PROCEDURES FOR INFANTS

The following procedures for infants (Procedures 139 to 141) and children (Procedures 142 and 143) are only guidelines for CPR and emergency treatment of an obstructed airway. You *must* successfully complete an approved course before you perform these procedures.

CPR AND OBSTRUCTED AIRWAY PROCEDURES FOR CHILDREN

A child is considered to be between 1 and 8 years of age. If the child is more than 8 years old, CPR and management of obstructed airway is done the same as for adults.

CPR FOR INFANTS

Note differences between CPR on infants and adults:

- CPR on infants is always performed by one person only.

- The ratio is always 1 rescue breath (ventilation) to 5 compressions.
- Breaths are given with rescuer's mouth covering infant's nose *and* mouth.

continues

PROCEDURE **139** *continued*

- Breaths must be *gentle*.
- Circulation is assessed by taking the brachial pulse rather than the carotid pulse.
- Chest compressions are administered by placing your index finger below an imaginary line between the nipples, with middle and ring fingers placed next to index finger. Do not compress over xiphoid process. Compress sternum only 1/2 to 1 inch at least 100 times per minute.

1. Determine unresponsiveness by tapping the shoulder (Figure 48-21A).

2. Call out for help. If a second rescuer is present, have him activate the EMS system.

3. Support infant's head and shoulders and place infant on his back on a firm surface.

4. Use the head tilt-chin lift technique to open the airway. Be careful not to tilt the head back too far (Figure 48-21B).

5. Maintain an open airway and place your head in position over infant's chest to look, listen, and feel for breathing (Figure 48-21C). If infant is breathing and there are no signs of trauma, place infant in recovery position.

6. If victim is not breathing, maintain open airway and give 2 slow breaths with your mouth completely covering victim's nose and mouth. The breaths must be gentle because of an infant's small size.

7. Determine lack of pulse by feeling for the brachial pulse with two fingers, while maintaining an open airway (Figure 48-21D).

8. If there is no pulse, begin chest compressions:

   - Draw an imaginary line between the nipples.

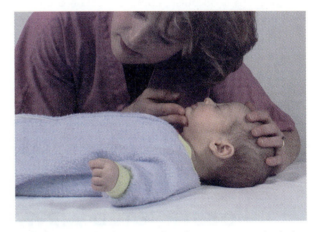

FIGURE 48-21C Place your head in position to look, listen, and feel for breathing.

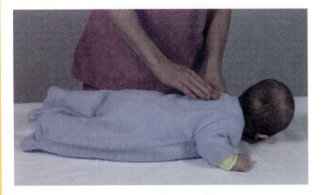

FIGURE 48-21A Determine unresponsiveness by tapping the shoulder.

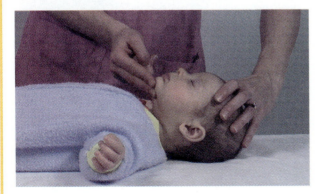

FIGURE 48-21B Open airway with head tilt-chin lift technique. Do not tilt head back too far.

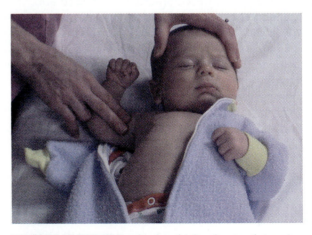

FIGURE 48-21D Take the brachial pulse to determine whether there is a pulse.

continues

PROCEDURE **139** *continued*

- Place your index finger below the imaginary line in the middle of the chest. Place your middle and ring fingers next to the index finger. Use these fingers to compress the sternum at that point (Figure 48-21E). *Do not compress over the xiphoid process.*
- Compress the sternum about 1/2 to 1 inch at least 100 times per minute.
- Give 1 rescue breath for every 5 compressions.

9. Do 20 cycles of compressions and rescue breaths.

10. After one minute of rescue support, check the brachial pulse.

11. If you are alone, activate the EMS system now.

12. If there is no pulse, continue rescue breaths and compressions.

13. Check for a pulse every few minutes. If pulse returns, check for breathing. If there is no breathing, give 1 rescue breath every 3

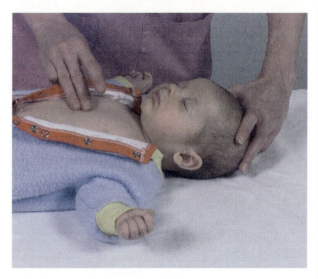

FIGURE 48-21E Use your middle and ring fingers to compress the sternum.

seconds (20 breaths per minute). Monitor the pulse. If breathing is present, place infant in recovery position, maintain an open airway, monitor breathing and pulse.

PROCEDURE **140**

OBSTRUCTED AIRWAY: CONSCIOUS INFANT

Perform this procedure only if the airway of the conscious infant is completely obstructed and someone has witnessed or strongly suspects that there is a foreign body obstruction. If the infant cannot breathe because of an infection, the infant should be rushed to the nearest life support facility. Procedures to clear the airway *should not be performed.* Allow the infant with respiratory distress to find and maintain the most comfortable position.

1. Determine whether there is airway obstruction by observing breathing difficulties, weak or absent cry, or ineffective cough.

2. Supporting infant's head and neck with one hand, position infant face down with head lower than trunk, over one arm (support your

arm on your thigh) and deliver up to 5 back blows (Figure 48-22A).

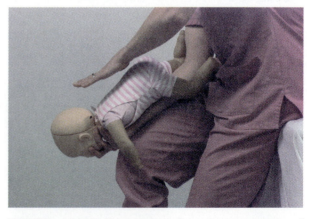

FIGURE 48-22A Place infant face down, with head lower than trunk, and deliver up to five back blows.

continues

PROCEDURE **140** *continued*

3. Supporting infant on your arm, turn infant face up and deliver up to 5 chest thrusts in midsternal region (using landmarks for positioning as for chest compressions) (Figure 48-22B). Do chest thrusts more slowly than chest compressions.

4. Repeat steps 2 and 3 until the foreign body is expelled or infant becomes unconscious.

If the Infant Becomes Unconscious

5. Call out for help. If someone responds, have that person call the EMS system. Place infant on back.

6. Perform tongue-jaw lift. Do not perform a

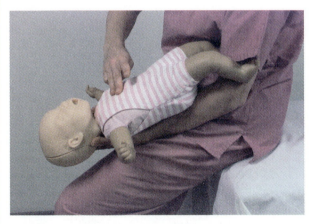

FIGURE 48-22B Turn infant face up and deliver up to five chest thrusts.

blind finger-sweep, but remove the foreign body if you can see it.

7. Open airway with head tilt-chin lift and try to give rescue breaths.

8. Reposition head and try again to give rescue breaths.

9. Deliver up to 5 back blows.

10. Deliver up to 5 chest thrusts.

11. Perform tongue-jaw lift and remove foreign body if you can see it.

12. Maintain open airway with head tilt-chin lift and try again to give rescue breaths.

13. Repeat steps 8 through 12 until successful.

14. If you are alone and your efforts are unsuccessful, activate the EMS system after trying to clear the airway for about one minute.

15. When obstruction is removed, check for breathing. If there is no breathing, give rescue breaths. If there is no pulse, give 2 breaths and start cycles of compressions and rescue breaths. If pulse is present, open airway with chin lift-head tilt and check for breathing. If there is breathing, place in recovery position. Monitor breathing and pulse while maintaining open airway. If no breathing, give 1 rescue breath every 3 seconds (20 breaths per minute). Monitor pulse.

PROCEDURE **141**

OBSTRUCTED AIRWAY: UNCONSCIOUS INFANT

1. Determine unresponsiveness as directed in Procedure 140.

2. Call out for help.

3. Support head and neck and turn infant on back on a firm, hard surface.

4. Use head tilt-chin lift method to open airway. Do not tilt head too far back.

5. Determine lack of breathing by maintaining open airway and looking, listening, and feeling for breathing.

6. Try to give rescue breaths by placing your mouth over infant's nose and mouth.

7. Reposition head, check mouth seal, and try again to give rescue breaths.

continues

8. Activate the EMS system. If someone else is available, have that person make the call.

9. Deliver up to 5 back blows.

10. Deliver up to 5 chest thrusts.

11. Do tongue-jaw lift and remove foreign body if you can see it.

12. Try to do rescue breaths again.

13. Repeat steps 9 through 12 until successful.

14. If you are alone and your efforts are unsuccessful, activate the EMS system after about one minute of effort.

15. Check for pulse and respirations when obstruction is removed.

16. If infant is breathing, place in recovery position. Maintain open airway and monitor pulse and breathing. If there is no breathing, give 20 rescue breaths per minute and monitor the pulse.

17. If there is no pulse, give 2 rescue breaths and start cycles of compressions and breaths. If there is a pulse, open airway and check for breathing.

P R O C E D U R E **142**

CPR FOR CHILDREN, ONE RESCUER

1. Establish unresponsiveness by tapping shoulder and calling name.

2. If another person is available, have that person activate the EMS system. If another person is not present, give one minute of rescue support and then activate the EMS system.

3. Use head tilt-chin lift method or jaw-thrust method to open airway. Check for breathing by looking, listening, and feeling. If victim is breathing or begins breathing, place child in recovery position.

4. If there is no breathing, give 2 slow breaths, taking 1 to 1-1/2 seconds per breath.

Observe chest for rising. Allow chest to deflate between breaths.

5. Assess for heartbeat by taking carotid pulse. If pulse is present but there is no breathing, do rescue breathing of 1 breath every 3 seconds (20 breaths per minute).

6. If there is no pulse, give 5 chest compressions (100 compressions per minute). Open airway and provide 1 slow breath. Repeat the cycle.

7. After about one minute of rescue support, check pulse. If there is no pulse, continue the cycle of 5 compressions to 1 breath.

P R O C E D U R E **143**

CHILD WITH FOREIGN BODY AIRWAY OBSTRUCTION

Conscious Child

1. Ask "Are you choking?"

2. Give abdominal thrusts.

3. Repeat thrusts until foreign body is removed or victim becomes unconscious.

Child Becomes Unconscious

4. If another person is present, have that person activate the EMS system.

5. Perform tongue-jaw lift. If you see the foreign body, perform a finger sweep to remove it.

continues

PROCEDURE **143** *continued*

6. Open airway and try to do rescue breathing. If still obstructed, reposition head and try to do rescue breathing again.

7. Give up to 5 abdominal thrusts.

8. Repeat steps 5 through 7 until effective. If victim is breathing or begins breathing, place in recovery position.

9. If airway obstruction is not relieved after about one minute, activate the EMS system.

Unconscious Child

1. Establish unresponsiveness. If another person is present, have that person activate the EMS system.

2. Open airway and try to ventilate. If unsuccessful, reposition head and try ventilations again.

3. Give up to 5 abdominal thrusts.

4. Perform tongue-jaw lift, remove foreign body only if you can see it.

5. Repeat steps 2 to 4 until effective. If child is breathing or resumes breathing, place in recovery position.

6. If airway obstruction is not relieved after about one minute, activate the EMS system.

OTHER EMERGENCIES

For some of the emergencies described here, a patient at home or in a long-term care facility may need to be transported to a hospital emergency room. Be sure, if the patient is at home, that you know:

- Initial emergency actions to perform
- How and when to notify the EMS system
- How and when to notify your supervisor
- How, when, and which family members to notify in the event of emergency

If the patient is in a long-term care facility, know the initial emergency actions to perform and the procedure to follow for emergencies.

BLEEDING

Remember that if the person is conscious, the extent of injuries is likely to be far less severe than if the person is unconscious. With the unconscious person, the next imminent threat to life is the loss of blood. Apply gloves and follow standard precautions if you see or suspect that the patient is bleeding. Bleeding is usually easy to see. Sometimes, however, the bleeding is internal. Internal bleeding will only be shown by the signs of shock (described in the next section). Examine the person for evidence of bleeding. Take the following steps to prevent additional loss:

- Identify the area that is bleeding.
- Have the victim apply continuous pressure over the bleeding area, if able.
- If the victim is not able, apply continuous, direct pressure over the bleeding area with a pad or even your hand, if necessary (Figure 48-23).
- Call for help.

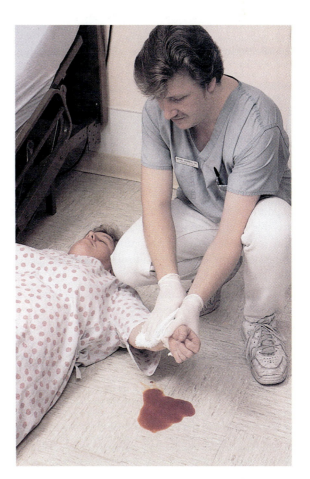

FIGURE 48-23 Apply direct pressure over bleeding area with a pad or your hand.

- If seepage occurs, increase the padding and pressure.
- If there are no broken bones and there is no pain, raise the wounded area above the level of the heart, but do not release pressure. This will help to reduce bleeding.

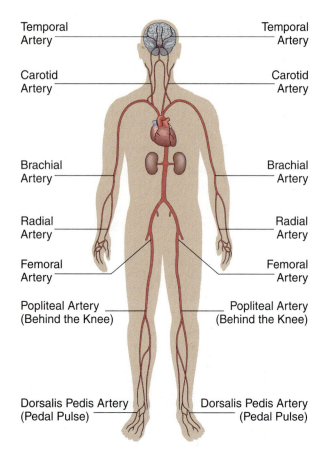

Temporal Artery

Temporal Artery

Carotid Artery

Carotid Artery

Brachial Artery

Brachial Artery

Radial Artery

Radial Artery

Femoral Artery

Femoral Artery

Popliteal Artery (Behind the Knee)

Popliteal Artery (Behind the Knee)

Dorsalis Pedis Artery (Pedal Pulse)

Dorsalis Pedis Artery (Pedal Pulse)

FIGURE 48-24 Pressure may be applied over appropriate pulse points.

- Support the elevated area.
- Use binding of some kind to hold the padded pressure if there is bleeding from more than one area.
- If you have learned the location of the major blood vessels that control blood flow to an area, and direct pressure seems ineffective, apply pressure over the appropriate pulse point to control **hemorrhage** (heavy bleeding) (Figure 48-24).
- Keep the person comfortably warm and quiet until help arrives.

Note: Persons who are bleeding are often very frightened. Their anxiety contributes to the development of shock. Continuous reassurance is essential.

SHOCK

Shock is defined as a disturbance of the oxygen supply to the tissues and return of blood to the heart. It can follow:
- Any severe injury
- Cardiac arrest
- Acute hemorrhage
- Severe pain
- Excessive loss of body fluids (as in severe burns)

Signs and Symptoms of Shock

Early signs and symptoms include:

- Pale, cold skin that is moist to the touch
- Complaints of weakness
- Weak, rapid pulse
- Rapid and irregular breathing
- Restlessness and anxiety
- Perspiration

Later signs of shock include:
- Mottled skin
- Lack of response
- Sunken eyes with pupils that are dilated, and vacant expression
- Loss of consciousness
- Drop in body temperature

Preventive Measures

Anxiety aggravates the situation, but shock can be prevented if steps are taken early. Prevention of shock includes controlling situations that could trigger it.
- Call for help—activate the emergency medical system.
- Keep the person lying down and quiet.
- Maintain normal body temperature. Provide light warmth if needed.
- Position person with the feet and legs slightly higher than body and head (Trendelenburg position), unless contraindicated by specific injury. This assures improved circulation to vital organs.
  - Burned areas should be elevated unless it causes the person pain.
  - If fractures are involved, make sure the part is splinted (braced) before positioning the person to prevent shock.
- Intravenous fluids to improve circulatory volume and low volumes of oxygen will be given.
  - This equipment will be readily at hand in a care facility.
  - In the community, the emergency personnel answering the call will bring the supplies necessary to manage fluid and oxygenation.
- Continue to monitor pulse and respirations.

Unless shock is controlled, death can occur. Until help arrives, your care can often make the difference between life and death.

FAINTING

When the blood supply to the brain is reduced for a short time, the person loses consciousness. This is called *fainting*. Fainting is usually a temporary condition. It is corrected as soon as blood flow to the brain is restored.

Unfortunately, when consciousness is lost, the person is likely to fall and injuries can occur. Patients who are ambulating for the first time should be assisted. If fainting occurs and the patient falls, do not try to hold the patient upright.

Ease the patient to the floor to prevent injury. Assist patients who are *feeling* faint to a safe position.

The patient who is sitting and feels faint, light-headed, dizzy, and nauseated should be encouraged to lower her head between her knees. Pallor, cold skin, perspiration, or visual changes also signal fainting. To provide assistance to a fainting person, the nursing assistant should:

- Help the patient to assume a protected position, sitting or lying down
- Loosen tight clothing
- Position head lower than heart to encourage cerebral blood flow
- Allow person to rest for at least 10 minutes
- Maintain normal body temperature
- Call for additional help
- Monitor pulse and respirations

HEART ATTACK

Heart attacks can occur in any age group, but the high-risk group includes those who:

- Are overweight
- Smoke
- Have atherosclerosis
- Remain immobile for long periods
- Are older
- Have diabetes
- Have a history of heart disease

Signs and Symptoms

Signs and symptoms of heart attack include:

- Crushing pain that can radiate up the jaw and down the arm, or heaviness in chest
- Perspiring, skin cold and clammy
- Nausea and vomiting
- Pale to grayish color of the face
- Difficulty breathing or absence of breathing
- Loss of consciousness
- Irregular pulse or loss of pulse (the loss of heart function is called cardiac arrest)

At other times, the pain of the attack may resemble indigestion and the person remains conscious. Do not be fooled into thinking that the degree of pain indicates the severity of the attack. Both victims need immediate attention.

Action

In the health care facility:

- Immediately signal for help.
- Stay with the patient if the patient is conscious.
- Help keep the patient calm.
- Elevate the head of the bed to assist breathing.
- Provide oxygen, if available.

If the patient is unconscious:

- Check for breathing and heartbeat.
- If necessary, institute CPR (if you have been trained) until a professional takes charge.

In the community, and if the person is conscious, proceed as follows.

1. Assess the situation.
2. If possible, activate the emergency medical system.
3. Allow the person to sit up or assume a position of comfort. Loosen clothing about the neck.
4. Keep onlookers away.
5. Provide fresh air but keep the person comfortably warm.
6. Monitor pulse and respirations.
7. Be prepared to initiate CPR.

In the community, if the person is unconscious, follow steps 1 and 2. Then:

3. Check for breathing and heartbeat.
4. If heartbeat is present but breathing has ceased, establish an open airway and institute mask-to-mouth resuscitation.
5. If breathing and heartbeat have ceased (cardiac and respiratory arrest), institute CPR until a professional takes charge.

BRAIN ATTACK

A brain attack (cerebral vascular accident or CVA), also called a stroke, occurs when there is interference with normal blood circulation to the brain. It usually is caused by a clot that has lodged in a cerebral vessel or by a blood vessel that has ruptured.

Signs and Symptoms

The person with a severe brain attack usually:

- Experiences seizure activity
- Loses consciousness
- Experiences difficulty breathing
- Develops paralysis on one side of the body and of the muscles on either side of the face
- Has unequal pupil reaction

The patient with a less severe brain attack may experience:

- Disorientation
- Dizziness
- Headache
- Slurred speech
- Memory loss
- Loss of consciousness

Action

First aid includes:

- Maintaining an airway

- Providing mask-to-mouth breathing as needed
- Administering CPR, if needed (by a trained, qualified individual)
- Positioning the victim on one side so fluids will drain from the mouth
- Maintaining normal body temperature
- Keeping the person quiet until help arrives or transportation to a medical facility can be arranged

SEIZURES

Seizures or convulsions are sometimes seen when there is:
- Drug overdose
- Head injury
- Degenerative brain disease
- Stroke
- Infectious disease and fevers
- Tumors
- Hypoglycemic reactions
- Seizure disorder. Seizure disorder now is largely controlled with medication, but unusual stress, missed medication doses, and other factors can cause a convulsion

Signs and Symptoms

Seizures do not always follow the same pattern. Their range may be:
- A momentary loss of contact with the environment *(petit mal),* in which there are no random or uncontrolled movements but the person seems to stare blankly.
- A *grand mal* form in which:
  - consciousness is lost.
  - the person falls.
  - the person becomes rigid.
  - uncontrolled voluntary movements occur.
  - frothing at the mouth occurs.
  - the person becomes cyanotic.
  - the person loses control of bladder and/or bowel function.

Gradually the seizure lessens and the person recovers. The person is usually:
- Confused
- Disoriented for a period of time
- Very tired

Action

If you witness a seizure, take the following steps:
- Wear gloves and apply standard precautions, because there is a high probability of contact with blood and body fluids when caring for a patient with a seizure.
- Do not restrain the person's movements.
- Protect the person from injury. For example, move any objects that might break or cause bruising.

- Loosen clothing around the neck.
- Maintain an airway by positioning. Do not try to put anything in the mouth.
- Cradle the person's head.
- Observe the seizure.

After seizure activity stops:
- Turn the person to the side so fluid or vomitus can drain freely after the movements subside.
- Give mask-to-mouth resuscitation if breathing is not resumed following the seizure.
- Allow the person to rest undisturbed.
- Stay with the person but summon medical assistance.
- Report and record seizure activity: time, length of seizure, body parts or activity involved.

ELECTRIC SHOCK

Electric shock can occur in the:
- community, when high-tension wires are knocked down in accidents or storms, or when electrical appliances are misused or malfunction.
- health facility, because of frayed wires and faulty outlets or fixtures.

Severe burns and cardiac and respiratory arrest can result from electric shock. You must protect yourself as you try to rescue the victim.

Action

- Turn off the electricity at the terminal source, such as at a fuse box, before touching the victim, if possible.
- If the source of electricity cannot be controlled, try to move the victim away with some nonconductive material. Dry wood (a broom handle, for example) is a good nonconductor.
- Once free of the electrical source, check the victim for breathing and pulse.
- Summon medical help.
- Administer CPR, if necessary.
- Once breathing and heart function are restored, check for burns and other injury. Keep the person lying down and comfortable.
- Give first aid for burns or other injuries.

BURNS

Burns result in loss of skin integrity. They may be caused by heat, chemicals, or radiation. There is a high risk of infection with any burn. Burns are classified as partial thickness or full thickness, depending on the degree of injury. Partial thickness burns are:
- First-degree burns—involve only the top layer (epidermis) of skin. There is redness, temporary swelling, and pain. There is usually no permanent scarring.

- Second-degree burns—involve both epidermis and dermis. The skin color may vary from pink or red to white or tan. Blistering, pain, and some scarring occur.

Full thickness burns are:

- Third-degree burns—involve epidermis, dermis, and subcutaneous tissue. The tissue is bright red to tan and brown. There may be no pain initially because nerve endings have been destroyed. Later, pain and scarring will result.

Emergency Treatment for Burns

1. Call the nurse immediately.
2. If the patient's clothing is on fire, use a coat or blanket to smother the flames.
3. Cool water may be applied to lower skin temperature and to stop further tissue damage. Remove wet clothing (follow nurse's instructions).
4. Third-degree burns usually require extensive treatment.

ORTHOPEDIC INJURIES

Orthopedic injuries include injuries to bones, joints, muscles, and ligaments.

- A **fracture** is a break in a bone.
- A **sprain** is an injury to a ligament caused by sudden overstretching. A sprained ankle may occur, for example, if a person falls and turns the ankle quickly while falling. Swelling may be noted shortly afterward.
- A **strain** is excessive stretching of a muscle that results in pain and swelling of the muscle. You may strain the muscles in your back if you use incorrect lifting and moving techniques.
- A **dislocation** occurs in a joint, when one bone is displaced from another bone. This can occur in a paralyzed arm that is allowed to hang without support. The

weight of the arm pulls the upper arm bone out of position in the shoulder joint. A dislocation can also be caused by improperly lifting a patient under the arms.

Treatment for Orthopedic Injuries

If you suspect a patient has suffered a fracture:

- Stay with the patient.
- Do not attempt to move the patient.
- Call the nurse immediately.

If a fracture is suspected, x-rays will be taken of the injury. If a fracture is present, the physician will put a cast on the affected extremity, place the patient in traction, or do surgery.

If you suspect that a patient has suffered a sprain, strain, or dislocation, notify the nurse at once. You may be instructed to:

- elevate the injured extremity.
- apply ice packs to the area.
- after 24 hours, you may be instructed to apply warm packs to the area.

ACCIDENTAL POISONING

Immediate attention is needed if a patient is the victim of accidental poisoning. All potentially harmful substances must be kept in locked cupboards. If you suspect that a poisoning has happened:

- Call the nurse immediately.
- Try to determine what the patient has taken and save the container.
- The nurse may administer a substance that will cause vomiting. (Not all substances can be safely removed from the patient's body by vomiting.)
- Know where to find the telephone number for the regional poison control center.

REVIEW

A. True/False.

Mark the following true or false by circling T or F.

1. T F You need no special training to give CPR.
2. T F CPR is needed if breathing and circulation fail.
3. T F The Heimlich maneuver is used to stop bleeding.
4. T F The person in shock should be kept quiet and lying down.
5. T F When controlling bleeding, the bleeding part should be elevated.
6. T F Vomiting should be induced on anyone who swallows a poisonous substance.
7. T F Immediate treatment for burns may include applying cold water to lower skin temperature.
8. T F A dislocation occurs when one bone is displaced from another bone.
9. T F For orthopedic injuries, immediate treatment includes the application of warm packs.
10. T F Third-degree burns only involve the epidermis.

B. Matching.

Choose the correct term from Column II to match each phrase in Column I.

Column I

Column II

11. _____ person needing first aid

12. _____ excessive bleeding

13. _____ care given when victim has no breathing or heartbeat

14. _____ signaled by a drop in blood pressure

15. _____ emergency care

a. arrest

b. first aid

c. victim

d. CPR

e. contraindicated

f. hemorrhage

g. splintered

h. shock

C. Multiple Choice.

Select the one best answer for each question.

16. An organization that offers instruction in CPR is the
    a. American Diabetes Association.
    b. American Association of Nurses.
    c. Association for the Blind.
    d. American Heart Association.

17. First aid is care given
    a. immediately to victims of injury.
    b. immediately to victims of sudden illness.
    c. if medical help is delayed.
    d. all of these.

18. Which of the following is a life-threatening situation requiring intervention? A person who
    a. broke a finger.
    b. fell and bruised a knee.
    c. is in shock.
    d. is coughing.

19. The first step you should take when arriving on the scene of an accident is to
    a. stop a passerby.
    b. assess the situation.
    c. move the victims to one side.
    d. help the victims get up and walk.

20. To assist a person who has fainted,
    a. help the person to stand up and walk to circulate the blood.
    b. cover the person with several blankets.
    c. loosen tight clothing.
    d. position the person's head higher than the heart.

21. To assist the person experiencing a seizure, you should
    a. keep the person as active as possible.
    b. restrain the person's movements.
    c. keep the head straight.

d. maintain an airway and protect the person from injury.

22. You suspect that a patient is in shock because the
    a. blood pressure is elevated.
    b. face is flushed.
    c. skin is cold and clammy.
    d. pulse is full and bounding.

23. The overstretching of a ligament can result in a
    a. fracture.
    b. sprain.
    c. strain.
    d. dislocation.

24. For one-person CPR, the ratio of chest compressions to ventilations is
    a. 15 compressions to 2 ventilations.
    b. 5 compressions to 1 ventilation.
    c. 5 compressions to 2 ventilations.
    d. 15 compressions to 1 ventilation.

25. If a victim of cardiac arrest resumes breathing but is unconscious, you should place the victim
    a. in recovery position.
    b. on his back.
    c. on his abdomen.
    d. in a chair.

26. The first action to take when someone is choking and is conscious is to tell the person what you are going to do and then
    a. slap the person on the back.
    b. give abdominal thrusts.
    c. begin artificial respirations.
    d. begin chest compressions.

27. The priorities of an emergency are
    a. airway.
    b. breathing.
    c. circulation.
    d. all of these.

28. When a person suffers cardiac arrest,
    a. the heart has stopped beating.
    b. the respirations have ceased.
    c. clinical death has occurred.
    d. all of these.

29. In the health care facility, you would initiate CPR for cardiac arrest unless
    a. the patient has a DNR order.
    b. you think the patient would not want to be revived.
    c. the patient is very old.
    d. all of these.

30. If you are working in a patient's home and CPR is initiated, you must
    a. call the EMS system yourself if you are alone.
    b. drive the patient to the closest hospital.
    c. do CPR for 20 minutes and if the patient does not respond, call the EMS system.
    d. go next door to have the neighbor call the EMS system.

31. CPR on an infant is always done with a ratio of
    a. 1 ventilation to 5 compressions.
    b. 5 ventilations to 1 compression.
    c. 15 ventilations to 1 compression.
    d. 15 compressions to 2 ventilations.

32. The procedure for obstructed airway on a conscious infant is to position the infant and
    a. deliver 5 abdominal thrusts followed by 5 back blows.
    b. deliver 5 back blows followed by 5 chest thrusts.
    c. perform a blind finger-sweep.
    d. perform 2 ventilations followed by 5 compressions.

33. When performing CPR on a child, the procedure is
    a. done as it is on an adult.
    b. done as it is on an infant.
    c. done with a ratio of 1 ventilation to 5 chest compressions.
    d. done with a ratio of 2 ventilations to 15 chest compressions.

34. During CPR on a child, the pulse is assessed by taking the
    a. carotid pulse.
    b. brachial pulse.
    c. radial pulse.
    d. femoral pulse.

35. The preferred treatment for external bleeding is to
    a. apply continuous, direct pressure.
    b. apply a tourniquet.
    c. apply pressure to pulse points.
    d. apply a heat pack.

D. Nursing Assistant Challenge.

You and a friend are driving home from work. A car immediately ahead of you goes through a stop sign and is hit on the passenger side by a car going through the intersection. You and your friend park your car to see what you should do in this emergency. The people in the other car are conscious, alert, and deny having any injuries. The passenger in the car that ran the stop sign is unconscious and begins to vomit. You see blood coming from the person's right arm. The driver is conscious but dazed and seems to be disoriented. List, in sequence, the actions you would take.

Moving Forward

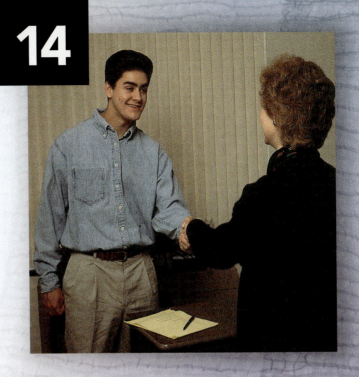

UNIT 49

Employment Opportunities and Career Growth

Employment Opportunities and Career Growth

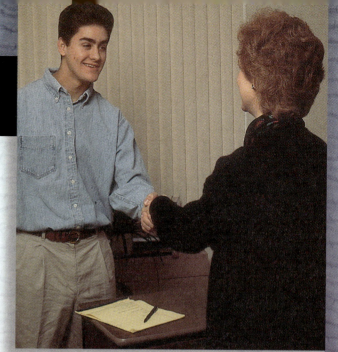

As a result of this unit, you will be able to:

- Spell and define terms.
- List nine objectives to be met in obtaining and maintaining employment.
- Follow a process for self-appraisal.
- Name sources of employment for nursing assistants.
- Prepare a résumé and a letter of resignation.
- List the steps for a successful interview.
- List the requirements that must be met when accepting employment.
- List steps for continuing development in your career.

VOCABULARY

Learn the meaning and the correct spelling of the following words and phrases:

job interview   networking   reference   résumé

INTRODUCTION

Having completed a training program to be a nursing assistant, you are now ready to look for employment. You will want to be as successful as an employee as you were as a student. If you meet the objectives presented in this unit of study, the task will be made much easier.

Searching for and obtaining a job requires several steps:

- Completing a self-appraisal
- Searching for employment opportunities
- Assembling a résumé
- Validating your references
- Making specific applications for work
- Participating in interviews
- Deciding whether to take the job

OBJECTIVE 1: SELF-APPRAISAL

The first objective is to determine your personal assets and limitations that could influence your choice of employment. To do this:

- Divide a piece of paper into three columns.
- Title one column *assets,* one *limitations,* and one *solutions.*
- Review all of the positive contributions you can make to an employment situation and list them. For example:
  - Your preference in the care of certain patients
  - Your caring attitude
  - Special skill you have with particular patients
  - Your personal appearance
- Honestly review all the limitations that might make certain employment less obtainable. For example, consider:
  - Home responsibilities
  - Specific hours you can work
  - Transportation problems
  - Physical limitations
- Think of possible solutions so that you reduce the number of limitations. The fewer limitations you have at the beginning of your job search, the more you expand the possibilities for employment.

Make your lists, review them, and add to them over several days.

OBJECTIVE 2: SEARCH FOR ALL EMPLOYMENT OPPORTUNITIES

Having thought through your assets and limitations and found as many solutions to the limitations as possible, you are ready to search for employment. Possible sources for the search process are all the agencies or facilities that employ nursing assistants:

- Physicians' offices
- Blood banks
- Clinics
- Hospices
- Homes for aged or disabled
- Nursing homes
- Hospitals
- Home health care agencies
- Rehabilitation centers
- Telephone directory—select facilities that meet your specific needs for available transportation or specific type of care
- Classified ads found in the newspaper
  - Look for facilities in your area.
  - Consider the type of work you are willing to do.
  - Consider the shifts that have openings.
  - Note the person to contact for an interview or additional information.
- Facility in which you received your clinical experience
  - Administrators sometimes offer jobs to new nursing assistants who trained in their facility.
  - Job openings may be posted on the employee bulletin board.
- Friends and colleagues
  - Friends may know of job openings.
  - Colleagues may put you in touch with others who have potential job connections (Figure 49-1).
  - A current term for these activities is **networking**.

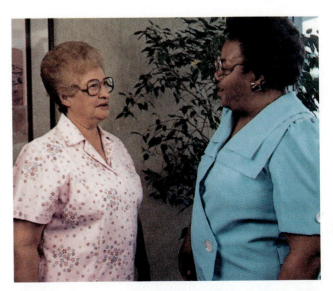

FIGURE 49-1 Friends and classmates are valuable sources of information about potential jobs.

OBJECTIVE 3: ASSEMBLE A PROPER RÉSUMÉ

A résumé is a written summary of work and educational history. You should:

- Prepare several copies
- Always keep a copy for yourself
- Type the résumé for a neat appearance
- Carry a copy whenever you seek employment
- Use the résumé as a ready reference when you fill out forms
- Update the résumé regularly

The résumé should be carefully prepared to include:

- Your name, address, and telephone number
- Your educational background
  - List your most recent education first.
  - Give dates.
  - Include a brief summary of the content.
- Your work history over the last five years, especially if it gives evidence of successful experiences in the same or related areas as the job for which you are applying
- Proof of being on the State Nurse Aide Registry
- List of any continuing education classes you have attended
- Other experiences you have had; include jobs that show initiative, reliability, trustworthiness, and worthwhile ways you have spent your time
- References—a list of three people who know you and can verify your abilities
- Some personal information that indicates your interests and activities

It is not necessary to include the following in your résumé, although some of this information may be shared during the interview:

- Age
- Marital status
- Religion
- Sex
- Height
- Weight

OBJECTIVE 4: VALIDATE REFERENCES

References are people who know you and who would be willing to comment, either in writing or verbally over the telephone, about you and your abilities. Be sure to include accurate titles, names, addresses, and telephone numbers when listing references.

Anyone you use as references:

- should give you permission to use their names (Figure 49-2).

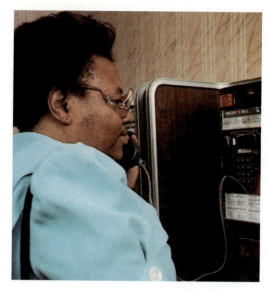

FIGURE 49-2 Get permission before using names for references.

- should know you well enough to make an honest evaluation.
- should not be related to you.
- may need to have their memories refreshed about dates of employment or experiences you have stated in your résumé.

OBJECTIVE 5: MAKE SPECIFIC APPLICATIONS FOR WORK

Handle this part of the job search process in a businesslike way:

- Select three facilities that interest you most.
- Call and ask for the director of nursing or personnel department.
- Tell the person who answers that you are interested in learning if there are any openings for a nursing assistant, and if so, what application procedure is to be followed.
- Be prepared to answer questions about your preparation and experience. Have your résumé in your hand.
- Make an appointment for an interview, if possible. A job interview is an opportunity for the person applying for a job and the employer's representative to learn about each other. Each person has the opportunity to ask questions to determine if the job seeker has qualifications that match the needs of the job available.
- Fill out an application form (Figure 49-3). Use your résumé to be sure you complete the form. Make sure the information is accurate, spelled correctly, complete, and neat.
- Learn the names of the persons to whom you speak.
- Thank the person speaking with you by name.

Repeat the steps until you land the job.

EMPLOYMENT APPLICATION
(PLEASE TYPE OR PRINT IN INK)

CHARTER SUBURBAN HOSPITAL
16453 South Colorado Avenue
Paramount, California 90723

PERSONAL DATA

LAST NAME	FIRST		TELEPHONE ( )	DATE

ADDRESS	STREET	CITY	STATE	ZIP	HOW LONG?

PREVIOUS ADDRESS	STREET	CITY	STATE	ZIP	HOW LONG?

OTHER NAMES UNDER WHICH YOU HAVE WORKED	HOW WERE YOU REFERRED TO US FOR EMPLOYMENT?

POSITION DESIRED:

1ST CHOICE: 2ND CHOICE:

DATE YOU CAN START:

SHIFT YOU CAN WORK:

☐ DAYS ☐ P.M.s ☐ NIGHTS ☐ WEEKENDS

ARE YOU APPYING FOR: ☐ FULL-TIME ☐ PART-TIME

☐ ON CALL/FLOAT ☐ TEMPORARY

SOCIAL SECURITY NUMBER	DO YOU HAVE THE LEGAL RIGHT TO WORK IN THIS COUNTRY? ☐ YES ☐ NO	ARE YOU UNDER 18 YEARS OLD? ☐ YES ☐ NO

LIST FRIENDS & RELATIVES (STATE RELATIONSHIP) EMPLOYED BY THIS HOSPITAL

TRANSPORTATION AVAILABLE?

☐ YES ☐ NO

HAVE YOU EVER BEEN CONVICTED OF A FELONY? IF YES, DESCRIBE THE CIRCUMSTANCES:

(A FELONY CONVICTION WILL NOT AUTOMATICALLY DISQUALIFY YOU FOR EMPLOYMENT) _____

EDUCATION

	NAME AND LOCATION	CIRCLE LAST YEAR COMPLETED	DATE LAST ATTENDED	MAJOR FIELD OF STUDY	DIPLOMA OR DEGREE RECEIVED
HIGH SCHOOL		1 2 3 4	✗		
COLLEGE OR UNIVERSITY		1 2 3 4			
PROFESSIONAL TRAINING		YEARS ATTENDED			
GRADUATE SCHOOL					
OTHER					

OFFICE SKILLS   (CLERICAL APPLICANTS ONLY)

☐ TYPING_____ WPM
☐ SHORTHAND/SPEEDWRITING _____ WPM
☐ 10 KEY ADDING MACHINE

☐ DICTAPHONE
☐ KEYPUNCH
☐ PBX

☐ MEDICAL TERMINOLOGY
☐ OTHER_____

PROFESSIONAL LICENSURE

TYPE	LICENSE NUMBER	STATE	EXPIRATION DATE

AP1018

FIGURE 49-3 Complete the application form neatly, correctly, and completely. *Courtesy of Charter Suburban Hospital*

EMPLOYMENT (LIST MOST RECENT FIRST)

MAY WE CONTACT PRESENT EMPLOYER? ☐ YES ☐ NO

FROM MO YR / TO MO YR	EMPLOYER'S NAME	POSITIONS & DUTIES	PRESENT OR LAST SALARY	REASON FOR LEAVING
STREET ADDRESS / CITY / STATE				
PHONE NO. ( ) / SUPERVISOR'S NAME & TITLE				
FROM MO YR / TO MO YR	EMPLOYER'S NAME			
STREET ADDRESS / CITY / STATE				
PHONE NO. ( ) / SUPERVISOR'S NAME & TITLE				
FROM MO YR / TO MO YR	EMPLOYER'S NAME			
STREET ADDRESS / CITY / STATE				
PHONE NO. ( ) / SUPERVISOR'S NAME & TITLE				
FROM MO YR / TO MO YR	EMPLOYER'S NAME			
STREET ADDRESS / CITY / STATE				
PHONE NO. ( ) / SUPERVISOR'S NAME & TITLE				
FROM MO YR / TO MO YR	EMPLOYER'S NAME			
STREET ADDRESS / CITY / STATE				
PHONE NO. ( ) / SUPERVISOR'S NAME & TITLE				

DO YOU HAVE A MEDICAL/PHYSICAL CONDITION WHICH COULD LIMIT YOUR JOB PERFORMANCE?

☐ YES ☐ NO, IF "YES", PLEASE EXPLAIN: _____

_____

_____

I CERTIFY THAT ALL STATEMENTS MADE ON THIS APPLICATION ARE TRUE AND THAT ANY MISSTATEMENTS MAY BE CAUSE FOR TERMINATION OR DENIAL OF EMPLOYMENT WITH CHARTER SUBURBAN HOSPITAL. PERMISSION IS GRANTED TO INVESTIGATE AND VERIFY EMPLOYMENT AND EDUCATION. I UNDERSTAND THAT EMPLOYMENT WITH CHARTER SUBURBAN HOSPITAL IS CONTINGENT UPON PASSING AN ANNUAL HEALTH ASSESSMENT THEREAFTER. CHARTER SUBURBAN HOSPITAL IS AN EQUAL OPPORTUNITY EMPLOYER.

_____   _____

SIGNATURE   DATE

FIGURE 49-3 *continued*

OBJECTIVE 6: PARTICIPATE IN A SUCCESSFUL INTERVIEW

Approach the interview in three steps.

1. Preparation
   - Plan what you will wear.
   - Do not overdress, but be neat and clean.
   - Check your clothes for loose or lost buttons or stains.
   - Be sure to take a bath and use deodorant.
   - Brush your teeth.
   - Make sure your fingernails are short and clean.
   - Polish your shoes.
   - Make sure your hair is neat.
   - If you have a beard or a mustache, be sure it is trimmed.
   - Do not chew gum.
   - Prepare a list of questions you want to ask.
   - Have your résumé in hand.
2. Actual interview
   - Be on time.
   - Offer a firm handshake.
   - Stand until you are invited to sit.
   - Remember that you are "selling" yourself.
   - Be careful of body language.
   - Share information willingly with the interviewer.
   - Use your list to learn information important to you such as:
     - Responsibilities (ask for a job description)
     - Hours of work
     - Uniform regulations
     - Opportunities for future assistance or financial aid to further your education
     - Starting salary
     - Fringe benefits such as health insurance
     - Schedule of raises
   - At the end of the interview, thank the interviewer, whether you are hired or not. Leave a copy of your résumé for future reference.
3. After the interview, when you get home
   - Write a short thank-you note to the person who interviewed you (Figure 49-4), thanking her for her time and the opportunity to be considered for the job.
   - Review the interview in your mind. Plan changes you would make to improve future interviews.

OBJECTIVE 7: ACCEPT A JOB

Before accepting a job, think carefully about your employer's expectations of your abilities and job performance. If you accept the job, you must be prepared to follow the policies and procedures of the facility. For example, if the interviewer told you that nursing assistants are scheduled to work every other weekend, do not take the job unless you are willing to do this. There are certain specific requirements you will have to complete as you begin your job, as we discuss in this section.

Orientation

Orientation is designed to help you safely perform the duties listed in your job description. It is mandatory and all new employees are required to attend. Keep in mind that even if you were hired to work an evening or night shift, orientation classes may be held during the day. Orientation generally consists of two parts. You will spend at least a day in the classroom learning about the policies and procedures of the employer (Figure 49-5). You will be given employee handbooks that you can refer to in the future. Information presented during the class may include:

- Policies for scheduling and making assignments
- What to do for fire and other emergencies
- How and when performance evaluations are completed
- The organizational chart of the facility
- Safety policies and procedures

A clinical orientation is provided on the nursing unit. An instructor, another nurse, or an experienced competent nursing assistant will work with you the first few days so that you may learn

- The routine of the unit
- The location of equipment and supplies
- How to do specific procedures as required by the employer

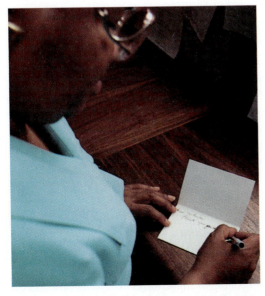

FIGURE 49-4 Write a thank-you note to the interviewer.

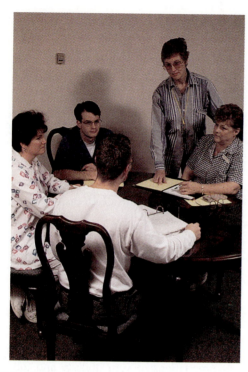

FIGURE 49-5 Orientation is an important part of your employment.

Health and Safety Requirements

State and federal regulations require new employees to:

- Obtain a physical examination within a specified number of days (some employers will require this before you begin work).
- Receive a two-step Mantoux (tuberculosis) test within a specified number of days (this too may be required before you begin work).
- Indicate whether they wish to receive the hepatitis B vaccine. Health care employers are required by law to offer this vaccination without cost to direct care employees. It is the employee's choice whether to take the vaccine. If the employee refuses it at the time of orientation, it can be given at another time if the employee changes her mind.

Some employers require employees to wear back supports while working. These are generally issued to you by the employer.

Health Care Worker Background Check

Some states require that a criminal background check be performed on all health care workers. If you work in one of these states, the procedure should be explained to you during the interview.

Drug Testing

Many employers require that drug testing be performed before you begin work. This procedure too should be explained during the interview.

Uniform Requirements

Most health care employers have uniform codes that indicate:

- Color and style of uniform to be worn on duty
- Acceptable jewelry that can be worn with the uniform
- Type of shoes and stockings that are safe to wear
- Acceptable hairstyles and make up (including whether nail polish is permitted)

Remember that these policies are for purposes of safety and infection control. Some employers will issue the uniforms to you either at no charge or for a charge that is deducted from your paycheck over a period of time.

OBJECTIVE 8: KEEP THE JOB

You can make your new position secure if you:

- Arrive on time prepared to work
- Follow the policies and procedures outlined in your orientation
- Follow the rules of ethical and legal conduct
- Recognize your limitations and seek help
- Have an open and positive attitude

OBJECTIVE 9: CONTINUE TO GROW THROUGHOUT YOUR CAREER

You will continue to grow if you take advantage of each new experience and opportunity you find.

- Keep your certificate current.
- Seek out knowledgeable staff members and watch and learn by their example.
- Do not be afraid to ask questions at appropriate times.
- Use the nursing medical literature to learn more about the patients' conditions.
- Participate in care conferences with an open mind so that each conference can be a learning experience for you.
- Complete 24 hours of continuing education each year (Figure 49-6).
- Investigate the possibilities of advancing your formal education by:
  - Enrolling in general education courses offered at the high school or college in your area.
  - Taking courses in communication, listening, English, and psychology.
  - Participating in in-service education programs at your facility or at nearby hospitals.
  - Enrolling in minicourses offered by hospitals on subjects of general public interest, such as hypertension, weight control, and diabetes.

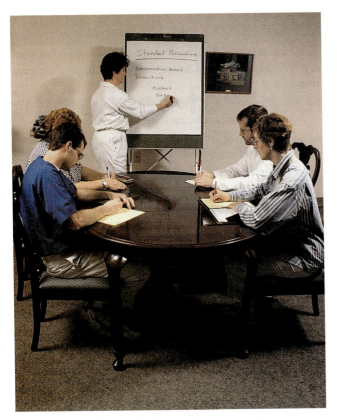

FIGURE 49-6 Take advantage of staff development programs to advance your education.

— Selecting books at the library that pertain to health issues.

— Researching programs that can prepare you for professional advancement into the ranks of LVN or RN.

OBJECTIVE 10: RESIGN PROPERLY FROM EMPLOYMENT

When you are ready to leave your present situation, you should do so pleasantly and properly.

- Give as much notice as possible—usually equal to the time of the pay period.
- Submit a letter of resignation and include:
  — Date
  — Salutation (greeting) to the director of nursing
  — Brief explanation of your reasons for leaving

 Note: Even if you feel upset by something that happened, make your reasons positive in nature.

  — Date your resignation is to be effective
  — Thank-you for the opportunity to have worked and grown with the experience of working in that facility
  — Your signature

REVIEW

A. True/False.

Mark the following true or false by circling T or F.

1. T F The employer may ask your religion during an interview.
2. T F In making a self-appraisal, you only need to list the things you could offer an employer.
3. T F What you wear to an interview is not important.
4. T F The availability of transportation should be considered when you are choosing a job.
5. T F The interview should provide you with information about the exact responsibilities you will have.
6. T F Checking for job possibilities with the administrator of the facility in which you had your clinical experience is proper.
7. T F If you fail to get the job after the interview, there is nothing left for you to do about the situation.
8. T F At the end of every interview, you should thank the interviewer, even if you did not get the job.
9. T F Participation in care conferences can be a way to continue to grow.

10. T F When resigning, give ample notice.

B. Multiple Choice.

Select the one best answer for each question.

11. The first step in finding a job is
    a. making phone calls.
    b. doing a self-assessment.
    c. looking in the paper.
    d. writing letters to friends.

12. Jobs can be found through
    a. classified ads.
    b. networking with friends.
    c. telephone directories.
    d. all of these.

13. A compilation of your work history is called a/an
    a. résumé.
    b. interview.
    c. summary.
    d. none of these.

Indications: Not routinely indicated for health care workers in the United States.

Major precautions: Vaccine safety in pregnant women has not been evaluated.

Special considerations: May be useful in certain outbreak situations.

Name: Polio vaccine

Primary/booster dose schedule: Two doses given 4-8 weeks apart followed by 3rd dose 6-12 months after 2nd dose.

Indications: Health care workers in close contact with persons who may be excreting virus and laboratory personnel who may be exposed to the virus.

Major precautions: Allergic reaction after receiving streptomycin or neomycin, pregnancy.

Special considerations: Use only inactivated polio vaccine for immunocompromised persons or workers who care for these patients.

Name: Rabies vaccine

Primary/booster dose schedule: Two different vaccines are given one each on days 0, 7, 21, or 28. Booster doses based on frequency of exposure.

Indications: Workers in contact with rabies virus or with infected animals in diagnostic or research activities.

Major precautions: None.

Special considerations: None.

Name: Tetanus and diphtheria (Td)

Primary/booster dose schedule: Two doses 4 weeks apart, 3rd dose 6-12 months after 2nd dose, booster every 10 years.

Indications: All adults, tetanus prophylaxis in wound management.

Major precautions: First trimester of pregnancy, history of neurological reaction or allergic reaction or severe local reaction.

Special considerations: None.

Name: Typhoid vaccine

Primary booster/dose schedule: One dose, booster doses depend on route of administration and rate of exposure.

Indications: Workers in laboratories who frequently work with Salmonella typhi.

Major precautions: History of severe local or systemic reaction, certain types of the vaccine should not be given to immunocompromised persons.

Special considerations: Vaccine should not be considered as an alternative to proper procedures.

Name: Vaccinia vaccine (smallpox)

Primary/booster dose schedule: One dose, boosters every 10 years.

Indications: Laboratory workers who work with animals or cultures with these viruses.

Major precautions: Pregnancy, presence or history of eczema, immunocompromised persons.

Special considerations: Vaccine may be considered for health care workers who have direct contact with contaminated dressings or other infectious material from volunteers in clinical studies involving the virus.

Postexposure Prophylaxis

Postexposure prophylaxis refers to actions that are taken after an employee is exposed to an infectious disease while working in the health care setting. The purpose of these measures is to prevent further transmission of infection. Postexposure prophylaxis through antibiotics or vaccines may be required for these diseases: diphtheria, hepatitis A, hepatitis B, meningococcal disease, pertussis (whooping cough), rabies and varicella-zoster virus. Work restrictions may be imposed on an employee after exposure or infection with infectious disease. Decisions on work restrictions are based on how the disease is transmitted and the epidemiology of the disease. Work restrictions may include any or all of these restrictions:

- patient contact.
- contact with patient's environment.
- food-handling.
- care of high-risk patients.
- care of infants, newborns.
- immunocompromised patients and their environments.
- performance of invasive procedures.
- exclude from duty (exclusion from the health care facility and from any health care activities outside the facility, no contact with susceptible persons in facility or in the community).
- Exposure or infection with any of these diseases may require work restrictions:
  - conjunctivitis (eye infection)
  - hepatitis A
  - hepatitis B
  - hepatitis C
  - herpes simplex
  - human immunodeficiency virus (HIV)
  - measles
  - rubella
  - streptococcal infection group A
  - varicella zoster
  - cytomegalovirus infections
  - diarrhea
  - diphtheria
  - enteroviral infections
  - meningococcal infections
  - mumps
  - pediculosis (lice)
  - pertussis

— scabies
— tuberculosis
— viral respiratory infections

Health Counseling

Health care workers should receive counseling regarding:

- the risk and prevention of infections acquired while working.
- the risk of illness or other problems after exposure to infectious disease.
- actions to take after exposure to infectious disease including postexposure prophylaxis procedures.
- possible consequences of exposure or diseases for family members, patients and other workers both inside and outside the health care facility.

Records

Employers must maintain records for all employees regarding medical evaluations, immunizations, exposures, postexposure prophylaxis, screening tests, and exposure to bloodborne pathogens. Employees have the right to review these records and to expect that all information in file is kept confidential. Information cannot be disclosed or reported without the written consent of the employee to any person within or outside the work place except as required by law.

INFECTIONS/INFECTIOUS DISEASES

Several infectious diseases are described in this section in addition to those included in the text on pages 125-128. Remember that standard precautions are followed with *all patients*. Isolation precautions may also be required. Follow your employer's procedures and policies. Anyone exposed to any of these diseases should report this fact to the proper facility authority before going to work. Work restrictions may be imposed, depending on the disease.

Conjunctivitis

Conjunctivitis (pink eye) is an infection of the clear membrane that covers the front of the eye and the inside of the eyelid. It may be caused by either bacteria or a virus. The eye is inflamed and there may be a purulent discharge. Contaminated hands are a major source of transmission. Handwashing, glove use, and disinfection of instruments can prevent transmission.

Cytomegalovirus

Cytomegalovirus (CMV) may be found in health care institutions, in infants and young children infected with the virus, and in immunocompromised patients such as persons with AIDS. The disease is transmitted through close, intimate contact, through contact with secretions or excretions like saliva or urine, or through the hands.

Diphtheria

Diphtheria is currently a rare disease in the United States since immunizations are given during infancy. It is caused by bacteria, affects the lining of the throat, and is highly contagious. The disease is transmitted by contact with respiratory droplets or contact with skin lesions of infected patients.

Acute Gastrointestinal Infections

Infections of the gastrointestinal tract may be caused by bacteria, virus, or protozoa. Symptoms include vomiting, diarrhea, or both, with or without fever, nausea, and abdominal pain. The microorganisms are transmitted through contact with infected individuals, or from consuming contaminated food, water, or other beverages. The most common gastrointestinal infection is that caused by Salmonella.

Herpes Simplex

The herpes simplex virus causes infections of the fingers and around the mouth (cold sores). The virus also causes genital herpes. There have been no reports that workers with genital herpes have transmitted the disease to patients. Transmission occurs through contact with lesions or secretions such as saliva, vaginal secretions, or amniotic fluid. Exposed areas of the skin are the most likely sites of infection, especially when cuts, abrasions or other skin lesions are present.

Measles

Measles is caused by a virus and is characterized by a rash on the body and fever. It is highly contagious. Measles is transmitted by large droplets during close contact with infected persons and by the airborne route. Workers born after 1957 should be considered immune to measles if they have had physician-diagnosed measles or appropriate vaccine on or after their first birthday, or have been proven immune through testing. Persons born and immunized between 1957 and 1984 were given only one dose of vaccine during infancy and may require a second dose. Persons born before 1957 are generally considered to be immune.

Meningococcal Disease

Transmission of meningococcal disease occurs through droplets during contact with respiratory secretions or through handling laboratory specimens. Transmission in health care settings is uncommon.

Mumps

Mumps (infection of parotid glands) is caused by a virus and is transmitted by droplets through contact with respiratory secretions, including saliva. Vaccination prevents mumps transmission. Workers are considered immune if they have had physician-diagnosed mumps, appropriate vaccination after their first birthday, or have been proven immune through testing. Persons born before 1957 may be considered immune.

Parvovirus

Parvovirus is the cause of erythema infectiosum (Fifth disease), a common rash illness that is usually acquired during childhood. The virus is transmitted through contact with infected persons, fomites, or large droplets. Transmission to workers from infected patients appears to be rare.

Pertussis

Pertussis (whooping cough) is caused by bacteria and is highly contagious. Symptoms include cough, mild fever, and loss of appetite. Transmission occurs by contact with respiratory secretions or large droplets from the respiratory tracts of infected persons.

Poliomyelitis

The last cases of acquired poliomyelitis were reported in 1979. Poliomyelitis is caused by a virus and is transmitted through contact with feces or urine of infected persons but can be spread by contact with respiratory secretions and in rare cases, through feces.

Rabies

Human rabies occurs primarily from exposure to rabid animals. Theoretically, rabies may be transmitted to health care workers from exposures to saliva from infected patients, but no cases have been documented to prove this.

Rubella

Rubella (three-day measles) is characterized by a rash and is transmitted by contact with droplets from the nose and throat of infected persons. Rubella is usually a mild disease but can cause congenital defects in the fetus of a pregnant woman. Persons are considered susceptible to rubella if they have not had appropriate immunization or if laboratory tests do not give evidence of immunity.

Scabies and Pediculosis

Scabies is caused by a mite that burrows into the skin, leaving "tracks". This results in intense itching. Scabies is easily transmitted through skin-to-skin contact. The disease is treated with applications of topical creams or lotions (scabicides).

Pediculosis (lice) may infest the human body, the human head, or the pubic area. Head lice are transmitted by head-to-head contact with infested fomites such as combs or brushes. Body lice are usually associated with poor personal hygiene and unclean environments and are transmitted by contact with the skin or clothing of an infested person. Pubic lice can also be found in the axilla, eyelashes, or eyebrows. Transmission is primarily through intimate or sexual contact.

Staphylococcus aureus

Staphylococcus aureus (staph) is a common bacterium that can cause infections in the skin, the lungs, the blood, and the urinary bladder. Food poisoning is frequently caused by staph. The major sources of staph are infected and colonized patients. A colonized patient is one who harbors the microorganism but has no symptoms. The most common sites are the nose, hands, axilla, perineum, and throat. Transmission of the bacteria usually occurs through the hands of the workers which can become contaminated by contact with colonized or infected body sites of patients. Staph infections are treated with antibiotics. In the last few years staph microorganisms have become resistant to many antibiotics. Methycillin staphylococcus aureus (MRSA) is an example. Infection with a resistant microorganism can be a dangerous situation for patients who are already at risk for infections.

Streptococcus, group A

Group A Streptococcus (GAS) can cause infections in the throat (strep throat), the skin, the blood, and other body organs. GAS can be transmitted from patients to health care workers after contact with infected secretions.

Vaccinia

The World Health Organization (WHO) declared the world free of smallpox in 1980. The smallpox vaccine is still available in the United States. Laboratory workers who are in contact with certain viruses need to be vaccinated every 10 years. Susceptible persons may acquire vaccinia from a recently vaccinated person through contact with the vaccination site for 2-21 days after vaccination. This can be prevented by covering the site and with thorough handwashing after contact with the site.

Varicella

Varicella (chickenpox) is caused by a virus and is characterized by blister like skin lesions. Herpes zoster (shingles) is caused by the same microorganism. Herpes zoster occurs in persons who have had chickenpox. The virus lies dormant in the body and later erupts in the form of shingles. The virus is transmitted by contact with infected lesions and in health care facilities. Airborne transmission has occurred from patients with chickenpox or shingles to susceptible persons who had no direct contact with the infected patient. Tests are available for determining a person's immunity to varicella. A vaccine was licensed for use in 1995.

Viral Respiratory Infections

Included in this group of infections are influenza and respiratory syncytial virus (RSV). There are several different viruses that can cause respiratory infections. Transmission is by person to person contact with an infected individual and by droplets. This may be from patients to workers, from workers to patients and between workers. Visitors may also be a source of infection. Persons at risk for complications include the elderly, residents of long-term care facilities, persons with chronic lung or heart problems, and persons with diabetes. Influenza vaccine given to health care workers before the beginning of the flu season can help reduce the risk of infection.

PREGNANT HEALTH CARE WORKERS

Pregnant health care workers are generally no more or no less at risk for acquiring work-related infections than are other workers. However, infections are of special concern to female health care workers of childbearing age for several reasons. Some infections may be more severe during pregnancy and some infections may affect the fetus. Women of childbearing age are strongly encouraged to receive immunizations for vaccine-preventable diseases before they are pregnant.

LATEX HYPERSENSITIVITY

The use of latex gloves has increased tremendously since the use of standard precautions has become routine in all health care settings. Along with increased use has come increased cases of hypersensitivity (allergic reactions) to latex among health care workers. However, less than 1% of the population is affected by latex allergy. Catheters, tubing, and condoms are other devices that also may contain latex and cause reactions in persons who are hypersensitive to latex. Latex contains proteins that may cause allergy. Persons who have hay fever, hand dermatitis, and allergies to foods such as bananas, avocados, kiwi fruit, and chestnuts have an increased risk for latex hypersensitivity. Local symptoms of allergy include itching, rash, and hives of the latex-exposed areas. Systemic symptoms include runny nose, sneezing, conjunctivitis, and asthma. Angioedema and anaphylactic reaction may occur in some cases. Tests are available to determine sensitivity to latex. Hypersensitive persons should use non-latex (vinyl) gloves or liners in the gloves that prevent the latex from coming in contact with the skin. Powder used for glove lubricant may contribute to sensitization so use of powder-free latex gloves may prevent symptoms of allergy.

Workplace restriction or reassignment may be necessary for workers with systemic symptoms of latex allergy.

AMERICANS WITH DISABILITIES ACT

The Americans with Disabilities Act affects infection control policies for health care workers as well as other disabilities. An employer can evaluate an applicant for their qualifications to perform the tasks required of the job for which they are being considered. The applicant may be asked about the ability to perform specific job functions but may not be asked about the existence, nature, or severity of a disability. Applicants with certain communicable diseases who are otherwise qualified for the job may justifiably be denied employment until they are no longer infectious.

INFECTION CONTROL PRACTICES

Unit 12 in the text describes the measures that are used to prevent the spread of infection. Remember that *standard precautions are used for **all patients**.* Special precautions are implemented when a patient has a known infectious disease. These precautions are based on the means by which the disease is transmitted. In addition to contact transmission, droplet transmission, and airborne transmision, there is common vehicle transmission (microorganisms transmitted by contaminated items such as food, water, medications, devices, and equipment) and vectorborne transmission (occurs when vectors such as mosquitoes, flies, rats, and other vermin transmit microorganisms).

The fundamentals of infectious disease prevention include: handwashing, gloving, patient placement, transport of infected patients, use of personal protective equipment, correct handling of equipment, supplies, and linens. These procedures are explained in Unit 12.

Glossary

abbreviation   shortened form of a word or phrase.

abdomen   area of the trunk between the thorax and the pelvis.

abduction   movement away from midline or center.

abuse   improper treatment or misuse.

accelerated   increased or faster motion, as in pulse or respiration.

acceptance   coming to terms with a situation and awaiting the outcome calmly; final stage of dying which some people, but not all, reach.

accommodation   adjustment.

acetone   colorless liquid produced during the metabolism of fats because glucose cannot be oxidized in the blood; has a sweet, fruity odor; appears in blood and urine of persons with diabetes.

acidosis   pathological condition resulting from accumulation of acid or depletion of alkaline reserves in the blood and body tissues.

acquired immune deficiency syndrome (AIDS)   a progressive disease of the immune system caused by the human immunodeficiency virus; initially an extremely high mortality rate was the norm for the disease; now combination drug therapy can slow the disease process and lengthen life expectancy of those infected with HIV.

activities of daily living (ADL)   the activities necessary to fulfill basic human needs.

acupuncture   placement of metal needles in the body to treat disease.

acute disease   disease that comes on suddenly, requires urgent treatment, and is usually resolved.

acute illness   illness that comes on suddenly; requires intense, immediate treatment.

adaptations   adjustments.

adaptive device   item altered to make it easier to use by those with functional deficits to perform any activity of daily living.

Addison's disease   disease caused by underfunctioning of the adrenal glands.

adduction   movement toward midline or center.

ADL.   *See* **activities of daily living**

admission   procedure carried out when a patient first arrives at a facility.

adolescence   teenage years.

adoptive parent   person who is a parent through a legal adoption procedure.

adrenal glands   endocrine glands; one is located on the top of each kidney; secrete hormones including epinephrine.

advance directive   document signed before the diagnosis is made of a terminal illness when the individual is still in good health, indicating the person's wishes regarding care during dying.

advocate   one who promotes the welfare of another.

afterbirth   *See* **placenta**

agency   business or company.

agent   person or substance by which something is accomplished.

agitation   mental state characterized by irregular and erratic behavior.

aiding and abetting   not reporting dishonest acts that are observed.

AIDS.   *See* **acquired immune deficiency syndrome**

airborne precautions   procedures used to prevent the spread of airborne pathogens.

airborne transmission   method of spreading disease by breathing tiny pathogens that remain suspended in the air for long periods of time.

akinesia   difficulty and slowness in carrying out voluntary muscular activities.

alcoholism   a dependency on alcohol.

alignment   keeping a patient's body in the proper position. *See* **body alignment**

allergen   substance that causes sensitivity or allergic reactions.

allergy   abnormal and individual hypersensitivity.

alopecia   absence of hair where hair normally grows.

alveoli   tiny air sacs that make up most of the lungs.

Alzheimer's disease   neurological condition in which there is a gradual loss of cerebral functioning.

ambulate   to walk.

ambulation   the process of walking.

AM care   care given in the early morning when the patient first awakens.

amenorrhea   without menstruation.

amino acids   basic components of proteins.

amniocentesis   transabdominal perforation of the amniotic sac to obtain a sample of the amniotic fluid.

amniotic fluid   fluid in which the fetus floats in the mother's womb.

amniotic sac   sac enclosing the fetus and amniotic fluid.

amputation   removal of a limb or other body appendage.

amulet   charm used to ward off evil.

anaphylactic shock   extreme, sometimes fatal, sensitivity or allergic reaction to a specific antigen.

anaphylaxis   severe, sometimes fatal, sensitivity reaction.

anatomic position   standing erect, facing observer, feet flat on floor and slightly separated, arms at sides, palms forward.

anatomy   study of the structure of the human body.

anemia   deficiency of quality or quantity of red blood cells in the blood.

aneroid gauge   device for measuring and registering blood pressure.

anesthesia   loss of feeling or sensation.

aneurysm   sac formed by dilation of the wall of a blood vessel (usually an artery); filled with blood.

anger   feeling of hostility, rage.

angina pectoris   acute pain in the chest caused by interference with the supply of oxygen to the heart.

anorexia   lack or loss of appetite for food.

anterior   in anatomy, in front of the coronal or ventral plane.

antibiotic   medication used to treat bacterial infection.

antibodies   proteins produced in the body in response to invasion by a foreign agent (antigen); react specifically with the foreign agent.

anti-embolism hose   elasticized stockings used to support the leg blood vessels.

antigen   marker on cells that identifies cell as self or nonself; antigens on foreign substances that enter the body, such as pathogens, stimulate the production of antibodies by the body.

apathy   indifference; lack of emotion.

Apgar score   method for determining an infant's condition at birth by scoring heart rate, respiratory effect, muscle tone, reflex irritability, and color.

aphasia   language impairment; loss of ability to comprehend normally.

apical pulse   pulse rate taken by placing stethoscope over tip of heart.

apnea   period of no respiration.

appliance   device used with colostomy or ileostomy to collect drainage from a stoma.

approaches   actions used by health care team to help resolve a patient's problems; steps taken to reach a goal.

Aquamatic K-Pad®   commercial unit for applying heat or cold.

arrest   to stop suddenly.

arteriosclerosis   general term meaning a narrowing of the blood vessels, which can result in subsequent tissue hypoxia and degeneration and hardening of the arterial walls and sometimes of the heart valves.

artery   vessel through which oxygenated blood passes away from the heart to various parts of the body.

arthritis   joint inflammation.

ascites   fluid accumulation in the abdomen.

asepsis   without infection.

aspirate   to withdraw.

aspiration   drawing of foreign materials into the respiratory tract.

assault   attempt or threat to do violence to another.

assessment   act of evaluating.

assignment   specific list of duties; tells you which patients you will care for during your shift and the specific procedures to be performed.

assimilate   to absorb.

assisted living   situation in which a person primarily cares for himself or herself but has some help in meeting health care needs; may reside in a facility that provides health care supervision.

assistive devices   equipment used to help people be more effective in their physical activity.

asthma   chronic respiratory disease characterized by bronchospasms and excessive mucus production.

atelectasis   collapse of lung tissue.

atheroma   degeneration or thickening of artery walls due to formation of fatty plaque and scar tissue.

atherosclerosis   degenerative process involving the lining of arteries, in which the lumen eventually narrows and closes; a form of arteriosclerosis.

atrium   one of the two upper chambers of the heart.

atrophy   shrinking or wasting away of tissues.

attitude   an external expression of inner feelings about self or others.

aura   peculiar sensation preceding the appearance of more definite symptoms in a convulsion or seizure.

auscultatory gap   sound fadeout for 1–15 mm Hg (mercury) pressure, after which sound begins again; sometimes mistaken for the diastolic pressure.

autoclave   machine that sterilizes articles.

autoimmune   presence of antibodies against component(s) of body.

autonomic nervous system   portion of the nervous system that controls the activities of the organs.

autonomy   self-determination.

autopsy   examination of body after death to determine cause of death.

axilla   armpit.

axon   extension of neuron that conducts nerve impulses away from the cell body.

bacillus (plural bacilli)   rod-shaped bacterium.

bacteremia   bacterial infection in the bloodstream; also known as *septicemia*.

bacterium (plural bacteria)   a form of simple microbes.

balance bar   section of an upright scale that holds the weights used to determine a patient's weight.

bargaining   stage of the grieving process in which the individual seeks to make a deal or form a pact that will delay death.

baseline   measurement of patient's vital signs or other body functions upon admission; future measurements are compared to baseline measurements to track the patient's progress.

baseline assessment   initial observations of the patient and his or her condition.

battery   an unlawful attack upon or touching of another person.

belief   idea based on commonly held opinions, knowledge, and attitudes.

benign   nonmalignant (tumor).

benign prostatic hypertrophy   noncancerous enlargement of prostate gland.

bile   substance produced by the liver that prepares fats for digestion.

biohazard   laboratory specimens or materials, and their containers contaminated by body fluids; these have the potential to transmit disease.

biological parent   natural parent who contributed sperm or an ovum to the development of the fetus.

biopsy   removal and examination of a piece of tissue from a living body.

bisexuality   having sexual interest in both genders.

blood pressure   pressure of blood exerted against vascular walls.

body alignment   position of a human body in which the body can properly function.

body core   center of the body (internal).

body language   use of facial expression, body positions, and vocal inflections to convey a message.

body mechanics   using muscles properly to move or lift heavy objects. *See also* **ergonomics**

body shell   outer surface of the body.

bolus   soft mass of food that is ready to be swallowed.

Bowman's capsule   tubule surrounding the glomerulus of the nephron.

box (square) corner   one type of corner used in the making of a hospital bed.

brachial artery   main artery of the arm.

bradycardia   unusually slow heartbeat.

braille   method of communication used by persons with visual impairments, who use fingertips to feel a series of raised dots representing letters and numbers.

brain attack   interference with the supply of blood to the brain; also known as *stroke* or *cerebral vascular accident.*

brain stem   base of the brain; enlarged extension of spinal cord, located in cranium; includes medulla oblongata, diencephalon, pons, and midbrain.

bridging   supporting the body on either side of an affected area to relieve pressure on the area.

bronchi   tubal structures connecting the trachea to the lungs.

bronchioles   smaller subdivisions or branches at end of the bronchi, located in the lungs.

bronchitis   inflammation of the bronchi.

burnout   loss of enthusiasm and interest in an activity.

bursae   small sacs of fluid found around joints.

bursitis   condition in which the bursae become inflamed and the joint becomes very painful.

cachexia   state of malnutrition, emaciation, and debility, usually in the course of a prolonged illness.

capillary   hairlike blood vessel; link between arterioles and venules.

carbohydrates   energy foods; used by the body to produce heat and energy for work.

carbon dioxide   gas that is a waste product in cellular metabolism.

carcinoma   malignant tumor made up of connective tissue enclosing epithelial cells.

cardiac arrest   sudden and often unexpected stoppage of effective heart action.

cardiac cycle   all (mechanical and electrical) events that occur between one heart contraction and the next.

cardiac decompensation   another name for congestive heart failure.

cardiac muscle   muscle that forms the heart wall.

cardiopulmonary resuscitation (CPR)   emergency medical procedure undertaken to restart and sustain heart and respiratory functions.

care plan   nursing plan for care of a resident in a long-term care facility.

care plan conference   meeting of members of an interdisciplinary health care team to develop approaches and a plan of care.

caries   tooth decay or cavities.

carrier   person who hosts infectious organisms without having symptoms of disease.

cartilage   type of body tissue.

cataract   opacity of the lens of the eye, resulting in loss of vision.

catastrophic reaction   severe and unpredictable violent behavior of a person with dementia.

catheter   tube for evacuating or injecting fluids.

causative agent   etiology of a specific disease process.

cavity   enclosed area; space within the body that contains organs.

celibate   has no sexual intercourse.

cell   basic unit in the organization of living substances.

cellulose   basic substance of all plant foods, which can supply the body with roughage.

Celsius scale   scale for measuring temperature.

centimeter   one-hundredth of a meter.

central venous (CV) catheter   tube inserted into large vein in area of clavicle.

cerebellum   portion of the brain lying beneath the occipital lobe; coordinates muscular activities and balance.

cerebrospinal fluid (CSF)   water cushion protecting the brain and spinal cord from shock.

cerebrovascular accident (CVA)   more commonly called *brain attack* or *stroke*; disorder of the blood vessels of the brain resulting in impaired cerebral circulation and often causing motor and cognitive deficits.

cerebrum   largest part of the brain, consisting of two hemispheres separated by a deep longitudinal fissure; controls all mental activities.

cervical traction   use of weights to apply traction in area of cervical vertebrae.

cesarean   method of delivering fetus through surgical incision in abdominal wall and uterus.

chain of infection   process of events involved in the transmission and development of an infectious disease.

chancre   shallow, craterlike lesion; primary lesion of syphilis.

charting   entering information (documentation) in a patient's medical record (chart).

chemical restraint   use of medications to control behavior.

chemotherapy   use of medications to treat disease.

Cheyne-Stokes respiration   periods of apnea alternating with periods of dyspnea.

CHF.   *See* **congestive heart failure**

chlamydia   type of sexually transmitted disease.

cholecystectomy   surgical removal of a diseased gallbladder and stones.

cholecystitis   inflammation of the gallbladder.

cholelithiasis   formation of stones in the gallbladder.

chronic   persisting over a long period of time.

chronic disease or **illness**   incurable illness or disease, but treatable; requires ongoing care.

chronic obstructive pulmonary disease (COPD)   any condition, such as emphysema or bronchitis, that interferes with normal respiration over a long period of time.

chronologic   in sequential order by date or age.

chyme   semiliquid form of food as it leaves the stomach.

chymopapain   an enzyme used to dissolve the protein in a ruptured disc.

CircOlectric® bed   special kind of bed used when a patient cannot be turned within the bed.

circumcision   removal of the end of the prepuce by a circular incision.

clear liquid diet   diet of water and high-carbohydrate fluids given every 2 to 4 hours.

client   person receiving care; depending upon the health care setting, also known as *patient* or *resident.*

client care record   documentation of care provided in the home situation.

Client's Rights   document spelling out rights of persons receiving home health care.

climacteric   menopause; the combined phenomena accompanying cessation of the reproductive function in the female or reduction of testicular activity in the male.

clinical thermometer   instrument used to measure body temperature.

clitoris   small, cylindrical mass of erotic tissue; part of the external female reproductive organs analogous to the penis in the male.

closed bed   bed with sheets and spread positioned to the head of the bed; unoccupied.

closed (oblique) fracture   fracture in which bones remain in proper alignment.

coccus (plural cocci)   round bacteria.

cochlea   spiral-shaped organ in inner ear that receives and interprets sounds.

cognitive impairment   deficit in intellect, memory, or attention.

coitus   sexual intercourse; copulation.

colon   large intestine.

colony   group of organisms derived from a single organism.

colostomy   artificial opening in the abdomen for the purpose of evacuation of feces.

colostrum   secretion from the lactiferous glands of the mother before the onset of true lactation two or three days after delivery of a baby.

colporrhaphy   suturing of the vagina; surgical procedure used to tighten vaginal walls.

combining form   word part that can be used with other word parts to form a variety of new words.

comminuted fracture   fracture in which the bone is broken or crushed into small pieces.

communicable disease   disease caused by pathogenic organism; can be transmitted from person to person, either directly or indirectly.

communication   exchange of messages.

community   people who live in a common area and share common health needs.

compensate   to seek a substitute for something unattainable or unacceptable.

complication   situation that makes original condition more serious.

compound (open) fracture   fracture in which part of the broken bone protrudes through the skin.

compression fracture   break in a bone with crushing of the bone fragments.

concurrent cleaning   daily, routine cleaning of patient unit.

condom   latex sheath that fits over the penis; used for urinary drainage when connected to a urinary collection bag.

confidential   keeping what is said or written to oneself; private; not shared.

congenital   condition present at birth.

congestive heart failure (CHF)   condition resulting from cardiac output inadequate for physiological needs, with shortness of breath, edema, and abnormal retention of sodium and water in body tissues.

conjunctiva   mucous membrane that lines the eyelids and covers the eye.

connective tissue   tissue that holds other tissues together and provides support for organs and other body structures.

connective tissue cells   cells that form connective tissue.

constipation   difficulty in defecating.

constriction   narrowing; compression.

contact precautions   practices used to prevent spread of disease by direct or indirect contact.

contact transmission   spread of disease by direct or indirect contact with infected person or contaminated objects.

contagious   communicable or easily spread.

contagious disease   disease that is communicable; disease that is caused by a pathogenic organism.

contaminated   unclean; impure; soiled with microbes.

contamination   process of exposing articles to known pathogens.

continent   able to control elimination of feces and urine.

continuum   continuous related series of events or actions.

contracture   permanent shortening or contraction of a muscle due to spasm or paralysis.

contraindicated   not recommended; disallowed; situation in which a remedy or treatment is not called for because of the patient's condition.

convulsion   involuntary muscle spasm.

COPD.   *See* **chronic obstructive pulmonary disease**

coping   handling or dealing with stress.

cornea   transparent portion of the eye through which light passes.

coronary embolism   blood clot lodged in a coronary artery.

coronary occlusion   closing off of a coronary artery.

coronary thrombosis   blood clot within a coronary vessel.

corporal punishment   use of painful treatment to correct behavior.

cortex   outer portion of a kidney.

countertraction   providing opposing balance to traction; used in reduction of fractures.

Cowper's glands   pair of small glands that open into the urethra at the base of the penis; part of the male reproductive system.

CPR.   *See* **cardiopulmonary resuscitation**

critical list   list that patients are placed on when they are dangerously or terminally ill.

cross-trained   educated in many different skills across (health care) disciplines.

crust   scab made of dried exudate.

CSF.   *See* **cerebrospinal fluid**

culture   views and traditions of a particular group.

culture and sensitivity   test to determine type of microorganisms causing a disease and the specific antibiotics that can be used to treat the disease.

Cushing's syndrome   condition that results from an excess level of adrenal cortex hormones.

cutaneous membrane   skin.

cuticle   base of the fingernail.

CVA.   *See* **cerebrovascular accident**

CV catheter.   *See* **central venous catheter**

cyanosis   dusky, bluish discoloration of skin, lips, and nails caused by inadequate oxygen.

cyanotic   relating to the condition of cyanosis.

cystitis   inflammation of the urinary bladder.

cystocele   bladder hernia.

cystoscopy   procedure that uses an instrument (cytoscope) for visualization of the urinary bladder, ureter, and kidney.

D & C.   *See* **dilatation and curettage**

dangling   sitting up with legs hanging over the edge of the bed.

debilitating   weakening.

debride   to remove foreign material and necrotic tissue.

defamation   something harmful to the good name or reputation of another person; slander.

defecation   bowel movement that expels feces.

defense mechanism   psychological reaction or technique for protection against a stressful environmental situation or anxiety.

degenerative joint disease (DJD)   deterioration of the tissues of the joints.

dehydration   excessive water loss.

delusion   false belief.

dementia   progressive mental deterioration due to organic brain disease.

dendrite   branch of a neuron that conducts impulses toward the cell body.

denial   unconscious defense mechanism in which an occurrence or observation is refused recognition as reality in order to avoid anxiety or pain.

dentures   artificial teeth.

depilatory   substance used to remove body hair.

depressant   drug that slows down body functions.

depression   morbid sadness or melancholy.

dermal ulcer   pressure sore; pressure ulcer.

dermis   layer of tissue that lies under the epidermis.

development   gradual growth.

developmental milestones   achievement of specific skills at a particular age level.

developmental tasks   in psychology, normal steps in personality development.

diabetes mellitus   disorder of carbohydrate metabolism.

diagnosis related groups (DRGs)   method used by Medicare to determine number of hospital days required by specific illnesses.

dialect   local terminology and usage of a group's common language.

dialysis   movement of dissolved materials through a semipermeable membrane, passing from an area of higher concentration to an area of lower concentration; means of cleansing waste or toxic materials from the body.

diaphoresis   profuse sweating.

diastole   period during which the heart muscle relaxes and the chamber fills with blood.

diastolic pressure   blood pressure during period of cardiac ventricular relaxation.

diathermy   treatment with heat.

digestion   process of converting food into a form that can be used by the body.

digital thermometer   hand-held, battery-operated device that registers temperature and displays reading as numbers.

dilatation and curettage (D & C)   procedure in which cervical canal is expanded and tissue is scraped from the lining of the uterus.

dilation stage   stage of labor in which the opening to the cervix enlarges.

diplo-   arranged in pairs, such as diplococci (bacteria that are arranged in groups of two).

dirty   anything that has been exposed to pathogens.

disability   persistent physical or mental deficit or handicap.

discharge   procedure carried out as a patient leaves the facility.

disease   definite, marked process of illness having characteristic symptoms.

disinfection   process of eliminating pathogens from equipment and instruments.

dislocation   displacement of the ends of a joint.

disorientation   loss of recognition of time, place, or people.

disposable   not reusable after one use.

disruption   interference with the normal progress of events.

distal   farthest away from a central point, such as point of attachment of muscles.

distention   the state of being stretched out (distended).

disuse osteoporosis   loss of calcium from bones due to immobility or inactivity.

diuresis   increase in output of fluids by the kidneys.

diverticula   small blind pouches that form in the lining and wall of the colon.

diverticulitis   inflammation of diverticula.

diverticulosis   presence of many diverticula.

DJD.   *See* **degenerative joint disease**

DNR   do not resuscitate when cardiac and respiratory arrest occur.

document   legal record; recording observations and data about a patient's condition.

dorsal   posterior or back.

dorsal lithotomy position   position in which the patient is on the back with knees flexed and well separated; feet are usually placed in stirrups.

dorsal recumbent position   position in which the patient is flat on the back with knees flexed and slightly separated, with feet flat on bed.

dorsiflexion   toes pointed up.

douche   irrigation of vaginal canal with medicated or normal saline solution.

drainage   systematic withdrawal of fluids and discharges from wounds, sores, or body cavities.

draw sheet   sheet folded under the patient, extending from above the shoulder to below the hips.

DRGs.   *See* **diagnosis related groups**

droplet precautions   procedures used to prevent spread of disease by droplets in air.

droplet transmission   a method of spreading infection by inhaling the droplets of a patient's respiratory secretions. The droplets do not travel more than three feet from the source patient.

duodenal resection   surgical removal of a portion of small intestine (duodenum).

duodenal ulcer   ulcer on the mucosa of the duodenum due to the action of gastric juice.

durable power of attorney for health care   document stating that a person appointed by the patient can make health care decisions when the patient is unable to do so for himself or herself.

dyscrasia   abnormality or disorder of the body.

dysentery   infection in lower bowel.

dysmenorrhea   painful menstruation.

dyspnea   difficult or labored breathing.

dysuria   painful voiding.

edema   excessive accumulation of fluid in the tissues.

efface   thinning of the cervix during labor.

ejaculatory duct   part of male reproductive system extending down from the seminal vesicles to the urethra.

elasticity   ability to stretch.

electric bed   bed operated by electricity.

electronic thermometer   battery-operated clinical thermometer that uses a probe and records the temperature on a viewing screen in a few seconds.

embolus   mass of undissolved material carried in the bloodstream; frequently causes obstruction of a vessel.

emergency   situation requiring immediate attention or medical treatment.

emergency care   medical treatment and nursing care provided to emergency patients.

Emergency Medical Services (EMS)   treatment and care

provided by specially trained health care personnel during emergencies.

emesis   vomiting.

emotional lability   unstable emotional status with frequent changes in emotions and mood.

emphysema   chronic obstructive pulmonary disease in which the alveolar walls are destroyed.

EMS.   *See* **Emergency Medical Services**

endocardium   lining of the heart.

endocrine gland   gland that secretes hormonal substances directly into the bloodstream; ductless gland.

endometrium   mucous membrane lining the inner surface of the uterus.

endoscope   instrument for examining the interior of the body.

enema   injection of water and/or medications into the rectum and colon; used to help the bowels eliminate feces.

engagement   time when fetus moves downward in the uterus in preparation for delivery (dropping).

enteral feeding   giving nutrition through a tube inserted into the digestive tract.

environmental safety   adaptation of the environment to prevent incidents and injuries.

epidermis   top layer of skin.

epididymis   elongated, cordlike structure along the posterior border of the testes, in the ducts of which sperm is stored.

epidural catheter   tube inserted into spinal area for delivery of medication.

epilepsy   noninfectious disorder of the brain manifested by episodes of motor and sensory dysfunction, which may or may not be accompanied by convulsions and unconsciousness.

episiotomy   incision of the perineum at the end of the second stage of labor to avoid tearing of the perineum.

epithelial cells   structures that form protective coverings (epithelial tissue) and sometimes produce body fluids.

epithelial tissue   structure formed from epithelial cells; protects, absorbs and produces fluids, excretes wastes.

ergonomics   process of adapting the environment and using techniques and equipment to prevent worker injuries.

erythrocyte   red blood cell.

eschar   slough of tissue produced by burning or by a corrosive application.

essential nutrients   foods required for normal growth and development and to maintain health.

estrogen   hormone produced by the ovaries.

ethical standards   guides to moral behavior.

ethnic   relating to customs, languages, and traditions of specific groups of people.

ethnicity   special groupings within a race.

etiology   cause of a disease.

eustachian tube   auditory tube; leads from the middle ear to the pharynx.

evaluation   judgment.

eversion   turning outward.

exchange list   list of measured foods that allows equivalent exchanges between foods within a designated food group.

excoriation   superficial loss of substance, such as that produced by scratching the skin.

excrete   to eliminate wastes from body.

expectorate   to spit (to bring up sputum).

expiration   exhalation.

exposure incident   an occurrence during which there is possible personal contact with infectious material.

expressive aphasia   inability to use verbal speech.

expulsion stage   stage of labor and delivery during which the fetus is expelled.

extension   movement by which the two ends of any jointed part are drawn away from each other.

face shield   type of personal protective equipment; protects mucous membranes of eyes, nose, and mouth from pathogens.

facility (health care)   an agency that provides health care.

Fahrenheit scale   system used in the United States and England to express temperature.

fallopian tube.   *See* **oviduct**

false imprisonment   unlawfully restraining another.

family   group of persons (usually related by blood or marriage) with common values and traditions.

fasting   not eating.

fat   nutrient used to store energy.

fecal   pertaining to feces (solid waste from digestive tract).

feces   stool; semisolid waste eliminated from the body.

fetal monitor   device used to register activity and health status of unborn fetus during labor.

fetoscopy   examination of the fetus while in the uterus.

fetus   child in the uterus from the third month to birth.

first aid   emergency care and treatment of an injured person before complete medical and surgical care can be secured.

fistula   abnormal communication between two hollow organs or between a hollow organ and the exterior.

flagged   marked in a special way to call attention to it.

flatulence   excessive gas in the stomach and intestines.

flatus   gas or air in the stomach or intestines; air or gas expelled by way of any body opening.

flexion   decreasing the angle between two bones.

flora   normal population of organisms found in a given area.

flow sheet   clinical record of ongoing patient care and progress.

fluid balance   balance between fluid intake and fluid output.

Foley catheter   indwelling catheter placed in the urinary bladder to remove urine continuously.

fomite   any object contaminated with germs and thus able to transmit disease.

footboard   appliance placed at the foot of the bed so the feet rest firmly against it and are at right angles to the legs.

foot drop   tightening of leg muscles that causes the foot to point downward.

force fluids   notation meaning that the patient must be encouraged to take as much fluid as possible.

foreskin   prepuce; loose tissue covering the penis and clitoris.

foster parent   parent figure assigned by an agency.

Fowler's position   position in which the patient lies on the back with back rest elevated 45 to 60 degrees.

fracture   break in the continuity of bone.

full liquid diet   diet consisting of all types of fluids.

full weight bearing   able to stand on both legs.

fundus   portion of uterus above the point of entrance of the oviducts.

fungus (plural fungi)   class of organisms to which molds and yeasts belong.

fusion   combination into a single unit.

gait   manner of walking.

gait belt   belt placed around the patient's waist to assist in ambulation.

gait training   teaching patient to walk.

gastrectomy   surgical removal of part or all of stomach.

gastric resection   surgical removal of part of stomach.

gastric ulcer   erosion of lining of stomach.

gastroscopy   procedure to examine the inside of the stomach, using a scope for visualization.

gastrostomy feeding   nutrition given through a tube inserted into the stomach through the abdominal wall.

gatch bed   bed fitted with a jointed back rest and knee rest; patient can be raised to a sitting position and kept in that position.

general anesthetic   medication that induces a state of unconsciousness and reduces or eliminates ability to feel pain.

genetic   pertaining to or carried by a gene or genes.

genitalia   reproductive organs.

geriatrics   care of the elderly.

gestational age   age of development of a new individual within the uterus from conception to birth.

global aphasia   loss of all language ability.

glomerulus   blood vessels that branch to form a ball of capillaries in the cortex of the kidney.

glucagon   hormone produced by pancreas that increases blood sugar level.

glucose   simple sugar; also called *dextrose*.

glycogen   polysaccharide that is the chief carbohydrate storage material.

glycosuria   sugar in the urine.

goal   an outcome resulting from implementation of a care plan.

goggles   type of personal protective equipment used with standard precautions to protect the eyes.

gonads   reproductive organs; ovaries and testes.

gonorrhea   sexually transmitted disease that causes an acute inflammation.

graduate   container marked for milliliters, used to measure liquids.

graft   body tissue used for transplantation.

grand mal seizure   major epileptic seizure attended by loss of consciousness and convulsive movements.

greenstick fracture   breaking of a bone on one side only; most often seen in children.

grievance   situation in which consumer feels there are grounds for complaint.

growth   physical changes that take place in body during development.

halitosis   bad breath.

handicap   inability of person to fulfill a normal role due to disability.

hand-over-hand technique   method in which an instructor or caregiver places his or her hand over the hand of a learner or patient to guide an activity.

harvest   to remove donor organs.

health   state of physical, mental, and social well-being.

health care consumer   person requiring health care services.

health maintenance organization (HMO)   one type of prepaid health insurance provider.

heart block   condition in which conduction of electrical impulses from atrium to ventricles is impaired and pumping action of heart is slowed down (change in rhythm of heart).

Heimlich maneuver   procedure that uses abdominal thrusts to relieve obstruction in the trachea.

hematuria   blood in the urine.

hemianopsia   visual impairment due to stroke; affects one-half of visual field in one or both eyes.

hemiplegia   paralysis on one side of the body.

hemodialysis   method for circulating blood through semipermeable membranes to remove liquid body wastes.

hemoptysis   expectoration of blood.

hemorrhage   escape of blood from blood vessels.

hemorrhoids   varicose veins in the rectum.

HEPA.   *See* **high efficiency particulate air respirator**

hepatitis   inflammation of liver.

hernia   protrusion or projection of a stomach organ through the wall or cavity that normally contains it.

herniorrhaphy   surgical operation for hernia.

herpes simplex II   an acute infectious viral disease.

heterosexuality   sexual attraction between persons of opposite genders.

high efficiency particulate air (HEPA) respirator   a mask used by health care workers that prevents the spread of airborne infection.

high Fowler's position   position in which back rest of bed is elevated to 90 degrees, with patient on back.

HIV.   *See* **human immunodeficiency virus**

HMO.   *See* **health maintenance organization**

home health aide   nursing assistant who works in a client's home to provide health care services.

home health assistant   nursing assistant who practices under supervision in a client's home.

homemaker aide   person hired to perform light housekeeping tasks in a client's home.

homemaker assistant   person who provides home management help to a client in the client's home.

homosexuality   sexual attraction between persons of the same gender.

hormone   secretion of endocrine gland; substance produced by an endocrine gland.

hospice   special facility or arrangement to provide care of terminally ill persons.

hospice care   health care for persons who are dying.

hospital   facility for care of the sick or injured.

host   animal or plant that harbors another organism.

human immunodeficiency virus (HIV)   virus that causes acquired immune deficiency disease (AIDS).

hydrochloric acid   acid produced by the stomach.

hydronephrosis   increased pressure of urine on the kidney cells that results in their destruction.

hyperalimentation   technique in which high-density nutrients are introduced into a large vein.

hypercalcemia   excess calcium in the bloodstream.

hyperglycemia   excessive level of blood sugar.

hypersecretion   excessive secretion.

hypersensitivity   state of altered reactivity in which the body reacts to a foreign agent more strongly than normal or in an abnormal way.

hypertension   high blood pressure.

hyperthyroidism   excessive functioning of the thyroid gland.

hypertrophy   increase in the size of an organ or structure that does not involve tumor formation.

hypochondriasis   abnormal concern about one's health.

hypoglycemia   abnormally low level of sugar in the blood.

hyposecretion   less than normal production of secretions.

hypotension   low blood pressure.

hypothermia   greatly reduced temperature.

hypothermia-hyperthermia blanket   a fluid-filled blanket, the temperature of which can be raised or lowered.

hypothyroidism   condition due to deficiency of thyroid secretion, resulting in a lower basal metabolism.

hypoxia   lack of adequate oxygen supply.

hysterectomy   surgical removal of the uterus.

ice bag   type of cold treatment.

IDDM.   *See* **insulin-dependent diabetes mellitus**

ileostomy   incision in the ileum.

immune response   response of the body to elements recognized as nonself, with the production of antibodies and rejection of the foreign material.

immunity   ability to fight off infectious disease; state of being protected from a disease.

immunization   process of making a person more resistant to an infectious agent.

immunosuppression   condition in which the immune system is unable to respond to the challenge of infectious disease.

impaction   condition of being tightly wedged into a part (as feces in the bowel).

implementation   putting into effect.

incarcerated (strangulated) hernia   abnormal constriction of part of the intestinal tract that has herniated.

incentive spirometer   apparatus used to encourage better ventilation.

incident   unexpected situation that can cause harm to a patient, employee, or visitor.

incident report   summary of information about an incident.

increment   amount of increase in measurements.

incubation   development of bacteria in body between time of exposure and onset of signs and symptoms.

indwelling catheter   Foley catheter that remains in the patient's bladder to drain urine.

infarction   death of tissue.

infection   invasion and multiplication of any organism and the damage this causes in the body.

infectious   capable of transmitting disease.

inferior   below another part.

inflammation   tissue reaction to injury, either direct or referred.

informed consent   permission given after full disclosure of the facts.

initiative   action of taking the first step or initial action.

insertion   distal point of attachment of skeletal muscle.

inspiration   drawing of air into the lungs; inhalation.

insulin   active antidiabetic hormone secreted by the islets of Langerhans in the pancreas.

insulin-dependent diabetes mellitus (IDDM)   form of diabetes mellitus that requires insulin administration as part of the therapy.

intake and output (I&O)   recording of the amount of fluid ingested and the amount of fluid expelled by a patient.

integument   the skin.

intention tremor   involuntary movement of muscles (particularly hands) that increases when the patient attempts to use the muscles.

interdisciplinary health care team   group of professionals from different health care disciplines who each contribute their expertise to the care of a single patient.

intermediate care   health care provided to persons with medically stable conditions.

intermittent care   care given periodically, at intervals.

interpersonal relationships   how people interact with each other.

intervention   actions that influence the eventual outcome of a situation.

intimacy   feelings of closeness and familiarity.

intracranial pressure   pressure exerted within the cranium.

intravenous infusion   nourishment given through a sterile tube into a vein.

intravenous pyelogram (IVP)   x-ray of urinary tract following injection of dye into vein.

invasion of privacy   taking liberties with the person or personal rights of another.

invasive   characterized by invading or spreading.

inversion   turning inward.

involuntary muscle   muscle not under conscious control, mainly smooth muscle.

involuntary seclusion   separation of patient from other patients and people, against the patient's will.

involution   reduction in the size of the uterus following delivery.

I&O.   *See* **intake and output**

iodine   element needed for proper function of the thyroid gland.

iris   colored portion of the eye.

ischemia   deficient blood supply to body tissues.

ischemic   having inadequate blood flow to an area.

islets of Langerhans   cells in the pancreas that produce insulin.

isolation   place where a patient with easily transmitted disease is separated from others.

isolation technique   special procedures carried out to prevent the spread of infectious organisms from an infected person.

isolation unit   used for patients with communicable illness, for protection of other patients, staff, and visitors.

isolette   environmentally controlled unit used to house a newborn infant.

IVP.   *See* **intravenous pyelogram**

job interview   discussion between employer and potential employee.

Kardex   type of file in which nursing care plans are kept.

ketosis   abnormal levels of ketones in the blood; complication of diabetes mellitus.

kidney   glandular, bean-shaped organ, purplish-brown in color, situated in back of the abdominal cavity, one on each side of the spinal column; excretes waste matter in the form of urine.

kilogram   metric unit of weight measurement, equal to 1,000 grams or 2.2 pounds.

knee-chest position   position in which the patient is on the abdomen with knees drawn up toward the abdomen and with legs separated; arms are brought up and flexed on either side of the head, which is turned to one side.

labia majora   two large, hair-covered, liplike structures that are part of the vulva.

labia minora   two hairless, liplike structures found beneath the labia majora.

labor   physiologic process by which the fetus is expelled from the uterus at term.

laceration   accidental break in skin, an injury.

lacrimal gland   produces tears.

lactation   secretion of milk.

laminectomy   surgical excision of rear part of one or more vertebrae, usually to remove herniated disk or lesion.

larynx   organ located at upper end of trachea; part of airway and organ of voice (voice box).

lateral   away from the midline.

legal custody   condition of having the responsibility for another person (including the right to consent to hospitalization and to give permission for procedures).

legal guardian   person who has the legal right to make decisions for another person.

legal standards   guides to lawful behavior.

lesions   abnormal changes in tissue formation.

leukemia   malignant disease of the blood-forming organs, characterized by abnormal proliferation and distortion of the leukocytes in the blood and bone marrow.

leukocyte   white blood cell.

leukorrhea   white vaginal discharge.

Lhermitte's sign   sharp, electrical-type sensation felt down spine when head is flexed; found in patients with multiple sclerosis.

liable   legally responsible.

libel   any written defamatory statement.

licensed practical nurse (LPN); licensed vocational nurse (LVN)   graduate of a one-year certificate program, who must pass a state exam before being permitted to practice nursing.

life-sustaining treatment   treatment given to a critically ill or injured patient to maintain life and prevent death.

ligament   band of fibrous tissue that holds joints together.

lithotripsy   the crushing of calculi such as kidney stones.

living will   document describing the wishes of a terminally ill person, relating to health care.

local anesthetic   substance that blocks pain receptors or sensation in a specific area.

lochia   discharge from the uterus of blood, mucus, and tissue during the puerperal period.

long-term care   health care given to a person in a facility or the person's home for an extended period of time.

LPN.   *See* **licensed practical nurse**

lumpectomy   excision of abnormal tissue, such as a "lump" in the breast.

LVN.   *See* **licensed vocational nurse**

lymph   fluid found in lymphatic vessels.

lymphatic vessel   vessel that conveys electrolytes, water, and proteins.

macular degeneration   vision impairment due to damage to the macula located at the back of the eye, generally related to aging.

macule   flat, discolored spot on the skin.

maladaptive behavior   inappropriate reaction due to mental breakdown.

malignant   cancerous.

mammogram   x-ray examination of the breasts.

managed care   methods used by insurance companies to reduce health care costs.

mastectomy   excision of the breast.

masturbation   sexually stimulating self.

Material Safety Data Sheet (MSDS)   information provided by manufacturers about hazardous products; includes health hazards, safe use guidelines, and emergency procedures for chemical exposure.

mechanical lift   apparatus used to assist in lifting and transferring a patient.

medial   close to the midline of the body or structure.

Medicaid   federal- and state-funded program that pays medical expenses for those whose income is below a certain level.

medical asepsis   procedures followed to keep germs from being spread from one person to another.

medical chart   patient record containing all information about that patient.

medical diagnosis   name of disease; determination made by a physician.

Medicare   federal program that assists persons over 65 years of age with hospital and medical costs.

medulla   forms part of the brain stem; also, the middle area of the kidney.

membranes   tissue sheets that line the body cavities.

memo   brief, written communication to relay information.

meninges   three-layered serous membranes covering the brain and spinal cord.

meningitis   inflammation of the meninges.

menopause   period when ovaries stop functioning and menstruation ceases; female climacteric.

menorrhagia   excessive bleeding during menstruation.

menstruation   loss of an unneeded part of the endometrium following the release of an ovum and lack of conception.

mental illness   behavioral maladaptations.

metabolism   sum total of the physical and chemical processes and reactions taking place in the body.

metastasize   to spread (cancer) to other body parts.

methicillin-resistant *Staphylococcus aureus* **(MRSA)**   bacteria resistant to most antibiotics.

metrorrhagia   abnormal discharge from the uterus.

MI.   *See* **myocardial infarction**

microbe   tiny organism that can be seen only with a microscope.

microorganism   tiny organism that can be seen only with a microscope, particularly bacteria.

mineral   inorganic chemical compound found in nature; many minerals are important in building body tissues and regulating body fluids.

mitered corner   one type of corner used in making a facility bed.

mobility   ability to move or to be moved easily from place to place.

mobility skills   ability to move about in bed, out of bed, and walking.

mold   organism in fungus family.

morbidity   state of being diseased; conditions inducing disease.

mores   customs of ethnic groups.

moribund   dying.

mortality   incidence of death in a population.

MRSA.   *See* **methicillin-resistant** *Staphylococcus aureus*

MSDS.   *See* **Material Safety Data Sheet**

mucous membrane   epithelial tissue that produces fluid called mucus; lines body cavities that open to the outside of the body.

mucus   secretion of mucous membranes; thick, sticky fluid.

multiple sclerosis   disease characterized by hardened patches scattered throughout the brain and spinal cord that interfere with the nerves in those areas.

muscle cells   form muscle tissue; have ability to shorten or lengthen and to change their shape and the position of parts to which they are attached.

muscle tissue   tissue that has the ability to shorten and lengthen.

myocardial infarction (MI)   formation of an infarct in the heart muscle due to interruption of the blood supply to the area.

myocardium   heart muscle.

N95 respirator   mask with small, tightly woven pores that protects the wearer from airborne infection.

NACEP.   *See* **Nurse Aide Competency Evaluation Program**

narcotic   drug that relieves pain and produces sleep.

nasal cannula   tubing inserted into nostrils to administer oxygen.

nasogastric feeding (NG feeding)   nourishment given through a tube inserted through the nose into the stomach.

nasogastric (NG) tube   soft rubber or plastic tube that is inserted through a nostril into the stomach.

nebulizer   device used to apply a liquid in the form of a fine spray or mist; may be used to administer medication.

necrosis   tissue death.

negligence   failure to give care that is reasonably expected of a nursing assistant.

neonate   newborn baby.

neoplasm   new growth; tumor.

nephritis   inflammation of the kidney.

nephron   microscopic kidney unit that produces urine.

nerve   bundle of nerve processes (axons and dendrites) that are held together by connective tissue.

nerve cells   carry electrical messages to and from different parts of body.

nervous tissue   highly specialized tissue capable of conducting nerve impulses.

networking   communication between individuals with a common interest or goal.

neuron   cell of the nervous system.

neurotransmitter   chemical compound that transmits a nervous impulse across cells at a synapse.

NG.   *See* **nasogastric feeding; nasogastric tube**

NIDDM.   *See* **non–insulin-dependent diabetes mellitus**

no-code order   an order not to resuscitate a patient.

non–insulin-dependent diabetes mellitus (NIDDM)   diabetes controlled by diet and sometimes oral medication, for which insulin is not needed.

noninvasive   remaining localized and not spreading.

nonpathogen   microorganism that does not produce disease.

nonverbal communication   communication transmitted without spoken words, such as by facial expression and body language.

nonweight bearing   unable to stand or walk on one or both legs.

nosocomial   pertaining to or originating in a facility.

nosocomial infection   infection acquired in a facility.

NPO   nothing by mouth.

Nurse Aide Competency Evaluation Program (NACEP)   test taken by the nursing assistant which, when passed successfully, entitles the nursing assistant to certification.

nurse's notes   section of medical record in which nursing staff records procedures, medications, and observations.

nursing assistant   person who helps, under supervision, with the care of the sick and infirm.

nursing diagnosis   statement of a patient's problems leading to nursing interventions.

nursing process   framework for nursing action.

nursing team   members of the nursing staff who provide patient care.

nutrient   nourishing substance or food.

nutrition   process by which the body uses food for growth and repair and to maintain health.

nystagmus   constant involuntary movement of eyeball.

obese   overweight.

objective observation   observation made through the senses of the observer.

oblique fracture.   *See* **closed fracture**

OBRA.   *See* **Omnibus Budget Reconciliation Act**

observation   noticing something.

obstetric, obstetrical   pertaining to pregnancy, labor, and delivery.

obstruction   blockage in a passageway.

occult blood   small quantity of blood that can be detected only by microscope or chemical means.

occupational exposure   coming into contact with infectious materials during the performance of a person's job.

Occupational Safety and Health Administration (OSHA)   federal agency that makes and enforces regulations to protect workers.

occupational therapy   therapeutic use of work and activities to help patients regain self-care skills.

OJD.   *See* **osteoarthritic joint disease**

Omnibus Budget Reconciliation Act (OBRA)   law that regulates the education and certification of nursing assistants in acute care and long-term care facilities.

oncology   study of cancer.

oophorectomy   surgical excision of an ovary.

open bed   bed with top bedding fanfolded to bottom, ready for occupancy.

open (compound) fracture   fracture in which part of the broken bone protrudes through the skin.

open reduction/internal fixation (ORIF)   surgical procedure to reduce a fractured bone. The skin is opened and the fracture realigned and held in place by screws, plates, and pins.

operative   pertaining to an operation.

ophthalmoscope   instrument for examining the eyes.

oral hygiene   care of the mouth and teeth.

oral report   verbal report.

orchiectomy   excision of one or both of the testes.

organ   any part of the body that carries out a specific function or functions, such as the heart.

organism   any living thing, plant or animal.

organizational chart   guide for communication; spells out lines of authority.

ORIF.   *See* **open reduction/internal fixation**

orifice   body opening such as the nose or mouth.

origin   proximal point of attachment to skeletal muscle.

orthopedic   concerning the prevention or correction of deformities (orthopedics).

orthopnea   need to sit upright in order to breathe without difficulty.

orthopneic position   position in which a patient, supported by pillows, leans on the overbed table.

orthoses   braces or splints used to immobilize an extremity and to maintain its position.

OSHA.   *See* **Occupational Safety and Health Administration**

ossicles   any small bones, such as one of the three bones in the ear.

osteoarthritic joint disease (OJD)   degenerative disease of joints.

ostomy   suffix meaning "to create a new opening"; for example, colostomy.

otitis media   inflamed condition of the middle part of the ear.

otosclerosis   formation of bone in the inner ear that causes the ossicles to become fixed.

otoscope   instrument used to examine the ear.

ovaries (singular **ovary**)   endocrine glands located in the female pelvis; female gonads.

oviduct   tube in body between ovary and uterus through which ovum travels; part of female reproductive system.

ovulation   lunar monthly ripening and discharge of an ovum from the cortex of the ovary.

ovum (plural **ova**)   female egg.

oxygen   gas that is essential to cellular metabolism and life.

oxygen concentrator   device that removes impurities from room air and concentrates oxygen to be delivered to a patient.

oxygen mask   device to administer oxygen through nose and mouth; placed over patient's face.

pacemaker   artificial device placed in the body to regulate the heartbeat.

PACU.   *See* **postanesthesia care unit**

pallor   less color than normal for the skin.

panhysterectomy   removal of the entire uterus.

Pap smear   simple test used to detect cancer of the cervix.

papule   solid, elevated lesion of the skin.

PAR.   *See* **postanesthesia recovery**

paralysis   loss or impairment of the ability to move parts of the body.

paranoia   state in which one has delusions of persecution and/or grandeur.

paraplegia   paralysis of lower portion of the body and of both legs.

parasite   organism that lives within, upon, or at the expense of another organism known as the *host*.

parathormone   hormone produced by parathyroid glands that regulates calcium and phosphorus levels in the blood.

parathyroid glands   two pairs of endocrine glands situated on posterior of thyroid gland; produce the hormone parathormone.

Parkinson's disease   neurological disorder due to deficiency of dopamine, a neurotransmitter; progressive disease characterized by stiffness of muscles and tremors.

partial weight-bearing   unable to bear full weight on one or both legs.

PASS   acronym for fire extinguisher use meaning: *P*ull the pin; *A*im the nozzle; *S*queeze the handle; *S*weep back and forth.

pathogen   microorganism or other agent capable of producing a disease.

pathology   disease.

patient   person who needs care; *see also* **resident** and **client**.

patient-controlled analgesia (PCA)   administration of pain-relieving medication controlled by the patient, using a special device; amount of medication to be delivered is preset by the nurse.

patient focused care   attention given to mental, physical, and emotional aspects of a person's being.

Patient's Bill of Rights   document developed by the American Hospital Association that describes the basic rights to which a patient is entitled.

PCA.   *See* **patient-controlled analgesia**

pediatric   patient from birth to 18 years of age.

pelvic belt traction   special form of traction in which a belt, secured around a person's hips, is attached to ropes, pulleys, and weights.

pelvic inflammatory disease (PID)   inflammation of the pelvic organs.

pelvis   lower portion of the trunk of the body; basin-shaped area bounded by the hip bones, the sacrum, and the coccyx.

penis   male organ of copulation and urinary elimination.

pepsin   enzyme produced in the stomach that begins protein digestion.

perceptual deficit   inability to reason, think systematically, make judgments, or use common items.

percussion hammer   instrument used to test reflexes.

pericardium   membrane that surrounds the heart.

perineal care   cleansing of genital and rectal areas.

perineum   in the male, the area between the anus and scrotum; in the female, the area between the anus and vagina.

perioperative   occurring in association with an operative procedure.

peripheral   pertaining to the outside or outer part.

peripheral intravenous central catheter (PICC)   intravenous line inserted into a vein in the arm and threaded through to a larger vein.

peristalsis   progressive, wavelike movement that occurs involuntarily in hollow tubes of the body, especially the alimentary canal.

peritoneal dialysis   removal of liquid waste by washing chemicals through the abdominal cavity.

peritoneum   serous membrane lining the walls of the abdominal and pelvic cavities.

personal protective equipment (PPE)   equipment such as waterproof gowns, masks, gloves, goggles, and other equipment needed to protect a person from infectious material.

personal space   physical closeness that a person is comfortable with during interactions with others.

personality   sum of the behavior, attitudes, and character traits of an individual.

petit mal seizure   type of epileptic attack that is generally short in nature; "absence" attack.

PFR95 respirator   mask with very tiny pores that prevents the wearer from breathing in infectious airborne microorganisms.

phagocyte   white blood cell that destroys substances such as bacteria, protozoa, and cells.

phantom pain   pain experienced in a body part that has been removed from the body as if the part were still attached.

pharynx   muscular, membranous tube between mouth and esophagus; throat.

phlebitis   inflammation of a vein.

physiatrist   medical doctor specializing in rehabilitation.

physical abuse   mistreatment by hitting or other physical contact.

physical restraint   device used to prevent a patient from moving about or having access to his or her own body.

physical therapy   structured exercise that assists patients to regain mobility skills.

physiology   the science that deals with the functioning of living organisms.

PICC.   *See* **peripheral intravenous central catheter**

PID.   *See* **pelvic inflammatory disease**

piggyback   procedure used to administer medication through a vein.

pigmentation   coloration of an area by pigment.

pineal body   pea-sized endocrine gland located in the brain.

pituitary gland   "master" endocrine gland located in brain at base of skull (attached to hypothalamus); produces hormones that regulate growth and reproduction.

pivot   to twist or turn in a swiveling motion.

placenta   structure within the womb through which the unborn child is nourished; the afterbirth.

placental stage   period of the delivery process during which the afterbirth is expelled from the uterus.

planning   establishing possible solutions for a patient's problems (as determined by nursing diagnoses).

plantar flexion   extending the foot in a downward movement.

plasma   liquid portion of blood.

pleura   membranes that surround the lungs.

PM care   care given to prepare a patient or resident for sleep.

pneumonia   inflammation and infection of the lungs.

polydipsia   excessive thirst.

polyphagia   excessive ingestion of food.

polyuria   excessive excretion of urine.

port   opening.

portal of entry   area of body through which microbes enter and cause disease.

portal of exit   area of body through which disease-producing organisms leave the body.

position sense   ability to know one's position in space, including how extremities are positioned.

postanesthesia care unit (PACU)   room where patients receive immediate care following surgery.

post-anesthesia recovery (PAR)   area where patients are taken after surgery to recover from anesthesia.

posterior   back or dorsal.

postmortem   after death.

postmortem care   care given to the body after death.

postoperative   after surgery.

postpartum   after parturition; after birth.

potentially infectious material   material or equipment that could be a source of disease-producing organisms.

pound   unit of measurement of weight, equivalent to 16 ounces or 453.6 grams.

PPE.   *See* **personal protective equipment**

preadolescence   years between the ages of 12 and 14.

predisposing factor   condition that contributes to the development of disease.

prefix   term that is placed before a word that changes or modifies the meaning of the word.

prenatal   before birth.

preoperative   period before surgery.

pressure ulcer   ulceration due to ischemia; pressure sore.

private room   room in a health care facility that contains only one patient at a time.

probe   as used in this text, a long, slender part of an instrument; that portion of the electronic or tympanic thermometer placed into the patient.

procedure   series of steps outlining how and in what order and manner to do something.

proctoscopy   inspection of the rectum using a proctoscope.

progesterone   hormone produced by female ovaries.

prognosis   probable outcome of a disease or injury.

projection   unconscious defense mechanism by which an individual denies his or her own emotionally unacceptable traits and sees them as belonging to another.

pronation   placing or lying in a face-downward position; as applied to the hand, indicates the palms facing backward.

prone   position in which the patient is on the abdomen, spine straight, legs extended, and arms flexed on either side of the head.

prostatectomy   removal of all or part of the prostate gland.

prostate gland   gland of male reproductive system that surrounds the neck of the urinary bladder and the beginning of the urethra.

prosthesis   artificial substitute for a missing body part, such as dentures, hand, leg.

protein   basic material of every body cell; an essential nutrient.

protocol   standards of procedure and care developed for preparation of a patient for diagnostic tests.

protozoan (plural protozoa)   microscopic unicellular organism.

proximal   closest to the point of attachment.

psychiatric   relating to mental illness.

psychological abuse   mistreatment by threatening, belittling, or otherwise causing mental or emotional harm or upset.

puberty   condition or period of becoming capable of sexual reproduction.

pubic   concerning the pubes.

pulse   wave of blood pressure exerted against the walls of the arteries in response to ventricular contraction.

pulse deficit   difference between contractions of the heart and pulse expansions of the radial artery.

pulse oximetry   procedure for measuring level of oxygen in arterial blood.

pulse pressure   difference between the systolic and diastolic pressures.

pupil   circular opening in center of iris; regulates light entering eye.

push fluids   to encourage a patient to drink additional fluids.

pustule   circumscribed pus-containing lesion of the skin.

pyelogram.   *See* **intravenous pyelogram (IVP)**

pyloric sphincter   muscle at the exit point of the pylorus.

quadrant   one of the four imaginary sections of the surface of the abdomen.

quadriplegia   paralysis of all four limbs.

quickening   first movement of fetus in uterus that is felt by the mother.

race   classification of people according to shared physical characteristics.

RACE   acronym relating to fire emergency procedure, meaning: *R*emove patient from danger; *A*ctivate alarm; *C*ontain fire; *E*xtinguish fire.

radial deviation   wrists are turned toward the thumb side.

radial pulse   pulse that can be measured by palpating the radial artery.

radiation therapy   treatment of cancer with radiation.

radical mastectomy   removal of entire breast and lymph nodes.

rales   abnormal respiratory sound heard in auscultation of the chest.

range of motion (ROM)   series of exercises specifically designed to move each joint through its full range.

rate   valuation based on comparison with a standard.

reaction formation   repressing the reality of an anxiety-producing situation; the individual exhibits behaviors that are exactly opposite to the real feelings.

reality orientation   techniques used to help a person remain oriented to environment, time, and self.

receptive aphasia   inability to understand written or spoken language.

recovery room   location where surgical patients are taken after surgery; they return to their rooms when their conditions stabilize.

rectocele   protrusion of part of the rectum into the vagina.

references   in a résumé, statements about abilities and characteristics; persons who give such statements.

reflex   activity performed without conscious thought.

registered nurse (RN)   specially educated person who is licensed to plan and direct the nursing care of patients.

regress   to move in a backward fashion.

rehabilitation   process of assisting ill or injured person to attain optimal level of well-being and function.

reminiscing   thinking and talking about the past.

renal calculi   kidney stones.

renal colic   spasm in an area near the kidney, accompanied by pain.

repression   involuntary exclusion from awareness of a painful experience or conflict-creating memory, feeling, or impulse.

reservoir   storage area; biologically, an animal or source that maintains infectious organisms that periodically can be spread to others.

resident   person being cared for in a long-term care facility; *see also* **client** and **patient.**

Resident's Rights   document that spells out rights of residents receiving care in long-term care facilities.

respiration   process of taking oxygen into the body and expelling carbon dioxide.

respiratory arrest   cessation of breathing.

restorative   returning to pre-existing level or status.

restorative care   care given by interdisciplinary health care team to assist a patient to reach optimal level of ability.

résumé   short account of a job applicant's career and qualifications.

retention   inability to excrete urine that has been produced.

retinal degeneration   breakdown and functional loss of the nervous layer of the eye.

retrograde pyelogram   backward-moving x-ray picture of ureter and renal pelvis.

rheumatoid arthritis   autoimmune response that results in inflammation of the joints.

rhythm   the repeat interval of measured time or movement.

rigor mortis   rigidity of skeletal muscles, developing six to ten hours after death.

risk factor   specific behaviors or conditions that promote certain diseases.

ritual   ceremonial acts that reinforce faith.

RN.   *See* **registered nurse**

ROM.   *See* **range of motion**

rooming-in   practice of having mother and baby share a single room after delivery.

rotation   act of turning about the axis of the center of a body, as in rotation of a joint.

rubra   unusual redness or flushing of the skin.

Sacrament of the Sick   last rites given by clergy to a person who is terminally ill (dying).

salpingectomy   surgical removal of the fallopian tubes.

sarcoma   connective tissue tumor, often highly malignant.

scope of practice   extent or range of permissible activities.

scrotum   saclike pouch that holds the male gonads.

sebaceous gland – gland that produces a lubricating substance for hairs.

self-care deficit   inability to perform an activity of daily living.

self-esteem   feeling of confidence about oneself.

self-identity   personal knowledge of who one is; personal view of self.

semicircular canal   three tubes in the inner ear containing fluid; the function is concerned with balance and detecting motion.

semi-Fowler's position   position in which the patient is on the back with knees slightly flexed, and head of bed is elevated 30 to 50 degrees.

seminal vesicles   pair of accessory male sex glands that open into vas deferens before it joins the urethra; they secrete fluid into seminal fluid.

semiprivate room   room in a health care facility that is shared by two patients.

semiprone   patient is positioned between side and abdomen.

semisupine   patient is positioned between side and back.

sensitivity   ability to be aware of and appreciate personal characteristics of others; state of acute or abnormal response to stimuli or allergens.

seropositive   state in which antibodies to HIV exist in the bloodstream.

serous membrane   tissue that produces serous fluid, covers organs, and lines closed body cavities.

sexual abuse   use of physical means or verbal threats to force a person to perform sexual acts.

sexuality   maleness or femaleness of an individual.

sexually transmitted disease (STD)   disease that is passed from one individual to another through sexual contact.

sharps   needles, knife blades, etc.; items that can cut or puncture skin.

shearing   force on skin over bone when skin remains at point of contact while bone moves; causes damage to skin.

shift report   information about patients passed from outgoing shift to oncoming shift.

shock   condition in which there is a disruption of the circulation that results in a dangerously low blood pressure and an upset of all bodily functions.

side rails   sliding metal bars that may be pulled up on each side of the bed to prevent the patient from falling out of bed.

sigmoidoscopy   direct examination of the interior of the sigmoid colon.

sign   any objective evidence of an abnormal nature in the body or its organs.

sign language   communication for the hearing impaired, which uses gestures and signs made with the fingers and hands.

simple fracture   fracture that does not produce an open wound in the skin. *See* **closed fracture**

simple goiter   thyroid gland hyperplasia unaccompanied by other signs or symptoms.

simple mastectomy   removal of the breast tissue without removal of the underlying muscles.

Sims' position   position in which the patient is on the left side with left leg extended and right leg flexed; left arm is extended and brought behind back; right arm is flexed and brought forward.

singultus   hiccup.

sitting transfer   moving patient from one surface to another with patient sitting.

skeletal muscle   muscle that is attached to bone and provides voluntary movement.

skilled care   health care provided to persons who require professional services over a period of time.

skilled care facility   long-term care facility.

slander   false oral statement that injures the reputation of another person.

smooth muscle   muscle located in internal organs, responsible for involuntary movement.

soft diet   intake consisting of low-residue, mildly flavored, easily digested foods.

source   person who has an infection that can be spread to others.

spasticity   continuous resistance to stretching by a muscle due to abnormally increased tension.

spatial-perceptual deficit   inability to distinguish between left and right and up and down.

speculum   instrument used to dilate a body opening.

speech therapy   treatment to assist a patient to regain communication skills.

sperm   male reproductive cell.

sphygmomanometer   instrument for determining arterial pressures; blood pressure gauge.

spica cast   body cast.

spinal anesthesia   technique of providing anesthesia by introducing drugs into the spinal canal.

spirillum (plural **spirilla**)   spiral-shaped bacteria.

spirituality   feeling of wholeness resulting from filling the human need to feel connected to the world and to a power greater than oneself.

splint   type of orthosis used to maintain position and prevent contractures of arm and hand.

sprain   injury to ligament, resulting in pain and swelling.

sputum   matter brought up from the lungs; phlegm.

stable   health condition is steady, predictable, without complications.

staff development   process used to educate staff in health care facilities.

standard   guide for performance by which performance is measured.

standard precautions   practices used in health care facilities to prevent the spread of infection via blood, body fluids, secretions, excretions, mucous membranes, and nonintact skin.

standing transfer   patient is moved from one surface to another while standing.

staphylo-   prefix meaning "in clusters."

status   condition or state of health.

status epilepticus   serious condition in which one epileptic-type seizure follows another.

STD.   *See* **sexually transmitted disease**

stepparent   person who is married to a child's natural parent.

stereotype   rigid beliefs based on generalizations.

sterile   absence of all microorganisms; incapable of reproducing sexually.

sterile field   area considered free of all microbes.

sterility   inability to produce offspring.

sterilization   process that renders an individual incapable of reproduction; process of cleaning equipment to remove all microbes and make equipment sterile.

stertorous   snoring-type respirations.

stethoscope   instrument used in auscultation to make audible the sounds produced in the body.

stimulant   agent that produces stimulation or elicits a response.

stimulus   'anything that provokes a response in a cell, tissue, or other structure.

stoma   artificial, mouthlike opening.

stool   another name for feces.

strain   injury to a muscle, resulting in pain.

strepto-   prefix meaning "in chains."

stressors   situations, feelings, or conditions that cause a person to be anxious about his or her well-being.

stroke   cerebrovascular accident or brain attack; damage to the blood vessels of the brain.

Stryker frame   special kind of bed used when a patient cannot be turned within the bed.

subacute care   transitional care provided after discharge from acute care.

subcutaneous tissue   connective tissue located under the dermis; attaches skin to muscle.

subjective observation   observation based on ideas perceived only by the individual involved.

sudoriferous gland   gland that secretes perspiration.

suffix   term added to the end of a word that changes or modifies the meaning of the word.

suicide   self-destruction; killing oneself.

sundowning   behavior in which a person becomes more agitated and disoriented during the evening hours.

superimpose   put on top of something else.

superior   toward the head; upward.

supination   act of turning the palm upward.

supine position   lying with the face upward.

supplement   to add; nutrients given in addition to meals, usually high in protein.

supportive care   care given to a dying patient that avoids prolonging life but provides comfort measures only.

supportive device   used to help maintain a patient's body in a specific position.

suppository   medication used to help the bowels eliminate feces.

suppression   consciously refusing to acknowledge unacceptable feelings and thoughts.

surgical bed   bed prepared for a patient returning from surgery.

surgical mask   mask worn by health care workers during surgery, sterile procedures, and work in a droplet precautions room.

symbols   signs, pictures, or other characters used to communicate.

symmetry   matching or correspondence in size, form, and arrangement.

sympathectomy   excision or interruption of a sympathetic nerve.

symptom   any perceptible change in the body or its function that indicates disease or the phases of disease.

synapse   space between the axon of one cell and the dendrites of others.

synovial membranes   tissues that produce synovial fluid and line joint cavities.

syphilis   infectious, chronic, venereal disease characterized by lesions that may involve any organ or tissue; usually exhibits cutaneous manifestations; relapses are frequent; may exist asymptomatically for years.

system   group of organs organized to perform a specific body function or functions; for example, the respiratory system.

systole   contraction or period of contraction of cardiac muscle.

systolic pressure   blood pressure exerted during the contraction phase of the ventricles.

tachycardia   unusually rapid heartbeat.

tachypnea   pattern of rapid, shallow respirations.

talisman   object used to ward off evil.

tasks   accomplishments throughout life that lead to healthy participation in society; work to be done.

tasks of personality development   growing stages through which personality is formed, as described by Erickson.

TED hose   support hose.

tendon   fibrous band of connective tissue that attaches skeletal muscle to bone.

TENS.   *See* **transcutaneous electrical nerve stimulation**

terminal   final; life-ending stage.

testes   male gonads; reproductive glands located in the scrotal sac.

testosterone   hormone produced by the testes.

tetany   nervous condition characterized by intermittent toxic spasms that are usually paroxysmal and involve the extremities.

THA.   *See* **total hip arthroplasty**

theft   taking anything that does not belong to you; stealing.

therapeutic diet   treatment through specifically planned nutrition.

therapy   treatment designated to eliminate disease or other bodily disorder.

thermal blanket   large, fluid-filled blanket used to raise or lower a patient's temperature.

thrombocyte   blood platelet that is formed in the bone marrow and is important in blood clotting.

thrombophlebitis   development of venous thrombi in the presence of inflammatory changes in the vessel wall.

thrombus (plural **thrombi**)   blood clot.

thyrocalcitonin   hormone produced in thyroid gland.

thyroid gland   endocrine gland situated in base of neck; has two lobes, one on either side of trachea; produces hormones thyrocalcitonin and thyroxine.

thyroxine   hormone of the thyroid gland that contains iodine.

TIA.   *See* **transient ischemic attack**

time/travel records   records kept of the time spent with clients and the distance traveled between client locations.

tissue   collection of specialized cells that perform a particular function; piece of paper used for cleansing (for example, toilet tissue, facial tissue).

toddler   stage of childhood from 1 to 3 years of age.

total hip arthroplasty (THA)   surgical replacement of hip joint with a prosthesis.

total parenteral nutrition   meeting an individual's entire nutritional needs by providing high-density nutrients directly into the bloodstream.

toxin   microbe that produces poisons that travel to the central nervous system and cause damage.

trachea   windpipe.

tracheostomy   opening made into anterior trachea.

traditions   customs and practices followed by a culture and passed from generation to generation.

transcutaneous electrical nerve stimulation (TENS)   use of electrical stimulation to relieve pain.

transfer   procedure followed when changing a patient's location.

transfer belt   gait belt used to assist and support patients during ambulation.

transient ischemic attack (TIA)   temporary reduction of flow of blood to the brain.

transitional care   subacute care given after acute care.

transmission   transfer from one place or person to another.

transmission-based precautions   isolation practices that prevent the spread of infection by interrupting the way in which the disease is spread.

trapeze   horizontal bar suspended overhead down the length of the bed.

trauma   wound or injury.

tremor   involuntary trembling.

Trendelenburg position   position in which the patient has the head lower than the feet.

trichomonas vaginitis   inflammation of vaginal tissues with vaginal discharge caused by a protozoan.

trimester   period of three months.

trochanter roll   rolled sheet or bath blanket placed under the patient extending from waist to mid-thigh; positioned against the hip to prevent lateral hip rotation.

tubercle   small, rounded nodule formed by infection with *Mycobacterium tuberculosis*.

tuberculosis disease   condition occurring when tuberculosis bacteria enter body and damage tissue.

tuberculosis infection   condition in which tuberculosis bacteria enter body but are walled off and contained and do not cause disease.

tumor   neoplasm.

turning (moving) sheet.   *See* **draw sheet**

tympanic membrane   membrane serving as the lateral wall of the tympanic cavity and separating it from the external acoustic meatus (outer ear).

tympanic thermometer   device used to measure temperature at the tympanic membrane in the ear.

ulcer   open sore caused by inadequate blood supply and broken skin.

ulcerative colitis   inflammation of the colon resulting in the formation of ulcers.

ulnar deviation   with hand in supination, lateral movement of the wrist.

ultrasound   high-frequency sound waves (mechanical radiant energy of a frequency greater than 20,000 cycles per second) used for noninvasive imaging and other procedures.

umbilical cord   attachment connecting the fetus with the placenta. It is severed artificially at the birth of the child.

umbilicus   depressed scar marking the site of entry of the umbilical cord in the fetus.

unilateral neglect   patient ignores one side of body, such as the affected side after a stroke.

upper respiratory infection (URI)   infection involving the organs of the upper respiratory tract.

ureter   narrow tube that conducts urine from the kidney to the urinary bladder.

urethra   mucus-lined tube conveying urine from the urinary bladder to the exterior of the body; in the male, the urethra also conveys the semen.

urgency   need to urinate.

urgent care   care that must be given right away to prevent loss of life.

URI.   *See* **upper respiratory infection**

urinalysis   laboratory analysis of urine.

urinary bladder   receptacle for urine before it is voided.

urinary incontinence   inability to control urination.

urinary meatus   external opening to urethra.

uterus   organ of gestation; womb.

vaccine   artificial or weakened antigens that help the body develop antibodies to prevent infectious disease.

vagina   tube that extends from the vulva to the uterine cervix; female organ of copulation that receives the penis during sexual intercourse.

vaginal examination   examination of vaginal and pelvic organs.

validation therapy   techniques used to help individuals feel good about themselves.

vancomycin-resistant enterococci   type of bacteria resistant to most antibiotics.

varicose vein   enlarged vein in the leg due to an impaired valve in the vein.

vas deferens   tube that carries sperm from the epididymis to the junction of the seminal vesicle; ductus deferens.

vasoconstriction   decrease in the inner diameter of the blood vessels.

vasodilation   dilation of the blood vessels.

vector   carrier, such as an arthropod, that transmits disease.

vein   vessel through which blood passes on its way back to the heart.

venereal wart   viral condition that can be sexually transmitted.

ventilation   process of breathing in oxygen and breathing out carbon dioxide.

ventral   front; anterior.

ventricle   small cavity or chamber, as in the brain or heart.

verbal abuse   use of speech to humiliate, threaten, or cause fear or anxiety in another person.

verbal communication   transmitting messages using words.

vertebrae   bones surrounding the spinal cord; the backbone or spine.

vertigo   sensation of rotation or movement of or about the person.

vesicle   blister-like skin lesion.

victim   someone who is injured unexpectedly, as in an accident.

virus   tiny living organisms by which some infectious diseases are transmitted.

visceral muscles   muscles that operate without conscious control.

vitality   exuberant physical and mental strength; capacity for endurance.

vital signs   measurements of temperature, pulse, respiration, and blood pressure.

vitamin   general term for various, unrelated organic substances, found in many foods in small amounts, that are necessary for normal metabolic function of the body.

vocal cords   tissue that stretches across larynx and produces vocal sounds.

void   to release urine from the bladder.

volume   capacity or size of an object or of an area; measure of the quantity of a substance.

voluntary muscle   muscle attached to bones and under voluntary control.

vulva   external female genitalia.

vulvovaginitis   inflammation of the external female reproductive structures (vulva and vagina).

ward   patient unit for three or more people.

warm soak   method of applying moist heat.

weight-bearing   able to stand on one or both legs.

wet compress   method for applying moist heat or cold.

wheal   localized area of edema on the body surface, often associated with severe itching.

word root   word form whose basic meaning can be used in forming new words by combining with prefixes or suffixes.

work practice controls   procedures used to prevent the spread of disease.

yeast   one type of fungus.

Index

Note: References in **bold type** are to nursing assistant procedures. References in *italics* are to nontext material.

Abbreviations, 41, 43, 44
ABCs (emergency priorities), 633
Abdominal cavity, 49, *50*
Abdominal regions, 47
Abdominal thrusts, 642
Abduction, 486
Ability, 583
Abuse, 34–36, 430
Accelerated, 243
Acceptance, 385, 386–87
Accidents, 405. *See also* Emergencies; Incidents preventing, 163–65. *See also* Patient safety; Safety
Accuracy, 16, 427
   in blood pressure readings, 250
   in charting/documentation, 89
   in observations, 54, 84
Ace bandages, 366, 479
Acetone, 506
Acidity, 59, 121
Acquired immune deficiency syndrome (AIDS), 118, 125–26, *409*, 436, 574
Activities, 102, 583
   children, 615, 617
   elderly, 406
   patients with dementia, 411
   physical, 99
Activities of daily living (ADL), 581, 584–85
   for Alzheimer's patients, 411
   assistance with, 398, *399*
   relearning, 519
Acupuncture, 109
Acute care facilities, 267
Acute disease, 55
Acute illness, 4
Adaptability, 428
Adaptation, 373, 374
Adaptive devices, 333, 582, 586
Addison's disease, 503
Adduction, 486, *487*
ADL. *See* Activities of daily living
Administrators, 11
Admission, 263–66
   child, 601, **602**
   procedure, **264–65**
   surgical patients, 357, 358
Admission form, 265, *266*
Adolescence, 96
Adolescents, 617–18
Adoptive parent, 601
Adrenal (suprarenal) glands, *501*, 502, 503, *547*
Adulthood, 96
Advance directives, 23, 387–88
Aerosol therapy, 466
African Americans, 106, *107*, 108, *110*
African sleeping sickness, 118

Afterbirth. *See* Placenta
Age
   blood pressure and, 247
   heat and cold applications, 339
   pulse rate and, 241
   respiration rate and, 244
Age groups, 93
Agencies, home health care providers, 417–18
Agent, 119, 388
Aging. *See also* Elderly
   developmental stages, 93–97, 601–2
   emotional adjustments to, 400, 402–3
   integumentary system changes, 447–48
   mental changes, 408
   physical changes, 400, *401*
   as risk factor, 54, 397
Agitation, 380–81, 412
Agnosia, 584
Aiding and abetting, 33
AIDS. *See* Acquired immune deficiency syndrome
Air, 459
   movement in room, 162
   negative pressure, 138
   temperature, 162, 461
Airborne precautions, 138
Airborne transmission, 120, 137
Airway
   maintaining, 522
   obstruction/occlusion of, 641, **643–44**, **646–49**
   opening, 635
Akinesia, 520
Alarms, 334
Alcohol, 377
Alcoholics Anonymous, 376
Alcoholism, 375–76
Allergens, 448, 460–61
Allergies, 56, 121, 134, 448, 492
Alopecia, 442
Alternating-pressure mattress, 272, 453, 454, *455*
Alveoli, 459, 461
Alzheimer's disease, 73, 408–14
AM care, 303, 406
Ambulate, 212
Ambulation. *See also* Gait
   assisting with, *99*
   safety in, 405
   after surgery, 368, 370
   with tubes, *370*
   unassisted, 175
Ambulatory units, 279
Amebiasis, 118
Amenorrhea, 572
American Heart Association, 635
American Red Cross, 635
Amino acids, 321
Amniocentesis, 591
Amniotic fluid, 590
Amniotic sac, 569, 590

Amputation, *58*, 195, 212, 493, 582
Amulets, 109
Analgesia, 440
Anaphylactic shock, 448, 492
Anatomic position, 45–46
Anatomy, 45
Anemia, 59, 480
Aneroid gauge, 247, *248, 250*, 252
Anesthesia, 356
Anesthetics, 356–57, 440
Anger, 385, 386
Angina pectoris, 474, 478
Angiogram, 481
Anorexia, 442
ANS. *See* Autonomic nervous system
Anterior, *46*, 47
Antibiotics, 122, 417
Antibodies, 59, 122, 470
Anticoagulants, 310, 376
Anticonvulsants, 376
Antidiabetic drugs, 376
Anti-embolism stockings, 365, **366–67**, 479
Antigens, 122
Antihypertensives, 247, 377
Anxiety, 99
    bleeding and, 650
    children, 613, 614
    in elderly, 402
    patients with dementia, 412
    re transfers, 264
Aorta, 470, 471
Apgar score, 592, 596
Aphasia, 72–73, 519, 520
Apical pulse, 241–42, **243**, 608
Apnea, 243
Appendicitis, 340
Appendix, 533
Appetite, 403, 584
Appliance, 625
Approaches, 77, 584
    burn management, 455–56
    communication, 70
    home health care, 419
Apraxia, 584
Aquamatic K-Pad®, 339, **343–44**, 345
Aqueous humor, 515
Arachnoid mater, 513
Arguing, 374, 381, 413
Arms, 47
    alignment, *188*, 189
    angle, 214, 216
    bandaging, 368
    for blood pressure measurement, 249, 250
Arteries, 247, *248*, 470, 471–72, *473, 650*
Arterioles, 470
Arthritis, 212, 488
Arthroscopy, 498
Artificial eye, 524, **525**
Ascites, 479
Asepsis, 131–32, 133, 156
Asian/Pacific ethnic group, 106, *107*, 108, *110*
Aspiration, 179, 334, 356. *See also* Choking
Assault, 34

Assessment, 77, *81*, 350. *See also* Physical examinations at admission, 263
    emergency situation, 634, 635
    form, *78–80*
    for home health care, 419, 427
    of mental state, 376
    pressure ulcer risk, 450
Assignment sheet, *67*
Assignments, 14, 66, 622
    home health care, 424
    managing, 421
    questions about, 18, 263
Assimilated, 506
Assistants, 168
    for logrolling, 186
    for patient transfers, 199, 200–201, 202–6
    wheelchair positioning, 219–20
Assisted living, 397
Assistive devices, 213–17, 378
Asthma, 460–61
Atelectasis, 363, *364*, 465
Atheromas, 474
Atherosclerosis, 474, 476
Atrium (pl. atria), 470
Atrophy, 182, 493
Attachment, points of, 47
Attitude, 16, 17, 18, 36
Audiometry, 528
Auditing, 420
Aura, 522
Aural temperature, 226
Auscultatory gap, 250
Authority
    higher, 14–15
    lines of, 14, 66
    of nursing assistant, 18, 420, 589, 621
Autoclave, 155
Autoimmune reactions, 56
Autonomic nervous system (ANS), 514, 521
Autonomy, 613
Autopsy, 392–93, 409
Awakening patient, 303
Axilla, 288
Axillary temperature, 226, **233, 235**, 608
Axons, 510

Bacillus (pl. bacilli), 117
Back supports, 168, 664
Background checks, 664
Backrubs, 83, 290, 308–10
    giving, **309–10**
Bacteremia, 121, 404
Bacteria (sing. bacterium), 117–18, 119, 460
Bacterial infections, 122, 124
Badges, 19
Balance, 195, 212, 213, 217, 221, 516
Balance bar, 255
Bandages, elasticized, 367–69, 479. *See also* Dressings
Baptist (religion), 327, *389*
Bargaining, 385, 386
Barrier equipment. *See* Personal protective equipment
Baseline, 254, 263, 450
Basinless bath, 283, 291

Bath blankets, 284
    for trochanter roll, 187, 312–13
Bath mitt, 288
Bathing, 99, 283–84, 406, 453, *585. See also* Grooming;
        Hygiene
    assistive devices for, 405
    bed bath, 277, **286–90**
    elderly, 407
    partial bath, **291**, 406
    perineal care, 292–94
    special-care patients, 283, 287–88
    tub bath/shower, **284–85**
Bathrooms, cleaning, 284, 431–32
Bathtub, transferring into and out of, **208–9**
Battery, 34
Bed bath, 277, **286–90**
Bed cradle, 182, 312, 454
Bed rails. *See* Side rails
Bedmaking, 272–80
    occupied bed, 277–80
    orthopedic patients, 491
    surgical bed, **279–80**
Bedpans, 99, 537
    giving and receiving, **313–15**
Beds, 161–62, 271–72
    head position, 190
    low position, 175, 180
    numbering, 161
    restraint attachment to, 162, *178*
    special, 271, 454–56, 473, 488
    surgical, **279–80**, 360
    work height, 168, 180
Bedside table, 161, 163
Bedsores. *See* Pressure ulcers
Bedtime care, 303
Behaviors
    agitation, 380–81, 412
    changes in, 405
    coping, 373, 374
    defensive, 373–74
    demanding, 374–75
    description of, 35
    effect of stress on, 17
    maladaptive, 376–81
    observations re, 85
    understanding, 374
Belongings, 265, 267, 268, 358–59
Below-the-knee amputation (BKA), 493
Benign prostatic hypertrophy, 571
Benign tumors, 59
Bile, 533, 534
Bilirubin, 596
Biohazardous waste, 136
Biological parent, 601
Biopsy, 462, 574
Birth, 590, 591
Bisexuality, 101
BKA. *See* Below-the-knee amputation
Bladder. *See* Urinary bladder
Blame, 376
Blanching, 340
Bleeding, 516, 649–50. *See also* Hemorrhage
Blindness, 524

Blood, 470
    abnormalities, 480–81
    contact with, 133
    gases in, 470
    occult, 537, **622–23**
    spills, 136
    viscosity, 247
Blood cells, 59, 470
Blood chemistry, 551
Blood clots. *See* Thrombus
Blood flow, 472
Blood glucose monitoring, 506–7
Blood pressure, 247–52. *See also* Hypertension
    children, 609
    measuring, **250–51**, 556, **609**
    measurement equipment, 247–48
Blood samples, *54*, 57
Blood tests, 56, 574
Blood transfusions, 126, 572
Blood vessels, 247, 459, 470, 471–72
Body alignment, 178, 182
Body core, 225, 345, 346
Body fluids, 133, 136–37, 329
Body language, 17, 18, 65–66, 374. *See also* Communication;
        Nonverbal communication
    pain demonstration through, *55*, 65
Body mechanics, 168, 181–82, 272, 284
Body odors, 18
Body organization, 45, 47–50
Body parts, 44, 45–47
Body shell, 226, 447
Body temperature, 225–26
    children, 596, **607–8**
    controlling, 345–47
    core, 345, 346
    measuring, 226, 228, 229–37, **607–8**
    pulse rate and, 241
    recording, 232, 233
    respiration rate and, 244
Bolus, 532
Bone marrow, 498
Bones, 484–85
Bony prominences, 309, 449
Boredom, 102, 380
Bowel movement, 313. *See also* Feces
Bowel retraining, 520, 535, 582
Bowman's capsule, 548
Box (square) corner, 274
Brachial artery, 248
Bradycardia, 241
Braille, 72
Brain, 510, 511–12, 514, 515
    damage, 436, 634–35
Brain attack, 474, 475, 517, 651–52. *See also* Stroke
Brain stem, 512
Breast care, 595
Breast-feeding, 611
Breast self-examination, 574, **575**
Breast tumors, 572
Breathing. *See* Respiration
Bridging, 313, 454, 455
Bronchi, 459
Bronchioles, 459

Bronchitis, 460, 461
Brushing teeth, 304–7
Buccal cavity, *50*
Buddhism, 110, *111*, 327, *389*
Bulb, 226
Burnout, 19
Burns, 179, 455–56, 650, 652–53
   beds for, 271
   electrical, 652
Burping infants, 610–12
Bursae, 485, 488
Bursitis, 488
Business services, 6

Cachexia, 59
Calcium, 323, 324, 583, 584
   endocrine system regulation of, 502, 503
Calorie-restricted diets, 328
Calories, 322, 325, 403
Cancer, 56, 448. *See also* Neoplasms; Oncology; Tumors
   blood, 481
   gastrointestinal tract, 533–34
   larynx, 462
   of testes, 571
Candida albicans, 118, 572
Canes, 213, 214–16
Cannula, 441
Capillaries, 59, 470
Carbohydrates, 321, 403, 532
   metabolism of, 503–4
   sources, 505, 506
Carbon dioxide (CO_2), 242, 459
Carcinomas, 59
Cardiac arrest, 387, 634–35
Cardiac catheterization, 57
Cardiac cycle, 471
Cardiac decompensation, 479
Cardiac monitoring, 436
Cardiac muscle, 48, 486
Cardiopulmonary resuscitation (CPR), 387, 635, 644
   on adult, **635–41**
   on child, **648**
   on infant, **644–46**
   two-person, 638, **639–41**
Cardiovascular system, *48*, *401*, 470–72, 584. *See also*
   Circulatory system
Cardiovascular disease, 327–38, 408, 472
Care plan, 68, 77, *82*, 427
   bed position, 272
   communication approaches, 70
   home health care, 419
   seclusion in, 35
Care plan conference, 13, 77, *81*, 427
Care provider specialists, 10–12
Career growth, 664–65
Caregivers, 419, 602. *See also* Nursing assistant
Caries, 304
Carriers, 119, 121
Cars, transfers into and out of, **209**
Cartilage, 484, 488
Cases, 119
Casts, 489–90
CAT scan. *See* Computerized axial tomography scan

Cataracts, 524
Catastrophic reactions, 410, 412
Catheter care, 404, 557–61
   bag position, 557, 560
   indwelling, **558–59**
Catheters, 99, 362, 557–65
   ambulation with, 560–61, 563
   disconnecting, **561–62**
   irritation from, 450, 453, 463
   leg-bag connection, **563–64**
   nasal, 464
Catholicism, Roman, 110, *111*, 327, *389*
Caucasians, 106, *107*, 108
Causative agent, 119
CAUTION (cancer signs), 59
Cavities, 49–50
CBC. *See* Complete blood cell count
CDC. *See* Centers for Disease Control
Celibate, 101
Cells, 47, 48, 58, 59, 459, 470
Cellulose, 321
Celsius (centigrade) scale (C), 225
Centers for Disease Control (CDC), 138
Centimeters (cm), 254
Central nervous system (CNS), 510–14
Central venous (CV) catheter, 438
Cerebellum, 512
Cerebrospinal fluid (CSF), 511, 513–14, 528
Cerebrovascular accident (CVA), 516, 517, 651. *See also* Brain
   attack; Stroke
Cerebrum, 511–12
Certification, 11, 664
Cervical traction, 491
Cervix, 569, *570*, 591, 592
Cesarean section, 594
Chain of command, 14–15
Chain of infection, 119–20, 132
Chair scales, 254, 256–57
Chancre, 573
Chapels, 103
Chaplain, 11, 102, 388. *See also* Clergy
Charge nurse, 13, 14
Chart. *See* Medical record
Charting, 44–45, 86–89. *See also* Documentation
Chemical restraints, 34, 177, 380
Chemicals, hazardous, 169
Chemotherapy, 58, 442
Chest drainage, 363
Chest thrusts, 642
Chewing, 325
Cheyne-Stokes respirations, 243
CHF. *See* Congestive heart failure
Chickenpox, 118, 138
Children, 323, 601–19. *See also* Infants
   airway obstruction, clearing, **648–49**
   body temperature, 225, 346, 596, **607–8**
   CPR for, 644, 648
   growth and developmental stages, 93–96, 601–2
   neoplasms in, 58
   pulse rate, 241, 242, **608–9**
   as surgical patients, 357
Chlamydia, 574
Choking, 179, 641–44, 646–49

Cholecystectomy, 534–35
Cholecystitis, 534
Cholelithiasis, 534
Cholesterol, 403
Choroid layer, 515
Christian Science (religion), 327, *389*
Chronic disease, 55, 397
Chronic illness, 4, 417
Chronic obstructive pulmonary disease (COPD), 460–61
Chronologic, 400
Church of Christ (religion), *389*
Chyme, 533
Chymopapain, 492
Cigarette drain, 362
Cilia, 121
CircOlectric® bed, 271, 456, 488
Circulation to tissues, 453
Circulatory system, 84, 120, 460. *See also* Cardiovascular system
Circumcision, 596, 597
Clean, 132
Clean technique, 132
Cleaning
    bathrooms, 284, 431–32
    breasts, 595
    concurrent, 163
    after elimination, 313, 315, 317. *See also* Perineal care
    in home health care, 162, 431, 432
    method of, 131
    stethoscope, 249
    terminal, 273
    thermometer, **237–38**
Cleanliness, 127, 162. *See also* Hygiene
Clear liquid diet, 324, 325
Clergy, 32, 33, 102–3, 111
Client, 4, 417, 418–19
Client care records, 420–21, *422–23*
Client's Rights in Home Care, 23, 27, 420
Climacteric, 571
Clinical thermometers, 226–38
Clinics, 4, 350
Clinitron® bed, 455, 456
Clitoris, 569, *570*
Closed bed, 273–77
Closed fractures, 488
Clothing, 108, 297, 298
    fit, 175, 405
CMET (fracture check), 489
CNS. *See* Central nervous system
Coccidioides immitis, 126
Coccidioidomycosis, 126
Coccus (pl. cocci), 117
Cochlea, 516
Cognitive impairments, 519
Cohorting, 137
Coitus, 101
Cold applications, 339–42
    applying cold pack (disposable), **342**
    applying ice bag, **340–41**
Colon, 533, 534
Colonies (bacterial), 117
Colostomy, 534, 625–27
Colostrum, 590, 595
Colporrhaphy, 571

Combining forms (words), 41–43
Comfort devices, 312–13
Comminuted fractures, 488
Commodes, 99, **316–17**, 479
Communicable, 137
Communication, 6, 17, 65–66, *101*, 103. *See also* Body language
    guidelines for, 108–9
    impairments, 70
    with infants, 603
    after laryngectomy, 462
    patient, 23, 70–73
    technology for, 69
    staff, 66–69. *See also* Documentation; Reports
Community, 4
Compensation, 374, 479
Complaints, 100, 101, 263
Complete blood cell count (CBC), 481
Complications, 55, 519, 581, 582
    from inactivity, 583–84
    from incorrect positioning, 182
    from infections, 404
    after surgery, *363–64*
Compound fractures, 488
Compresses, wet, 340, 343, 345
Compression fractures, 488
Computerized axial tomography (CT or CAT) scan, 56, 462, 498, 528, 551, 574
Computers, 69
Concurrent cleaning, 163
Conditions, 55, 77, 109
    baseline, 263
    debilitating, 400
Condom (urinary drainage), 561, **562–63**
Confidence, 357, 388
Confidentiality, 23, 32, 36, 102
Congenital abnormalities, 55
Congestive heart failure (CHF), 479
Conjunctiva, 515
Conjunctivitis, 574
Connective tissue, 48, 510
Consent, 23, 34
    to restraints, *176*, 177
Consistency in care, 23, 375, 378, 520, 584, 586
    for infants, 602–3
Constipation, 403, 535, 537, 590
    mental disorders and, 376, 380
Consumers, 23
Contact precautions, 140–41
Contact transmission, 120, 137
Contagious, 124
Contagious diseases, 137
Containers, 329–30
Contaminated items, 131, 132, 144
Contamination, 119, 405
Continuum, 97
Contraction, 487
Contractures, 182, 312, 493, 581, 583
    from burns, 455–56
Contraindicated, 448
Conversion, 374
Convulsions, 517, 522. *See also* Seizure disorder
Cooperation, 16

COPD. *See* Chronic obstructive pulmonary disease
Coping, 373, 374, 376, 414
Cornea, 515
Coronary embolism, 478
Coronary occlusion, 478
Coronary thrombosis, 478
Corridor rails, 175, 213
Cortex (kidney), 547
Coughing, 121, 361, 363–65, 641
    assisting in, **364–65**
    in elderly, 404
    encouraging, 465
Countertraction, 490
Course of disease, 54, 55, 58
Courtesy, 16, 18, 263, 424. *See also* Respect
Cowper's glands, 568
CPR. *See* Cardiopulmonary resuscitation
Cradle hold, *597*
Cranial cavity, 50
Cranial nerves, 510
Cribs, **605–6**, 613
Critical care department, 5
Critical care nursing, *517*
Critical list, 388
Cross-training, 13
Croupette, 464
Crusts, 448
Crutches, 213, 214
Cryptosporidiosis, 127
Cryptosporidium, 127
CSF. *See* Cerebrospinal fluid
CT scan. *See* Computerized axial tomography scan
Cuff, 247, 248
Culture, 97, 106
    communication across, 73
    food preferences, 99
    pain response and, 85
    sensitivity to, 106–12
Culture and sensitivity tests, 122, 405
Cultures (tests), 57, 462, 574
Cushing's syndrome, 503
Custody, 601
Cutaneous membrane, 49. *See also* Skin
Cuticle, 289
CV. *See* Central venous catheter
CVA. *See* Cerebrovascular accident
Cyanosis, 242, 340, 479
Cyanotic, 447
Cystitis, 548
Cystocele, 571
Cystoscopy, 57, 549, 551, 574

D & C. *See* Dilatation and curettage
Dangling, 368, **369–70**
Data collection, 77, 265, 601
Databases, 69
Day care, 279, 417
Death, 19, 32, 385, 634
    attitudes toward, 388
    physical changes before, 390–91
    preparation for, 387
    from shock, 650
    signs of, 391

Debilitating, 400
Debriding, 453
Decision making, 23, 387–88
    children, 615, 617, 618
    family members and, 107
    patient involvement in, 31, 586
Defamation, 34
Defecation, 325, 533. *See also* Elimination; Excretion
Defense mechanisms, 373–74
Defenses against disease, 59, 121–22
Degenerative joint disease (DJD), 488
Dehydration, 326, 329
Delivery, 590, 591–93
Delusions, 381
Demanding patients, 374–75
Dementia, 405, 408–9, 521. *See also* Alzheimer's disease
Demonstration, 586
Dendrites, 510, 515
Denial, 374, 385–86
Dentures, 228, **307–8**, 358, 408
Departments, 45, 66
Dependability, 16
Depilatory, 358
Depressants, 247
Depression, 376–79, 380
    in elderly, 402–3
    from inactivity, 584
    in Parkinson's disease, 521
    signs of, 65
    as stage of grieving, 385, 386
Dermal ulcers. *See* Pressure ulcers
Dermis, 447, 451
Development, 93–97, 601–2
Developmental milestones, 602, *603*
Developmental tasks, 601–2, 613, 615, 616
Diabetes mellitus, 326–27, 503–7
Diabetic diet, 326–27
Diagnosis, 10, 44
    medical, 56, 85
    nursing, 77, *81*, 350
Diagnosis-related groups (DRGs), 264, 267, 417
Diagnostic services, 5
Diagnostic tests and techniques, 4, 5, 56, 448, 462. *See also* Tests and testing
    cardiovascular problems, 481
    endocrine problems, 506
    gastrointestinal problems, 537
    musculoskeletal problems, 498
    nervous system problems, 528–29
    reproductive system problems, 574
    urinary problems, 551
Dialect, 108
Dialysis, 441–42
    peritoneal, 436, 442
    renal, 549, 556–57
Diaphragm, *50*, 459
Diarrhea, 118, 535
Diastole, 247
Diastolic pressure, 248
Diathermy, 342
Dietary department, 5, 324
Dietitian, 5, 10, 11
Diets, 322, 326–28

control of, 324
diabetic, 504–5
for elderly, 403
newborn, 94
types of, 324–26
Digestion, 321
Digestive system, 84–85, *401. See also* Gastrointestinal system
Digestive tract, 321. *See also* Gastrointestinal system
Digital thermometers, 226–27
Digitalis, 377
Dignity, 18, 33, 391, 412, 414, 586
Dilatation and curettage (D & C), 574
Dilation, 59
Dilation stage, 592
Diplo-, 117
Direct contact, 140
Direction. *See* Supervision of nursing assistants
Dirty, 132
Disability, 582
Discharge, 264, 267–68, 436
mother and infant, 598–99
planning, 267, 357, 418
time of, 4, 417
Discs, 492–93
Disease, 45, 54–55, 109
affecting mobility, 195
blood pressure and, 247
cardiovascular system, 327–38, 408, 472
causes of, 54, 109, 110
chronic, 4, 55, 397, 417
communicable (contagious), 137
course of, 54, 55, 58
defenses against, 59, 121–22
progression of, 54
pulse rate and, 241
resistance to, 404
respiration rate and, 244
risk factors. See Risk factors
sexually transmitted, 573–74
terminal, 385
transmission of, 120, 573
tuberculosis, 124
Dishes, 144, 150, 154
Disinfectants, 155
Disinfection, 131, 155. *See also* Infection control
reusable equipment, 154
thermometers, 237–38
Dislocation, 653
Disorientation, 73, 175, 379–80
from inactivity, 584
from infection, 405
Displacement, 374
Disposable, 144
Disruption, *364*
Distal, 47
Distention, *363*
Distractions, 175
Distress signal, 641
Disuse osteoporosis, 583
Diuretics, 247, 254, 376, 377
Diverticula, 403
Diverticulitis, 403
Diverticulosis, 403

DJD. *See* Degenerative joint disease
DNR (do not resuscitate), 388, *634, 635*
Document, 86
Documentation, 69, 86–89
of home health care, 420
of need for restraints, 175
neurosurgical watch, 517, *518*
of observations, 84, 86–87, 263
pressure ulcers, *451*
temperatures, 238
Dorsal, *46, 47*
Dorsal cavity, 49, 50
Dorsal lithotomy position, 352
Dorsal recumbent position, 350
Dorsiflexion, 212, 497
Douche, vaginal, 574, **576–77**
Drainage, 330, 362–63, 549
checking tubes, 361
after childbirth, 594–95
from ostomies, 625, 627–28
urinary. *See* Urinary drainage
Draping, 350–52
Draw sheet, 182, 183, *219*
grasping, 202, 203
Dressing patient, 297, **298–300**, *585*
Dressings, 361, 362
dry sterile (DSD), 453
DRGs. *See* Diagnosis-related groups
Drip rate, 439
Droplet precautions, 138, 140
Droplet transmission, 120, 137
Drug abuse, 19
Drug interactions, 380
Drug testing, 664
Drugs
administration methods, 442
alcohol interaction with, 375–76
blood pressure and, 247
depression-causing, 377
hypoglycemic, 505
pulse rate and, 241
respiration rate and, 244
DSD. *See* Dressings
Duodenal resection, 534
Duodenal ulcers, 534
Dura mater, 513
Durable power of attorney for health care, 388
Dye studies, 57, 481, 537, 551. *See also* Diagnostic tests and techniques; Imaging; Tests and testing
Dying, 385–87. *See also* Death; Hospice care
Dyscrasias, 472
Dysentery, 118
Dysmenorrhea, 572
Dyspnea, 243, 460, 479
Dysuria, 548

Ear, 408, 516, 524–26
Eastern Orthodox Christian, 327, *389*
Eating, *585. See also* Diets; Food; Food service
assisting patient in, **331–33**
blood pressure and, 247
independence in, 403
preparing patient for, 331

ECG. *See* Electrocardiogram
Edema, 85, 329, 479, 516
Education
    CPR, 635
    of health care workers, 3, 68, 112, 436, 664–65
    in-service, 399
    patient, 4, 357, 465, 504
    pediatric patients, 615, 618
EEG. *See* Electroencephalogram
Effaces, 592
Efficiency, 427
Ejaculatory duct, 568
EKG. *See* Electrocardiogram
Elasticity, 247
Elasticized bandages, 367–69, 479
Elasticized stockings, **366–67**, 479
Elder abuse, 430
Elderly, 397, *398*, 400–408. *See also* Aging
    emotional adjustments, 402–3
    infections in, 403–5
    needs, 3, 403, 406
Electric bed, 271
Electric shock, 652
Electrical activity, recording, 57
Electrocardiogram (EKG or ECG), 57, 471, 481
Electroencephalogram (EEG), 528
Electrolytes, 455, 503
Electromyelogram (EMG), 57, 498
Electronic speech, 462
Electronic thermometers, 226, *227*, 228, **233–35**, 608
Electronic wheelchair scales, 257
Elimination. *See also* Excretion
    helping with, 99, 313–17
    regularity of, 625
    through skin, 447
e-mail, 69
Embolus (pl. emboli), *364*, 365, 478, 584
Emergencies, 168, 633–34, 649
    body's response to, 514
Emergency care, 4, 634
Emergency department, 5
Emergency Medical Services (EMS), 420, 633
Emergency numbers, 430
Emergency procedures, 166, 649
Emesis, 330. *See also* Vomiting
EMG. *See* Electromyelogram
Emotional needs, 100–102
Emotional stress, 100, 120, 247, 263, 357, 571
Emotions
    blood pressure and, 247
    control of, 16
    lability, 519
    pulse rate and, 241
    reactions to illness, 613–14, 615, 616–17
    respiration rate and, 244
Empathy, 16, 17
Emphysema, 461
Employee manuals, 68
Employee safety, 168–71, 218
Employment, 418, 659, 663, 664–65
EMS. *See* Emergency Medical Services
Encephalitis, 118
Endocardium, 470

Endocrine glands, 501
Endocrine system, *48*, 85, *401*, 501–2
Endometrium, 569, *570*
Endoscope, 591
Endurance, 195, 212, 213, 217
Enemas, 99, 351, 537–43
    cleansing, 551
    commercially prepared, **541–42**
    pre-surgery, 357
    soap solution, **538–40**
Energy, 321, 459
Engagement, 591
Entamoeba coli, 119
Enteral feeding, 334, 438
Environment, 161, 586
Environmental procedures, 135–37
Environmental safety, 161
Environmental services, 6, 11
Enzymes, 532
Epidermis, 447, 451
Epididymis, 568
Epidural anesthetic, 592
Epidural catheter, 440
Epilepsy, 522. *See also* Seizure disorder
Episcopalianism, *389*
Episiotomy, 592
Epithelial cells, 48, 49
Epithelial tissue, 48, 49
Equipment
    assembling, 180
    checking before use, 204, 213, 257, 284
    cleaning, 163
    dedicated, 150
    disposable, 141, 144, 227, 268, 339, 340, 342, 537–38
    for home health care, 428, *429*
    for isolation unit, 151
    for measurements, 225
    for physical examinations, 352, 353
    operating, 272, 350, 489
    repair, 163
    reusable, **151**, 339, 340
Ergonomics, 168
Erikson, Erik, 97
Erythrocytes, 470
Eschar, 455
Escherischia coli, 122
Escorts, 263
Esophageal speech, 462
Esophagus, 532
Essential nutrients, 321–22, 324
Estrogen, 502, 568
Ethical standards, 31–33, 34
Ethics committees, 31
Ethics in health care, 4, 31–33
Ethnicity, 73, 106
Etiology, 54
European Americans, *110*
Eustachian tubes, 516
Evaluation, 77. *See also* Assessment
    of home care, 427
    for rehabilitation, 584
Eversion, 496
Exchange list, 327, 504–5

Excoriations, 448
Excretion, 329. *See also* Defecation; Elimination
Excretions, 48, 133
Exercise, 127, 212, 484
    blood pressure and, 247
    for diabetes, 505
    by elderly, 404, 405–6
    postoperative, 357, 363–66
    pulse rate and, 241
    range-of-motion. *See* Range-of-motion exercises
    respiration rate and, 244
    warm-ups, 168, *170*
Exhalation (expiration), 242, 460
Expectoration, 466
Expiration (exhalation), 242, 460
Exposure incident, 133
Expressive aphasia, 520
Expulsion stage, 592
Extended family, 107
Extension, 485, *486*
Extremities, 47
Extremity restraint, 611–12
Eye contact, 108, 112
Eyes, 408, 515–16
    artificial, 524, **525**
    care for neonates, 593, 596, 597
    disorders, 524, 574
    socket care, **525**
Eyewear. *See* Goggles; Personal protective equipment

Face shield, 134, 135, 142
Facilities, 3, 417, 581
    diets. *See* Diets
    hazards in, 169. *See also* Patient safety
    infections in, 122, 127–28, 132, 357–58
    orientation, 663
    policies, 622
    types of, 4, 581
Fahrenheit scale (F), 225
Fainting, 284, 478, 650–51
Fallopian tubes, 569, *570*
Falls, 217–18, 405
    avoiding, 429
    causes of, 405, 650–51
False imprisonment, 34
Family, 601
    of Alzheimer's patient, 409, 410
    of dying patient, 389–90, 393
    grief process and, 387
    home health care and, 419, 424
    as interdisciplinary health care team member, 10
    needs of, 17
    organization of, 106–7
    patient admission and, 263
    of rehabilitation patient, 583
    siblings, 603–4, 615
Fanfolding, 277
Fantasy, 374, 603, 615
Fasting, 247
Father, 107, 593
Fatigue, 120
    CHF patients, 479, 480
    from diabetes, 504

    in MS, 522
Fats, 321, 403, 532
Fax machines, 69
Fear, 100, 101
    bleeding and, 650
    children's, 615, 617
    position changes, 271
    of PPE, 137–38
    of surgery, 356, 357
Feces, 313, 532, 537, 625. *See also* Enemas; Stool specimens
Federal regulations, 13, 14
Feil, Naomi, 414
Fetal monitor, 592
Fetoscopy, 591
Fetus, 573, 590
Fever, 121, 346, 404, 447
Fiber, dietary, 321
Finger sweep, 643–44
Fire, 166–68. *See also* Burns
    oxygen precautions, 167, 310, 462
First aid, 634
First-degree burns, 455, 652
Fistula, 441–42
Fit testing, 138, *139*
Flagged, 238
Flatulence, 403
Flatus, 534, 537
Flatus bag, 543, **544**
Flexion, 182, 485, *486*
Flora, 121
Flossing teeth, 305, **307**
Flotation mattress, 454, 455
Flow sheets, 86–90
Flu. *See* Influenza
Fluid balance, 329
Fluid intake, 329, 548. *See also* Intake and output
    by elderly, 403, 404
    encouraging, 99, 127, 331
Fluids. *See* Body fluids
Fluoroscopy, 56, 481
Foley catheters, 623, 557, 571
Fomites, 119
Food, 321, 532. *See also* Diets; Eating; Nutrients; Nutrition
    religious restrictions on, 111
    serving. *See* Food service
Food groups, 322–24, 327
Food guide pyramid, 322
Food intake, *85*, 322, 326
    alternative routes, 334, 438
Food management, 432
Food service, 5, 98–99, 131, 324
    isolation unit, **149–50**
    presentation, 403
    supplements and snacks, 328–29
Foot care, 406–7, 477, 506
Foot drop, 312. *See also* Contractures
Football hold, *597*
Footboard, 182, 312, 479
Footrest, 312
Force fluids, 329
Foreskin, *568*, 596
Foster parent, 601
Fowler's position, 183, 190, 454

Fractures, 488–90, 583, 653
Friction, 450, 452
Fruit group, 322, 323
Frustration, 73, 100, 374, 402
 role in disorientation, 380
 spinal cord injuries, 523
 stroke recovery, 520
Full liquid diet, 324, 325
Full thickness burns, 653
Full weight-bearing, 195
Function, observations re, 85
Functional abilities, regaining, 517, 519
Functional deficits, 398
Functional nursing, 13
Fundus, 569, 595
Fungal infections, 126–27
Fungi (sing. fungus), 118, 119
Fusion, 492

Gait, 212, 213–14
 three-point, 214, **215**, **216–17**
 two-point, 214, 216, 217
Gait belt, 195, 213
Gait training, 212
Gallbladder, 533
Gallbladder (GB) series, 537
Ganglia, 510
Gangrene, 474
Gas exchange, 459
Gases, 242, 459, 470. *See also* Oxygen
Gastrectomy, 534
Gastric resection, 534
Gastric ulcers, 534
Gastroenteritis, 128
Gastrointestinal (GI) series, 537
Gastrointestinal (GI) system, 48, 120, 532–33. *See also* Digestive
 system
 disorders, 533–36
 inactivity and, 584
Gastroscopy, 537
Gastrostomy feeding, 334
Gatch bed, 271
Gatch handles, 161, 162
Gauges, 247, *248*, 250, 252
Gel packs, 339, 341
General anesthetics, 356, 594
General diet, 324
Genetic defects, 55
Genital herpes, 573
Genitalia, 569
 bathing, 285, 290. *See also* Perineal care
Genitourinary system, 49, 84, 120, 547–51, 584
Gentleness, 17, 379
Geriatric, 582. *See also* Elderly
Geri-chairs, 452, 454. *See also* Wheelchairs
Gestational age, 591
Giardia lamblia, 127
Giardiasis, 127
Glands, 49, 447, 501–2
 adrenal, *501*, 502, 503, *547*
 prostate, *547*, 568, 571
Glass (broken), 165
Glass clinical thermometers, 226, 227–28

 cleaning, **237–38**
 taking temperatures with, **229–30**, **232**, **233**
Global aphasia, 520
Glomerulus, 548
Glove use, 132, 134, 141, 146, 181
 bathing, 284, 286
 drainage tubes, 362
 elimination assistance, 313
 I&O, 330, *331*
 temperature taking, 233, 235
 weight measurements, 255
Gloves, 142
 changing, 135, *142*
 disposal of, 135, 142, 146
 putting on, 144–46
 removing, 146–48
Glucagon, 502, 505, 533
Glucose, 503–4
Glycogen, 504
Glycosuria, 504
Goals, 586
 of care, 31, 581
 functional, 584
 patient, 77
Goggles, 134, 135, 142
Goiter, simple, 503
Gonads, 502
Gonorrhea, 118, 573
Gown, 141–42
 changing on patient with IV, **439–40**
 putting on, **144**, 145
 removing, 147–49
 use, 134, 135, 141
Graduate, 330
Graft, 442, 556
Grain group, 324
Grand mal seizures, 522, *523*, 652
Greek Orthodox, 327, *389*
Greenstick fractures, 488
Grief, stages of, 385–87
Grievances, 23
Groin temperature, 226, **233**
Grooming, 18–19, 131, 408, 664. *See also* Bathing; Hygiene
 patients, 101, 411
Group insurance plans, 7
Growth, 93–97, 602, 618
Guardian, 601
Guidelines
 activities of daily living (residents with dementia),
  411
 adolescent safety, 619
 agitated patient, managing, 381
 ambulation, 213, 370
 bathing, 284, 407
 bedmaking, 272
 blood pressure measurement preparations, 249
 charting, 89
 communicating with patients, 70
 cultural sensitivity, 112
 depressed patient, assisting, 378
 dressing and undressing patient, 298
 emergency, responding to, 633
 environmental procedures, 135–37

hearing aid care, 526
incontinent patient care, 550
infant safety, 612
infection prevention, 127
intravenous line, caring for patients with, 439
liability avoidance, 420
linen handling, 272
medical asepsis, 131
medication self-administration, supervising, 430
nursing assistants generally, 14–15
patient transfers, 194
peripheral vascular disease, caring for patients with, 477
preschooler safety, 615
pressure ulcer prevention, 452–53
preventing falls, 175
reality orientation, 380, 413
restorative programs, implementing, 586
restraint use, 178
school-age child safety, 617
shaving safety, 310
staff interpersonal relationships, 18
standard precautions, 134–35
THA, caring for patients with, 492
thermometer use, 228
toddler safety, 614
warm and cold treatments, 339–40
weight and height measurements, 255
wheelchair safety, 218

Hair, 442, 447
Hair care, 283, 290, 311–12, 407–8
    facial hair, 408. See also Shaving
    shampoos. See Shampoos
Halitosis, 304
Hallways, 163
Hand and nail care, **295**, 406
Handicap, 582
Hand-over-hand technique, 411, 586
Handwashing, **132–33**, 180, 181, 403
Harvesting (organs), 392
Hazards in workplace, 169
Head, heat applications on, 339, 343
Health, 31, 45, 109, 373
Health care, 3, 4
    consumers, 4, 23, 28
    cost, 4, 7, 264, 266, 436
    cultural differences re, 107, 108, 109
    paying for, 397–98, 418, 430
Health care facilities. See Facilities
Health care workers
    education, 3, 68, 112, 436, 664–65
    immunizations, 122, *123*
    specialties, 5–6
Health maintenance organizations (HMOs), 7
Hearing. See Ear; Senses
Hearing aids, 525–26
    applying/removing, **526–28**
Hearing-impaired patients, 70–71, 175, 525–26
Heart, 49, 242, 470–71
    condition of, 195
    disorders, 478–80
    rate. See Pulse
    sounds, 241–42, 248

Heart attack, 478, 651
Heart block, 480
Heart rate. See Pulse
Heat, 226, 321, 447. See also Body temperature; Temperature
Heat applications, 339–40, 342–45
    cautions, 342–43
    warm moist compress, **345**
    warm soak, **344**
Height, 254, **256**, **257**, *258*
    abbreviations for, 45
    by age, *94*
Heimlich Maneuver, 642–63
HemaCombistix®, 554, **556**
Hematest®, **623**
Hematuria, 548
Hemianopsia, 519
Hemiplegia, 519
Hemoccult®, **622–23**
Hemodialysis, 441–42
Hemoptysis, 124, 479
Hemorrhage, 247, 339, *364*, 650
Hemorrhoids, 571
HEPA. See High efficiency particulate air filter mask
Hepatitis, 118, *123*, 125, 128, 664
Heredity, 55, 247
Hernia, 534
Herniorrhaphy, 534
Herpes, 118
Herpes simplex II, 573
Heterosexuality, 101
Hiccups, *363*
Hierarchy of needs, 97–98
High efficiency particulate air (HEPA) filter mask, 138, *139*
High Fowler's position, 183, 190, 465, 479
Hinduism, 110, *111*, 327, *389*
Hip
    rotation, 187, *188*
    surgery, 195, 491–92
Hispanics, 106, *107*, *110*
HIV. See Human immunodeficiency virus
HMO. See Health maintenance organizations
Hoarding, 413
Home health aide, 427
Home health assistant, 427
Home health care, 4, 23
    bathroom safety, 207
    heat and cold applications, 339
    new mother, 599
    providers, 417–18
    team, 418–19, 427
Homemaker aide, 427
Homemaker assistant, 427
Homemaker tasks, 428, 431–33
Homosexuality, 101
Honesty, 33–34, 427
    with children, 614, 615
    from patient, 23
Hope, 378, 424
Horizontal recumbent position, 350–51
Hormones, 501, 510, 568
Hospice care, 4, 390, 417, 436
Hospital stay length, 4, 264, 267, 593, 595
Hospitals, 3–6, 23, 417

Host, 120
House diet, 324
Housekeeping, 420, 427, 431–33
Housekeeping department, 6, 163
Human immunodeficiency virus (HIV), 125–26. *See also*
    Acquired immune deficiency syndrome
Humidifiers, 461, 462, **464**
Huntington's disease, 212, 408
Hydrochloric acid (HCl), 121, 532, 534
Hydronephrosis, 549
Hygiene, 101, 406, 479, 618. *See also* Bathing; Grooming; Oral
    hygiene
Hyperalimentation, 334, 438
Hypercalcemia, 503
Hyperglycemia, 505–6
Hypersecretion, 501, 502
Hypersensitivity reactions, 56. *See also* Allergies
Hypertension, 250, 476–77
Hyperthermia, 346
Hyperthyroidism, 502
Hypertrophy, 479, 503
Hypochondriasis, 380–81
Hypoglycemia, 505
Hypoglycemic drugs, 505
Hyposecretion, 501, 503
Hypotension, 250
Hypothermia, 340, 345–46
Hypothermia-hyperthermia blankets, 339, 345, **347**
Hypothyroidism, 503
Hypoxia, *364*, 479
Hysterectomy, 572

Ice bags, 339, 340–41
IDDM. *See* Insulin-dependent diabetes mellitus
Identification, 374
    of neonate, 593, 596
    of patient, 332
Ileostomy, 534, 627–29
Illness. *See* Disease
Imaging, 5, 56–57, 462. *See also* Diagnostic tests and
    techniques; Dye studies; Tests and testing; Ultrasound
Imbalance, 56, 109, 121
Immune response, 59, 122
Immune system compromise, depression, impairment, or
    suppression, 118, 122, *123*, 448, 460
Immunity, 122, 573
Immunizations, 122
Immunosuppression, 118, 122, *123*, 448, 460
Impaction, 535, 540, 550
Implementation, 77, *83*, 427
Inactivity, 99, 583–84
Incarcerated (strangulated) hernia, 534
Incentive spirometer, 465–66
Incident report, 163, *164–65*
Incidents, 163, 175, 421
Incontinence
    fecal, 519, 535
    patients with dementia, 411
    urinary, 404, 550–51, 584
Increments, 255
Incubation, 119
Independence
    promoting patient's, 212, 357, 375, 403, 586–87

for toddlers, 613
Inderal, 377
Indigestion, 651
Indirect contact, 140
Indwelling catheters, 557
    care, 557, **558–59**
    connecting leg bag, **563–64**
    disconnecting, **561–62**
Infants, 94–95, 602–12. *See also* Children
    airway obstruction, clearing, **646–48**
    bottle-feeding, **610**
    burping, 610, **611–12**
    CPR for, 644–46
    feeding, 610–11
    holding and handling, 597, 604
Infarction, 478
Infection control, 127, 131–57, 403, 417. *See also* Standard
    precautions
    in home health care, 430
    manual, 68
    rules for, *154–55*
Infections, 56, 117–19
    bacterial, 122, 124
    bladder, 584
    catheters, 561, 623
    chain of, 119–20, 132
    chlamydia, 574
    defenses against, 121–22
    in elderly, 403–5
    fungal, 126–27
    local, 339
    lungs, 124, 460, 584
    nosocomial, 132, 357–58
    from pressure ulcers, 452
    preventing, 127, 404–5. *See also* Infection control
    protozoal, 127
    resistance to, 120
    respiratory arrest from, 646
    respiratory tract, 120, 460, 584
    signs of, 404
    in skull, 516
    surgical, 358
    tuberculosis, 124–25
    types of, 121
    viral, 125, 460
    of wounds, *364*
Infectious, 120
Inferior, *46*, 47
Inflammation, 56, 59, 121, 339, 516
    in elderly, 404
    of meninges, 524
Influenza, 118, *123*, 125, 128
Information
    baseline, 84
    discussing, 32, 70, 225, 424
    for EMS response, 633
    from patient, 23, 32
    for surgical patient, 357
Information gathering, 77, 265, 601
Informed consent, 23, 34
Inhalation (inspiration), 242, 460
    anesthetics, 356
Initiative, 615

Insertion, 487
Insight, 427
Inspiration (inhalation), 242, 460
Insulin, 326, 502–5, 533
Insulin-dependent diabetes mellitus (IDDM), 504
Insurance, 4, 7, 267, 418
  equipment, 430
  home health care, 420
  long-term care, 397
Intake and output (I&O), 329–31, 480
Integrity, 34. *See also* Ethics in health care; Honesty
Integument, 447
Integumentary system, *48*, 84, *401*, 447–56. *See also* Pressure
    ulcers; Skin
Intention tremor, 521
Intercostal muscles, 459
Interdisciplinary health care team, 10–12, 582, 583
Intermediate care, 397
Intermittent care, 418
Intermittent partial pressure breathing (IPPB), 464, 466
International time, 89, *90*
Interpersonal relationships, 16–18
Interventions, 77
Intestines, 532, 533
Intimacy, 100–101
Intracranial pressure, 516–17
Intravenous (IV) infusions, 334, 356, 361–62
  bathing patient on, 287–88
Intravenous pyelogram (IVP), 551
Intravenous therapy, 437, 439
Invasion of privacy, 36
Inversion, 496
Involuntary muscle, 486
Involuntary seclusion, 35
Involution, 595
Iodine, 502, 503
IPPB. *See* Intermittent partial pressure breathing
Iris, 515
Ischemia, *55*, 478
Islam, 110, *111*, 327, *389*
Islets of Langerhans, 502
Isolation, 137–39
Isolation technique, 141, 154–55
Isolation unit, 141, 150
Isolette, 596, *597*
IV. *See* Intravenous infusions
IVP. *See* Intravenous pyelogram

Jacket restraint, 611
Jackson-Pratt (J-P) drain, 362
Jaundice, 596
Jehovah's Witness, *389*
Jewelry, 18
Job applications, 660, *661–62*
Job description, 420
Job hunting, 659–63
Job interview, 660, 663
Joints, 485, 487, 488, 515
  change in mobility, *84*
Judaism, 110, *111*, *389*, 596
  diet, 326, 327
Judgment, 374

Kaposi's sarcoma, 448
Kardex, 77, *83*
Ketosis, 503
Ketostix® strip test, **507**
Kidney stones, 503, 549
Kidneys, 48, 327–28, 547
Kilograms (kg), 254
Kitchens, cleaning, 432
Knee-chest position, 351
Kubler-Ross, Elizabeth, 385

Labia majora, 569
Labia minora, 569
Labor and delivery, 590, 591–93
Laboratory tests. *See* Tests and testing
Lacerations, 179
Lacrimal glands, 516
Lactation, 595
Lamaze method, 591
Laminectomy, 492
Language, 108
Large intestine, 533
Laryngoscopy, 57
Larynx, 459, 460, 462
Lateral, 46
Lateral position, 183, 189, 454
Latter Day Saints (Mormon), 327
Laundry, 6, 272, 433
Laws, 33, 589
  health and safety, 4, 664
  long-term care, 399
Leg bags, 563, **563–65**
Leg exercises, 365–66
Legal custody, 601
Legal guardian, 601
Legal standards, 31, 33–36
Legs, 47, 368
Lesions, *55*, 448
Leukemia, 481
Leukocytes, 470
Leukorrhea, 573
Lhermitte's sign, 521
Liability, avoiding, 31, 420
Liable, 31
Libel, 34
Licensed practical nurse (LPN), 10, 11, 12
Licensed vocational nurse (LVN), 10, 11, 12
Licensing, 11, 12, 417
Life
  quality of, 31, 32, 581
  respect for, 31
Life support, 635
Life-sustaining treatment, 387–88
Life-threatening emergencies, 634
Lifting, 168, *169*
Lifting patients, 183
Lifting sheet. *See* Draw sheet
Lifts, 166, 168. *See also* Mechanical lifts
Ligaments, 485, 487
Lighting, 162, 175, 405
Linens
  changing, 272–73, **605–6**. *See also* Bedmaking
  checking, 278

Linens *(cont.)*
    crib, 605–6
    handling, 131, 272
    handling soiled, 135, 150–51, 154, 272, 279
    in isolation unit, **152–53**
    smoothness, 272
Lines of authority, 14, 66
Liquid diets, 325
Listening, 70, 99, 101, 374
Lithotripsy, 549
Liver, 125, 533
Living will, 388
Lobes, 501
    brain, 511, *512*
    liver, 533
Local anesthetics, 356–57, 440
Lochia, 595
Logrolling patient, **186**
Loneliness, 380
Long-term care, 4, 397–98, 417
Long-term care facilities, 267, 397–98
Losses, 376, 378, 402, 414
Low-fat/low-cholesterol diets, 328
LPN. *See* Licensed practical nurse
Lumpectomy, 572
Lungs, 49, 459, 460
    atelectasis, 363, *364*, 465
    infections, 124, 460, 584
Lutheran, *389*
LVN. *See* Licensed vocational nurse
Lymph, 470
Lymph nodes, 470
Lymphatic vessels, 470

Macular degeneration, 524
Macules, 448
Magnetic resonance imaging (MRI), 56–57, 462, 528, 551, 574
Maintenance department, 6
Maladaptive behaviors, 376–81
Malaria, 118
Malignant tumors, 59, 461–62
Malnutrition, 403, 404
Mammograms, 574
Managed care, 4
Mantoux test, 124, 664
Manuals, 68
Masks, 142
    fit testing, 138
    oxygen, 436–64
    putting on, **144**
    removing, 147–48
    types of, 138, *139*
    use, 134, 135
Maslow, Abraham, 97–98
Massage, 453
Mastectomy, 572
Masturbation, 101
Material Safety Data Sheet (MSDS), 169, *171*
Mattresses, 453, 454
Maturity, 96, 427
Meal trays, 324, 331. *See also* Food service
    for isolation units, **149–50**

Meaning, 65. *See also* Communication
Measles, *55*, 118, *123*, 138
Measurement, 45, 329. *See also* Vital signs
    equipment for, 225
    weight and height, 254–58
Meat group, 324
Mechanical lifts, 194, 204–6, 207, 254
Medial, 46
Medic Alert® identification, 503
Medicaid, 7, 397–98, 418
Medical asepsis, 131–32, 133
Medical care, 417
Medical chart. *See* Medical record
Medical department, 5
Medical diagnosis, 56, 85
Medical history, abbreviations for, 45
Medical record, 23, 68–69, 77
    as legal document, 86, 89, 90
Medical records department, 6
Medical science, 45
Medical terminology, 41–45, 45–47
Medicare, 7, 267, 398, 418, 420, 430
Medication
    effect of, 175
    preoperative, 358, 359
    self-administration, 430, 505
    for surgery, 356
Medulla (kidney), 547
Medulla oblongata, *511*, 512
Membranes, 49. *See also* Mucous membranes
Memos, 67–68
Meninges, 49, 511, 513
Meningitis, 524
Menopause, 570, 571
Menorrhagia, 572
Menstruation, 569–70
Mental condition, 195, 212, 361, 583. *See also* Alzheimer's disease; Dementia; Disorientation
Mental health, 373, 402
Mental illness, 376–81
Menu planning, 432–33
Mercury, 226, 228, 230, 247
Metabolic imbalances, 56
Metabolism, 226
    alcohol's effect on, 376
    diabetes and, 503–4
    fats, 328
    slowing, 346
Metastasis, 59
Methicillin-resistant *Staphylococcus aureus* (MRSA), 122, *124*, 128
Metric system, 254
Metrorrhagia, 572
MI. *See* Myocardial infarction
Microbes, 117, 121, 122
Microorganisms, 117
Micturition. *See* Urination
Midbrain, *511*, 512
Middle age, 96
Middle Eastern ethnic group, 106, *107*
Midline, 46
Milk, yogurt, cheese group, 322, 323–24
Minerals, 322, 403, 493

Mitered corner, 274
Mobility, 175, *585*. *See also* Ambulation; Range-of-motion
    exercises
    impairment, 194
    joint, *84*
    regaining, 520
Mobility skills, 6, 520, 581
Modems, 69
Moisture, 157
    in heat and cold applications, 339, 340, 342, 344
    in oxygen therapy, 462
Molds, 118
Monitoring patients, 175, 179
    in bandages, 369
    heat and cold applications, 340–47
    postsurgery, 360
    on stretchers, 203
    during transfer, 264
    in wheelchairs, 221
Morbidity, 503
Mores, 106
Morgue kits, 391, *392*
Moribund, 391
Morning care, 303, 406
Mortality, 503
Mother, 107, 602
    child's attachment to, 93, 95
Motor nerves, 510
Motor skills, 95, 602, 615
Mouth, 532. *See also* Oral care; Oral hygiene
Mouthpieces, 635, 636
Moving patients, 183, 185
MRI. *See* Magnetic resonance imaging
MRSA. *See* Methicillin-resistant *Staphylococcus aureus*
MS. *See* Multiple sclerosis
MSDS. *See* Material Safety Data Sheet
Mucolytics, 466
Mucous membranes, 49
    as body defense, 59, 121
    contact with, 133
    in digestive tract, 532
    disease and infections via, 120, 573
    eye, 515
Mucus, 49, 59, 243
Multiple sclerosis (MS), 212, 521–22
Multiskilling, 13
Mumps, 118, *123*
Muscle cells, 48
Muscle tissue, 48
Muscles, 48, 484, 486–88
    of breathing, 460
    intercostal, 459
    rigidity, 520
Musculoskeletal system, *49*, 84, *401*, 484–88
    disorders, 488–93, 582
    exercising, 493–98
    inactivity and, 583
Mycobacterium tuberculosis, 124
Myelin, 510, 521
Myelogram, 528
Myocardial infarction (MI), 474, 478–79
Myocardium, 470
Myths, 376

N95 respirator, 138, *139*
NACEP. *See* Nurse Aide Competency Evaluation Program
Nail care, 283, 289–90, 295, 406–7, 477
Nails, 447
Narcotic, 440
Nasal cannula, 463
Nasal cavity, *50*
Nasogastric (NG), 334
Nasogastric tubes, *450*, 534
Nasopharynx, 516
National Council of State Boards of Nursing, Inc., 13
National Institute for Alcohol Abuse, 375
Native Americans, 106, *107*, 108, *110*
Nausea, *363*
Navel. *See* Umbilicus
Nebulizers, 466
Neck, 494
Necrosis, 449
Needles, 135
Needs, 93, 97–99, 101
    gratification methods, 402
Negligence, 33
Neisseria gonorrheae, 118, 573
Neonatal and infant period, 93–94
Neonatal care, 595–97
Neonate, 94, 592
Neoplasms, 56, 58–59. *See also* Cancer; Tumors
    malignant, 59, 461–62
Nephritis, 548
Nephrons, 548
Nerve cells, 48
Nerves, 471, 492, 510
Nervous system, *49*, 84, *401*, 510–16
    depressants, *375*
    disorders, 516–28, 582
    in newborn, 94
Nervous tissue, 48
Networking, 659
Neurological trauma, 516–18
Neurons, 510
Neurotransmitters, 510, 520
NG. *See* Nasogastric
NIDDM. *See* Non–insulin-dependent diabetes mellitus
Night lights, 162
No-code order, 388, *634*, 635
Noise, 99, 162, 175
    blood pressure measurement and, 249
    disorientation and, 380
    as risk factor, 405
Non–insulin-dependent diabetes mellitus (NIDDM), 504
Nonintact skin, 131, 133, 154. *See also* Skin breakdown
Nonpathogens, 117
Nonverbal communication, 65–66, 72, 108, 410. *See also* Body
    language; Communication
Non–weight-bearing, 195
Nose, 408, 459, 515
Nosocomial infections, 132, 357–58
Nourishments, 127, 328–29. *See also* Diet; Eating; Food;
    Nutrition
NPO (nothing by mouth), 331, 357, 534
Nuclear family, 107
Nurse Aide Competency Evaluation Program (NACEP), 13
Nurse's notes, 89

Nursery, 5, 594
Nurses' station, 77, *83*
Nursing assistant, 3, 13, 16, 238, 417
  adjustments to job, 16, 18
  assignment handling, 14
  care goals, 19
  certification, 13
  characteristics of, 16, 399–400, 427–28, 436, 659
  education and training, 12, 13–14, 15, 399
  employment sources, 659
  ethics and, 31–33
  grooming, 18–19, 131, 664
  home health care work, 418, 419, 424, 428–29
  information gathering by, 77
  legal issues and, 33–36
  names for, 12
  personal health, 125, 127, 128, 168–69
  PPE for tasks, *143*
  qualifications, 633
  regulation of, 13–14
  skilled care facility work, 399–400
  supervision of, 3, 15, 339, 420, 621, 622
  tasks permitted, 15, 16, 621, 622
  as team member, 10, 11, 12
Nursing care, 12–13, 45
  consistency in. *See* Consistency in care
  dying patients, 388
  patients with dementia, 410–14
Nursing diagnosis, 77, *81*, 350
Nursing Home Reform Act, 399
Nursing physical assessment, 350
Nursing process, 77
Nursing team, 10, 12, 14
Nutrients, 321–22, 324, 470
Nutrition, 48, 321, 403, 452. *See also* Diet; Eating; Food;
  Nourishments
Nystagmus, 521

Obesity, 247, 403, 449. *See also* Weight
Objective observations, 83, 85
Oblique fractures, 488
OBRA. *See* Omnibus Budget Reconciliation Act
Observational skills, 427
Observations, 16, 77–86
  at admission, 263
  during care, *83*, 283, 285, 303
  cold application area, 340, 341
  drainage, 362–63
  food intake, 326, 332, 333
  fractures, 489
  for home health care, 420–21, 427
  of mental health, 376
  of mouth and teeth, 308
  of paranoid behaviors, 381
  reporting, 16, 85–86, 127
  of skin, 308–9, 407, 448, 452
  use of, 54, *81*
Obstetric departments, 5
Obstetrical, 590
Obstructions, 56
Occult blood, 537, **622–23**
Occupational exposure, 133
Occupational Safety and Health Administration (OSHA), 169

Occupational therapist, 10, 11, 406, 419
Occupational therapy, 6, 520, 582
Odors, 18
Oil glands, 447
OJD. *See* Osteoarthritic joint disease
Old age, 97
Omnibus Budget Reconciliation Act (OBRA), 13, 14, 23, 33,
  175, 399
Oncology, 436, 442
One-glove technique, 142, 313
Oophorectomy, 572
Open bed, **277**
Open fractures, 488
Open reduction/internal fixation, 491
Operating rooms, 5
Operative care, 357, 360
Ophthalmoscope, 353
Oral care, 283, 290, **304–5**
  denture care, 307–8, 408
  for tube-fed patients, 334
Oral hygiene, 304–7, 408
Oral reports, 86
Oral temperature, 226, **229–30**, 233–34, 608
Oral thermometers, 226, 228
Orbital cavity, *50*
Orchiectomy, 571
Orders, 10
  abbreviations for, 44–45
  discharge, 267, 268
  DNR/no-code, 388, *634*, 635
  enemas, 537
  equipment, 430
  heat and cold applications, 339, 340, 342
  home health care, 418, 419, 430
  obeying, 16
  restraints, 34, 178, 362, 379
  telephone, 66
Organisms, 117
Organization, 427, 604
Organizational chart, 66
Organs, 47, 48, 50, 512
  donation, *389*, 392
  transplant, 557
Orientation
  to job, 663
  of new patient, 265
Orifices, 362
Origin, 487
Orthopedic, 212
Orthopedic injuries, 653
Orthopedic surgery, 5
Orthopnea, 479
Orthopneic position, 183, 190, 465, 479
Orthotist, 11
Oscillating bed, 473
OSHA. *See* Occupational Safety and Health Administration
Ossicles, 516
Ossification, 94
Osteoarthritic joint disease (OJD), 488
Osteoporosis, 583
Ostomy, 625–29
Otitis media, 524–25
Otosclerosis, 525

Otoscope, 353
Outpatient facilities, 4
Output, 329. *See also* Intake and output
Ovaries (sing. ovary), 48, *501*, 502, 569, *570*
Overbed table, 161
Oviducts, 569
Ovulation, 569
Ovum (pl. ova), 502, 568
Oxygen (O₂), 98, 447, 459. *See also* Respiration
Oxygen concentrator, 464
Oxygen precautions, 167, 310, 462
Oxygen tent, 464
Oxygen therapy, 462–64, 479

Pacemakers, 480
PACU. *See* Postanesthesia care unit
Pain
    blood pressure and, 247
    as cancer sign, 59
    effect on sleep, 99
    heat applications, 342
    management, 436, 440
    observations re, 85
    perception of, 356, 404
    phantom, 493
    relief, 357, 388, 592
    reporting, *58*, 85, 362
    showing, *55*, 65
Palliative care, 58, 387
Pallor, 447
Pancreas, 48, *501*, 502, 533
Panhysterectomy, 572
Pap smear, 574
Papoosing, 598
Papules, 448
PAR. *See* Postanesthesia recovery room
Paralysis, 195, 510, 517
Paranoia, 381
Paraplegia, 521, 523
Parasites, 118
Parasympathetic fibers, 514
Parathormone, 502, 503
Parathyroid glands, 502, 503
Parents, 591. *See also* Father; Mother
    separation from, 613–14, 616
Parkinson's disease, 212, 408, 520, 521
Partial bath, **291**, 406
Partial weight-bearing, 195
PASS (fire extinguisher use), 168
Pastoral care, 6. *See also* Clergy; Religion
Pathogens, 117, 119, 121, 132. *See also* Bacteria; Infection
        control; Infections
Pathology, 5
Patience, 17, 36, 100
Patient, 3, 4, 17
    admitting. *See* Admission
    communicating with, 70–73. *See also* Body language;
        Communication
    as health care team member, 10, 11
    in isolation, 137–38
    physical condition of, 195
    problems, 17
    relationship with, 17, 103, 400

surgical. *See* Surgical patients
    as unique individual, 32, 101, 102, 112, 374, 379
    view of nursing care, 12, 13
    as whole person, 583
Patient care items, handling, 135
Patient comfort, 16, 32, 303. *See also* Backrubs; Grooming
    bathing, 283
    dying patient, 387, 388, 391
    postsurgery, 363
    privacy and, 350
Patient concerns, 436
Patient-controlled analgesia (PCA), 440
Patient focused care, 3, 13, 31, 77
Patient history, 56
Patient identification, 180
Patient needs, 17, 98–103, 583
    communication, 70
    elderly, 400, 402
    specific, 357
Patient rights, 17, 23–28
Patient safety, 16, 175
    adolescents, 619
    bathtub/shower, 207
    children, 601
    disoriented patients, 379
    in home, 419
    infants, 612
    long-term care, 405
    oxygen use, 167, 310, 462
    during physical exam, 352
    preschoolers, 615
    school-age children, 617
    shaving, 310
    toddlers, 613, 614
    transfers, 194
    wheelchairs, 218
Patient Self-Determination Act of 1990, 387
Patient unit, 161, 271
    entering, 180
    for isolation, 141
    for surgical patient, 360
Patient's Bill of Rights, 23, 25–26
Patient's property, 265, 267, 268, 358–59
Pattern (of disease), 54, 55, 58
PCA. *See* Patient-controlled analgesia
Pediatric patients. *See* Children
Pediatric units, 5, 601
Pediatrics, 582
Pelvic belt traction, 491
Pelvic cavity, *50*
Pelvic inflammatory disease (PID), 573, 574
Pelvis (kidney), 547
Penis, *568*, 569. *See also* Perineal care
Penrose drain, 362
Pepsin, 532
Perceptual deficits, 584
Percussion hammer, 353
Perfumes, 18
Pericardium, 49, 470
Perineal care, **292–94**, 404, 595
Perineum, 292
Perioperative care, 357
Peripheral intravenous central catheter (PICC), 438

Peripheral nervous system (PNS), 510, *511*
Peripheral vascular disease, 472–73, 477
Peristalsis, 532, 533, 584
Peritoneal cavity, *50*
Peritoneal dialysis, 436, 442
Peritoneum, 49
Perseveration, 410, 412
Personal care, 101, 131, 155. *See also* Bathing; Grooming; Hygiene
Personal protective equipment (PPE), 133, 135. *See also* Gloves; Gown; Masks
    applying, 143
    for isolation, 137–38, 141
    removing, 143, **147–49**
    use, 141–49, 180, 181
Personal space, 107–8, 112
Personality, 97, 400, 519
Personality conflicts, 19
Petit mal seizures, 522, 652
PFR95 respirator, 138, *139*
Phagocytes, 121
Phantom pain, 493
Pharmacist, 5, 10, 11
Pharmacy services, 5
Pharynx, 459, 532
Phenylketonuria (PKU), 54, 597, *598*
Phlebitis, 475
Phocomelia, *55*
Phosphorus, 502
Physiatrists, 582
Physical abuse, 35
Physical activity, 99
Physical examinations, 45, 56, 350–53, 591
    assisting with, **353**
    for employment, 664
Physical restraints, 34, 177
Physical therapist, 10, 11, 419
    ambulation evaluation by, 212
    exercises by, 493
    prosthesis training, 493
    transfer method decision by, 194
Physical therapy, 6, 520, 582
Physician, 10, 11, 14
    diagnosis by, 56
    home health care role, 419
Physicians' offices, 4, 350
Physiology, 45
Pia mater, 513
PICC. *See* Peripheral intravenous central catheter
PID. *See* Pelvic inflammatory disease
Piggyback, 437
Pigmentation, 407
Pillaging, 413
Pillows, 312–13, 454, 455
Pineal body (gland), 501–2
Pituitary gland, 501, *511*
Pivot, 198
PKU. *See* Phenylketonuria
Placenta, 569, 590
Placental stage, 593
Places, abbreviations for, 45
Planning care, 77, 427. *See also* Care plan
Plantar flexion, 497
Plasma, 470

Platelets, 470
Play, 614, 615
Play therapy, 357, 617
Pleura, 49, 460
PM care, 303
Pneumocystis carinii, 460
Pneumonia, 363, 460, 584
PNS. *See* Peripheral nervous system
Poisoning, 179, 653
Polydipsia, 504
Polyphagia, 504
Polyuria, 504
Pons, *511*, 512
Pores, 447
Port, 623
Portal of entry, 120
Portal of exit, 120
Position of patient, 180
    basic, 183
    changing, 183, 452
    maintaining, 181, 187
    pulse rate and, 241
    respiration rate and, 244
Position sense, 519
Positioning patient, *313*, 453–54
    for breathing ease, 462, 465
    for enemas, 537, *538*
    fainting, 651
    at head of bed, **185**
    infants, 611
    for perineal care, 292, 293, 294
    for physical examination, 350–52
    for spinal puncture, 528–29
    with THA, 491–92
    turning, **183–85**, 186
    for urination, 206
Postanesthesia care unit (PACU), 360
Postanesthesia recovery (PAR) room, 5
Posterior, *46*, 47
Postmortem, 385
Postmortem care, 391–93
Postoperative care, 357, 360–70, 436
Postpartum, 590
Postpartum care, 594–95
Postpartum unit, 5
Posture, 181, 520, *521*
Potentially infectious material, 133, *136*, 137
Pounds (lb.), 254
PPE. *See* Personal protective equipment
Practice, scope of, 15
Preadolescence, 96
Precautions, 131, 137. *See also* Oxygen precautions; Standard precautions; Transmission-based precautions
Predisposing factors, 54. *See also* Risk factors
Prefix, 41, 43
Pregnancy, 323, 571, 573, 590
Prenatal, 590
Prenatal care, 4, 590–91
Preoperative care, 357
Preschoolers, 95, 603, 615–16
Prescriptions. *See* Orders
Pressure relief, 220–21, 313, 452
    mechanical aids for, 453, 454–55

Pressure ulcers, 182, 449–53, 581, 582
    inactivity and, 583, 584
    infection from, 404
    stages, 450–52
Preventive care, 4
Primary nursing, 12
Principal, 388
Privacy
    during bathing, 285
    for elimination, 313
    invasion of, 36
    protecting, 36, 102, 633
    providing, 180, 350
    for religious acts, 111, 112, 389
    respecting, 101
    right to, 23
Private room, 161
Probe (thermometer), 226, 228
Procedures, 179–80
    advanced, 621, 622
    beginning (preprocedure) actions, 179–80
    completion actions, 180–81
    doing as taught, 420
    permitted, 542, 543
Proctoscopy, 537
Progesterone, 502, 568
Prognosis, 54, 58
Progression, 93
Projection, 374
Pronation, 496
Prone position, 183, 187–88, 351
Prostate gland, *547*, 568, 571
Prostatectomy, 571
Prosthesis, 212, 358, 491, 493
Protein, 321, 403, 532
Protestantism, 110, *111*
Protocols, 56
Protozoa (sing. protozoan), 118, 119, 460
Protozoal infections, 127
Proximal, 47
Pseudomonas aeruginosa, 122
Psychiatric hospitals, 5
Psychiatrist, 377
Psychological abuse, 35
Psychologist, 377
Puberty, 569
Pubic area, 289
Pudendal block, 592
Pulmonary artery, 470, 471
Pulmonary blood vessels, 459
Pulmonary emboli, *364*
Pulse, 241–42, **243**
    before ambulation, 370
    apical, 241–42, **243**, 608
    children, 241, 242, **608–9**
    CPR check for, 637, 645
    radial, 241, **242**, **243**, 470
    before transfers, 195
Pulse deficit, 242, *479*
Pulse oximetry, 437
Pulse points/sites, 241, *650*
Pulse pressure, 248
Pupils, 515, 517

Push fluids, 329
Pustules, 448
Pyelogram, 551
Pyloric sphincter, 532
Pyrexia, 346

Quadrants, 47
Quadriplegia, 521, 523
Quality assurance manual, 68
Quality of life, 31, 32, 581
Questions, 3. *See also* Information, discussing
    about assignments, 18, 263
Quickening, 590

Race, 106
RACE (fire emergency procedure), 167
Radial artery, 470
Radial deviation, 496
Radial pulse, 241, **242**, **243**, 470
Radiation, 58
Radiation therapy, 442
Radical mastectomy, 572
Radiology, 5, 462. *See also* Diagnostic tests and techniques;
        Imaging
Rails. *See* Corridor rails; Side rails
Rales, 243
Range-of-motion (ROM) exercises, 283, 290, 411, 453, 493
    passive, 182, **494–98**
    after surgery, 492
Rashes, *55*, 448
Razors, 310–11
RBC. *See* Red blood cells
Reaction formation, 374
Reality orientation, 379, 380, 413–14
Receptive aphasia, 520
Reconditioning, 582
Recording. *See also* Charting; Documentation; Reporting
    discharge information, 599
    height and weight, 254
Records. *See* Medical record
Recovery room, 360, 594
Recreation, 406
Rectal temperature, 226, **232**, **234–35**, 607
Rectal thermometers, 226, 228, 232
Rectal tube, 543, **544**
Rectocele, 571
Red blood cells (RBC), 470
References, 660
Referrals, 418
Reflexes, 94, 513, *514*
Regional caudal block, 592
Registered nurse (RN), 10–12, 14, 77, 263
    ambulation evaluation by, 212
    education and licensing, 12, 417
    home health care supervision by, 419
    hypothermia-hyperthermia blankets, 345, 347
    transfer method decision by, 194
Regress, 602, 613, 616
Regular diet, 324
Rehabilitation, 4, 6, 436–37, 581–82
    activities for, 406
    functional skills, 517, 519
    principles, 583
    stroke patients, 520

Rehabilitation hospitals, 5
Rehabilitation services, 6
Religion, 109–11. *See also* Spiritual needs
   death and, 388–89
   food restrictions, 326, 327
   respecting, 32, 102–3, 111, 388
Reminiscing, 414
Renal calculi, 503, 549
Renal colic, 549
Reporting, 86. *See also* Charting; Documentation; Recording
   abuse signs, 430
   approach effect, 77
   blood pressure changes, 252
   food intake, 404
   hyperthermia, 346
   hypothermia, 346
   IV therapy, 439
   observations, 16, 85–86, 127
   pain, *58*, 85, 362
   patient leaving facility, 267
   postsurgical complications, *363–64*
   pulse problems, 241
   repairs needed, 163
   shaving cuts, 311
   skin condition, 308–9, 310
   temperature changes, 229, 231, 238
Reports, 66, 86. *See also* Documentation
   chain of command, moving up, 14–15
   incident, 163, *164–65*
Repression, 373
Reproduction, 48
Reproductive system, *49*, 85, *401*, 568–71
   disorders, 571–74
Reserpine, 377
Reservoir, 119
Resident's Rights, 23, 24, 175
Residents, 4, 398
Resignation, 665
Resistance, 120
Respect, 16, 31
   for patients, 23, 33, 374, 413, 587
   for religion, 32, 102–3, 111, 388
Respiration, 48, 242–44, 460
   character of, 243
   counting, **244**, **609**
   deep, 361, 363–65
   exercises, **364–65**
   improving, 461
   positions to ease, 188, 190
   rate, 243–44, 609
   shallow, 243
   signs of, 635–36
   voluntary control of, 241, 243–44
Respiratory arrest, 634
Respiratory system, *49*, 84, *401*, 459–60. *See also* Lungs
   inactivity and, 584
   infections, 120, 460, 584
Respiratory therapist, 10, 11, 465
Restorative care, 13, 581, 584–87
Restraints, 34, 175, 177–79. *See also* Supportive devices
   attachment to bed, 162, *178*
   avoiding need for, 178–79
   consent for use, *176*, 177
   for disoriented patients, 379–80
   fit, 453
   for infants, 611–12
   unauthorized use, 34
Résumé, 660
Resuscitation devices, 135
Retention, 547
Retention catheters, 557
Retina, 515
Retinal degeneration, 524
Retraining (incontinence), 520, 535, 550, 582, 584
Retrograde pyelogram, 551
Retroperitoneal space, *50*
Rheumatoid arthritis, 488
Rhythm, 241, 243
Rights, 23
Rigor mortis, 391
Risk factors, 54, 120, 121, 397
   age as, 397
   atherosclerosis, 475
   for falls, 175, 405
   for heart attack, 651
Rituals, 110, 388–89
R.O. *See* Reality orientation
ROM. *See* Range-of-motion exercises
Roman Catholicism, 110, *111*, 327, *389*
Roman numerals, 45
Room. *See* Patient unit
Rooming-in, 593, 602, 603, 613
Roommates, 616
Rotation, 486
Roughage, 321
Rubella, *123*
Rubra, 447
Rules, obeying, 16

Sacrament of the Sick, 388–89, *390*
Saddle block, 592
Safety, 163. *See also* Accidents; Employee safety; Incidents; Patient safety
   in client's home, 428–30
Safety needs, 100
Salivary glands, 532
Salmonella, 124
Salpingectomy, 572
"Sandwich" generation, 96
Sarcomas, 59, 448
Scabies, 128
Scales, 254–58
Scarring, 455
School-aged children, 95–96, 616–17
Sclera, 515
Scope of practice, 15
Scrotum, 502
Second-degree burns, 455, 653
Secretions, 120, 133, 584
Security devices, 179
Security needs, 100
Security thermometers, 226
Seeing. *See* Eyes; Senses
Seizure disorder, 522–23, 652
Self-abuse, 430
Self-appraisal, 659

Self-care deficit, 584
Self-care skills, 6
Self-discipline, 427
Self-esteem, 100
    building, 378, 379
    children, 617
    of elderly, 402
    threats to, 373
Self-identity, 97
Semicircular canals, 516
Semi-Fowler's position, 183, 190, 351
Seminal vesicles, 568
Semiprivate room, 161
Semiprone position, 183, 188–89, 454
Semisupine position, 183, 187, *188*, 454
Senses, 84, 379, *401*, 447
    use in observing, 77, 83–84
Sensitivity, 17, 106, 357
    to cultural differences, 428
Sensitivity reactions, 121. *See also* Allergies
Sensory losses, 517, 521
Sensory nerves, 510
Sensory receptors, 515
Separation, 35
Septum, 470
Seropositive, 126
Serous fluid, 49
Serous membranes, 49
Serum, 59
Serving size, 322–23
Setup, 584–85
Seventh Day Adventist, 327
Sex, vital signs and, 241, 244, 247
Sexual abuse, 34–35
Sexuality, 100–101, 587, 615
Sexually transmitted diseases (STDs), 573–74
Shampoos, 285, **295–97**, 408
    dry, 311–12
Sharps, 135, 165, 380
Shaving, **310–11**
    before surgery, 358, **359–60**
Shearing, 449, 453
Sheath (for thermometer), 226–27, 228, **230–31**, 234
Sheets. *See* Draw sheet; Linens
Shelter, 98
Shift report, 66, 86
Shifts, 663
Shingles (herpes zoster), 125
Shock, 247, 351, *364*, 650
    anaphylactic, 448, 492
    electric, 652
    insulin. *See* Diabetes mellitus
Shoes, 213, 216, 298, 300
Short-term care, 4, 279
Shoulder hold, *597*
Siblings, 603–4, 615
Side rails, 162
    falls and, 405
    position, 175, *523*
    as restraints, 34, 177
Sigmoidoscopy, 57, 537
Sign language, 71
Signal devices, 163, 180, 284

answering, 313, 315
Signs, 54, 119, 634
Silence, 108
Simple mastectomy, 572
Sims' position, 183, 189–90, 351
Singultus, *363*
Sinuses, 459
Sitting position, 190
Sitting transfer, 194
Skeletal muscle, 48
Skeletal system, *49. See also* Musculoskeletal system
Skeleton, 484
Skilled care facilities, 3, 4, 23, 397, 398
Skin, *447. See also* Integumentary system
    as body defense, 59, 121
    breaks in, 131, 133, 154
    dryness, 408
    in elderly, 404
    functions, 49, 447
    irritation from stoma, 625, 627–28
    lesions, 407, 448–56. *See also* Pressure ulcers
    observing, 308–9, 407, 448, 452
    sense receptors in, 515
    surgical prep, 358
Skin breakdown (decubiti), 308. *See also* Pressure ulcers
    areas, 449–50
    bed linens and, 272
    preventing, 450, 452–53
    risk factors for, 406
Skin cancer, 407
Skin eruptions, 448
Skin injuries, 179
Skull, *485, 511, 512*
Slander, 34
Sleep, 99, 303
    adolescents, 618
    blood pressure and, 247
    medication for, 357
Sling scales, 254
Small intestine, 533
Smoking, 167, 430, 461, 462, 477
Smooth muscle, 48
Sneezing, 121
Soaks, warm, 343, **344**
Soap, 132
Social needs, 103
Social services, 6, 582
Social worker, *10*, 11, 267, 419
Sodium-restricted diet, 327–28
Soft diet, 324, 325–26
Sonograms, 56, *57*
Source, 119
Spasticity, 182
Spatial-perceptual deficits, 519
Specialties, 10–11, *12*, 582
Specimen collection, 56
    delivery to lab, 551, 554
    from isolation patient, **151–52**
    toilet tissue disposal, 314, 551, 554
Speculum, 353
Speech, 441, 462
Speech therapist, 10, 419
Speech therapy, 6, 520, 582

Sperm, 502, 568
Sphygmomanometers, 247–52
Spica cast, 489
Spills, 136, 163, 175, 284, 432
Spinal (lumbar) puncture, 528–29
Spinal anesthesia, 357, 361, 594
Spinal bed, 271
Spinal cavity, 50
Spinal cord, 510, 511, 512–13
    injuries, 523–24
Spinal nerves, 492, 510
Spirillum (pl. spirilla), 117
Spiritual needs, 102–3, 388. See also Religion
Spirituality, 109
Spleen, 470
Sprains, 653
Spreadsheet programs, 69
Sputum, 466
Sputum specimens, 57, **466–67**
Stable, 361
Staff development, 68, 436, 664–65
Stairs, 212
Standard precautions, 133–35, 138, 180, 181, 403–4
    for body excretion measurement, 330
    in emergencies, 633, 635, 641
    in home health care, 428
    for postpartum care, 594
    for seizures, 652
Standards
    of care, 56
    cultural, 106
    ethical/legal, 31
    of procedure, 56
Standing transfer, 194
Staphylo-, 117
Staphylococcus aureus, 118
State Nurse Aide Registry, 660
State regulations, 13
Status, 596
Status epilepticus, 522
STDs. See Sexually transmitted diseases
Stealing, 33
Stem, 226
Stepparent, 601
Stereotypes, 106, 376
Sterile, 156
Sterile field, 156–57
Sterile packages, 155–56
    opening, **156–57**
Sterile procedures, 557
Sterility, 573
Sterilization of equipment, 155. See also Cleaning; Disinfection
Sternal puncture, 57
Stertorous, 243
Stethoscope, 247, 249
Stimulants, 247
Stimulus, 487
Stoma, 462, 625. See also Ostomy
Stomach, 533
Stool. See Feces
Stool specimens, 57, 58, 537, 622
    collecting, **536–37**
Strains, 653

Strength, 195, 212, 217
Strepto-, 117
Streptococcus A, 124
Streptococcus hemolyticus, 117
Streptococcus pneumoniae, 460
Stress, 17
    emotional. See Emotional stress
    factors, 373, 374
    illness-created, 98, 373, 379
    reactions to, 400
    reducing, 19–20, 36, 374
    signs and symptoms of, 376
Stressors, 373, 374
Stroke, 212, 517, 519–20, 651. See also Brain attack
Stryker frame, 271, 456, 488
Subacute care, 397, 436
Subacute units, 267
Subcutaneous tissue, 447
Subjective observations, 83
Sucking, 610
Suffix, 41, 43
Sugars, 403
Suicide, 377–78
Sundowning, 409, 412–13
Superimposed, 402
Superior, 46, 47
Supervision of nursing assistants, 3, 15, 339, 420, 621, 622
Supervisors, 14, 419
Supination, 494
Supine position, 183, 187, 454
Supine recumbent position, 350–51
Supplements, 328–29. See also Diet; Nourishments; Nutrition
Support hose, 365, 366
Support systems, 377, 378
Supportive care, 58, 387
Supportive devices, 179, 182–83, 187
Supportiveness, 374, 520
Supports, 34. See also Restraints
Suppositories, 99, 542, **542–43**
Suppression, 373–74, 547
Surgery, 4, 58, 358
    diets following, 325
    hip, 195, 491–92
    orthopedic, 5, 212
Surgical asepsis, 156
Surgical bed, **279–80**, 360
Surgical checklist, 360
Surgical department, 5
Surgical masks, 142
Surgical patients, 356, 357–70, 594
    preparation, 357–60
Surgicenters, 4
Swallowing, 6, 179, 334
Sweat, contact with, 133
Sweat glands, 447
Swelling, 339
Symbols, 45, 65
Symmetry, 243
Sympathectomy, 477
Sympathetic fibers, 514
Sympathy, 17
Symptoms, 54, 119, 634
Synapses, 510

Syncope, 284, 478, 650–51
Synovial fluid, 49
Synovial membranes, 49
Syphilis, *409*, 573
Systems, 47, 48–49, 84
Systole, 247
Systolic pressure, 248

Tachycardia, 241
Tachypnea, 243
Tact, 17, 424
Tagged equipment, 163, *165*
Talismans, 111
Tasks, 93. *See also* Assignments
    developmental, 601–2
    permitted, 15, 16, 621, 622. *See also* Authority
    of personality development, 97–98
Teaching. *See* Education
Team nursing, 13. *See also* Interdisciplinary health care team
Tears, 121
Technology, 3, 4, 417
TED hose, 365, **366–67**, 479
Teeth, 532. *See also* Oral care
Telephone calls, 66, *67*, 618
Telephones, 180
Televisions, 163
Temperature
    abbreviations for, 45
    air, 162, 461
    body. *See* Body temperature
    as body defense, 122
    heat and cold applications for, 339
    room, 162, 284
    water, 283, 284
Tendons, 487
TENS. *See* Transcutaneous electrical nerve stimulation
Terminal, 385
Terminology, 41–45, 45–47
Testes (sing. testis), *501*, 502, 568, 571
Testicular self-examination, 571, 574
Testosterone, 502, 568
Tests and testing
    abbreviations for, 45
    for AIDS, 126
    blood, 56, 574
    culture and sensitivity, 122, 405
    diagnostic. *See* Diagnostic tests and techniques
    drug, 664
    invasive, 57
    laboratory, 56
    noninvasive, 56
    nursing assistant competency, 399
    occult blood, 622–23
    prenatal, 591
    results, 66
    skin, 448
    stool, 622–23
    tuberculosis, 124
    ultrasound, 56, 481, 537, 591
    urine testing, **507**, 554, **556**, 622
Tetany, 502, 503
THA. *See* Total hip arthroplasty
Theft, 33

Therapeutic diets, 325, 326–28
Therapies, 58, 377, 581. *See also* Treatment
Thermal blankets, 340
Thermal injuries, 179
Thermography, 56
Thermometers, *225*, 226–38
Thickeners, 329
Third-degree burns, 455, 653
Thoracic cavity, *50*
Thrombocytes, 470
Thrombophlebitis, 366
Thrombus (pl. thrombi), 365, 368, 474, 475, 584
Thymus gland, *501*
Thyrocalcitonin, 502
Thyroid gland, *501*, 502–3
Thyroidectomy, 502–3
Thyroxine, 502
TIA. *See* Transient ischemic attack
Time, 45, 89–90
Time management, 421, 613
Time/travel records, 420, *421*
Tinea capitis, 118
Tinea pedis, 118
Tipping, 33
Tissue fluid, 470
Tissues, 47, 48, 453
Toddlers, 95, 603, 612–15
Toilet, transferring on and off, 206–7
Toileting, 127, 175, *585*
    children, 613
    new mother, 595
    regularity in, 404
Tongue, 515, 532
Tonometry, 528
Toothettes®, 306, 308
Total hip arthroplasty (THA), 491–92
Total parenteral nutrition (TPN), 334, 438
Touch, 17, *73*, 586. *See also* Body language; Communication
    cultural differences re, 108
    making observations with, 83–84
    need for, 101
Toxins, 121, 517
Toxoplasmosis, 118
TPN. *See* Total parenteral nutrition
TPR (temperature, pulse, respiration), 244. *See also* Vital signs
Trachea, 459
Tracheostomy, 436, 440–41, 462
Trachoma, 574
Traction, 490–91
Traditions, 111
Transcutaneous electrical nerve stimulation (TENS), 440, *441*
Transfer belt, 195, **195–96**
Transferring patients, 194–95
    into and out of bathtub, **208–9**
    from bed to chair (one assistant), **196–98**
    from bed to chair (two assistants), **199**
    from bed to stretcher, **202–3**, 360
    into and out of car, **209**
    from chair to bed (one assistant), **200**
    from chair to bed (two assistants), **200–201**
    on and off commode, 316–17
    with mechanical lift, **204–6**
    standby assist for, **202**

Transferring patients *(cont.)*
  from stretcher to bed, **203–4**, 360
  on and off toilet, **206–7**
  unassisted, 175
  walkers and, 216
Transfers (within facility), 6, 263, 264, **267**
Transient ischemic attack (TIA), 476, 517–18
Transitional care, 436
Transmission-based precautions, 137–41
Transmission of disease, 120, 573. *See also* Infections
Transplacental infection, 120
Transportation, 418
Transporting patients
  for bathing, 284
  during home health care, 428, *429*
  isolation, 138, 141, 151, **153–54**
  during transfers, 264
  in wheelchairs, 218
Trapeze, 314, 315, 490
Trauma, 56
Treatment, 10, 23, *110*. *See also* Therapies
Tremors, 520, 521
Trendelenburg position, 351–52, 650
Treponema pallidum, 573
Trichomonas vaginalis, 573
Trichomonas vaginitis, 573
Trimesters, 590
Trochanter roll, 187, *188*, 312–13
Trust, 374, 381, 602
Tub bath/shower, **284–85**. *See also* Bathing; Hygiene
Tube feeding, 334
Tubercles, 124
Tuberculosis, 124–25
Tuberculosis disease, 124
Tuberculosis infection, 124–25
Tubes, 362–63. *See also* Catheters; Drainage; Intravenous infusions
  attachment to bed, 162
  handling, 439, 534, 571
  rectal, 543, **544**
Tumors, 56, 503, 517. *See also* Cancer; Neoplasms
  reproductive organs, 571, 572
Turning patients, **183–85**, 186
Turning sheet. *See* Draw sheet
Tympanic membrane, 516
Tympanic temperature, 226, **235–36**, 237
Tympanic thermometer, 226, 227, 227, 235–36, 608

Ulcerative colitis, 534
Ulcers, 534. *See also* Pressure ulcers
Ulnar deviation, 496
Ultrasound, 56, 481, 537, 591
Umbilical cord, 590, 596
Umbilicus, 47, 359
Unconsciousness, 649
Undoing, 374
Undressing patient, **298–300**, *585*
Uniforms, 18–19, 664
Unilateral neglect, 519
Unit. *See* Patient unit
Upper respiratory infection (URI), 460
Upright scale, 254, 255–56
Ureters, 547, *570*

Urethra, 547, *568*, 569, *570*
Urgency, 537
Urgent care centers, 4
URI. *See* Upper respiratory infection
Urinals, 99, 313, **315–16**
Urinalysis, 548, 551, 574
Urinary bladder, 547, *568*, *570*
  control, 519. *See also* Incontinence
  infections, 584
  retraining, 520, 550, 582
Urinary drainage, 99, 557–65, 623–25
  check, **558**
  emptying unit, **560**, **564–65**
  external, 561, **562–63**
Urinary incontinence, 404, 550–51, 584
Urinary meatus, 547, 569
Urinary retention, *363*
Urinary system, *49*, 84, 547–51, 584
Urinary tract infections, 404, 405
Urination, 206, 313, 595
Urine specimens, 57, 547, 551–56
  from catheter, 554
  clean-catch, 405, **553**
  fresh fractional, **554**
  from closed drainage system, 623, **624–25**
  routine, **551–52**
  24-hour, 554, **555–56**
Urine, observing, *84*, 316
Urine testing, **507**, 554, **556**, 622
U.S. Department of Agriculture, 322
Uterus, 569, *570*, 590, 595

Vaccines, 59, 122, 664
Vagina, 569, *570*
Vaginal douche (nonsterile), **576–77**
Vaginal examination, 592
Validation therapy, 414
Valves, 470–71
Vancomycin-resistant enterococci (VRE), 122
Varicella zoster, *123*
Varicose veins, 475–76, *477*
Vas deferens, 568
Vasoconstriction, 340
Vasodilation, 342
Vectors, *120*
Vegetable group, 322, 323
Veins, 470, *474*, 475–76, *477*
Venereal warts, 574
Ventilation, 460
Ventilator weaning, 436
Ventral, *46*, 47
Ventral cavity, 49, 50
Ventricle, 470
  brain, *511*, 513
Verbal abuse, 34
Verbal communication, 65
Verbal cues, 585
Vernix caseosa, 596, *597*
Vertebrae, 484
Vertigo, 368, 521
Vesicles, 448
Vibrios, *117*
Victim, 633, 634

Viral infections, 125
Viruses, 118, 119, 125–26, 460
Visceral muscle, 486
Visitors, 103, 127, 138, 180, 181
    after birth, 593
    for children, 616
    parents, 614
    during patient admission, 263
    surgical patients, 360
Visualization procedures (direct), 57, 462, 498, 537
Visually impaired patients, 71–72, 175, 524
Vital signs, **150**, 225. *See also* Blood pressure; Body temperature;
        Pulse; Respiration
    children, 607–9
    at patient admission, 265
    after surgery, 361
Vitality, 402
Vitamins, 321–22, 403, 533
Vitreous humor, 515
Vocal cords, 460
Voice production, 459, 460. *See also* Speech
Voiding, 551. *See also* Urination
Volume, 45, 329
    of respiration, 243
Volume studies, 462
Voluntary muscle, 486
Volunteers, 6, 11, 102, 103
Vomiting, 334, 356, 361, *363*, 644
    infants, 610
    for poisoning, 653
VRE. *See* Vancomycin-resistant enterococci
Vulva, 569
Vulvovaginitis, 572

Walkers, 213, 216–17
Walking. *See* Ambulation
Wandering, 411, 412
Wards, 161
Waste
    in blood, 470
    carbon dioxide, 459
    dialysis of, 441–42
    disposal of, 135–36, 165
    formation of, 533, 547, 548
    solid. *See* Feces
Watch, 18, 145, 148, 150
Water, 180, 331, 533. *See also* Fluid intake
    temperature, 283, 284
WBC. *See* White blood cells
Weighing patients, 255–58
    children, **604–5**
    patient in bed, **257–58**
    with upright scale, **255–56**
Weight, 45, **254–58**
    by age, *94*
    diet and, 328
    in elderly, 403
    loss, 59, 584
    TPN patients, 438
Weight-bearing, 195, 492
Wheals, 448
Wheelchairs, 218
    exercises, 220–21
    positioning in, 219–20
Whirlpool bath, 283
White blood cells (WBC), 470
Windows, 162
Withdrawal, 403
    from alcohol, 376
Womb. *See* Uterus
Word parts, 41–45
Word processing, 69
Word roots, 41
Work practice controls, 133
Worry. *See* Anxiety; Fear
Wound management, 436

Xiphoid process, 642
X-rays, 56, 462. *See also* Imaging; Radiology

Yeasts, 118